Medication Guide

For Patient Counseling

Medication
Guide
for Patient Counseling

DOROTHY L. SMITH, Pharm. D.

Director of Clinical Affairs
American Pharmaceutical Association
Washington, D.C.

Formerly Associate Professor of Clinical Pharmacy
Faculty of Pharmacy
University of Toronto, Toronto, Ontario

SECOND EDITION

LEA & FEBIGER · 1981 · PHILADELPHIA

Lea & Febiger
600 Washington Sq.
Philadelphia, Pa. 19106
U.S.A.

Library of Congress Cataloging in Publication Data

Smith, Dorothy L.
  Medication guide for patient counseling.

  Bibliography: p.
  Includes index.
  1. Drugs. 2. Drugs—Administration. 3. Counseling.
4. Medical personnel and patient. I. Title. [DNLM:
1. Drugs—Administration and dosage—Outlines. 2. Patient
compliance. 3. Patient education—Outlines. 4. Professional-
patient relations. WB 340 S645m]
RM300.S63   1981   615.5′8   81-6053
ISBN 0-8121-0791-8   AACR2

First edition, 1977
Reprinted 1978

PRINTED IN THE UNITED STATES OF AMERICA
Print Number 3   2   1

Preface

I have always felt that if a medication is important enough to be prescribed for a patient, it is important enough to be explained to the patient. Health practitioners who accept this philosophy are frequently faced with the dilemma of how much time they can feasibly spend counseling a patient. Repeated explanations of basic instructions take precious minutes; however, the lack of adequate instruction may have a negative effect on the physician-patient relationship, may contribute to patient noncompliance with the drug regimen, and may result in unnecessary telephone calls and visits by the patient. It became clear to me that a preprinted set of general medication instructions which the practitioner could verbally transmit and/or hand to the patient would help to overcome this problem.

The second edition of Medication Guide for Patient Counseling has been prepared for all health professionals who are involved with the prescribing, dispensing, and administering of medications. The book contains a comprehensive set of medication instructions for almost all of the medications available in the United States and Canada. The book is unique in that it also contains specific instructions pertaining to the method of administration and storage for individual commercial products available in the United States and Canada. The medication instructions have been translated from medical terminology into language that the majority of patients can understand. The specific content and organization of the medication instructions are outlined in detail in the section entitled "How To Use The Written Medication Instructions." The individual drug monographs in this edition have been completely updated, and it is hoped that the new format will make the information easier to use.

It is the intent of this book to provide pharmacists, physicians, dentists, and nurses with a reference guide which can be used during the education of the patient regarding his medications so that he is able to become a more active and reliable partner in his drug therapy. The drug monographs contain the pertinent information that should be conveyed to the patient; however, the practitioner must also be skillful in the utilization of the various communication techniques if he is to be successful in modifying behavior and effectively educating the patient. The introductory chapter, "The Patient and His Medications," has been completely revised and expanded to include new information regarding patient education, basic interviewing techniques, as well as some practical suggestions for handling difficult patient situations. Several general recommendations pertinent to the safe use of all prescription and nonprescription medications are included in the section entitled, "GENERAL PATIENT INSTRUCTIONS: HOW TO USE YOUR MEDICINES SAFELY." Every patient should be familiar with this basic information, and the practitioner may wish to consider using this information in the preparation of brochures that could be distributed to his patients. An Appendix of pertinent patient education material also has been included in this edition.

The inclusion of a drug monograph in the guide does not imply that the Editor or the Editorial Advisory Board endorses the therapeutic efficacy of the medication. Many drugs and drug combinations designated as therapeutically ineffective or irrational by the American Medical Association Council on Drugs have already been excluded. However, a few of these preparations have been included owing to the frequency with which they are prescribed. Until such preparations are no longer prescribed by physicians, it seems rational that patients should be adequately instructed.

Considerable care has been taken to ensure the accuracy and completeness of the information contained in the drug monographs. Reference has been made to authoritative published sources of information as well as to the package inserts of the individual pharmaceutical companies. The individual drug monographs have also been extensively reviewed by an Editorial Advisory Board composed of physicians and pharmacists actively practicing in various specialty areas in the United States and Canada. Their comments and recommendations have been invaluable and have been incorporated into the monographs.

It shall always be the legal and professional responsibility of the practitioner to review the medication profile of the patient for individual problems. In no way is this book designed to reduce the responsibility of the physician, dentist, pharmacist, and nurse in the patient care system. The book has been designed as a guide to assist them in patient education, and there will always be a need for professional judgment as it applies to the individual patient. The contents of the drug monographs are not intended to take the place of the patient's doctor or other health professional, and the practitioner may wish to add or delete instructions that apply to the specific patient. The editor and publisher cannot be responsible for errors in publication or any consequences arising from the use of the information contained herein.

Since the first edition of the book was published in 1977, the acceptance of it by the health professions has been very fulfilling. The professional journal reviews have been very kind, and the book has been accepted in several colleges of pharmacy in the United States and Canada. This response has been gratifying, but is not the sole reason for the decision I made to prepare the second edition. Every person who has been involved with the publication of a book will understand how the manuscript dominates one's life during its preparation. I had been trying to decide whether I was personally willing to spend the time that would be required to update the book. I walked into a community pharmacy approximately one year ago and saw a pharmacist using the book prior to counseling a patient. The pharmacist later told me that she found the book very helpful to her in her practice. I made the decision that day to agree to update the book because I saw the book being used for its original intent. Twelve months later, I do not regret the decision I made and I hope that other health professionals will find the information helpful to them in their practices.

Patient noncompliance with medications is a problem that cannot be solely solved by any of the health professions. It will require a concerted effort by physicians, dentists, pharmacists, and nurses on both an individual and an interdisciplinary level. The second edition of this book is offered in the hope that it will help to improve collaboration between the health professions and help to increase patients' understanding of their medications.

DOROTHY L. SMITH

Washington, D.C.

Acknowledgments

T HE SECOND edition of this book would not have been possible without the help of my friends, family, and colleagues and I would like to express my sincere appreciation to all of them. I am deeply indebted to Mrs. Betty Crichton for her invaluable assistance throughout the entire preparation of the manuscript. Her enthusiasm and dedication were instrumental in the completion of the manuscript.

Grateful acknowledgment is expressed to the Faculty of Pharmacy of the University of Toronto and to Miss Amy Ho for their assistance in the preparation of the manuscript. I would also like to thank Mrs. Eva Janecek, Mrs. Peggy Holloway, Mrs. Diana Petre, and Miss Janice Smith for their assistance in the tedious job of preparing this manuscript for press as well as my friends who helped to proofread the manuscript and who donated many hours of their free time. I would like to thank Mr. James R. Boyd, Managing Editor of FACTS AND COMPARISONS and Mr. Jim Knox, Managing Editor of COMPENDIUM OF PHARMACEUTICALS AND SPECIAL-TIES for their assistance in providing me with information on newly-released and deleted commercial products. Grateful appreciation is extended to the many medical directors of the pharmaceutical companies who have cooperated by supplying requested information.

A very special thank you goes to all the members of the Medical Advisory Board and the Pharmacy Advisory Board for their valuable review of the written medication instructions as well as their cooperation in helping me to meet the publication deadlines. Any suggestions for improvement which the users of this book wish to make will be gratefully received and considered for any future editions.

It has been a pleasure working with Lea & Febiger and I look forward to a continued good relationship. I am grateful to Mrs. Lenora Hume, Copy Editor, Mr. Thomas Colaiezzi, Production Manager, and Mr. Martin C. Dallago and Mr. R. Kenneth Bussy, Executive Editors, Lea & Febiger, for the professional manner in which they handled the manuscript through its many stages. Finally, I would like to express heartfelt thanks to my family and friends for their encouragement and support during the preparation of this second edition. A very special thank you goes to my mother, Mrs. Edna Smith, who proofread the entire set of galley proofs for me and made it possible for the book to be printed on time. The work has been tedious and demanding at times, but because of these people, it has also had many enjoyable moments. I hope that the many hours we spent "burning the midnight oil" will in turn be useful to you and your patients.

D.L.S.

Medical Advisory Board

RICHARD E. ELLIS, M.D., M.P.H.

Associate Professor, Department of Family Practice, University of Texas Health Science Center at San Antonio, San Antonio, Texas

RORY M. FISHER, M.B., F.R.C.P. (Ed)(C)

Head, Department of Extended Care, Sunnybrook Medical Centre; Associate Professor, Department of Medicine and Department of Family and Community Medicine, Faculty of Medicine, University of Toronto, Toronto, Ontario

STEPHEN HAMBURGER, M.D.

Director, Internal Medicine Residency Program, Truman Medical Center, Kansas City, Missouri; Associate Professor of Medicine, University of Missouri-Kansas City, Kansas City, Missouri

JOHN R. HILDITCH, M.D., C.C.F.P.

Associate Professor, Department of Family and Community Medicine, Faculty of Medicine, University of Toronto, Toronto, Ontario

ROBERT S. HILLMAN, B.S., M.D., F.A.C.P.

Professor of Medicine, School of Medicine, University of Washington, Seattle, Washington

ROBIJN KERST HORNSTRA, M.D., F.A.P.A.

Director, Training and Education, Western Missouri Mental Health Center and Associate Director, Greater Kansas City Mental Health Foundation; Professor of Psychiatry, University of Missouri-Kansas City School of Medicine, Kansas City, Missouri

DOUGLAS H. JOHNSON, M.D., C.C.F.P.

Head, Department of Family and Community Medicine, Sunnybrook Medical Centre; Professor, Department of Family and Community Medicine, Faculty of Medicine, University of Toronto, Toronto, Ontario

ALLAN KNIGHT, M.D.C.M., F.R.C.P.(C), F.A.C.P.

Head, Division of Clinical Immunology, Sunnybrook Medical Centre; Associate Professor, Department of Medicine, Faculty of Medicine, University of Toronto, Toronto, Ontario

RICHARD A. MacLACHLAN, M.D., C.C.F.P.

Director, Cowie Hill Family Medicine Centre; Lecturer, Department of Family Medicine, Faculty of Medicine, Dalhousie University, Halifax, Nova Scotia

JOHN W. NORRIS, M.D., M.R.C.P., F.R.C.P.(C)

Division of Neurology, Sunnybrook Medical Centre; Associate Professor of Medicine, Department of Medicine (Neurology), Faculty of Medicine, University of Toronto, Toronto, Ontario

DAVID OSOBA, B.Sc., M.D., F.R.C.P.(C)

Head, Medical Oncology, Ontario Cancer Treatment and Research Foundation, Toronto-Bayview Clinic and Sunnybrook Medical Centre; Associate Professor, Department of Medicine, Faculty of Medicine, University of Toronto, Toronto, Ontario

RAYMOND E. RECORD, M.D.

Professor and Chairman, Department of Ophthalmology, College of Medicine, University of Nebraska, Omaha, Nebraska

PAUL W. ROBERTS, M.D., C.C.F.P. (C)

Family Physician, Department of Family and Community Medicine, Sunnybrook Medical Centre; Associate Professor, Department of Family and Community Medicine, Faculty of Medicine, University of Toronto, Toronto, Ontario

ROGER WM. RODGERS, M.D.

Bay Area Oncology Hematology Clinic, 12 Professional Park, Webster, Texas; Clinical Assistant Internist, Hematology Section, Department of Medicine, M.D. Anderson Hospital and Tumor Institute, Houston, Texas; Clinical Consultant in Medical Oncology, University of Texas Medical Branch, Galveston, Texas

JOHN F. ROGERS, M.D.

Staff Physician, North Carolina Memorial Hospital; Assistant Professor, Departments of Medicine and Pharmacology, School of Medicine, The University of North Carolina at Chapel Hill, Chapel Hill, North Carolina

SAMUEL R. SCOTT, B.S., M.D.

Associate Professor of Medicine, Head, Division of General Internal Medicine, Department of Medicine, University of Kentucky, Lexington, Kentucky

R. GARY SIBBALD, B.Sc., M.D., F.R.C.P.(C) (Med.), F.R.C.P.(C) (Dermat.), M.A.C.P., DIP. A.A.D.

Staff Physician, Department of Medicine, Toronto General Hospital; Lecturer in Medicine, Department of Medicine, University of Toronto, Toronto, Ontario

RICHARD B. SIMPSON, B.Sc., M.D., C.C.F.P., DIP. A.B.F.P.

Assistant Professor, Department of Family and Community Medicine, Faculty of Medicine, University of Toronto, Toronto, Ontario

DIANA STEELE, B.MED.Sc., M.D., C.C.F.P.

Staff Physician, Department of Family Practice, Toronto General Hospital; Lecturer, Department of Family and Community Medicine, Faculty of Medicine, University of Toronto, Toronto, Ontario

Pharmacy Advisory Board

JOEL O. COVINSKY, Pharm.D.

Docent Clinical Pharmacist, Section Clinical Pharmacology, Truman Medical Center; Associate Professor, Schools of Pharmacy and Medicine, University of Missouri-Kansas City, Kansas City, Missouri

GERALDINE A. DONOHUE, B.S.P., R.N.

Assistant Professor of Pharmacy, College of Pharmacy, University of Saskatchewan, Saskatoon, Saskatchewan

R. LEE EVANS, B.S.Ph., Pharm.D.

Associate Professor of Clinical Pharmacy, Head, Section of Ambulatory Care, School of Pharmacy and Associate Professor of Medicine, Department of Psychiatry, School of Medicine, University of Missouri-Kansas City, Kansas City, Missouri

THOMAS A. GOSSEL, B.S., M.S., Ph.D.

Associate Professor of Pharmacology and Chairman, Department of Pharmacology and Biomedical Sciences, College of Pharmacy, Ohio Northern University, Ada, Ohio

DICK R. GOURLEY, B.S., Pharm.D.

Associate Professor and Chairman, Department of Pharmacy Practice, University of Nebraska Medical Center, College of Pharmacy, Omaha, Nebraska

SANDRA H. HAK, B.S.Pharm.

Assistant Director, Pharmacy Department, Orange-Chatham Comprehensive Health Services, Inc.; Clinical Instructor, School of Pharmacy, University of North Carolina at Chapel Hill, Chapel Hill, North Carolina

DAVID W. HAWKINS, B.S.Pharm., Pharm.D.

Associate Professor of Pharmacy and Assistant Professor of Pharmacology and Family Practice; College of Pharmacy, The University of Texas at Austin and the University of Texas Health Science Center at San Antonio, San Antonio, Texas

DENNIS K. HELLING, B.S., Pharm.D.

Head, Division of Clinical/Hospital Pharmacy, College of Pharmacy, University of Iowa; Associate Professor, College of Pharmacy, University of Iowa, Iowa City, Iowa

LINDA R. HENSMAN, B.Sc.Phm., Pharm.D.

Assistant Director of Pharmacy, Department of Pharmacy, Burnaby General Hospital, Burnaby, British Columbia

STEPHEN G. HOAG, B.Sc. (Pharm.), M.Sc. (Clin.Pharm.), Ph.D. (Clin.Pharm.)

Associate Professor and Chairman, Department of Pharmacy Practice, College of Pharmacy, North Dakota State University, Fargo, North Dakota

JOHN IAZZETTA, B.Sc., Pharm.D.

Clinical Coordinator, Drug Information Centre, Department of Pharmacy, Sunnybrook Medical Centre; Assistant Professor of Clinical Pharmacy, Faculty of Pharmacy, University of Toronto, Toronto, Ontario

MARY ANNE KODA-KIMBLE, Pharm.D.

Associate Clinical Professor of Pharmacy and Vice Chairwoman, Education, Division of Clinical Pharmacy, School of Pharmacy, University of California, San Francisco, California

DAVID W. LOVE, M.Sc.

Assistant Director of Pharmacy for Ambulatory Care Services; Associate Professor of Pharmacy, College of Pharmacy, University of Kentucky, Lexington, Kentucky

THOMAS J. MATTEI, Pharm.D.

Associate Director of Pharmacy, Mercy Hospital; Associate Professor of Clinical Pharmacy, School of Pharmacy, Duquesne University, Pittsburgh, Pennsylvania

JAMES M. McKENNEY, B.S.(Math.), B.S.(Pharm.), Pharm.D.

Coordinator, Ambulatory Clinical Services, Medical College of Virginia Hospital; Associate Professor and Director, Doctor of Pharmacy Program, School of Pharmacy, Medical College of Virginia, Virginia Commonwealth University, Richmond, Virginia

DONALD C. McLEOD, M.Sc. (Pharm.)

Associate Professor and Chairman, Division of Pharmacy Practice, College of Pharmacy, Ohio State University, Columbus, Ohio

KENNETH J. MICHALKO, B.Sc.Phm., Pharm.D.

Supervisor, Clinical Services and Education, Pharmacy Department, Toronto General Hospital; Assistant Professor of Clinical Pharmacy, Faculty of Pharmacy, University of Toronto, Toronto, Ontario

JUDITH M. OZBUN, B.S. (Pharm.), M.S. (Hosp. Pharm.)

Associate Professor of Pharmacy Practice, North Dakota State University, Fargo, North Dakota

Henry A. Palmer, B.S. (Pharm.), M.S. (Pharm.), Ph.D.

Assistant Dean for Clinical Affairs and Associate Clinical Professor, School of Pharmacy, University of Connecticut, Storrs, Connecticut

Nicholas G. Popovich, B.Sc., M.Sc., Ph.D.

Associate Professor of Clinical Pharmacy, Purdue University School of Pharmacy and Pharmaceutical Sciences, West Lafayette, Indiana

Debra J. Ricciatti-Sibbald, B.Sc.Phm.

Research Assistant, Division of Dermatology, Toronto General Hospital, Toronto, Ontario

Joseph A. Romano, B.Sc., Pharm.D.

Associate Professor of Pharmacy Practice and Acting Chairman, Department of Pharmacy Practice (1980–81), Associate Dean of Pharmacy, School of Pharmacy, University of Washington, Seattle, Washington

David K. Solomon, B.S., Pharm.D.

Director of Pharmacy Services, Detroit Receiving Hospital and University Health Center; Associate Professor of Clinical Pharmacy and Director, Graduate Studies in Hospital Pharmacy, College of Pharmacy and Allied Health Professions, Wayne State University, Detroit, Michigan

Susan K. Steinberg, B.Sc.Phm., M.Sc.Phm.

Clinical Coordinator, Extended Care Pharmacy Services, Sunnybrook Medical Centre; Assistant Professor of Clinical Pharmacy, Faculty of Pharmacy, University of Toronto, Toronto, Ontario

J. Richard Wuest, B.S., M.S., Pharm.D.

Director of Professional Experience Programs; Associate Professor of Clinical Pharmacy, College of Pharmacy, University of Cincinnati Medical Center, Cincinnati, Ohio

Editorial and Research Assistants

ELIZABETH F. CRICHTON, B.Sc.Phm.

Supervisor, Ambulatory Patient Pharmacy, Sunnybrook Medical Centre; Tutor of Clinical Pharmacy, Faculty of Pharmacy, University of Toronto, Toronto, Ontario

PEGGY R. HOLLOWAY, M.Sc.Phm.

Senior Pharmacist, Clinical Institute, Addiction Research Foundation; Assistant Professor of Clinical Pharmacy, Faculty of Pharmacy, University of Toronto, Toronto, Ontario

EVA JANECEK, B.Sc.Phm.

Pharmacist, Addiction Research Foundation; Tutor of Clinical Pharmacy, Faculty of Pharmacy, University of Toronto, Toronto, Ontario

Contents

Medication Guide

For Patient Counseling

The Patient
and His Medications

I. Patient Education

Patient noncompliance with medication regimens remains one of the major unsolved therapeutic problems confronting health professionals today. Effective medical treatment of a patient is based upon an accurate diagnosis and an optimum course of therapy, which usually involves a medication regimen For too long, health professionals have assumed that patients will take their medications according to instructions and that they require no other information than what appears on the label However, it has been estimated that at least 30% of patients in most studies fail to comply with the physician's medication instructions and one-third of the studies report a noncompliance rate of 50% or higher.[1]

No drug is effective unless it is properly prescribed and dispensed, and accurately administered.[2,3] This chain of responsibilities demands knowledge on the part of the physician, the dentist, the nurse, the pharmacist—and the PATIENT. Unfortunately, we have often forgotten the educational requirements of the patient and have overlooked the significance of his contribution to the drug therapy. Through the effective use of communication techniques, we must motivate the patient so that he is able to participate maximally in his drug therapy. We must recognize that the patient is a decision-making individual who has the prerogative of deciding which aspects (if any) of his therapeutic regimen he will follow. Drug defaulting is not a question of obeying, but rather of understanding. Not until the patient learns and is motivated to take "the right drug—at the right time in the right amounts"[4] will it be possible for rational drug therapy to become a reality of our ambulatory health care system.

The four health professionals who have an opportunity to educate the patient about his prescribed medications are the physician, the dentist, the nurse, and the pharmacist. When the physician or dentist hands a prescription to the patient, he has a unique opportunity to explain the reason(s) he is prescribing the medication and why it is important for the patient to have the prescription filled and to take it according to the instructions. It is extremely important for the physician and dentist to convince the patient that the medication is necessary to treat his condition, since one of the most common errors made by patients is never having the prescription filled.[4] Before a patient is discharged from a hospital, the nurse, in cooperation with the physician and the pharmacist, can conduct an educational program to prepare the patient for his ambulatory drug regimen. Since it is usually the nurse who is charged with the responsibility for administering the medications to the patient in the hospital setting, an educational program or self-administration program should be conducted during the hospitalization. The public health nurse and the office nurse are also asked numerous questions about medications by their patients, and their success in teaching the patient about his drugs can have a favorable impact. The pharmacist also has a key role to play in drug counseling. The pharmacist is the last person of the health team to have contact with the patient before he becomes independent in the administration of his medications. The pharmacist is in an ideal position to reinforce the instructions of the physician and to answer any questions the patient may have about his drug regimen. The level of anxiety of most patients has decreased by the time they reach the pharmacy and they are in a more receptive state for learning about their drugs. Since it is unlikely that the patient will have remembered all the medication instructions he received from the physician, the pharmacist has an excellent opportunity to examine the patient's memory, to repeat the prescription instructions, and to reinforce the patient's faith in the prescribed therapy. The pharmacist is also able to correlate the instructions with each drug by showing the patient the actual pharmaceutical preparation. In addition, the pharmacist is able to closely monitor the nonprescription medications the patient may be taking and to evaluate any implication they may have on the prescribed medication regimen. In summary, patient noncompliance with medication regimens is a serious problem which presents a challenge to physicians, dentists, nurses, and pharmacists.

Whenever a medication is prescribed for a patient, it will have some effect on his life-style and require some type of behavioral change. There are basically three factors which will determine whether a patient will comply with the prescription instructions (Fig. 1)[5]:

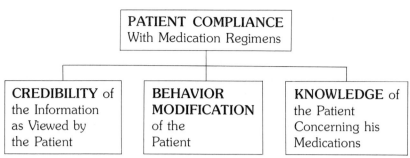

Figure 1. *Three primary factors affecting patient compliance with medication regimens.*

A. Credibility of the Information

Every patient has his own concept of health, illness, and drugs. We must remember that the patient has to decide whether he needs the prescribed drugs and whether he believes the medication will produce a beneficial effect.[6-9] A belief in the efficacy of the prescribed medications correlates positively with regular administration by the patient.[10] A health professional can spend hours teaching a patient about his medications; however, the patient must be convinced that he needs the medications and that the information he has been given is credible. Otherwise, he will resist all efforts to teach him. Since learning requires emotional readiness,[11-13] a realistic goal cannot be set without considering the patient's desires. The patient must believe that the psychologic, financial, and physiologic costs of taking the prescribed medication are less than the perceived benefits. In other words, the patient also weighs the risks against the benefits!

B. Behavior Modification

Every drug regimen necessitates some behavioral change on the part of the patient in order to adapt the drug regimen to his daily routine. The patient is most likely to comply with those aspects of the regimen which are the least disruptive of his normal routine. It is for this reason that the design of the drug regimen is so important and that once-daily dosing schedules or schedules which do not require great changes in the lifestyle of the patient meet with the greatest success.[14,15] Because it is not always realistic to expect a patient to consistently take his medications at the indicated times, the practitioner and patient should negotiate a schedule which is acceptable both to the patient and to the therapeutic goals of the practitioner.[16] For example, a patient who has been prescribed an antibiotic "q6h" may completely eliminate the nighttime dose because of the inconvenience of setting an alarm which would wake him up. It would be more acceptable to both the patient and the physician if the dosage schedule were adjusted slightly so that the patient could take the last dose before retiring. Rigid dosage schedules will be rejected by the patient, and thus the practitioner must develop **practical** schedules based upon his therapeutic acumen and the patient's needs.

In order to persuade the patient to make the necessary changes in his daily routine, the practitioner must establish a good rapport with the patient through the effective use of communication techniques. The patient must accept his medical condition and assume some responsibility in his drug therapy. He should be encouraged to ask questions, and the autonomous, independent patient should be made to feel that he is a partner in planning the schedule. In contrast, the extremely anxious patient should be reassured in order to reduce his fear and anxiety to a level that can be constructive in motivating him to comply with the prescription instructions.[17,18] Compliance from a patient's point of view is a series of trade-offs between his daily routine and the restrictions imposed upon him by the drug regimen.[19] In other words, the patient **must be motivated** to participate in his drug treatment. Pharmacists and physicians can be strong motivating forces and should consider patient education as a type of CLINICAL NEGOTIATION.[16]

C. Knowledge of the Patient Concerning His Medications

One of the major reasons for medication errors made by the ambulatory patient is his lack of understanding of the instructions.[4,20-22] Failure is inevitable if the patient does not understand the information presented to him. Directions on the prescription label are almost always incomplete and do not provide enough information for a person responsible for treating himself or a family member.[5,7] Prescription instructions must be more specific, and care should be taken to adapt them to the daily activities of the patient.

It has been demonstrated in the literature that improved educational techniques can significantly improve patient compliance with drug regimens[23-26] and that the frequency of medication errors decreases as the amount and clarity of the instructions increase.[27] Patient recall of information is poor and they remember approximately 50% of the information given to them by the physician.[28,29] Patients tend to remember those instructions which are stated first and those which are more strongly emphasized. Very high and very low levels of anxiety are associated with low levels of recall. Patients are generally anxious when they are with the physician and especially after they learn the diagnosis. Perhaps this is the reason that patients remember the diagnoses better than the treatment instructions. Patients also remember the instructions that are personally most important to them. This can be in sharp contrast to the instructions that the physician and pharmacist consider the most important. In addition, the patient is usually not encouraged to actively participate during the stage regarding treatment. This is in contrast to the diagnostic stage in which the patient describes his symptoms, answers questions, and allows the physician to examine him. The active participation of the patient may have a direct positive influence on his recall of information, and the use of written medication instructions can reinforce the verbal instructions the patient has received.

The long-term effect of verbal counseling on the management of chronic diseases has been disappointing. The effect of education on hypertensive patients has been demonstrated to significantly improve compliant behavior while counseling was being provided, but failed to produce a lasting benefit after the counseling was discontinued.[30,31] McKenney et al. reported that during their patient counseling program, the percentage of hypertensive patients who were compliant with their therapy increased from 25% to 79%.[31] However, six months after the program was discontinued, only 25% of the patients were compliant with their therapy. The results of these studies suggest that patient education should be a continuous process.

In summary, more time must be spent explaining to patients the therapeutic benefits as well as the limitations of the prescribed drug therapy. Patients must be told of the importance of the drug therapy as well as the potential consequences if the medications are not used correctly. Communicating prescription instructions to patients is clearly a professional responsibility, and efforts should be taken to make the information concise, precise, and readily understandable to the patient. This information must be presented in a manner which the patient can understand and incorporate into his daily routine. If this does not occur, the patient has merely received "information" and has not been "educated" because the latter implies understanding and behavioral change.[32]

II. General Techniques of Interviewing

"He didn't listen or give me enough time."
"He belittled me, treated me like a child, made light of my problem."
"I was just another patient. He never remembered my name."
"I couldn''t understand him. He never explained anything."
"He had bad personal habits or mannerisms, was too familiar,

was cold and callous, was too impressed with his own importance."

These were the most frequently occurring complaints of patients who were unsatisfied with their relationships with their doctors[33] and the majority of these unsatisfied patients reported that they would rather switch than fight for their doctor's attention. One of the recommendations of the professional practice consultant was:

Listen to your patients with your eyes as well as your ears. Don't be immersed in the case history file or keep glancing at your watch. It's not a matter of how much time you give the patient but more a matter of attitude . . . Treat the patient as a person.

Few persons are born with the ability to communicate skillfully, and it is a common misconception that the awarding of a professional degree also confers the ability to communicate effectively. This skill is not guaranteed by any degree and is gained only through practice and experience. Every health practitioner involved in the provision of health education should be familiar with the various communication techniques and should be able to adapt them to his purposes.

The quality of the practitioner-patient relationship can determine whether the patient will believe that the prescribed therapy is important enough to have the prescription filled. Only after the confidence of the patient has been gained will it be possible to effectively educate the patient and improve compliance.[34,35] Most patients take clinical abilities for granted and judge the health professional by other means. The health professional must demonstrate that he is genuinely interested in the patient and is not simply displaying curiosity. The patient also expects thoroughness and empathy. He must be made to feel completely accepted as a person rather than as a hospital file number. The method of interviewing a patient can vary, but the attitude toward the patient must be one of complete acceptance. Value judgments should never be made, and each patient must be respected for his particular beliefs.

Every practitioner brings to the interview a unique combination of abilities, values, and needs. The skilled interviewer is aware of his personal traits and should be able to prevent them from interfering with his patient relationships. The skilled interviewer maintains leadership throughout the consultation and consciously directs the interview by deciding when it is best to talk and when it is best to listen. Whenever possible, it is desirable to use the least amount of authority but still guide the interview and help the patient to make decisions regarding his drug therapy. Patients are more willing to modify their daily life-styles to accommodate a drug regimen IF they decide such changes are best for them. Only in this way will a patient seriously assume a personal respon-sibility in his treatment.

The ability to conduct a successful interview is an ART and is more than simply asking the patient a series of questions. Several general interviewing techniques can readily be applied to drug consultations. As the skill of the practitioner in utilizing these techniques increases, the time required to conduct the interview should proportionately decrease. Human behavior is too variable to be dealt with successfully by mechani-cally applying a set of rules. Therefore, the skilled interviewer has learned to modify these techniques according to the individual circum-stances.

During the first few minutes of the interview, the patient will judge the health professional in terms of his professional manner, which includes his physical setting, dress, and body language. The degree of clarity with which the patient is given insight into what the medication regimen in-volves is extremely important. Almost all people, regardless of their in-tellectual capacity, are naive and simplistic when dealing with their own health problems. Nothing should be assumed and the basic facts should be presented to each patient. In addition, patients quickly forget what they have been told and are easily confused when they are told too much at one time. Needless details and technicalities should be avoided as they may not be understood and could result in anxiety. Very often, patients retain only the information that **they** feel is important and in accordance with their own beliefs. Any instruction that requires the pa-tient to make a change in his daily schedule must be emphasized and re-emphasized. The practitioner must have an understanding of illness behavior and the social-psychologic factors of drug response. Once he is aware of the various factors involved in illness behavior, he can accept the anxiety, anger, or fear expressed by the patient and can conduct a more effective interview.

A. Verbal Communication

Questioning

Perhaps one of the most important interviewing skills to be learned is the fine art of questioning. Several types of questions can be used to determine the medication history of a patient. It is generally recom-mended that open-ended questions should be asked initially and increas-ingly directed and specific questions should be reserved until later in the interview.

OPEN-ENDED questions and phrases can be used to prompt the patient to open a topic for discussion or to continue speaking about a topic. Open-ended questions always require a few words to answer and cannot be answered with a "yes" or a "no." Questions such as "What medicines are you currently taking?" and "What good effects have you noticed since you started taking this drug?" will prompt the patient to provide additional information before you question him more actively. A maneuver such as, "You have been having ringing of the ears? Tell me a little more about it." may help the interviewer to extract important information. The skillful use of open-ended questions can provide useful information with a minimal amount of effort.

FACILITATION is very similar to open-ended questioning. It is a nondirective technique that can be used to encourage the patient to say more, but does not limit the area to be discussed. This technique may take the form of nonverbal behavior, such as nodding the head and urging the patient to continue, or use of such phrases as "Mmm-hmm," "I see," or "Uh-huh." In using this technique, it is critical that the interviewer listen to the patient and demonstrate concern.

REFLECTION is another technique that can be used to help the patient continue in his own style and focus on a particular point. It is a type of questioning in which the interviewer repeats the last few words of the patient in a questioning tone. For example, a patient may remark that "The rash was really bad yesterday." The practitioner could reflect on this statement by asking, "It was 'bad?'" This will encourage the patient to describe the rash in greater detail. Reflection is an extremely useful technique in the management of patients who are relatively nontalkative and who respond to every question with as few words as possible. By repeating the last words of the patient in a questioning manner, the practitioner can usually receive more information about that "red pill" the patient has been taking or "those yellow spots on the wall" that the patient has noticed. Almost every patient will respond favorably to this type of questioning because in hearing his own language repeated, he is reassured that the practitioner is listening to him.

If the interviewer remains uncertain about a particular fact, DIRECT questions can then be useful. A direct question asks for specific information and can usually be answered in one word or a short phrase. Examples of direct questions are: "Could you tell me more about the bleeding?" and "How soon after you took the drug did you develop the skin rash?" Another advantage of using this type of questioning is that the patient may learn to become more precise in his future descriptions. When using direct questions, it is important to phrase all questions briefly and simply and to ask only ONE question at a time. To string several questions together will only confuse both parties, and the patient may be uncertain which question he should answer first. When the patient does finally respond, the interviewer will not always be certain to which question he has responded!

10

Several types of questions can be used to determine the medication history of the patient, but it is a good general rule to avoid CLOSE-ENDED questions that can be answered by a "yes" or a "no." Such questions generally encourage the patient to prejudice his answer in order to meet the expectations of the practitioner, or give the patient an opportunity to avoid discussing an area. For example, the question "Have you taken your medication as it was prescribed?" will generally yield a positive response from the patient. The patient may indeed have been noncompliant with the therapeutic regimen, but because of guilt feelings responds positively with the hope that he will not have to discuss it any further. Another danger is that spontaneity is discouraged with this type of questioning, and the patient may fall into a pattern of waiting silently for the next question.

The interviewer should avoid designing questions which by their wording suggest the possible answer. For example, one should avoid asking a patient a SUGGESTIVE question such as "This drug sometimes causes nausea. Did you develop any nausea?" Instead, the question should be phrased as follows: "Did this medication agree with you?" or "Did you experience any side effects from this medication?" Another danger of using suggestive questions is that the patient may decide that one of the interviewer's possible answers sounds better than what he had originally intended to say!

Listening

In order to be a successful interviewer, one must listen to the patient. Active listening is probably one of the most difficult skills to learn. One of the reasons for this may be the fact that the average rate of speech is approximately 125 words per minute, and the average person thinks at a speed nearly four times faster.[36] As a result, the person on the listening side of the conversation has more time at his disposal and can easily be thinking about the next question he will ask. This is often apparent in students when they first begin conducting medication history interviews. They may have asked the patient every question perfectly; however, at the end of the interview, they cannot remember the responses the patients gave to those questions! Therefore, it is important to listen patiently and attentively during the interview and to appear unhurried. Through the skilled use of listening, the interviewer frequently obtains answers to many unasked questions, and these answers often suggest the best techniques for obtaining additional information.

Silence

Another technique closely related to listening is the use of silence. Skillfully used, silence can convey support and interest to the patient. It can encourage the patient to talk or can be used to slow the pace of the interview and to give the patient some time to consider a question.

If a patient falls silent, the practitioner should not become anxious but should consider remaining silent for a short time. In most instances, the patient will continue. He may simply have needed some time to formulate what he wanted to say. During periods of silence, the interviewer should convey interest in the patient. This can be accomplished by a nod of the head, by looking at the medication profile or by leaning forward in the chair. The effective use of silence can be negated if the interviewer looks away from the patient, begins writing in the patient profile or slumps back in the chair in an attitude of fatigue. If the patient fails to respond to the silence, some other form of questioning should then be used.

With experience, silence can be a very useful technique. However, if a practitioner overuses this technique, his patients may perceive him as being cold and distant. It is also unwise to use silence too frequently with overly talkative patients! In addition, if the patient feels that the practitioner is using silence because he is unsure of himself or because he is not listening, the patient will withdraw from the communication, and it may be very difficult to reestablish the patient relationship.

Confrontation

Confrontation is a technique that can be used when there are inconsistencies in the patient's behavior or statements. For example, a patient who appears disinterested when the pharmacist is explaining the proper use of his medications can usually be effectively confronted with a statement such as, "I get the feeling that you do not think your medications are important." If the patient has taken the time to bring the prescription to the pharmacy, he undoubtedly feels he should take the drug and confrontation can be used to help uncover the reasons for his unusual behavior. When confrontations are made in an interview, they should not be hostile accusations, but should reflect a sympathetic interest in the patient. The practitioner should convey the attitude that he is trying to understand the feelings, behavior, or previous statement of the patient.

Interpretation

It is sometimes necessary for the interviewer to link events or ascribe motives to a patient's response or behavior. The term used to describe this technique is interpretation, which is a type of confrontation based on inference rather than observation. For example, a patient may attribute recently occurring tinnitus to a recently prescribed medication, which has not been reported to cause this side effect. Upon questioning the patient further, the interviewer may learn that the patient has also been taking high doses of salicylates for the treatment of rheumatoid arthritis and this drug is more likely to be the cause of the tinnitus. One method of interpreting this information to the patient would be, "It sounds more likely to me that this problem (tinnitus) is due to your aspirin therapy." The interviewer would then take the appropriate steps to help solve this problem.

Empathy

Every patient attempts to maintain a positive self-image and is hesitant in divulging information that will expose his weaknesses or inability to perform certain tasks or to afford certain things, including medications. The practitioner should recognize that these defenses are normal, and he should try to be empathetic in his approach. This implies that the practitioner simply recognizes and accepts the patient's feelings and does not criticize or condone him. Empathy does not involve giving advice, being reassuring to a patient, or trying to do something about the patient's feeling or emotion. An example of an empathetic response would be, "The complicated schedule for this medicine must be difficult for you to manage." In many cases, a patient will then express his feelings more directly to the practitioner.

Reassurance

Reassurance is a technique that conveys understanding as well as approval of something the patient has described. Patients feel reassured when they are helped to work out their problems and when they feel they are completely understood by the interviewer. An example of a reassuring response would be: "I understand. The dizziness from this drug can be annoying during the first month." In order for a patient to be genuinely reassured, he must feel that the information is reliable and that the practitioner is competent and can be trusted.

It is extremely important not to falsely reassure a patient about his drug therapy. A patient should never be told that "everything will be all right" or that "this drug is safe." The practitioner can no more guarantee the desired therapeutic response than a surgeon can guarantee the success of an operation. In most cases, he should attempt to instill hope without being falsely optimistic. If a patient asks, "Is this drug any good?", it may be more appropriate to answer in the following manner: "This drug has helped many other people and we hope that it will also help you." Using this technique, the practitioner reduces the patient's fear, but does not falsely reassure him.

Summation

Summation is a technique that is useful in letting the patient know how the interviewer has understood his statements. It is a method of reemphasis whereby the interviewer can clarify a statement that the patient has made. An example of a summation response would be, "Now, as I understand it, you are having difficulty remembering to take your afternoon dose of the drug." Summation can be done periodically throughout the interview and should always be used at the termination of the session. It can be used to reinforce the important points of the interview so that both the patient and the interviewer leave with the same ideas and goals.

B. Nonverbal Communication

Some psychologists state that approximately 15% of a message is carried through words, another 30% in voice quality and intonation, and probably more than 50% through facial expression and body posture.[37] The way a person stands or sits and the manner in which he uses his arms, legs, and face to communicate are extremely important, and the practitioner should be familiar with the various nonverbal signals that imply anxiety, anger, or embarrassment. Most patients are preoccupied with their disease conditions. They may easily misinterpret what the practitioner is trying to say and become unduly upset. The interviewer must constantly be alert for any warning signs of poor communication and appropriately rephrase any misunderstood statements.

If the practitioner can successfully communicate a feeling of trust and respect by his nonverbal actions, the patient will become more responsive and less anxious. Patient rapport is partially established through eye contact; the interviewer should look directly—but should not stare—at the patient. The patient senses a feeling of interest if the practitioner maintains good eye contact during the interview. The practitioner should refrain from "reading" a list of questions since this will diminish the eye contact that can be established. In addition, if the interviewer looks out the window or at a spot on the floor instead of looking at the patient, he will soon notice that the patient will also begin looking at those same spots!

The tone and inflection of the voice are sometimes more important than the actual wording of a question. If the patient is asked a question in an accusing or suspicious tone, fear and suspicion could be aroused and it will be difficult to gain or maintain the cooperation of the patient. In addition, words can take on completely different meanings simply by the voice tone and volume. For example, a simple word such as "Oh" can infer such feelings as fear, surprise, exuberance, pleasure, awe, compassion, gratitude, pity, superiority, or understanding depending upon the manner in which it is said.

The body posture can also indicate the feelings of both the patient and the practitioner. There are always exceptions, but in general relaxed posture, open hands, a head nod, leaning forward, or turning toward the other person indicate openness and are positive nonverbal signals. In contrast, an averted glance, crossing of the legs, crossing of the arms tightly across the chest, wringing of the hands, nervous cough or nervous laugh, or turning of the body away from the other person signal negative feelings and the practitioner should immediately try to correct the problem. He may decide to rephrase the question or may decide to call this nonverbal behavior to the attention of the patient. For example, he may say, "You appear upset." or "It seems as though you are having trouble with some of these dosage times. What is unclear so far?"

An awareness of nonverbal communication is critical to a successful interview; thus, the practitioner should also become familiar with the various nonverbal signals he commonly uses. If he is having difficulty establishing satisfactory patient relationships, part of the problem may be the nonverbal communication he is conveying to the patient. The use of video tape equipment and an instant playback of a patient interview can help to increase the practitioner's awareness of his own nonverbal techniques and help him to correct any annoying mannerisms.

The practitioner often wonders whether he should take detailed notes during the interview. Some patients approve and look upon note-taking as a sign of interest; however, the majority of patients sense that they do not have the complete attention of the practitioner and their train of thought is broken. In addition, the participation of the interviewer is usually interrupted by notetaking, and as a result, communication is decreased. Practitioners who do take detailed notes usually find that they lose good eye contact with the patient. Some patients even stop speaking until the practitioner has recorded everything they have just said. In such cases, the practitioner is no longer guiding the interview and, instead, the patient has assumed the leadership. With increasing practice, the interviewer will learn to rely on mental notes. A word or two jotted down on a piece of paper will enable him to recall the entire context of the conversation. The interviewer should strive to take as few notes as possible and should prepare a detailed review immediately after the consultation.

The physical setting also has an effect on the success of the interview. Some degree of privacy and a relaxed atmosphere are essential. Since prescription medication is a private and personal matter, the consultation should be conducted in a private area. Most patients do not want other people to overhear the discussion and will speak more openly if privacy is assured. The ideal setting is a private office; however, other arrangements can also be effective. The patient has a right to feel that he deserves the undivided attention of the practitioner and will resent any interruptions or phone calls. The interviewer should instruct his receptionist and colleagues not to interrupt him during a consultation. Unless absolutely necessary, the practitioner should refrain from accepting telephone calls during the interview. The interview that is conducted in privacy without interruptions helps to improve rapport and assures the patient that the information will remain confidential to those involved in his medical care.[38] In terms of knowledge, patients who are educated in a private area have a better recall for both general and special medication instructions.[38] In addition, private medication counseling has a positive effect on patient compliance.[19,38] In summary, communication, patient comprehension, and compliance can be enhanced by an atmosphere that offers some measure of privacy.

Effective communication with a patient is not accidental. It must be learned and studied to be effective. Self-study is essential to the process of consultation, and the practitioner should evaluate his communication techniques after every interview. Did he use too many direct questions when silence would have prompted the patient more effectively? How could he have better handled the patient's question, "Can you imagine my other doctor being so stupid as to prescribe prednisone for ten years for my arthritis?" How could he have better handled his own feelings of anger and anxiety during the interview? As the practitioner repeats this type of evaluation after every interview, he will begin to develop self-confidence and techniques that reflect the intertwining of his own knowledge and communication skills.

III. The Drug Consultation

In addition to the general techniques of interviewing previously discussed, several communication techniques are specific to a drug consultation. The drug consultation has four primary objectives:

(1) to gather information about the medication history of the patient that is not available from other sources;

(2) to establish with the patient a relationship that will facilitate his therapy;

(3) to educate the patient in the proper use of his medications; and

(4) to support and direct the patient in his drug therapy.

In practice, the medication history and teaching components of the drug consultation are frequently separated by time intervals. If the patient is being admitted to the hospital, the medication history is acquired by the pharmacist, physician, or nurse. A few days prior to discharge, the patient should be instructed in the correct use of the medications he will be expected to take at home. In contrast to the hospitalized patient, the medication history of the ambulatory patient will initially be determined by the physician or dentist in the clinic or the pharmacist in the dispensary. The information obtained from the medication history will provide the basis of the medication profile maintained in the pharmacy, which must be continually updated with all prescription and nonprescription medications the patient is taking. Every time the patient receives a prescription for a medication, he should be instructed and educated accordingly.

The following protocol is designed to accommodate health practitioners involved in the care of the ambulatory patient; however, the principles can readily be applied to the hospitalized patient. The protocol outlines the types of questions that should be asked in order to obtain the complete medication history as well as the types of information that should be explained to the patient whenever a medication has been prescribed. With experience, the practitioner will undoubtedly revise the order of the protocol to suit the interview to the particular patient situation.

Introduce yourself to the patient and greet the patient by name. Be certain that you are interviewing the correct patient.

From the moment the practitioner introduces himself to the patient, he is being evaluated by the patient. It is at this point that the patient is deciding whether he will speak openly, and his decision is influenced by the professional behavior of the practitioner. This includes not only his personal appearance, but also his conduct and language. The practitioner should introduce himself to new patients and explain the purpose of the interview clearly. His opening remarks will set the tone of the professional relationship, and they should convey cordiality, interest, and respect. Since anxiety blocks communication, the patient must be put at ease. If this is effectively accomplished, the first barrier to patient communication has been broken.

The patient will also appreciate being greeted by name because it acknowledges an interest in him as a person. It is important that the practitioner is certain he is interviewing the correct patient. In a busy dispensary waiting area, it is not uncommon for a patient to mistakenly come forward when another patient's name is called! The patient may have difficulty hearing or a mental incapacity. If the practitioner has any doubt about the identity of a patient, he should always clarify the issue before proceeding any farther.

Determine the medication history of the patient.

The medication history of the patient is essentially obtained via a goal-directed method of communication in which the practitioner has the goal of **obtaining** information from the patient. The practitioner is basically interested in learning which medications (including nonprescription preparations) the patient has been taking as well as any allergic reactions or adverse effects the patient has ever experienced from drugs. The purpose of the medication history is to assist the physician, dentist, and pharmacist in selecting a drug regimen most suitable to the patient and to determine whether any medications (including nonprescription preparations) may have contributed to the present condition of the patient. The reporting of any drug allergies or adverse drug reactions will also enable the team to avoid the use of these drugs or to exercise extreme caution in their use.

The following questions are useful in obtaining the medication history from the patient:

What medications has the patient been taking?
For what medical reason has he been taking these drugs?

It is important to ask only one question at a time in language that the patient can understand. Patients similarly respond in common language and state, for example, "I've been taking a water pill for my blood pressure." Since generic and trade names are foreign nomenclature to patients, it is difficult for most patients to remember the exact names of their medications. In an attempt to describe a medication, the patient usually resorts to a physical description such as "a capsule that was black and yellow." A few patients may bring their medications to the hospital or the clinic, and the procedure of identification is facilitated by the label on the prescription vial. If the patient has removed his medication from the original container, the pharmacist can usually identify the drug by physical means or by contacting the pharmacist who dispensed the medication.

It is imperative that the nonprescription drug usage of the patient is also acquired. Most patients do not consider over-the-counter preparations as drugs and have to be specifically asked, "Are you regularly taking any drugs that can be purchased without a prescription?" A patient who does not feel that his nonprescription drug usage is important usually responds in a negative manner. The practitioner, upon asking the patient about specific types of preparations, such as cold remedies, laxatives, and headache remedies, often learns that the patient has been self-medicating with one or more of these remedies. It is important not to make the patient feel guilty at this point, but rather to explain the importance of nonprescription preparations to the prescribed drug regimen.

How often does he take these medications (dosage schedule)?

The practitioner is concerned with two types of dosage schedules: (1) the dosage schedule of nonprescription medications, which is com-

18

pletely determined by the patient, and (2) the dosage schedule of pre-scription medications. With respect to the use of nonprescription medi-cations, it is important that the interviewer determine whether the patient is self-medicating with a drug that is contraindicated or should be used with caution in his disease and/or with his prescription medications. Has the patient been self-medicating a condition that requires medical atten-tion? Laxatives, analgesics, and nasal decongestants are among the most frequently abused medications, and the interviewer should determine whether the patient has been taking such preparations in the recom-mended dose for the appropriate time period or whether he has been chronically abusing these preparations.

With respect to the prescribed medications, the interviewer is inter-ested in learning how closely the patient adheres to the recommended dosage schedule. If the patient has not been taking his medication at the correct times, the interviewer should attempt to determine the reason(s) the patient had for being noncompliant. Did the patient simply forget to take his drug? Did the patient have a conflict between his dosage sched-ule and his work schedule? Was it inconvenient for him to take the medi-cation at work? For example, liquid antacid preparations are usually more effective than the solid dosage forms; however, the latter may be more practical for the construction worker. Did the patient omit a dose because of side effects? Was the patient able to afford the medication? Was the patient convinced that he really needed the medication? If the patient does not feel that his medication regimen is important, he will probably be noncompliant. Behind every refusal to cooperate with the drug regimen, there is a reason. The practitioner must discover that reason and attempt to remove the barrier.

How many doses of the prescribed drug does he miss in one day? In one week?
How often does he take an "extra" dose?

Because of the high incidence of medication errors made by ambula-tory patients, it is important to ask patients, **"How many times** do you miss a dose?" rather than **"Do you ever** miss a dose?" Every patient occasionally forgets to take a dose at some time during his therapy; we are more concerned with patients who regularly skip one or more doses. Depending on the drug, it is important to decide **how many doses** the patient can miss before the problem becomes clinically significant. For example, the omission of one or two doses of antacid therapy in the treatment of peptic ulcer would not be as critical as the omission of one or two doses of anticoagulant therapy in the treatment of thrombo-phlebitis.

When a patient does confess to missed doses, do not put him on the defensive by asking, "Why didn't you take your drugs as they were prescribed?" Instead, ask the patient, "Was there any particular reason that you could not take the drug?" Using this approach, the practitioner can often uncover specific problems the patient had with the regimen and may learn, for example, that the patient has difficulty swallowing capsules or that the strawberry taste of the medication caused him to become nauseated. If the problem is one of forgetfulness, it is sometimes possible to design a once-daily dosage regimen to help improve compliance. Overdosing is just as critical as underdosing, and all patients should be asked how often they take an extra dose(s) of the medication. Some patients feel that if ONE tablet is good, TWO tablets will be twice as good and will bring about a quicker recovery!

Has he had any problems with his drugs?
If so, what?

The development of unpleasant side effects has been reported to be a deterrent to patient compliance.[39] However, it has more recently been suggested that a patient may consider side effects to be evidence that the drug is working and thus be more compliant with the regimen.[40] Annoying but minor side effects can often be managed by redesigning the method of administration or by simple techniques outlined in more detail in the specific drug monographs.

Is the patient allergic to any drugs?
If so, what symptoms did he experience?
How soon after he took the drug did the symptoms appear?

When questioning a patient about drug allergies, it is important to remember that many people say they are allergic when they are actually trying to say that the drug was not effective or that they experienced a side effect of the drug. The practitioner should determine whether the patient experienced a delayed or immediate type of allergic reaction and whether it was respiratory or dermatologic in nature. Some patients when questioned further had their "allergic" reactions even *before* they took the medication! Asking the patient if he has received the drug since that time will help to determine whether the patient has a true allergy. The seriousness of the "reaction" can often be determined by asking the patient whether he notified his physician or dentist or whether he treated himself at home. It is important to remember that some patients may be allergic to an excipient of a drug product (for example, chocolate) and may not be allergic to the specific drug. Because many patients do not understand what an allergic reaction entails, it is important that all of their remarks be carefully screened. If a patient is overly concerned about a drug allergy, he may be comforted by the explanation that, in most diseases, there are several alternative drugs which can be used if a patient is allergic to a medication.

Because of time limitations imposed on every interview, a questionnaire can be useful in obtaining the drug history from a patient (Fig. 2). The questionnaires can be completed by the patient on admission to the hospital, in the waiting room of the pharmacy, or in the office of the physician or dentist. It is extremely important that the questions and terminology be written in language that the patient can understand. If a questionnaire is well designed, it can save the practitioner a significant amount of time. The practitioner can pursue any additional information he requires to complete the medication history according to the information appearing on the questionnaire. The medication history of the patient should be updated every time the patient receives a prescription for a medication. In summary, a complete medication history can be an invaluable tool in the diagnosis and in the design of future drug regimens for every patient.

If the patient has never received the prescribed medication before, he should be given the following information in order to be able to assume responsibility for his drug therapy while ambulatory.

Name and purpose of the medication.

Many drugs can be used to treat several disease conditions, and the pharmacist working in a community setting usually does not have immediate access to the medical record of the patient. As a result, it is sometimes difficult for the pharmacist to know why a certain drug has been prescribed. This problem can often be overcome by asking the patient, "What did your doctor/dentist tell you about this medication?" Using this technique, the pharmacist can determine what information the physician/dentist has given to the patient. This technique enables the pharmacist to coordinate his instructions with those of the physician/dentist and to prevent alarming the patient by using the same terminology to describe the purpose of the medication. If, after asking this question, the pharmacist still does not know the medical condition for which the drug was prescribed, it is often helpful to ask, "Could you tell me why you went to see your doctor today? This drug has several uses, and in order for me to explain it to you, I have to know what your medical problem is." Patients always know the symptoms that prompted them to visit their

MEDICATION HISTORY

NAME: _____
          (FAMILY)   (FIRST)   (MIDDLE)

ADDRESS: _____

PHONE NO: _____ BIRTHDATE: _____

Please check *all* the medicines you are taking at present. This information is very important to your doctor and pharmacist.

Antibiotics (Penicillin, Sulfa, etc.)	☐
Anticoagulant (Blood Thinner)	☐
Asthma or Allergy Medicine	☐
Cough or Cold Medicine	☐
Nose Drops or Sprays	☐
Eye Medicine	☐
Ear Medicine	☐
Heart Medicine (Digitalis, Nitroglycerin)	☐
High Blood Pressure Medicine	☐
Water Pills (Diuretic)	☐
Potassium Supplement	☐
Diabetes Pills	☐
Insulin	☐
Birth Control Pills	☐
Hormones	☐
Cortisone Medicine (Prednisone)	☐
Epilepsy Medicine	☐
Thyroid Medicine	☐
Pain Medicine (at least once a week)	☐
Aspirin, Anacin, Bufferin, Alka-Seltzer, etc.	☐
Laxatives (at least once a week)	☐
Diarrhea Medicine	☐
Stomach or Ulcer Medicine	☐
Antacids	☐
Skin Medicine	☐
Vitamins	☐
Suppositories	☐
Reducing Medicine (to lose weight)	☐
Iron or Anemia Medicine	☐
Tranquilizers (Nerve Pills)	☐
Sleeping Pills	☐
"Natural (Herbal) Remedies"	☐

Are you taking any other medicine not listed above?   ☐ Yes ☐ No

Are you allergic to any of the following drugs?   ☐ Aspirin ☐ Penicillin ☐ Anesthetics ☐ Iodides ☐ Antihistamines ☐ Sulfa Drugs ☐ X-Ray Drugs
    ☐ Other Drugs

Have you ever had any unpleasant effects from drugs?   ☐ Yes ☐ No

Figure 2. *Medication history questionnaire.*

physician or dentist and usually remember what the physician told them regarding the diagnosis.

The purpose of a medication can be explained in terms of an organ, a disease, or a symptom. The choice of description depends on the terminology that would be best understood by the patient. For example, digoxin is best understood when it is described as a drug for the heart (organ). In contrast, probenecid is best described as a medication used in the treatment of gout (disease), and imipramine can be described as a drug used to help decrease anxiety and tension (symptoms). Always explain the purpose of a drug to the patient in language that the patient can understand. For example, it is normally less disconcerting to the patient to explain digoxin as "a drug for the heart" rather than as "a cardiotonic glycoside." The use of medical terminology usually is not understood by the patient and may even frighten him. An exception would be the student or colleague of the health sciences who understands medical terminology and who would be insulted if he felt he was being "talked down to."

Dosage schedule.

Prescription instructions should be written as specific as possible. Such written instructions as "Take as directed" are inadequate,[41] as they can easily be misinterpreted by the patient. In order for the patient to assume responsibility for his drug therapy, it is essential that the dosage schedule be designed to be consistent with the patient's daily activities and that the patient understand the importance of the assigned dosage times.

A label reading "Take 1 capsule four times daily" is also an inadequate instruction. Mazullo, Lasagna, and Griner, in 1974,[22] studied the variations in interpretation of prescription instructions by patients. Sixty-seven patients were asked to read ten prescription labels and to describe how he/she would take the medication. Only 35.8% of the patients indicated they would take tetracycline every six hours around the clock for a total of 4 doses daily when they interpreted the label "Take 1 capsule every 6 hours." Twenty-five percent of the patients said they would not take a night-time dose because they conceived the "day" as being 18 hours of working time and divided the time into three six-hour periods and omitted the fourth dose. For an antiarrythmic drug such as procainamide whose plasma half-life is short and whose constant blood levels may be critical, the deletion of a dose may spell therapeutic failure. It is accepted that penicillin G should be taken on an empty stomach to facilitate absorption. When patients were asked to interpret the label, "Penicillin G—Take 1 tablet three times a day and at bedtime," 89.5% indicated they would take the drug *with* meals and at bedtime. A more appropriate instruction would have been "Take 1 tablet 30 minutes before meals and at bedtime on an empty stomach," since 91% of the patients interpreted this correctly. Some drugs are best taken on a full stomach in order to decrease gastrointestinal irritation. Fifty percent of the patients interpreted the instruction "with meals" to mean to take the drug before meals and some patients would have taken it one hour before meals. A more appropriate instruction would have been, "Take immediately after food."

In summary, misinterpretation by patients of instructions on prescription labels is an important factor in noncompliance. There is definitely a need to explain the dosage instructions and to adapt the dosage schedule to the daily activities of the patient. A simple method of determining the daily schedule of the patient is to ask the patient what time he arises and when he eats his meals. It is also important not to ask too much of the patient. For example, if the pharmacist recommends that the last daily dose of an antibiotic be taken at 2 AM, how many patients will simply omit that dose and take the medication "q8h" rather than "q6h"? Any therapeutic regimen necessitates some behavioral change on the part of the patient, and he is most likely to comply with those aspects of the therapy which are least disruptive of his normal routine. Asking for the impossible will only result in discouragement and withdrawal.

One problem particularly common with antibiotic therapy is premature discontinuation of the medication. Patients should be told how long to take the antibiotic and that the disappearance of symptoms does not necessarily mean that the drug should be stopped. The maximum daily dose of any medications prescribed on a "pro re nata" basis should also be interpreted for the patient.

Method of administration.

Another important aspect of the consultation is teaching the patient the proper method of administration of the medication. Many patients fail to respond to a therapeutic regimen simply because they have not administered their medication(s) correctly. Among the many pharmaceutical preparations that require special methods of administration are ophthalmic, otic, and nasal preparations; sublingual and buccal tablets; respiratory inhalers; vaginal tablets and creams and rectal suppositories. Diagrams and teaching models can be extremely useful in instructing the patients in this psychomotor stage of learning. For example, a diagram of an ophthalmic solution being instilled into the eye can often help the patient to learn the correct method of administration. When the medication is being dispensed, the patient sometimes asks the pharmacist to instill the first dose. As long as the medication will not interfere with the patient's trip home, a more effective teaching approach would be for the pharmacist to decline and to encourage the patient to instill the first dose of the solution under his supervision. If the pharmacist instills the first dose of the solution, there is no guarantee that the patient will learn the correct technique. However, by explaining the proper method and then observing the patient as he instills the solution, the pharmacist is able to detect and help correct any mistakes the patient is making. In order to maximize this type of teaching, a mirror should be available in the counseling area of the dispensary.

Diagrams of the respiratory system and a sample inhaler are extremely useful in teaching patients the proper method of administering a medication by means of a respiratory inhaler. In order to deliver an accurate dose, most aerosol inhalers must be shaken prior to use and some inhalers must also be inverted. Respiratory inhalers require special care, and a sample inhaler should be available to demonstrate its proper use and cleaning.

Whenever a medication is dispensed, the pharmacist must ensure that the patient knows how to administer it correctly. An excellent technique of assessing the comprehension of the patient is to ask him to repeat the administration instructions.

Pertinent side effects which the patient can recognize and manage (if appropriate).

One area of the medication consultation that requires extreme care is the selection of side effects a patient should know in order to use a drug most effectively and with the least anxiety. Patients should only be informed of those side effects they can recognize and for which they can take the appropriate precautionary measures. For example, if the patient is prescribed an antihypertensive medication that commonly causes orthostatic hypotension, he should be warned to get up slowly in the morning and to dangle his feet over the edge of the bed for a few minutes. If a drug commonly causes photosensitization, the patient should be advised to avoid undue exposure to the sun, to wear appropriate clothing, and to wear sunglasses if necessary. Every patient receiving a medication that commonly causes drowsiness, dizziness, or blurred vision should be advised to exercise caution in driving an automobile or operating electrical equipment until his response to the drug has been determined. Patients should be told whether food or an antacid should (or should not) be taken at the same time as the medication.

It is important not to frighten the patient, but it is also important that the patient be warned of possible side effects, which otherwise could cause undue alarm. For example, drug-induced urine color changes can often cause undue alarm and patients should be informed of the possibility of such changes before they occur. Some side effects, such as xerostomia, are simply annoying to the patient and can often be managed by means of simple techniques. This helps to prevent premature discontinuation of the therapy by the patient.

The patient should be advised to avoid drugs and foods that have been reported to interact significantly with the prescribed medication. In addition, many drugs can interact with alcohol, and probably the most clinically significant alcohol interactions occur with disulfiram and with central nervous system depressants. As little as seven milliliters of ethanol can produce a mild reaction in patients receiving disulfiram.[42] Many oral liquid pharmaceuticals contain ethanol, and patients should be advised to avoid these preparations. Patients receiving central nervous system depressants should be advised of the possibility of potentiation of drowsiness and to avoid alcoholic beverages. Many deaths have resulted from the combined use of central nervous system depressants and alcohol, and yet the problem is frequently overlooked in practice.

The placebo component of drug response and the power of suggestion must never be underestimated. If the patient were told that the drug may cause a headache, "9 times out of 10" that patient would develop a headache and discontinue taking the medication. The only time a patient should be forewarned of a headache is when the headache is predictable, as with isosorbide dinitrate, and treatable. Similarly, every oral medication is capable of causing some degree of gastrointestinal upset, and patients should be advised of the possibility of nausea, vomiting, and diarrhea only when it is critical to the success of the drug therapy. An example of the latter case is the patient receiving digoxin who should be told to contact his physician if he loses his appetite or develops nausea, vomiting, or diarrhea.

The patient should also be informed of the dangers of self-medication. The patient must realize that some preparations contain drugs that can sometimes negate the desired therapeutic effect of their prescribed medication. For example, results of several well-documented clinical studies indicate that patients receiving oral anticoagulants should avoid salicylates.[42] These patients should be cautioned against using all nonprescription products containing salicylates and, if in doubt, to ask their pharmacist. Depending on the specific diagnosis of the patient, undesirable side effects from over-the-counter products should be discussed. For example, a patient with acne vulgaris should be advised to avoid sleep aids containing bromides, since bromides can aggravate the skin condition.

In summary, through the careful selection of side effects and recommendations for the appropriate precautions, the patient is made a more active partner in his drug therapy, and needless accidents or more severe adverse effects can often be prevented. The practitioner must evaluate each patient individually and decide how much information the patient

26

should be given. In most cases, an intelligent, interested patient can be helped to use his medication more reliably if he is given this information; however, extremely anxious or hypochondriacal patients could become unduly concerned. Both the physician and the pharmacist should have some method of informing each other if they feel a patient should not be counseled in the normal manner.

Pertinent adverse effects which should prompt the patient to notify his physician.

Patients are admitted to hospitals every year because of adverse drug reactions. It will never be possible to completely eliminate these adverse effects; however, they are frequently preceded by signs or symptoms that can be recognized by the patient at home and can prompt him to contact his physician earlier. For example, clindamycin-induced pseudomembranous colitis is preceded by diarrhea, and the earlier the diagnosis is made, the more favorable the prognosis. Unless the patient was told to contact the physician if he developed diarrhea, he would probably attribute the diarrhea to something he ate or to "flu." Patients can be informed of contraindications to continued use without frightening them. At the same time careful use of medications can be encouraged.

Storage instructions.

In general, a cool dry place is the best storage place for most medications. It is important to remind the patient that the traditional bathroom medicine cabinet often becomes hot and steamy and is not the ideal storage area for medications. Some medications, such as nitroglycerin, require special methods of storage which should be carefully explained to the patient. In addition, if a patient takes his medication exactly according to the dosage schedule in the proper manner, but takes a deteriorated drug because of improper storage, the dosage regimen becomes ineffective and perhaps dangerous.

The physician and nurse should stress the importance of having the prescription filled, and the pharmacist should explain the procedure for having the prescription refilled (if applicable), at the proper intervals.

Ask The Patient If He Has Any Questions

It is extremely important to give the patient an opportunity to ask questions regarding any of the information he has just been given about his drug therapy. Many patients will also ask questions regarding other medications they have been taking. Very often, the practitioner gains information about problems the patient is having with his present drug regimen or nonprescription drug usage. This portion of the drug consultation can sometimes become the most informative and should be present during every consultation. It is essential that the practitioner maintain control of the interview at this stage. This is sometimes difficult when the patient is exceedingly talkative and relates everything except the pertinent information. It is at times like this that the patient must be reminded that the purpose of the interview is to discuss the drug regimen.

Terminating the interview

The interview should be closed with the same concern and thoughtfulness with which it was opened. The limitations on the interview as dictated by the clock make it important for the practitioner to terminate the interview skillfully and make the patient sense that it has come to a natural conclusion. The termination of an interview consists of three steps:[43]

1. a summary statement by the practitioner;
2. a prescription for action;
3. the physical parting.

The **summary statement** by the practitioner relates information that he has gained from the interview. This final statement should be positive without controversial or critical comments. The **prescription for action** stresses the responsibility of the patient in assuming management of his medication regimen. The **physical parting** is probably the most awkward and most difficult aspect of the interview.

If the interviewer terminates the interview abruptly, it is quite feasible that the patient will be insulted. Several techniques are useful in closing the interview. One method, which has previously been discussed, is to ask the patient if he has any questions. This technique will signal the patient that the purpose of this particular interview has been reached, and before the interview is completely terminated, the practitioner wants to know if the patient has understood all of the information presented. The more experienced interviewer will use nonverbal signals that the interview is completed. For example, he may close the patient's folder and lay his pen down on the desk; he may sit back in his chair as though he is ready to get up, or he may stand up. All of these nonverbal techniques communicate to the patient that the interview is about to be terminated. If neither of these techniques successfully communicates to the patient that the interview must be closed, it is usually helpful to say, "We're going to have to stop here, I'm afraid, unless there is something you particularly wanted to ask before we stop." The physical parting is completed when the practitioner opens the office door for the patient. The practitioner's final remarks should include a statement reminding the patient to contact him if he has any questions or problems relating to the drug regimen. Often the patient's last remarks will indicate what the interview has meant to him or the degree to which he intends to comply with the drug regimen.[44] Through the use of a few specific techniques, the practitioner can use the last few minutes of an interview to solidify the constructive rapport that has been established and set the stage for the patient to manage his own drug regimen.

SUBSEQUENT VISITS

If the patient has received the medication before and has previously been counseled, the interviewer should review the dosage schedule and ask the patient if he has any questions about the use of his medications. The interviewer should briefly review those aspects of the therapy that are particularly significant and update the medication history record. Through the application of the previously mentioned techniques of communication, he should evaluate the degree of compliance of the patient and the compatibility of the drug regimen with his life style. During subsequent visits, all patients should be monitored for drug response as well as the appearance of adverse effects. The absence of normally occurring side effects should also be a cue that the patient may not be taking his medication.

DOCUMENTATION

Immediately after the termination of an interview or consultation, any facts pertinent to the interview should be documented in the patient record. In addition, any telephone inquiries made by the patient regarding a symptom or possible adverse effect should be recorded. Such documentation will not only make it easier to provide optimum patient care, but it will also become a legal document in the event of a malpractice suit.

It has been suggested that malpractice suits are not the cause of but rather the result of the breakdown of the patient relationship in 90% of cases.[45] The "suit-prone" practitioner wants patients to look up to him and put their hopes in him. He tries to promise patients what they want and is afraid to admit to them or himself his own inabilities or inadequacies. This type of practitioner never warns patients of things that could go wrong.[45] In contrast, the "suit-prone" patient cannot accept the realistic limitations of modern health care and becomes upset over issues that most people would overlook. This patient is usually dependent, emotionally immature, rigid, quick to blame others, and incapable of accepting adult responsibility.[46] It is obviously to the advantage of the practitioner to be sensitive to the needs of the patient and to be completely familiar with the various components of the learning process and the appropriate use of interviewing techniques.

IV. Understanding "Problem" Patients

Every physician, nurse, pharmacist, and dentist finds that there are certain recurrent problem situations which they encounter with some of their patients. Many of these patients are often labeled as "problem" patients, and they arouse emotions ranging from anger to frustration to hopelessness in the practitioner. In order to maintain his own sanity as well as to provide effective patient care, the practitioner should try to understand why the patient is behaving in such a manner. He should also examine his own emotions in an effort to better understand his own reactions to certain types of patients.

Every patient who has been prescribed a medication is experiencing some degree of emotional stress. The most common reactions are fear and worry. The patient may be afraid of the unknown. If he is not routinely prescribed medications or if he is prescribed a new medication, he may become unduly worried about the effectiveness of the drug or the adverse effects it could cause. Other patients who have been prescribed analgesics or sedatives are afraid they could become addicted to the medication and often express this fear when they present the prescription to the pharmacist. Some of these patients may decide to take a lower dose or to take the drug less frequently than prescribed because of this fear. It is important that these patients understand why the drug has been prescribed and why they should take it according to the recommended schedule. Some patients are concerned that their illness will permanently disable them and other patients are confronted with the possibility of a surgical procedure or even death. There is a certain amount of financial worry associated with any illness, and a few patients never recover sufficiently to be able to return to their previous occupations. People with stoical personalities may find it difficult to accept the fact that they need a medication to help them overcome their illness. Illness can also cause some people to become unusually dependent and preoccupied with their illness. These are a few of the most common emotions which underly not only the placebo response of the patient to the drug, but also the manner in which the patient responds to the practitioner.

There are a few special communication techniques which are helpful in interviewing patients who are deaf or blind. Some elderly patients who are partially deaf are too proud to admit they have this problem. They may become upset if they do not hear you properly and misinterpret something you said. It is important to speak slowly and distinctly with these patients. If they cannot understand something, it may help to re-word the sentence because some sounds are easier to detect than others. If the patient is deaf, it may be necessary to write down all the questions and answers. Another approach is to give the patient a written questionnaire to complete. If the patient is able to lip-read, the practitioner should sit or stand directly in front of the patient and should not turn his head while speaking since the person must be able to see his lips in order to understand. A completely different approach is needed if the patient is blind. The interviewer should always speak to the blind patient as he is approaching him so that he is not startled. The blind person is acutely aware of sounds because his sense of hearing is usually hyper-developed in response to his loss of sight. The blind patient relates to his medication history in terms of touch, taste, and smell and may describe a round, film-coated, scored tablet as being "round and waxy with a line down the middle." The interviewer should similarly discuss the medications in these terms so that the patient can understand him. The ambulatory blind patient will find it helpful if the pharmacist dispenses his medications in different sizes of containers so that he can better identify them at home. It may also be helpful if the drug is identified with a dymo tape attached to the label. The blind patient can "read" such a label with his fingertips. Although deaf and blind people do need some assistance, they are not helpless and are never seeking pity. It is important that they be allowed to maintain as much independence as possible, and every effort should be taken to help them achieve greater security and independence.

Anger can be expressed by the patient in many forms. When confronted with direct hostility, the normal temptation of the interviewer is to respond with less understanding or an angry response. Such a response is nontherapeutic because counterhostility produces further anger in the patient and makes it difficult to maintain an effective relationship. It may help the practitioner to control his anger if he realizes that most criticisms and demands of patients are usually reflections of their fears and worries about their illnesses. One of the most common complaints that patients have about their medications is the cost. People do not want to spend money on prescription drugs and, as a result, pharmacists deal with many unwilling customers. It may help to explain to these patients how modern drugs can prevent many hospitalizations and decrease the number of days that people will have to stay away from work. Another useful technique is to break down the total cost of the prescription into the individual price for the tablet or capsule. A cost of 10 cents per tablet does not sound nearly as expensive as $12.00 for the one-month supply of medication. If the patient has a legitimate reason for being angry, the practitioner should not attempt to ignore the complaint. For example, if the patient is upset that he had to wait too long to have his prescriptions filled, the best response would be to agree with the patient and say "I am sorry you had to wait so long" or "I understand how you feel." It is advantageous to discuss the situation in a private area because anger can be contagious and could disrupt the other patients in the waiting area. If the interviewer does not understand why the patient is angry, he should use the various interviewing techniques previously discussed in an attempt to better understand the patient's frustration. Perhaps the most important concept for the practitioner to remember is to avoid responding to the angry outburst of the patient as a personal criticism. The anger is a symptom of the patient's illness and should be treated in a therapeutic manner.

What do you say to the patient who asks, "Am I going to die?" Most people feel uncomfortable with the topic of death and tend to hide behind an armor of professionalism.[47,48] However, the patient with a terminal illness is reaching out for understanding, appreciation, and someone who will listen to him.[49] Death is a difficult topic for every person to cope with. When a patient asks if he is dying, it is helpful to encourage him to discuss his fears. An appropriate response could be, "What makes you ask that?" As the practitioner becomes more aware of his own attitudes toward death, he will find that he has become more sensitive to the needs of the patient. If the person is religious, it will be easier because death means peace and passing into a better life.

Terminally ill patients have special emotional needs that must be dealt with. Kübler-Ross has described the five psychological stages of dying.[47] The first stage is denial and shock when patients are told that they have a serious illness. This is the stage in which the patient says, "No, it can't be me." This stage may last from a few seconds to a few months. Denial is a self-protective measure that gives the patient time to gain enough strength to cope. Health professionals should never prolong this denial stage because the patient may refuse treatment or may even become psychotic or suicidal.[50] When the patient can no longer continue to deny his prognosis, he will become critical, demanding, and difficult. This is the stage during which he freely displaces his anger. The practitioner should not respond with anger because the patient may repress any future anger and become extremely depressed. The third stage is the bargaining stage in which the patient may try to promise something in exchange for an extension of life. This is the "maybe, not me" stage, and the practitioner should be careful that he does not give the patient false hope. Instead, he should remain sensitive and understanding. The fourth stage is depression and preparatory grief. This is a very difficult stage in which the patient recognizes the progress of his illness and goes through his own mourning process. It is helpful to allow the patient to openly express his grief rather than saying "Don't cry. It isn't as bad as that." The final stage of acceptance is not reached by all patients; however, it is these patients who are able to "die with dignity." [50] They have accepted their prognosis, have decided to live their remaining days as fully as possible, and have been able to complete their responsibilities. The skillful practitioner will recognize that the patient is progressing through these various emotional stages and will provide appropriate counsel.

All patients with chronic diseases—especially alcoholism, diabetes, and tuberculosis—should be managed in a firm, explicit, and direct nature. The facts should be clearly explained. It should never be suggested that there are simple ways to treat these conditions and that the patient can make a choice and drift half-heartedly along. Such patients must accept the reality of what they are told and must learn to accept their responsibility. If the patient is constantly complaining, it may help to make a positive comment to him. For example, if the patient is complaining about the weather, it may help to say, "Yes, it is rainy today but yesterday was really a nice day, wasn't it?" A responsible family member is the best source of information for pediatric patients, patients in severe pain, and patients with psychiatric disturbances. Occasionally, the practitioner will encounter a paranoid patient who is distrustful, suspicious, and chronically angry. Such patients are very difficult to interview, and it is best to be friendly and firm with these patients. Sympathetic understanding usually arouses their suspicion and should probably not be used.

If a parent is having difficulty administering a medication to a child, there are a few techniques that may be helpful. It is easier to gain the cooperation of the child if the parent uses a positive approach. For example, children love to imitate and may be more cooperative if the parent says, "Here is your medicine. Drink it and I will give you some special medicine for your teddy bear." [51] Parents should not mix pediatric medications with infant formulas or foods because the taste of the drug may destroy the infant's or child's acceptance of those foods. There are also several oral syringes and special teaspoons which can be used as administration aides.

Health professionals are frequently troubled by the personal questions that patients ask them. They are often embarrassed and do not know whether to ignore the question or how to answer it. A patient may ask a personal question because he thinks this is socially acceptable or he may be curious about the person who is asking him confidential information. In some cases, the patient may actually be trying to introduce a problem of his own which he would like to discuss. The practitioner may redirect the question and respond "Why do you ask?" This will focus the attention back to the patient. Another technique would be to respond frankly and briefly and immediately redirect the interview back to the patient.

In summary, understanding is the key to communicating with "problem" patients. In trying to understand the person's behavior, the practitioner will find it helpful to look at the problem from the patient's point of view. Once he understands the reasons a patient is upset or not cooperative, he will be able to develop a true empathy with his patients.

V. Written Medication Instructions

Total patient recall is rare.[28,29] Patients know or retain very little knowledge about their medications by the time they arrive at the pharmacy. In one study of ambulatory patients, the average knowledge level of 109 patients upon arrival at the pharmacy was 26% of the total knowledge of which they should have been aware.[5] This represented all the information the patient could remember about his prescribed medication and the level at which he would assume responsibility for his drug therapy at home. The level of anxiety of most patients has decreased by the time they reach the pharmacy and they should be in a more receptive state for learning about their drugs. The study demonstrated that the average knowledge level seven days after the patients had been given verbal instructions by the pharmacist rose to 77%. The highest recall (89%) was achieved by those patients who had received both verbal and written instructions. The study also demonstrated that reinforcement of medication instructions can significantly improve patient recall. It was recommended that the pharmacist reinforce the verbal prescription instructions of the physician through a combination of verbal and written instructions.

Drug compliance can also be significantly improved by giving patients both written and verbal instructions. One study specifically compared the effects of no additional instructions, verbal instructions, written instructions, and a combination of written plus verbal instructions.[52] The highest rate of compliance occurred in those patients who received both written and verbal instructions. Similar results have also been reported by other investigators.[53-55] In summary, it appears that written instructions presented alone are not as effective in improving patient recall of the information or in improving patient compliance with the drug regimen. Printed information improves compliance **provided** there is verbal reinforcement.

Written medication instructions that have been properly designed can be very helpful to a patient who is receiving prescribed medications. The degree of clarity with which the patient is given insight into his drug regimen is extremely important. The patient generally wants enough information to help him complete the therapy as easily and safely as possible. Since failures of comprehension of the prescription instructions are at least as frequent as failures of volition,[56] the information must be presented to the patient in language that he can understand. It requires a special sensitivity and skill for the pharmacist to avoid medical terminology and to explain the drug therapy at approximately the sixth- to seventh-grade level of education.[58,59] If the written instructions are not meaningful to the patient, there is a high probability that the patient will never refer to them at a later date.[59] Great care must be taken during the preparation of written instructions, and the terminology must correspond to that used during the interview so that the patient does not become confused.

In summary, written medication instructions have several advantages:

1. Patient recall will gradually decrease over a period of time. Written instructions can be retained by the patient and referred to by the patient whenever he is in doubt at a later date. A combination of both written and verbal instructions has the advantage that if a patient forgets or becomes confused over the instructions that were previously outlined during the interview, he can readily refer to the supplementary sheet at home.
2. Written instructions help ensure that all patients receive complete and uniform information which is not dependent upon the memory or time of the health professional.
3. Written instructions help standardize patient information and can be used by health professionals as a method of reinforcing the verbal instructions. It is essential that there be a close liaison between physicians and pharmacists who are involved in such an education program.
4. In a pharmacy, many medications are mailed, delivered, or dispensed to someone other than the patient and the pharmacist has no verbal contact with the patient. In such cases, written instructions are very useful and can be forwarded with the medication.
5. Written instructions promote patient respect for medications.

In response to requests from pharmacists, physicians, and patients over the past three years, 96 written medication instruction sheets have been prepared for the most commonly prescribed medications in the United States and Canada (Fig. 3).[60] These written medication instructions are intended to be given to the patient at the time a medication is dispensed, or they can be read by the patient while the prescription is being filled. It was recognized that the format of the leaflets was a critical factor in patient acceptance. Color has been used and the graphics were carefully selected in order to increase the sensory feedback which is essential in the reading process.[57]

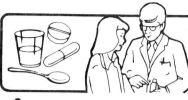

Digoxin

Common Trade Name:
Lanoxin

 This medicine is used to help make the heart beat strong and steady.

HOW TO USE THIS MEDICINE

 It is very important that you take this drug as your doctor has prescribed and that you do not miss any doses. Take this medicine at the same time every day and do not go without this medicine between prescription refills.

If this medicine causes stomach upset, take it with some food.

 If a dropper is used to measure the liquid dose and you do not fully understand how to use it, check with your pharmacist.

SPECIAL INSTRUCTIONS

 Some nonprescription drugs can aggravate your condition. Do not take any of the following products without the approval of your doctor: cough, cold or sinus products, asthma or allergy products and diet or weight reducing medicines.

 Most people experience few or no side effects from their drugs. However, any medicine can sometimes cause unwanted effects. Call your doctor immediately if you develop a slow or irregular pulse, nausea, vomiting, diarrhea (loose bowel movements), loss of appetite, unusual weakness, blurred vision or changes in colour vision.

These instructions may be altered by your doctor or pharmacist because of your medical condition or other drugs you may be taking.

Adapted from Smith, D. L.: Medication Guide for Patient Counseling.
Exclusive permission granted by Lea & Febiger. © 1980 ABP/PHARMEX

Figure 3. *Patient advisory leaflets.*

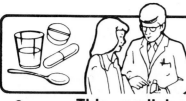

Fenoprofen

Common Trade Name:
Nalfon

This medicine is used to help relieve pain, redness and swelling in certain kinds of arthritis and other medical conditions.

The full effect of this medicine will not be noticed immediately but may take from a few days to 3 weeks.

HOW TO USE THIS MEDICINE

It is best to take this medicine on an empty stomach at least 1 hour before (or 2 hours after) food unless otherwise directed. If you develop stomach upset, take the drug with food or immediately after meals. Call your doctor if you continue to have stomach upset.

SPECIAL INSTRUCTIONS

In some people, this drug may cause dizziness or drowsiness. Do not drive a car or operate dangerous machinery or do jobs that require you to be alert until you know how you are going to react to this drug.

If you become dizzy, you should be careful going up and down stairs. Sit or lie down at the first sign of dizziness.

It is best not to drink alcoholic beverages while you are taking this medicine.

Most people experience few or no side effects from their drugs. However, any medicine can sometimes cause unwanted effects. Call your doctor if you develop a skin rash, "ringing" or "buzzing" in the ears, fast heart beats, swelling of the ankles, blurred vision, black stools or severe stomach pain.

These instructions may be altered by your doctor or pharmacist because of your medical condition or other drugs you may be taking.

Adapted from Smith, D. L.: Medication Guide for Patient Counseling.
Exclusive permission granted by Lea & Febiger. © 1980 ABP/PHARMEX

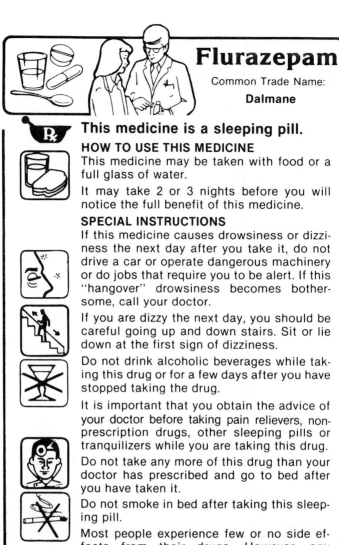

Flurazepam

Common Trade Name:

Dalmane

This medicine is a sleeping pill.

HOW TO USE THIS MEDICINE

This medicine may be taken with food or a full glass of water.

It may take 2 or 3 nights before you will notice the full benefit of this medicine.

SPECIAL INSTRUCTIONS

If this medicine causes drowsiness or dizziness the next day after you take it, do not drive a car or operate dangerous machinery or do jobs that require you to be alert. If this "hangover" drowsiness becomes bothersome, call your doctor.

If you are dizzy the next day, you should be careful going up and down stairs. Sit or lie down at the first sign of dizziness.

Do not drink alcoholic beverages while taking this drug or for a few days after you have stopped taking the drug.

It is important that you obtain the advice of your doctor before taking pain relievers, nonprescription drugs, other sleeping pills or tranquilizers while you are taking this drug.

Do not take any more of this drug than your doctor has prescribed and go to bed after you have taken it.

Do not smoke in bed after taking this sleeping pill.

Most people experience few or no side effects from their drugs. However, any medicine can sometimes cause unwanted effects. Call your doctor if you develop bothersome nightmares or sleepiness during the day.

Adapted from Smith, D. L.: Medication Guide for Patient Counseling.
Exclusive permission granted by Lea & Febiger. © 1980 ABP/PHARMEX

Figure 3. *Continued. Patient advisory leaflets.*

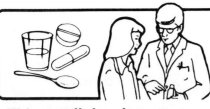

Propranolol

Common Trade Names:
Inderal

This medicine has many uses and the reason it was prescribed depends upon your condition. It is usually used to keep the heart beat slow and steady or to treat high blood pressure. Make sure you understand why you are taking it.

 Depending upon your doctor's instructions, this medicine can be taken with a glass of water before or after meals **or** on an empty stomach (1 hour before or 2 hours after meals). It is important to always take it in the same way each day.

 In some people this drug may cause drowsiness or dizziness. Do not drive a car or operate dangerous machinery or do jobs that require you to be alert until you know how you are going to react to this drug. If you become dizzy, you should be careful going up and down stairs. Sit or lie down at the first sign of dizziness.

 Some non-prescription drugs, especially cough and cold remedies, may aggravate your condition. Read the label of the product you select to see if there is a warning. If there is, check with your doctor or pharmacist before using it.

 It is recommended that patients receiving this drug should stop smoking.

 Call your doctor if you develop a skin rash or shortness of breath.

Do not stop taking this medicine suddenly without the approval of your doctor.

Adapted from Smith, D. L.: Medication Guide for Patient Counseling.
Exclusive permission granted by Lea & Febiger. © 1980 ABP/PHARMEX

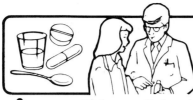

Phenytoin

Common Trade Name:

Dilantin

This medicine is used to help control convulsions or seizures.

HOW TO USE THIS MEDICINE

Take this medicine with food if it upsets your stomach. Call your doctor if you continue to have stomach upset.

If you were prescribed the **liquid medicine,** shake the bottle well just before using so that you can measure an accurate dose.

It is very important that you take this drug as your doctor has prescribed and that you do not miss any doses. Take this medicine at the same time every day and do not go without this medicine between prescription refills.

SPECIAL INSTRUCTIONS

Do not stop taking this medicine suddenly without the approval of your doctor.

In some people this drug may cause dizziness. Do not drive a car or operate dangerous machinery or do jobs that require you to be alert until you know how you are going to react to this drug. If you become dizzy, you should be careful going up and down stairs. Sit or lie down at the first sign of dizziness.

If this medicine is for a child, do not let him (her) climb trees, ride a bike, etc. until you can determine their reaction to the medicine. Children could hurt themselves if they participated in these activities and were dizzy.

Avoid swimming alone or high risk sports in which a sudden seizure could cause injury.

Figure 3. *Continued. Patient advisory leaflets.*

40

Phenytoin, continued

 Do not drink alcoholic beverages while taking this drug.

 It is important that you obtain the advice of your doctor before taking pain relievers, non-prescription drugs, sleeping pills or tranquilizers or medicines for depression while you are taking this drug.

 While taking this medicine, brush your teeth and gums regularly. The next time you visit your dentist, tell him you are taking this medicine. Call your doctor if your gums become red or swollen.

 Most people experience few or no side effects from their drugs. However, any medicine can sometimes cause unwanted effects. Call your doctor if you develop a skin rash, sore throat, fever, mouth sores, persistent headache, slurred speech, fast eye movements, joint pain, swollen glands or difficulty in walking.

 Carry a card in your wallet or wear a bracelet stating that you are taking this drug.

These instructions may be altered by your doctor or pharmacist because of your medical condition or other drugs you may be taking.

Adapted from Smith, D. L.: Medication Guide for Patient Counseling. Exclusive permission granted by Lea & Febiger. © 1980 ABP/PHARMEX

General Instructions for the Safe Use of Your Medicine

- Take your medicines exactly as your doctor has prescribed. Always read the prescription label carefully.
- Always tell your doctor and pharmacist if:
  - —you are allergic to any drugs or other substances or have had any unpleasant reactions to drugs.
  - —you have any other disease conditions.
  - —you are taking any other drugs—including those products you can buy yourself without a prescription (for example: aspirin, laxatives, vitamins, cough medicines).
  - —you are pregnant, plan to become pregnant or if you are breast-feeding.
  - —you are planning to have dental work or surgery.
  - —you are on a special diet.
  - —you have been unable to take all the medicine for some reason.
- Most people experience few or no side effects from their drugs. However, if you think the medicine is bothering you and causing unusual reactions, call your doctor or pharmacist.
- Call your doctor immediately if you think you may be allergic to a medicine or if you develop a skin rash, hives, itching, swelling of the face, or difficulty in breathing.
- DO NOT take or save old medicines. Throw them away.
- STORE your drugs in a cool, dry place—NOT in the bathroom medicine cabinet. Keep all drugs out of the reach of children.
- DO NOT share your drugs with other members of your family or friends. They should see their own doctor.
- DO NOT take any other drugs (including those you can buy without a prescription) without the consent of your doctor.
- If you have any questions about your drugs, ask your pharmacist or your doctor.

◄ Have all of your prescriptions filled at the same pharmacy ►

These instructions may be altered by your doctor or pharmacist because of your medical condition or other drugs you may be taking.

Adapted from Smith, D.L., Medication Guide for Patient Counseling.
Exclusive permission granted by Lea & Febiger. © 1979 ABP/PHARMEX

AREA BELOW FOR DRUG MANUFACTURER'S NAME, SPECIAL INSTRUCTIONS OR YOUR STORE NAME

Figure 3. *Continued. Patient advisory leaflets.*
These general instructions appear on the reverse side of every patient advisory leaflet.

In conclusion, written medication instructions do not negate the need for verbal communication with the patient. Written instructions can provide the knowledge component of the educational process. An equally important component of patient education is behavior modification, which is most effectively accomplished through verbal communication. Almost every patient will have questions relating to the application of the drug therapy to his own daily schedule, and such questions can only be answered on an individual basis. Therefore, written instructions should be used to complement and reinforce the verbal instructions communicated to patients.

VI. Conclusions

Through the effective use of communication techniques, we must motivate the patient so that he is able to participate maximally in his drug therapy. We must recognize that drug defaulting is not a question of obeying, but rather it is a question of understanding. The importance of educating patients regarding the proper use of their medications cannot be overemphasized and requires expansion of the traditional system whereby the physician or dentist hands the prescription to the patient and the patient hands the prescription to the pharmacist from whom he receives a medication in exchange. In this system, the only information a patient often receives is that which is written on the prescription label. Education of the patient is clearly a professional responsibility and must be incorporated into both stages of the prescription transaction.

It has been demonstrated that compliance with medication regimens can be improved through the utilization of both verbal and written instructions. The comprehensiveness of the drug consultation should depend on a variety of factors including the potential of the patient to comprehend the information. It is essential that the information be presented to the patient in a manner he can understand and incorporate into his daily routine. If this does not occur, the patient has merely received "information" and has not been "educated" because the latter implies both understanding and the appropriate behavioral change. The communication skills required by the practitioner to accomplish this goal can be learned only through practice and self-evaluation. With experience, each practitioner develops a personal style of interviewing which complements his individual personality. All medication consultations should be carefully planned in order to guide the patient through each of the three learning stages. The patient should be encouraged to ask questions and should be made to feel that his contribution to the drug therapy is extremely important. A verbal and/or written contract with the patient may help to reinforce this responsibility. The written medication instructions in this book have been designed as a guide to assist health professionals in patient education. There will always be a need for professional judgment as it applies to the individual patient regarding information provided either orally or in writing concerning prescribed medications.

Approximately 80% of all patients receive their medications on an ambulatory basis,[61] and if one of every two or three patients is noncompliant, it is difficult to justify the present method of treating ambulatory patients with therapeutic regimens. Patient noncompliance with medication regimens not only curtails the usual therapeutic benefits from the drugs prescribed, but the additional costs to the patient, the physician, the dentist, the pharmacist, and the government must be taken into account. It is hoped that through the cooperation of all health professionals involved, communication with the patient can be improved to the extent that the patient becomes a more reliable partner because he has been given the necessary information as well as assistance in adapting the drug regimen to his daily activities. The ultimate goal of every prescribing physician and dentist is that the patient receive the full benefits of the therapeutic program that he has designed. This goal can only be achieved if health professionals stress the educational component of every prescription and guide the patient toward more responsible drug use.

References

1. Davis, M. S.: Variations in patients' compliance with doctors' advice: an empirical analysis of patterns of communication. *Amer. J. Public Health,* *58:*274–288 (Feb.), 1968.
2. Millis, J. S.: Future health professional practice in America. *Amer. J. Hosp. Pharm.,* *3:*161 (Feb.), 1975.
3. Boyd, J. R., Covington, T. R., Stanaszek, W. F., and Coussons, R. T.: Drug defaulting. Part I: Determinants of compliance. *Amer. J. Hosp. Pharm.,* *31:*362–367 (Apr.), 1974.
4. Boyd, J. R., Covington, T. R., Stanaszek, W. F., and Coussons, R. T.: Drug defaulting. Part II: Analysis of noncompliance patterns. *Amer. J. Hosp. Pharm.,* *31:*485–491 (May), 1974.
5. Crichton, E. F., Smith, D. L., and Demanuele, F.: Patient recall of medication information. *Drug Intell. Clin. Pharm.,* *12:*591–599 (Oct.), 1978.
6. Kasl, S. A., and Cobb, S.: Health behavior, illness behavior and sick role behavior. I. Health and illness behavior. *Arch. Environ. Health,* *12:*246–266 (Feb.), 1966.
7. Rosenstock, I. M.: Patients' compliance with health regimens. *J. Amer. Med. Assoc.,* *234:*402–403 (Oct. 27), 1975.
8. Becker, M. H., and Maiman, L. S.: Sociobehavioral determinants of compliance with health and medical care recommendations. *Med. Care, 13:*10–24 (Jan.), 1975.
9. Morris, L. A., and O'Neal, E. C.: Judgements about a drug's effectiveness: The role of expectations and outcomes. *Drugs in Health Care, 2:*179–186 (Summer), 1975.
10. Becker, M. H., Drachman, E. H., and Kirscht, J. P.: A new approach to explaining sick-role behavior in low-income populations. *Amer. J. Public Health, 64:*205–216 (March), 1974.

44

11. Zifferblatt, S. M.: Increasing patient compliance through the applied analysis of behavior. *Prev. Med.,* *4:*173–182 (June), 1975.
12. Redman, B. K.: The Process of Patient Teaching in Nursing. Second edition. C. V. Mosby Company, St. Louis, 1972, pp. 22–87.
13. National High Blood Pressure Education Program: Patient behavior for blood pressure control. *J. Amer. Med. Assoc., 241*(23):2534–2537 (June 8), 1979.
14. Porter, A. M. W.: Drug defaulting in general practice. *Br. Med. J., 1:*218–222 (Jan.), 1969.
15. Report No. 148 of the General Practitioner Group: Dosage schedules in general practice. *Practitioner, 204:*719–723 (May), 1970.
16. Benarde, M. A., and Mayerson, E. W.: Patient-physician negotiation. *J. Amer. Med. Assoc., 239*(14):1413–1415 (April 3), 1978.
17. Smith, D. L.: Patient compliance with medication regimens. *Drug Intell. Clin. Pharm., 10:*386–393 (July), 1976.
18. Gillum, R. F., and Barsky, A. J.: Diagnosis and management of patient noncompliance. *J. Amer. Med. Assoc., 228:*1563–1567 (June 17), 1974.
19. Madden, E. E.: Evaluation of outpatient pharmacy counseling. *J. Amer. Pharm. Assoc., NA13*(8):437–443 (Aug.), 1973.
20. Schwartz, D., et al.: Medication errors made by elderly, chronically ill patients. *Amer. J. Public Health, 52:*2018–2029 (Dec.), 1962.
21. Latiolais, C. J., and Berry, C. C.: Misuse of prescription medications by out-patients. *Drug Intell. Clin. Pharm., 3:*270–277 (Oct.), 1969.
22. Mazullo, J. M., Lasagna, L., and Griner, P. F.: Variations in interpretation of prescription instructions. *J. Amer. Med. Assoc., 227:*929–931 (Feb. 25), 1974.
23. Malahy, B.: The effect of instruction and labelling on the number of medication errors made by patients at home. *Amer. J. Hosp. Pharm., 23:*283–292 (June), 1966.
24. Stimson, G. V.: Obeying doctor's orders: a view from the other side. *Soc. Sci. Med., 8:*97–104 (Feb.), 1974.
25. Sharpe, T. R., and Mikeal, R. L.: Patient compliance with antibiotic regimens. *Amer. J. Hosp. Pharm., 31:*479–484 (May), 1974.
26. Marsh, W. W., and Perlman, L. V.: Understanding congestive heart failure and self-administration of digoxin. *Geriatrics, 27:*65–70 (July), 1972.
27. Latiolais, C. J., and Berry, C. C.: Misuse of prescription medications by outpatients. *Drug Intell. Clin. Pharm., 3:*270–277 (Oct.), 1969.
28. Joyce, C. R. B., Caple, G., Mason, M., et al.: Qualitative study of doctor-patient communication. *Quart. J. Med., 38:*183–194, 1969.
29. Ley, P., and Spelman, M. S.: Communication in an outpatient setting. *Br. J. Soc. Clin. Psychol., 4:*115, 1965.
30. Wilber, J., and Barrow, J.: Reducing elevated blood pressure. *Minn. Med., 52:*1303–1306 (Aug.), 1969.
31. McKenney, J., Slining, J., Henderson, N., et al.: The effect of clinical pharmacy services on patients with essential hypertension. *Circulation, 48:*1104–1111 (Nov.), 1973.
32. Rosenberg, S. G.: Patient compliance or non-adherence. *Hosp. Form. Manag., 8:*6–12 (Nov.), 1973.
33. Lost patients: They'd rather switch than fight for attention. *The Cincinnati Enquirer,* July 5, 1970.
34. Francis, V., Lorsch, B. M., and Morris, M. J.: Gaps in doctor-patient communication. *New Engl. J. Med., 280:*535–540 (Mar. 6), 1969.
35. Waitzkin, H., and Stoeckle, J. D.: The communication of information about illness. *Adv. Psychosom. Med., 8:*180–215, 1972.
36. The act of listening. *The Royal Bank of Canada Monthly Letter, 60*(1):1–4 (Jan.), 1979.

37. Ventura, F. P.: Counselling the hearing-impaired geriatric patient. *Patient Counselling and Health Education,* First Quarter: 22–25, 1978.
38. Beardsley, R. S., Johnson, C. A., and Wise, G.: Privacy as a factor in patient counselling. *J. Amer. Pharm. Assoc., NS17*(6):366–368 (June), 1977.
39. Wynn-Williams, N., and Aris, M.: On omitting PAS. *Tubercle, 39:*338–342 (June), 1958.
40. Morris, L. A., and O'Neal, E. C.: Judgments about a drug's effectiveness: the role of expectations and outcomes. *Drugs in Health Care, 2:*179–186 (Summer), 1975.
41. Powell, J. R., Cali, T. J., and Linkewich, J. A.: Inadequately written prescriptions. *J. Amer. Med. Assoc., 226:*999–1000 (Nov. 19), 1973.
42. Hansten, P. D.: Drug Interactions. Fourth edition. Lea & Febiger, Philadelphia, 1979.
43. Froelich, R. E., and Bishop, M. F.: Medical Interviewing—A Programmed Manual. C. V. Mosby Company, St. Louis, 1969, pp. 47–48.
44. Davis, M. S.: Physiologic, psychological and demographic factors in patient compliance with doctors' orders. *Med. Care, 6:*115–122 (Mar.–Apr.), 1968.
45. Editorial: *Bull. Amer. Coll. Surgeons, 44:*137–140, 1959.
46. Blum, R. H.: The Management of the Doctor-Patient Relationship. McGraw-Hill, New York, 1960.
47. Kübler-Ross, E., Wessler, S. W., and Avioli, L. V.: On death and dying. *J. Amer. Med. Assoc., 221*(2):174–179 (July 10), 1972.
48. Ujhely, G. B.: The Nurse and Her Problem Patients. First edition. Springer Publishing Company, Inc., New York, 1963, p. 41.
49. Wagner, J., and Goldstein, E.: Pharmacist's role in loss and grief. *Amer. J. Hosp. Pharm., 34:*490–492 (May), 1977.
50. Bernstein, L., Bernstein, R. S., and Dana, R. H.: Interviewing: A Guide for Health Professionals. Second edition. Appleton-Century-Crofts, New York, 1974, p. 175.
51. Johnson, M. A.: Developing the Art of Understanding. Second edition. Springer Publishing Co., Inc., New York, 1972, p. 226.
52. Clinte, J., and Kabat, H.: Improving patient compliance. *J. Amer. Pharm. Assoc., 16:*74–85 (Apr.), 1976.
53. Mattar, M. E., Markello, J., and Yaffe, S. J.: Pharmaceutic factors affecting pediatric compliance. *Pediatrics, 55:*101–108 (Jan.), 1975.
54. Wandless, I., and Davie, J. W.: Can drug compliance in the elderly be improved? *Br. Med. J., 1:*359–361 (Feb. 5), 1977.
55. Dickey, F. F., Mattar, M. E., and Chudzik, C. M.: Pharmacist counseling increases drug regimen compliance. *J. Amer. Hosp. Assoc. 49:*85–88 (May 1), 1975.
56. Hulka, B.: Communication, compliance and concordance between physicians and patients with prescribed medications. *Amer. J. Public Health, 66:*847–853 (Sept.), 1976.
57. Griffith, H. W., Attarian, P. J., and Harrison, W. T.: Information for patient package inserts—I. *Drug Infor. J., 11:*35S–40S (Jan.), 1977.
58. Wingert, W. A., Grubbs, J. P., and Friedman, D. B.: "Why Johnny's parents don't read": An analysis of indigent parents' comprehension of health education materials. *Clin. Pediatr., 8:*655–660 (Nov.), 1969.
59. Hladik, W. B., and White, S. J.: Evaluation of written reinforcements used in counselling cardiovascular patients. *Amer. J. Hosp. Pharm., 33:*1277–1280 (Dec.), 1976.
60. Patient Advisory Leaflets, Pharmex Ltd., Willimantic, Connecticut, 1979, and Pharmasystems, Toronto, Canada, 1980.
61. White, K. L., Williams, T. F., and Greenberg, B. G.: The ecology of medical care. *New Engl. J. Med., 265:*885–892 (Nov. 2), 1961.

Organization and Use
of the Written
Medication Instructions

I̲n̲d̲i̲v̲i̲d̲u̲a̲l̲ patient monographs have been prepared for the majority of medications prescribed for ambulatory patients. Medications used solely within a hospital have been purposely omitted since the patient is not responsible for their correct administration. Only those prescription and nonprescription medications listed in FACTS AND COMPARISONS (United States) and the COMPENDIUM OF PHARMACEUTICALS AND SPECIALTIES (Canada) have been considered. The monographs are arranged alphabetically according to the generic name of the drug. The generic name is followed by an alphabetical listing of the Registered Trademarks of the commercial products available in the United States and Canada. Generic brands have not been included. Some drugs are subject to different legal restrictions in each country and it is the responsibility of the pharmacist to dispense the medications according to the specific legal requirements of his state or province.

The written medication instructions contained in this book have been designed to reinforce the verbal instructions of the practitioner and to help him provide the patient with basic information regarding the correct use of prescribed medications. Considerable care has been taken to translate the medical terminology into language which the majority of patients can understand. The Fry Readability Test and the SMOG Readability Test have demonstrated that the instructions are written at approximately the grade seven level and, therefore, should be meaningful to most adult patients.

The basic text of each monograph consists of the following information:

1. PURPOSE OF THE MEDICATION

In order for the patient to decide to participate in his drug therapy, he must understand the purpose of the medication as it relates to his diagnosis and he must also believe in the necessity of the prescribed therapy.

A general statement outlining the purpose(s) of the medication has been prepared and, in certain instances, the practitioner may wish to interpret the purpose of the drug in more specific terms. For medications that are used to treat a variety of disease conditions, only the practitioner will know the specific reason a patient is being prescribed such a medication. It is intended that the practitioner who is familiar with the condition of the patient will interpret the specific purpose of the drug to him. The written instructions refer only to approved uses and do not include the investigational uses of any drug.

HOW TO USE THIS MEDICINE

2. CORRECT METHOD OF ADMINISTRATION

Many patients fail to respond to a therapeutic regimen simply because they have not administered their medications correctly. Such pharmaceutical preparations as respiratory inhalers; ophthalmic, otic, and nasal preparations; sublingual and buccal tablets; vaginal tablets and creams; and rectal suppositories require special methods of administration which are included in the pertinent monographs. The recommendations of the pharmaceutical manufacturers have been the primary reference sources regarding the method of administration of the drugs.

One of the unique aspects of the book is the inclusion of SPECIFIC instructions for certain dosage forms of a commercial product that require individualization of the method of administration. For example, the enteric-coated preparations of salicylazosulfapyridine will have the following specific instructions:

☐ This medicine has a special coating and must be swallowed whole. Do not crush, chew, or break it into pieces. (**United States:** Azulfidine En-tabs; **Canada:** Salazopyrin En Tablets)

If the pharmacist wishes to dispense a commercial product that is not listed but which is a generic equivalent, he should check the dosage form he is dispensing for any special instructions that product may require. The pharmacist should also check for any additional ingredients that may require special instructions.

3. CORRECT TIMES OF ADMINISTRATION

General recommendations regarding the recommended times of administration in relation to food and daily activities have been prepared. The practitioner should assist the patient in correlating these general recommendations with the dosage schedule prescribed by the physician and should suggest specific times that the medication can be taken. The final dosage schedule should be one that is complementary to the daily activities of the patient.

SPECIAL INSTRUCTIONS

4. "SELECTED" SIDE EFFECTS AND ADVERSE EFFECTS

Every precaution has been taken not to frighten the patient. Only those side effects that occur most commonly and can be managed by the patient are included. Only those adverse effects that are potentially harmful, can be recognized by the patient, and should be reported to the physician are included.

As previously discussed, these instructions are intended to be used as an aid in patient education in order to help the patient use a drug most effectively and with the least amount of anxiety. The patient instructions have NOT been designed to be used for the purposes of informed consent, and it is for this reason that they do not discuss every possible adverse drug effect or contraindication to the use of a drug. If informed consent is required, it should be obtained by the physician before he writes the prescription and before the patient comes to the pharmacy. In the preparation of this book, it has been assumed that the decision to prescribe a particular drug has been made by the physician or jointly by the physician and patient and that informed consent has been received by the prescriber.

Careful selection of side effects and recommendations for the appropriate precautions allows the patient to become a more active partner in his drug therapy and can often prevent needless accidents or more severe adverse effects. This can be done without frightening the patient unnecessarily.

5. PRECAUTIONS AND SPECIFIC ACTIVITIES TO AVOID

Whenever possible, recommendations are made regarding precautionary measures that should be taken by the patient. Some drugs will initially cause minor side effects, such as drowsiness, and the patient should be advised to take the appropriate precautionary measures during the first few days of therapy. Other medications may produce irritating side effects after continued use. An example would be the dry mouth which can occur with many antipsychotic medications, and the patient should be informed of some of the simple methods he can take to reduce this uncomfortable feeling. It is always in the best interest of the patient to inform him of any special precautions he should take so that he does not accidentally injure himself or stop taking a medication because of a minor side effect. The recommendations in this book have been based upon the medical and pharmaceutical literature and have been carefully reviewed by the panel of practitioners on the Medical and Pharmacy Advisory Boards. It has been the intent to make these recommendations as practical as possible.

6. DRUG INTERACTIONS

Clinically significant drug-food, drug-alcohol, and drug-nonprescription medication combinations that should be avoided or used with caution are included. The monographs were designed to provide a basic list of instructions that could be used with almost every patient. For this reason, drug interactions between the prescribed medication and other prescription medications have not been included. It is the responsibility of the physician and pharmacist to review the individual drug therapy of each patient for such interactions. In addition, the exclusion of prescription drug interactions will prevent undue alarm on the part of the patient.

7. SPECIFIC METHODS OF STORAGE

Commercial products that require special methods of storage are individually listed. For example, the following instruction applies to the specific commercial preparations of amoxicillin:

☐ Store the bottle of medicine in a refrigerator unless otherwise directed. Do not freeze. Do not use after the expiration date. (**United States:** Amoxil, Larocin, Polymox Suspensions; **Canada:** Amoxican, Amoxil, Penamox, Polymox Suspensions; Polymox Pediatric Drops)

Contraindications to the use of prescription medications have not been included because there are instances in which medications have to be used even though their use is normally contraindicated. In these cases, the patient may become alarmed or lose confidence in his physician if he were given a set of instructions stating that the drug should not be used in his disease condition. It is the professional responsibility of the physician to weigh the risks against the benefits, and considerable discretion should be used in prescribing medications in such cases as pregnancy, severe debilitation, kidney and liver diseases, and allergy-prone patients. It is for this reason that precautions regarding breast-feeding, pregnancy, or symptoms of an allergy have not been routinely included in the monographs. Instead, general statements regarding these conditions appear in the "GENERAL PATIENT INSTRUCTIONS: HOW TO USE YOUR MEDICINES SAFELY." It is assumed that EVERY patient receiving a drug should be informed about these very basic precautions.

50

In order to facilitate rapid retrieval of all information pertinent to a specific drug and to facilitate the preparation of written instructions that can be distributed to the patient, the medication instructions have not been coded or grouped by therapeutic class. At the risk of being repetitious, the guide should be considerably more convenient to the practitioner. An Appendix has been included in this edition in order to help decrease duplication of some of the patient information.

In summary, the written medication instructions contained in this book are general in nature, and the practitioner may wish to vary or omit some of the information depending upon the individual needs and circumstances of the patient. These instructions should never take the place of verbal counseling, but they can reduce the number of times it is necessary to repeat instructions to the patient and can reinforce verbal counseling.

General References Used in the Preparation of the Written Medication Instructions

American Medical Association Council on Drugs: AMA Drug Evaluations. American Medical Association, Chicago, Illinois, Third edition, 1977.

American Hospital Formulary Service. American Society of Hospital Pharmacists, Washington, D.C.

American Pharmaceutical Association: Evaluations of Drug Interactions, American Pharmaceutical Association, Washington, D.C., Second edition, 1976.

Blacow, N. W., and Wade, A.: Martindale—The Extra Pharmacopoeia. 27th edition, Council of the Pharmaceutical Society of Great Britain, The Pharmaceutical Press, London, 1977.

Connaught Laboratories: Insulin and Insulin Preparations, A Handbook for Diabetic Patients. Twelfth edition, Connaught Laboratories Ltd., 1973.

Fuerst, E. V., and Wolff, L. V.: Fundamentals of Nursing. Fourth edition, J. B. Lippincott, Philadelphia, Pennsylvania, 1969.

Goodman, L. S., and Gilman, A.: The Pharmacological Basis of Therapeutics. Sixth edition, MacMillan Publishing Co. Inc., New York, 1980.

Govoni, L. E., and Hayes, J. E.: Drugs and Nursing Implications. Third edition, Appleton-Century Crofts, New York, 1978.

Hansten, P. D.: Drug Interactions. Fourth edition, Lea & Febiger, Philadelphia, 1979.

Harrison's Principles of Internal Medicine, Ninth edition, McGraw-Hill Book Company, New York, 1980.

Hart, F. D.: French's Index of Differential Diagnosis, Eleventh edition, John Wright & Sons Ltd., Bristol, 1979.

Kastrup, E. K., and Schwach, G. H.: Facts and Comparisons. Facts and Comparisons, Inc., St. Louis, Missouri, May, 1980.

Martin, E. W., et al.: Techniques of Medication. First edition, J. B. Lippincott Company, Philadelphia, Pennsylvania, 1969.

Mathemy, R. V., Nolan, B. T., Hogan, A. E., and Griffen, G. E.: Fundamentals of Patient Centered Nursing. Third edition, C. V. Mosby Company, St. Louis, Missouri, 1972.

Miller, R. R., and Greenblatt, D. J.: Handbook of Drug Therapy, First Edition, Elsevier North Holland, Inc., New York, 1979.

Rotenberg, G. N., and Hughes, F. N.: Compendium of Pharmaceuticals and Specialties. The Canadian Pharmaceutical Association, Toronto, Ontario, 1980.

General Patient Instructions: How to Use Your Medicines Safely

Prescription Medicine

1. Not all medical conditions require the use of medicines. Your doctor has carefully prescribed your medicines for you because he believes that they are the best possible treatment for your particular condition. In order for you to receive the greatest benefit from your drugs, it is essential that you take them *exactly* as your doctor has prescribed. This information is on the prescription label—**be sure to read the label carefully.** If you should have any questions about your medicines which the label does not answer, ask your pharmacist or your doctor.

2. Whenever you receive a medicine from a pharmacist, YOU SHOULD KNOW THE ANSWER TO THESE QUESTIONS:

   What is the name of the medicine?
   What is the purpose of the medicine?
   Are there any precautions you should be aware of while you are taking the medicine?
   Are there any other medicines you should not take at the same time?
   Is there any food or beverage you should avoid?
   How and when should you take the medicine?
   How long should you continue to take the medicine?
   Can the prescription be refilled and how?

3. Have all of your prescriptions filled at the same pharmacy so that the pharmacist can keep a complete record of your medicines. Do not go without medicine between prescription refills. Call your pharmacist 1 or 2 days before you will need the repeat of your prescription.

4. If you visit more than one doctor, tell each one what medicines you are taking. This should include prescription and nonprescription drugs as both could interfere with a new medicine that the doctor may prescribe for you. Always tell your doctor if you did not have a prescription filled or if you did not take your medicine. Otherwise, he may conclude that the medicine was not effective. It is important that you take the medicine your doctor has prescribed for you; only by taking it will you derive any benefit from your medicine.

5. In addition to their benefits, most drugs have additional minor actions. These are called side effects and are usually not detrimental to your health. You may not experience any side effects from a drug. Side effects vary from one patient to another, and at times a particular medicine produces an unpleasant side effect in one patient, whereas another medicine that is almost identical will have no unpleasant effect. If you think your medicine is causing a problem, call your doctor or pharmacist and let him know. He can tell you if the problem is due to the medicine and can make any necessary adjustments.

Allergies

6. Always tell your doctor and pharmacist if you are allergic to any drugs or other substances or if you have had any unpleasant reactions to drugs. Call your doctor immediately if you think you may be allergic to a medicine or if you develop a skin rash, itching, hives, swelling of the face, or difficulty in breathing.

7. Remember that the medicine you have received is specifically for you. DO NOT SHARE it with other members of your family or your friends who seem to have the same symptoms you have. They should see their own doctor who will decide which is the best treatment for them.

Nonprescription Medicine

8. Be careful in treating yourself with any **medicine you can purchase without a prescription** (for example, aspirin, laxatives, vitamins, or cough medicines). Always read the directions on the folder and if you do not understand them, consult your pharmacist. These medicines are usually designed to alleviate a symptom and they do not cure a disease. Do not continue using the medicine if the first few doses do not help to relieve the symptom. If a symptom is severe or persistent, check with your doctor.

9. If you are taking a drug that has been prescribed by your physician, always be careful in self-medicating with drugs you can purchase without a prescription (for example, cough syrups, laxatives, or nasal sprays). Some drugs can interact and cause unpleasant reactions. Always check with your pharmacist before you purchase these products.

Pregnancy and Breast-Feeding

10. Women who are **pregnant** or **breast-feeding** or who plan to become pregnant should not take any medicines or home remedies without consulting their doctor or pharmacist.

Children

11. Do not give any medicine to a **child** less than one year of age unless it has been prescribed by your doctor. Do not give any nonprescription drugs to children between 1 and 12 years of age unless the doses for the different age groups are listed on the package container.

Storage of Medicines

12. The way in which you store your drugs is important. Certain drugs require refrigeration. If this is the case, there will be a **Keep Refrigerated** label on the container. Do not store any medicines in the refrigerator unless specified by your pharmacist. A cool, dry, dark cupboard is the best storage for most other medicines. Remember that your bathroom medicine cupboard often becomes hot and steamy and is not the best place to store your medications. Above all, keep your medicines in a safe place and away from the reach or sight of small children.

13. Always keep your medicine in the container in which you received it from the pharmacist. Do NOT remove the label until all the medication is finished. The information on the label is necessary to properly identify the patient, the physician, the drug, the instructions for use, and the date the prescription was dispensed.

14. Over the years you may have had numerous drugs prescribed for you. If these drugs are discontinued by your doctor, destroy the remaining portion by flushing it down the toilet. By doing this you avoid building up a cupboard of old, outdated, and potentially dangerous drugs.

Medicine Card

15. It is recommended that you carry a **card** in your wallet that lists important facts about your health and your medicines. This allows you to have a complete list of your medicines if you should see another doctor. If you move to another neighborhood, you should carefully choose your new pharmacy and doctor. It is important that your new pharmacist and doctor are thoroughly familiar with the medicines you are taking and your medical history.

Written Medication Instructions

Acenocoumarol (*Oral Anticoagulant*)
    Canada: Sintrom

☐ This medicine is used to help prevent harmful blood clots from forming. It is commonly called a "blood thinner."

HOW TO USE THIS MEDICINE

☐ Take this medicine **exactly** as your doctor has prescribed. Try to take the medicine at the same time every day and do not miss any doses. Do not take extra tablets without your doctor's approval because overtreatment will cause bleeding.

☐ Regular blood tests, called "prothrombin times," are necessary in order for your doctor to prescribe the correct dose for you. Your dose may change from time to time depending on these tests.

☐ It is best to take this medicine with a glass of water. Do not take it with food or other drugs unless otherwise directed.

☐ If you forget to take a dose, take it as soon as possible. However, if it is almost time for your next dose, do not take the missed dose. Instead, continue with your regular dosing schedule. Record the date of the missed dose so that you can tell your doctor the next time you see him for a blood test. Call your doctor if you miss more than one dose.

SPECIAL INSTRUCTIONS

☐ Do not take any other drugs or stop taking any drugs you are currently taking without first consulting with your doctor. This even includes many products that you can buy without a prescription such as pain relievers and antacids. Always check with your pharmacist before you take or buy ANY nonprescription products.

56

- [ ] Do not take aspirin or medicines containing aspirin or salicylates. It is usually safe to take acetaminophen as a substitute for aspirin for occasional headaches and pain. Check with your pharmacist.

- [ ] It is best to avoid alcoholic beverages while you are taking this medicine because the combination may cause undesirable side effects. Ask your doctor if he feels it is safe for you to have an occasional drink.

- [ ] Do not eat unusually large amounts of leafy, green vegetables or change your diet without telling your doctor.

- [ ] If you have a tendency to cut yourself while shaving, you may wish to use an electric razor to avoid possible bleeding.

- [ ] Try to avoid contact sports or activities in which you could become injured because such injuries could result in internal bleeding.

- [ ] If your body gets more medicine than it needs, bleeding may occur. Call your doctor if you notice any of the following signs of bleeding which you cannot explain or are unusual for you: nosebleeds, bruising or heavy menstrual bleeding; bleeding from the gums after brushing the teeth, heavy bleeding from cuts, red or black stools, red or dark brown urine, or vomiting or coughing up blood. Your doctor will do some blood tests and adjust your dose.

- [ ] Women who are pregnant, breast-feeding, or planning to become pregnant should tell their doctor before taking this medicine.

- [ ] Most people experience few or no side effects from their drugs. However, any medicine can sometimes cause unwanted effects. Call your doctor if you develop stomach or back pain, unusual headaches, changes in eyesight, constipation or diarrhea, dizziness, a skin rash, sore throat, fever, mouth sores, a yellow color to the skin or eyes, or unusual tiredness.

- [ ] Carry an identification card indicating that you are taking this medicine. Always tell your pharmacist, dentist, and other doctors who are treating you that you are taking this medicine.

- [ ] Do not go without this medicine between prescription refills. Call your pharmacist 2 or 3 days before you will run out of the medicine.

- [ ] After you stop taking the medicine, it will take your body some time to return to normal. Your doctor or pharmacist will tell you how long you must follow these instructions AFTER you have stopped taking this medicine.

* * * * *

Acetaminophen (*Oral Analgesic-Antipyretic*)

United States: Apamide, Capital, Dapa, Datril, Datril 500 Extra Strength, Dolanex, Dularin Syrup, Febrogesic, G-1, HI-Temp, Liquiprin, Napap, Nebs, Phenaphen, SK-Apap, Tapar, Temlo, Tempra, Tylenol, Tylenol Extra Strength, Valadol

Canada: Atasol, Atasol Forte, Campain, Empracet, Paralgin, Pedia-
phen, Rounox, Tempra, Tylenol

☐ This medicine is used to help relieve pain and/or reduce fever.

☐ IMPORTANT: If you have ever had an allergic reaction to acetaminophen or
phenacetin, tell your doctor or pharmacist before you take any of this medicine.

HOW TO USE THIS MEDICINE

☐ This medicine may be taken with food or a full glass of water.

☐ If a dropper or a dispensing spoon is used to measure the dose and you do
not fully understand how to use it, check with your pharmacist. (**United
States:** Liquiprin, Proval, Tempra, Tylenol; **Canada:** Tempra, Tylenol)

☐ Children under 3 years of age should only be given this medicine with the
approval of the doctor. Children under 5 years of age should not be given
this medicine for more than 5 days in a row, and adults should not use this
medicine for longer than 10 days without the approval of their doctor.

SPECIAL INSTRUCTIONS

☐ Do not take any other medicines containing acetaminophen while you are
taking this medicine unless otherwise directed.

☐ Most people experience few or no side effects from their drugs. However,
any medicine can sometimes cause unwanted effects. Call your doctor if you
develop stomach pain, diarrhea, sore throat or fever, unusual weakness or a
yellow color to the skin or eyes, or easy bruising or bleeding.

☐ Call your doctor if the medicine does not relieve your symptoms.

☐ Store the medicine in a cool dark place.

*　*　*　*　*

Acetaminophen (*Rectal Analgesic-Antipyretic*)
United States: Aceta, Anuphen, Neopap Supprettes

☐ This medicine is used to help relieve pain and/or reduce fever.

☐ IMPORTANT: If you have ever had an allergic reaction to acetaminophen or
phenacetin, tell your doctor or pharmacist before you take any of this medicine.

HOW TO USE THIS MEDICINE

☐ Administration of Suppositories:
  • Remove the wrapper from the suppository.
  • Lie on your side and raise your knee to your chest.
  • Insert the suppository with the tapered (pointed) end first into the rec-
    tum.

58

- Remain lying down for a few minutes so that the suppository will dissolve in the rectum.
- Try to avoid having a bowel movement for at least one hour so that the drug will have time to work.

☐ Children under 3 years of age should only be given this medicine with the approval of the doctor. Children under 5 years of age should not be given this medicine for more than 5 days in a row, and adults should not use this medicine for longer than 10 days without the approval of their doctor.

SPECIAL INSTRUCTIONS

☐ Do not take any other medicines containing acetaminophen while you are using this medicine unless otherwise directed.

☐ Most people experience few or no side effects from their drugs. However, any medicine can sometimes cause unwanted effects. Call your doctor if you develop stomach pain, diarrhea, sore throat or fever, unusual weakness, a yellow color to the skin or eyes, or easy bruising or bleeding.

☐ Call your doctor if the medicine does not relieve your symptoms.

☐ Store the medicine in a cool, dark place.

*   *   *   *   *

Acetaminophen-Codeine-Caffeine (Oral Analgesic-Antipyretic-Antitussive)

Canada: (Atasol-8, -15, -30; Tylenol No. 1, No. 2, No. 3, No. 4)

Acetaminophen-Codeine

United States: Capital W/Codeine, Coastaldyne, Empracet with Codeine, Hasacode, Liquix-C, Phenaphen with Codeine, SK-APAP with Codeine, Tylenol with Codeine

Canada: Empracet-30, Rounox + Codeine

☐ This medicine is used to help relieve pain, fever, and certain types of coughs.

☐ IMPORTANT: If you have ever had an allergic reaction to phenacetin, caffeine, or codeine medicine, tell your doctor or pharmacist before you take any of this medicine.

HOW TO USE THIS MEDICINE

☐ This medicine may be taken with food or a glass of water.

☐ Do not take any more of this medicine than your doctor has prescribed. The drug could become habit-forming or you could take an overdose if you take it more often or longer than prescribed.

59

- [ ] If you are taking this medicine to help relieve pain, do not wait until the pain becomes severe. This medicine works best if you take it at the beginning of the pain. Call your doctor if you feel you need it more often than he prescribed.

SPECIAL INSTRUCTIONS

- [ ] Do not drink alcoholic beverages while taking this drug without the approval of your doctor.

- [ ] It is important that you obtain the advice of your doctor or pharmacist before taking ANY other medicines, including other pain relievers, sleeping pills, tranquilizers or medicines for depression, cough/cold or allergy medicines, or weight-reducing medicines.

- [ ] In some people, this drug may cause dizziness or drowsiness. Do not drive a car or operate dangerous machinery or do jobs that require you to be alert until you know how you are going to react to this drug.

- [ ] If you become dizzy, you should be careful going up and down stairs. Sit or lie down at the first sign of dizziness. Get up slowly if you have been lying or sitting down.

- [ ] If you do feel nauseated when you first start taking the medicine, it may help if you lie down for a few minutes.

- [ ] If you become constipated, try increasing the amount of bulk in your diet (for example, bran and salads), exercising more often, or drinking more water. Call your doctor if the constipation continues.

- [ ] Most people experience few or no side effects from their drugs. However, any medicine can sometimes cause unwanted effects. Call your doctor if you develop a sore throat or fever, unusual weakness, a yellow color in the skin or eyes or easy bruising or bleeding, shortness of breath, slow heartbeat, unusual nervousness, stomach pain, or difficulty in urinating ("passing your water").

- [ ] Store the medicine in a cool, dark place.

- [ ] Always tell your dentist, pharmacist, and other doctors who are treating you that you are taking this medicine.

* * * * *

Acetazolamide (*Oral Carbonic Anhydrase Inhibitor*)
United States: Diamox
Canada: Acetazolam, Diamox

- [ ] This medication will initially cause you to urinate (pass your water) more frequently and in larger amounts than usual. It is used to help rid the body of excess fluids and is also used in the treatment of glaucoma and epilepsy.

60

HOW TO USE THIS MEDICINE

☐ Take the medication at the same time every day. If possible, do not initially take this medication at bedtime in order to avoid having to urinate while trying to sleep.

☐ This medication must be swallowed whole. Do **not** crush, chew, or break it into pieces. (**United States:** Diamox Sequels; **Canada:** Diamox Sequels)

SPECIAL INSTRUCTIONS

☐ Women who are pregnant, breast-feeding, or planning to become pregnant should tell their doctor before taking this medicine.

☐ If you forget to take a dose, take it as soon as possible. However, if it is almost time for your next dose, do not take the missed dose. Instead, continue with your regular dosing schedule.

☐ Most people experience few or no side effects from their drugs. However, any medicine can sometimes cause unwanted effects. Call your doctor if you develop a skin rash, sore throat, fever, blurred vision, easy bruising, numbness of the hands or feet, drowsiness, unusual weakness, stomach pain, or vomiting.

*   *   *   *   *

Acetohexamide (Oral Hypoglycemic)
United States: Dymelor
Canada: Dimelor

☐ This medicine is used in the treatment of diabetes. When you have diabetes, the body either is not producing enough insulin or is not able to use what is produced. Insulin is needed for the body's proper use of food, especially sugar. In a diabetic, the sugar in the blood can build up to dangerous levels and is passed out in the urine. Your doctor has prescribed this medicine to help keep your blood sugar at nearly normal levels.

HOW TO USE THIS MEDICINE

☐ This medicine may be taken with food to help prevent stomach upset.

☐ It is very important that you take this medicine exactly as your doctor has prescribed. Do not miss any doses. Try to take this medicine at the same time every day. Do not take extra tablets without your doctor's approval.

☐ Do not take this medicine at bedtime unless your doctor tells you to.

☐ If you forget to take a dose, take it as soon as possible. However, if it is almost time for your next dose, do not take the missed dose. Instead, continue with your regular dosing schedule.

SPECIAL INSTRUCTIONS

☐ Women who are pregnant, breast-feeding, or planning to become pregnant should tell their doctor before taking this medicine.

☐ This medicine may make some people more sensitive to sunlight and sunlamps. When you begin taking this medicine try to avoid too much sun until you see how you are going to react. If your skin does become more sensitive to sunlight, tell your doctor and try to stay out of direct sunlight. While in the sun, wear protective clothing and sunglasses. You may wish to ask your pharmacist about suitable sunscreen products. Check with your doctor if you become sunburned.

☐ Most people experience few or no side effects from their drugs. However, any medicine can sometimes cause unwanted effects. Call your doctor if you develop a skin rash, sore throat, fever, mouth sores, dark-colored urine, a yellow color to the skin or eyes, easy bruising or bleeding, unusual tiredness, diarrhea, or light-colored stools.

GENERAL INSTRUCTIONS FOR DIABETIC PATIENTS

☐ Keep a regular schedule of daily activities. Eat, exercise, and take your insulin at approximately the same time every day.

☐ The diet that your physician has prescribed has been carefully planned especially for you. It is to your advantage to follow it very closely.

☐ Test your urine regularly for sugar and, if your doctor recommends, test it for acetone.

☐ Learn the signs of hypoglycemia (low blood sugar). When this happens, your urine sugar will be negative. Hypoglycemia may occur if you delay or skip a meal, exercise too much, become sick or emotionally upset, take too much insulin, drink alcohol, or take certain drugs. If you develop sweating, drowsiness, headache, unusual hunger, dizziness, nausea, nervousness, blurred vision, weakness, or shaking or trembling, eat or drink any of the following:

- 2 sugar cubes or 2 teaspoons of sugar in water
- 4 ounces orange juice
- 4 ounces regular ginger ale, cola beverages, or any other sweetened carbonated beverage. Do NOT use low-calorie or diet beverages.
- 2 to 3 teaspoons honey or corn syrup
- 4 Lifesaver candies

Artificial sweeteners are of no use. Call your doctor if this does not relieve your symptoms in about 15 minutes.

☐ Always carry sugar cubes or hard candy in case you have a hypoglycemic (low blood sugar) reaction.

☐ Before you purchase any nonprescription medicine (for example, cough and cold medicines), ask your pharmacist if the medicine is safe for diabetic patients to use. Some nonprescription medicines have very high sugar contents which could interfere with the control of your diabetes. Aspirin and medicines containing salicylates or vitamin C could affect your urine test results. Check with your pharmacist.

☐ Ask your doctor if it is safe for you to drink alcoholic beverages because the combination may cause low blood sugar as well as a pounding headache, flushing, upset stomach, dizziness, or sweating.

☐ Take special care of your feet.
- Wash your feet daily and dry them well.
- Check your feet daily for minor injuries. Bring these to the attention of your doctor immediately.
- Wear clean shoes and stockings and choose shoes that fit well.
- If you develop corns or calluses, soak your feet in lukewarm water for about 10 minutes. Then rub them off gently with a pumice stone. Never use a knife to cut corns or calluses on your feet. Do NOT use commercial corn removers or commercial arch supports.
- Soften dry skin by rubbing with oil or lotion.
- Trim your toenails straight across with a file or a nail cutter. Do not cut your own toenails if your eyesight is poor.
- Do not wear garters or socks with tight elastic tops. Do not sit with your knees crossed.
- Do not warm your feet with a hot water bottle or a heating pad. Use loose bed socks instead. If your feet are cold under normal conditions, tell your doctor. Your circulation may be poor and your doctor can offer advice.
- Call your doctor if you injure your toes or feet. Cuts and scratches in the diabetic can become infected easily and take longer to heal. Do not apply iodine or strong antiseptics to the feet at any time.

☐ Call your doctor immediately if you develop any of the following symptoms of hyperglycemia (high blood sugar): high urine sugar, acetone in urine, drowsiness, hunger, unusual thirst, fast breathing, nausea, confusion, a flushed dry skin, increase in urination ("passing your water"), or a fruity odor to the breath. These symptoms may occur if you are taking too little insulin, miss a dose, overeat, or if you have a fever or infection.

☐ Call your doctor if you become sick and have a fever, an infection, nausea, or vomiting.

☐ Carry an identification card or wear a bracelet indicating that you are a diabetic and that you are taking this medicine. Always tell your pharmacist, dentist, and other doctors who are treating you that you are taking this medicine.

*　*　*　*　*

Acetophenazine Maleate (*Oral Antipsychotic-Antianxiety*)
United States: Tindal

☐ This medicine is used to treat certain types of mental and emotional problems. Check with your doctor if you do not fully understand why you are taking it.

- ☐ IMPORTANT: If you have ever had an allergic reaction to a phenothiazine medicine, tell your doctor or pharmacist before you take any of this medicine.

HOW TO USE THIS MEDICINE

- ☐ This medicine may be taken with food or a full glass of water.

- ☐ Do not take this medicine at the same time as antacids or diarrhea medicine. Try to space them at least 1 hour apart.

- ☐ The effect of the medicine may not be noticed immediately, but may take from 2 to 4 weeks. Be patient. Take the medicine regularly and try not to miss any doses.

- ☐ Do not stop taking this medicine suddenly without the approval of your doctor.

SPECIAL INSTRUCTIONS

- ☐ If you forget to take a dose, take it as soon as possible. However, if it is almost time for your next dose, do not take the missed dose. Instead, continue with your regular dosing schedule.

- ☐ Any medicine has a few unwanted side effects. Because this medicine takes a few weeks to work, the side effects show the doctor that the drug is being absorbed. Many of these side effects will go away as your body adjusts to the medicine.

- ☐ Women who are pregnant, breast-feeding, or planning to become pregnant should tell their doctor before taking this medicine.

- ☐ In some people, this drug may cause dizziness or drowsiness. Do not drive a car or operate dangerous machinery or do jobs that require you to be alert until you know how you are going to react to the drug.

- ☐ If this medicine causes dizziness, you should be careful going up and down stairs and you should not change positions too rapidly. Get out of bed slowly in the morning and dangle your feet over the edge of the bed for a few minutes before standing up. Sit down or lie down at the first sign of dizziness. Tell your doctor you have been dizzy. Avoid hot showers and baths because they could make you dizzy.

- ☐ Do not drink alcoholic beverages while taking this drug without the approval of your doctor.

- ☐ This medicine may make some people more sensitive to sunlight and sunlamps. When you begin taking this medicine, try to avoid too much sun until you see how you are going to react. If your skin does become more sensitive to sunlight, tell your doctor and try to stay out of direct sunlight. While in the sun, wear protective clothing and sunglasses. You may wish to ask your pharmacist about suitable sunscreen products. Check with your doctor if you become sunburned.

☐ If your mouth becomes dry, suck a hard sour candy (sugarless) or ice chips, or chew gum. It is especially important to brush your teeth regularly if you develop a dry mouth.

☐ It is important that you obtain the advice of your doctor or pharmacist before taking **any** other medicines, including pain relievers, sleeping pills, other tranquilizers or medicines for depression, cough, cold, or allergy medicines, weight-reducing medicines, or laxatives.

☐ This medicine may cause your urine to turn pink, red, or red-brown in color. This is not unusual.

☐ In hot weather or during exercise, be careful not to become overheated. You may be more sensitive to heat since this medicine may affect the body's ability to regulate temperature.

☐ If you become constipated, try increasing the amount of bulk in your diet (for example, bran and salads), exercising more often, or drinking more water. Call your doctor if the constipation continues.

☐ Call your doctor if you develop a sore throat, fever, mouth sores, skin rash, changes in eyesight, rapid heart rate, a yellow color in the eyes or skin, unusual weakness or unusual movements of the face, tongue, or hands, or difficulty in urinating ("passing your water"). Also call your doctor if you become restless or unable to sit still or sleep.

☐ Carry an identification card indicating that you are taking this medicine. Always tell your dentist, pharmacist, and other doctors who are treating you that you are taking this medicine.

*　*　*　*　*

Acetylsalicylic Acid (*Oral Analgesic-Antipyretic-Anti-inflammatory*)

> **United States:** Aspirin, A.S.A., A.S.A. Enseals, Bayer Timed-Release, Children's Aspirin, Ecotrin, Measurin
>
> **Canada:** Acetal, Acetophen, Acetyl-Sal, Ancasal, Astrin, Cetasal, Coryphen, Ecotrin, Entrophen, Neopirine-25, Novaphase, Novasen, Rhonal, Triaphen-10

Acetylsalicylic Acid-Caffeine

> **Canada:** 217 Tablets, Children's 217 Tablets, Neopirine Co. No. 35

Acetylsalicylic Acid-Phenacetin-Caffeine

United States: APC, ASA Compound Pulvules, ASA Compound Tablets, Buffadyne, Empirin Compound Tablets, P-A-C Compound Capsules and Tablets

☐ This medicine is used to help relieve pain, reduce fever, and relieve redness and swelling in certain kinds of arthritis.

☐ IMPORTANT: If you have a stomach ulcer or if you have ever had an allergic reaction to aspirin, tell your doctor or pharmacist before you take any of this medicine.

HOW TO USE THIS MEDICINE

☐ This medicine may be taken with food or a full glass of water.

☐ Do not take this medicine if it smells strongly like vinegar since this means the aspirin is not fresh.

☐ The following medicine has a special coating to help prevent stomach upset. It must be swallowed whole. Do not crush, chew, or break it into pieces and do not take chipped tablets. (*United States:* A.S.A. Enseals, Bayer Timed-Release, Ecotrin, Measurin; *Canada:* Coryphen, Ecotrin, Entrophen, Novaphase, Triaphen-10)

☐ Do not take this medicine regularly for more than 10 days without consulting your doctor and do not administer it to children under 12 years of age for more than 5 days without your doctor's approval.

SPECIAL INSTRUCTIONS

☐ Women who are pregnant, breast-feeding, or planning to become pregnant should tell their doctor before taking this medicine.

☐ Do not take any other medicines containing aspirin while you are taking this medicine because it could result in too high a dose.

☐ If you are taking this medicine for arthritis, it is very important that you take it regularly and that you DO NOT MISS ANY DOSES. If you miss a dose, the level of the medicine in your body will fall and the drug will not be as effective. Only if the level of drug is high enough will the inflammation in your joints be decreased and further damage be prevented. If you forget a dose, take it as soon as possible. However, if it is almost time for your next dose, do not take the missed dose. Instead, continue with your regular dosing schedule.

☐ It is best not to drink alcoholic beverages while you are taking this medicine since the combination can cause stomach problems.

☐ Most people experience few or no side effects from their drugs. However, any medicine can sometimes cause unwanted effects. Call your doctor if you

66

develop "ringing" or "buzzing" in the ears, skin rash, stomach pain, red or black stools, dizziness, fever, sweating, wheezing, or shortness of breath.

☐ Call your doctor if the medicine does not relieve your symptoms.

* * * * *

Acetylsalicylic Acid (*Rectal Analgesic-Antipyretic*)
United States: ASA
Canada: Sal-Adult, Sal-Infant, Supasa

☐ This medicine is used to help relieve pain and reduce fever.

☐ IMPORTANT: If you have a stomach ulcer or if you have ever had an allergic reaction to aspirin, tell your doctor or pharmacist before you take any of this medicine.

HOW TO USE THIS MEDICINE

☐ Administration of Suppositories:
  • Remove the wrapper from the suppository.
  • Lie on your side and raise your knee to your chest.
  • Insert the suppository with the tapered (pointed) end first into the rectum.
  • Remain lying down for a few minutes so that the suppository will dissolve in the rectum.
  • Try to avoid having a bowel movement for at least one hour so that the drug will have time to work.

☐ Do not use this medicine for more than 10 days without your doctor's approval.

SPECIAL INSTRUCTIONS

☐ Do not take any other medicines containing aspirin while you are using this medicine because it could result in too high a dose.

☐ Women who are pregnant, breast-feeding, or planning to become pregnant should tell their doctor before taking this medicine.

☐ Most people experience few or no side effects from their drugs. However, any medicine can sometimes cause unwanted effects. Call your doctor if you develop "ringing" or "buzzing" in the ears, skin rash, stomach pain, red or black stools, dizziness, fever, sweating, wheezing, or shortness of breath.

☐ Call your doctor if the medicine does not relieve your symptoms.

* * * * *

Acetylsalicylic Acid-Barbiturate (*Oral Analgesic-Sedative*)
United States: Amytal & Aspirin, Salibar, Jr.
Canada: Nova-Phase with Pheno

Acetylsalicylic Acid-Barbiturate-Caffeine
Canada: Fiorinal

Acetylsalicylic Acid-Barbiturate-Caffeine-Phenacetin
United States: Buff-A Comp, Fiorinal

Acetylsalicylic Acid-Barbiturate-Caffeine-Phenacetin-Codeine
United States: Fiorinal with Codeine

Acetylsalicylic Acid-Barbiturate-Codeine
Canada: Fiorinal-C$\frac{1}{4}$, Fiorinal-C$\frac{1}{2}$

☐ This medicine is used to help relieve pain and tension.

☐ IMPORTANT: If you have ever had an allergic reaction to aspirin or a barbiturate medicine, tell your doctor or pharmacist before you take any of this medicine.

HOW TO USE THIS MEDICINE

☐ This medicine may be taken with food or a full glass of water.

☐ The following medicine has a special coating and must be swallowed whole. Do not crush, chew, or break it into pieces. (**Canada:** Nova-Phase with Pheno)

☐ Do not take any more of this medicine than your doctor has prescribed. The drug could become habit-forming or you could take an overdose if you take it more often or longer than prescribed.

☐ Do not take this medicine if it smells strongly like vinegar since this means that the aspirin in it is not fresh.

SPECIAL INSTRUCTIONS

☐ Women who are pregnant, breast-feeding, or planning to become pregnant should tell their doctor before taking this medicine.

- [ ] In some people, this drug may cause dizziness or drowsiness. Do not drive a car or operate dangerous machinery or do jobs that require you to be alert until you know how you are going to react to this drug.

- [ ] If you become dizzy, you should be careful going up and down stairs. Sit or lie down at the first sign of dizziness.

- [ ] Do not drink alcoholic beverages while taking this drug without the approval of your doctor.

- [ ] It is important that you obtain the advice of your doctor or pharmacist before taking ANY other medicines, including pain relievers, sleeping pills, tranquilizers or medicines for depression, or cough/cold or allergy medicines.

- [ ] If you become constipated, try increasing the amount of bulk in your diet (for example, bran and salads), exercising more often, or drinking more water. Call your doctor if the constipation continues, (**Canada:** Fiorinol-C)

- [ ] Call your doctor immediately if you think you may be allergic to the medicine or if you develop a skin rash, hives, itching, swelling of the face, or difficulty in breathing. If you cannot reach your doctor, phone a hospital emergency department.

- [ ] Most people experience few or no side effects from their drugs. However, any medicine can sometimes cause unwanted effects. Call your doctor if you develop bothersome sleepiness or laziness during the day, nightmares, staggering walk, unusual nervousness, a yellow color to the skin or eyes, easy bruising, a slow heartbeat, stomach pain, red or black stools, "ringing" or "buzzing" in the ears, or difficulty in urinating ("passing your water").

* * * * *

Acetylsalicylic Acid-Caffeine-Codeine (*Oral Analgesic-Antipyretic*)

> *Canada:* 222, 282, 292, 293, 294, Codophen-R, C3, C4, Neopirine Co. with Codeine, Phenacodein Tablets 002, Phenacodein Tablets 003

Acetylsalicylic Acid-Codeine

> *United States:* Ascriptin with Codeine, Codasa
>
> *Canada:* Ancasal Compound No. 1, Ancasal Compound No. 2, Ancasal Compound No. 3, Coryphen-Codeine, Entrophen with Codeine

Acetylsalicylic Acid-Acetaminophen-Codeine
Canada: Veganin

Acetylsalicylic Acid-Caffeine-Codeine-Phenacetin
United States: Anexsia with Codeine, Apa-Deine, APC with Codeine, ASA + Codeine Compound, Buff-A-Comp., Empirin Compound with Codeine, Monacet with Codeine, PAC Compound with Codeine, Salatin with Codeine

☐ This medicine is used to help relieve pain and fever.

☐ IMPORTANT: If you have a stomach ulcer or if you have ever had an allergic reaction to acetaminophen, phenacetin, aspirin, or codeine medicine, tell your doctor or pharmacist before you take any of this medicine.

HOW TO USE THIS MEDICINE
☐ This medicine may be taken with food or a glass of water.

☐ Do not take any more of this medicine than your doctor has prescribed. The drug could become habit-forming, or you could take an overdose if you take it more often or longer than prescribed.

☐ Children under 3 years of age should only be given this medicine with the approval of the doctor. Children under 5 years of age should not be given this medicine for more than 5 days in a row and adults should not take this medicine for longer than 10 days without the approval of their doctor.

☐ This medicine must be swallowed whole. Do not crush, chew, or break it into pieces. (*Canada:* 293, Entrophen with Codeine)

☐ Do not take this medicine if it smells strongly like vinegar since this means the aspirin is not fresh.

SPECIAL INSTRUCTIONS
☐ Women who are pregnant, breast-feeding, or planning to become pregnant should tell their doctor before taking this medicine.

☐ Do not drink alcoholic beverages while you are taking this medicine as this may cause dizziness and fainting.

☐ In some people, this drug may cause dizziness or drowsiness. Do not drive a car or operate dangerous machinery or do jobs that require you to be alert until you know how you are going to react to this drug.

☐ If you become dizzy, you should be careful going up and down stairs. Sit or lie down at the first sign of dizziness. Get up slowly if you have been lying or sitting down.

- ☐ It is important that you obtain the advice of your doctor or pharmacist before taking pain relievers, nonprescription drugs, sleeping pills, tranquilizers, or medicines for depression while you are taking this drug.

- ☐ Call your doctor immediately if you think you may be allergic to the medicine or if you develop a skin rash, hives, itching, swelling of the face, or difficulty in breathing. If you cannot reach your doctor, phone a hospital emergency department.

- ☐ Most people experience few or no side effects from their drugs. However, any medicine can sometimes cause unwanted effects. Call your doctor if you develop "ringing" or "buzzing" of the ears, stomach pain, red or black stools, dizziness, fever, sweating, unusual weakness, a yellow color to the skin or eyes, easy bruising or bleeding, severe constipation, or difficulty in urinating ("passing your water").

*   *   *   *   *

Acetylsalicylic Acid-Meprobamate-Caffeine (*Oral Analgesic-Muscle Relaxant*)
Canada: 217 MEP

Acetylsalicylic Acid-Meprobamate-Caffeine-Codeine
Canada: 282 MEP

- ☐ This medicine is used to help relieve pain and to relax muscles.

- ☐ IMPORTANT: If you have ever had an allergic reaction to aspirin, sleeping pills, or a tranquilizer, tell your doctor or pharmacist before you take any of this medicine.

HOW TO USE THIS MEDICINE
- ☐ This medicine may be taken with food or a glass of water.

- ☐ Do not take any more of this medicine than your doctor has prescribed. The drug could become habit-forming or you could take an overdose if you take it more often or longer than prescribed.

- ☐ Do not take this medicine if it smells strongly like vinegar since this means that the aspirin in the medicine is not fresh.

SPECIAL INSTRUCTIONS
- ☐ Women who are pregnant, breast-feeding, or planning to become pregnant should tell their doctor before taking this medicine.

☐ In some people, this drug may cause dizziness or drowsiness. Do not drive a car or operate dangerous machinery or do jobs that require you to be alert until you know how you are going to react to this drug.

☐ If this medicine causes dizziness, you should be careful going up and down stairs and you should not change positions too rapidly. Get out of bed slowly in the morning and dangle your feet over the edge of the bed for a few minutes before standing up. Sit down or lie down at the first sign of dizziness. Tell your doctor you have been dizzy. Avoid hot showers and baths because they could make you dizzy.

☐ Do not drink alcoholic beverages while taking this drug without the approval of your doctor.

☐ It is important that you obtain the advice of your doctor or pharmacist before taking *any* other medicines including pain relievers, sleeping pills, tranquilizers, or medicines for depression, coughs, colds, or allergies.

☐ If you become constipated, try increasing the amount of bulk in your diet (for example, bran and salads), exercising more often, or drinking more water. Call your doctor if the constipation continues. (*Canada:* 282 MEP)

☐ Call your doctor immediately if you think you may be allergic to the medicine or if you develop a skin rash, hives, itching, swelling of the face, or difficulty in breathing. If you cannot reach your doctor, phone a hospital emergency department.

☐ Most people experience few or no side effects from their drugs. However, any medicine can sometimes cause unwanted effects. Call your doctor if you develop a sore throat, fever or mouth sores, easy bruising or bleeding, nightmares or unusual nervousness, stomach pain, red or black stools, or "ringing" or "buzzing" in the ears.

* * * * *

Acrisorcin (*Topical Antifungal*)
United States: Akrinol

☐ This medicine is used to treat fungal infections of the skin.

HOW TO USE THIS MEDICINE

☐ Each time you apply the medicine, wash your hands and gently cleanse the skin area well with water unless otherwise directed by your doctor. Do not allow the skin to dry completely. Pat with a clean towel until almost dry.

☐ Apply a small amount of the drug to the affected area and spread lightly. Only the medicine that is actually touching the skin will work. A thick layer is not more effective than a thin layer. Do not bandage unless directed by your doctor.

□ Do not use the drug more frequently or in larger quantities than prescribed by your doctor.

SPECIAL INSTRUCTIONS

□ It is important to use **all** of this medicine, plus any refills that your doctor told you to use. Do not stop using it earlier than your doctor has recommended in spite of the fact that your symptoms seem to have improved. Otherwise, the infection may return.

□ If you forget to apply the medicine, apply it as soon as possible. However, if it is almost time for your next dose, do not apply the missed dose but continue with your regular schedule.

□ This medicine may make some people more sensitive to sunlight and sunlamps. When you begin taking this medicine, try to avoid getting too much sun until you see how you are going to react. If your skin does become more sensitive to sunlight, tell your doctor and try to stay out of direct sunlight. While in the sun, wear protective clothing and sunglasses. You may wish to ask your pharmacist about suitable sunscreen products. Check with your doctor if you become sunburned.

□ Do not apply cosmetics or lotions on top of the drug unless your doctor approves.

□ Keep this preparation away from the eyes. If you should accidentally get some in your eyes, wash it away with water immediately.

□ Call your doctor if the condition for which this drug is being used persists or becomes worse or if you develop a constant irritation such as itching or burning that was not present before you started using this medicine. Also, call your doctor if you develop blisters or hives.

□ Keep the medicine away from the eyes, nose, and mouth.

□ For external use only. Do not swallow.

* * * * *

Alfacalcidol (*Oral Vitamin D₃ Metabolite*)
Canada: One-Alpha

□ This medicine is used in the treatment of certain conditions to help restore to normal the calcium levels in the body.

□ IMPORTANT: If you have ever had an allergic reaction to a vitamin D medicine, tell your doctor or pharmacist before you take any of this medicine.

HOW TO USE THIS MEDICINE

□ It is very important that you take this medicine exactly as your doctor has prescribed and that you do not miss any doses. Try to take this medicine at the same time every day. Do not take extra tablets without your doctor's approval.

SPECIAL INSTRUCTIONS

☐ Do not take any nonprescription drugs while you are taking this medicine unless otherwise directed. This includes antacids containing magnesium and the prolonged use of mineral oil.

☐ Follow any diet that your doctor has prescribed, especially with respect to dairy products and calcium supplements.

☐ Do not take any other vitamin products containing vitamin D unless otherwise directed.

☐ Most people experience few or no side effects from their drugs. However, any medicine can sometimes cause unwanted effects. Call your doctor if you develop unusual weakness, headache, irregular pulse, nausea, vomiting, dry mouth, muscle or bone pain, constipation, a metallic taste in the mouth, or excessive thirst.

*   *   *   *   *

Allopurinol (*Oral Xanthine Oxidase Inhibitor*)
United States: Zyloprim
Canada: Alloprin, Purinol, Zyloprim

☐ This medicine is used in the treatment of gout and in other conditions in which the body has high levels of uric acid.

HOW TO USE THIS MEDICINE

☐ It is best to take this medicine with food or a glass of milk or after meals to help prevent stomach upset. Call your doctor if you continue to have stomach upset.

SPECIAL INSTRUCTIONS

☐ Women who are breast-feeding should tell their doctor before taking this medicine.

☐ If you forget to take a dose, take it as soon as possible. However, if it is almost time for your next dose, do not take the missed dose. Instead, continue with your regular dosing schedule.

☐ It is very important that you take this medicine exactly as your doctor prescribed and that you do not miss any doses. Otherwise, you cannot expect the medicine to help you.

☐ Try to drink at least 8 to 10 glasses of water or other liquids every day while you are taking this medicine unless otherwise directed by your doctor.

☐ Do not take vitamin C, vitamins with iron, or alcohol while you are taking this medicine without the approval of your doctor.

☐ In some people, this drug may cause drowsiness. Do not drive a car, operate dangerous machinery, or do jobs that require you to be alert until you know how you are going to react to this drug.

☐ Call your doctor immediately if you think you may be allergic to the medicine or if you develop a skin rash, hives, itching, swelling of the face or difficulty in breathing. If you cannot reach your doctor, phone a hospital emergency department.

☐ Most people experience few or no side effects from their drugs. However, any medicine can sometimes cause unwanted effects. Call your doctor if you develop a skin rash, sore throat or fever, unusual bruising or bleeding, weakness, a yellow color to the skin or eyes, low back pain, or pain when you urinate ("pass your water").

*   *   *   *   *

Alseroxylon (*Oral Antihypertensive*)
United States: Rautensin, Rauwiloid
Canada: Rauwiloid

☐ This medication is used to lower the blood pressure.

☐ Hypertension (high blood pressure) is a long-term condition, and it will probably be necessary for you to take the drug for a long time in spite of the fact that you feel better. It is very important that you take this medicine as your doctor has directed and that you do not miss any doses. Otherwise, you cannot expect the drug to keep your blood pressure down.

☐ IMPORTANT: If you have allergies, tell your doctor or pharmacist before you take any of this medicine.

HOW TO USE THIS MEDICINE
☐ Take this medicine with food, meals, or milk.

☐ Try to take the medicine at the same time(s) every day.

SPECIAL INSTRUCTIONS
☐ If you forget to take a dose, take it as soon as possible. However, if it is almost time for your next dose, do not take the missed dose. Instead, continue with your regular dosing schedule.

☐ Women who are pregnant, breast-feeding, or planning to become pregnant should tell their doctor before taking this medicine.

☐ In some people, this drug may cause dizziness or drowsiness. Do not drive a

car or operate dangerous machinery or do jobs that require you to be alert until you know how you are going to react to this drug.

☐ In a few people, this medicine may cause dizziness or fainting if you get up quickly from a lying or sitting position. Get up slowly, especially in the morning. It is advisable to dangle your feet over the edge of the bed for a few minutes before standing up. Sit or lie down at the first sign of dizziness. Tell your doctor that you have been dizzy.

☐ In order to help prevent dizziness and fainting, it is also recommended that you avoid strenuous exercise, standing for long periods of time (especially in hot weather), and hot showers or hot baths.

☐ If you develop a stuffy nose, tell your doctor.

☐ Some nonprescription drugs can aggravate your condition. Do not take any of the following without the approval of your doctor or pharmacist: cough, cold, or sinus products; asthma or allergy products, or diet or weight-reducing medicines.

☐ Most people experience few or no side effects from their drugs. However, any medicine can sometimes cause unwanted effects. Call your doctor if you develop severe diarrhea (loose bowel movements); stomach pain; a skin rash; nightmares; depression or loss of appetite; swelling of the legs or ankles; sudden weight gain of 5 pounds or more; chest pains; or difficulty in breathing.

☐ Carry an identification card indicating that you are taking this medicine. Always tell your pharmacist, dentist, and other doctors who are treating you that you are taking this medicine.

☐ Do not stop taking this medicine without your doctor's approval and do not go without medication between prescription refills. Call your pharmacist two or three days before you will run out of the medicine.

* * * * *

Aluminum Carbonate (*Oral Antacid*)
United States: Basaljel

Aluminum Hydroxide-Sucrose
Canada: Basaljel

☐ This medicine is an antacid which is used to reduce the amount of phosphate in the body and to prevent phosphate stones. It is used in the treatment of chronic kidney conditions.

HOW TO USE THIS MEDICINE

☐ For LIQUID MEDICINE
   • Shake the bottle well before using so that you can measure an accurate dose.

☐ For CAPSULES and TABLETS
   • Take as directed by your doctor.

SPECIAL INSTRUCTIONS

☐ Do not take this medicine more often than recommended by your doctor.

☐ Most people experience few or no side effects from their drugs. However, any medicine can sometimes cause unwanted effects. Call your doctor if you develop stomach pain which lasts for more than 3 days, loss of appetite, constipation, tremors, weakness, or bone pain.

*   *   *   *   *

Aluminum Hydroxide (*Oral Antacid*)

United States: Alu-Cap, Alu-Tab, Amphojel, Dialume
Canada: A-H Gel, Alu-Tab, Amphojel, Basaljel, Chemgel Antacid

☐ This medicine is an antacid which is used to reduce the acidity of the stomach contents to help relieve the symptoms of heartburn as well as in the treatment of peptic ulcer, "reflux" or hiatal hernia. It is also used to reduce the amount of phosphate and to prevent phosphate stones in certain types of conditions.

HOW TO USE THIS MEDICINE

☐ For LIQUID MEDICINE
   • Shake the bottle well before using so that you can measure an accurate dose. The dose may be followed with a sip of water. (**United States** and **Canada:** Amphojel Suspension)
   • Store in a cool place, but do not freeze.

☐ For CHEWABLE TABLETS
   • The tablets may be chewed or dissolved slowly in the mouth. Follow with a glass of water. Do not swallow the tablets. (**United States:** Amphojel; **Canada:** Amphojel, A-H Gel, Chemgel)
   • Place the tablet on the tongue and sip one-half glass of water as you let the tablet dissolve. (**Canada:** Amphojel)

SPECIAL INSTRUCTIONS

☐ Do not take this medicine more often than recommended by your doctor.

☐ If you are taking this medicine because you have an ULCER, you will have to

77

have this antacid very often. This is because your stomach must not be without food or this medicine for usually more than 2 hours at a time. You must follow any diet prescribed by your doctor and continue to take this medicine even if your pain fades. If you stop the antacid too early, your ulcer may not be fully healed and could quickly return. It is best to avoid smoking as well as coffee, tea, alcohol, spices, and aspirin because all of these agents can irritate the stomach. Check with your pharmacist before you take any nonprescription drugs.

☐ If you are taking this medicine because you have REFLUX or HIATAL HERNIA, it is usually best to avoid overeating, to limit the amount of fluids you drink during a meal, to reduce the amout of fats you eat, and to keep your shoulders elevated about 30° in bed.

☐ Most people experience few or no side effects from their drugs. However, any medicine can sometimes cause unwanted effects. Call your doctor if you develop stomach pain which lasts more than 3 days, loss of appetite, tremors, weakness, or bone pain.

* * * * *

Aluminum Oxide Compound (*Topical Acne Therapy*)
United States: Brasivol, Epi-Clear Scrub Cleanser
Canada: Brasivol

☐ This medication is used in the treatment of acne.

☐ This medication is used in place of ordinary soaps and cleansers.

HOW TO USE THIS MEDICINE
☐ For CLEANSER
  • Apply the medicine to the skin with water and rub gently with the fingertips for 15 to 20 seconds.
  • Rinse thoroughly with hot water.

GENERAL INSTRUCTIONS FOR ACNE PATIENTS
☐ Avoid greasy hair oils and creams.

☐ Try to keep your hands away from your hair and face.

☐ Shampoo your hair frequently—at least once or twice a week. Keep your hair brushed back off the face.

☐ Remember to keep your brush and comb clean with regular washing.

☐ Get plenty of exercise, fresh air, and sleep and eat a balanced diet.

☐ Do not squeeze or pick the blemishes.

SPECIAL INSTRUCTIONS

☐ Call your doctor if the condition for which this drug is being used persists or becomes worse or if you develop a constant irritation such as itching or burning that was not present before you started using this medicine.

☐ IMPORTANT: If you have ever had an allergic reaction to acne or skin medicine, tell your doctor or pharmacist before you use any of this drug.

☐ Discontinue use of this medication if excessive drying or skin irritation occurs.

☐ For external use only.

*   *   *   *   *

Amantadine HCl (*Oral Antiparkinsonian-Antiviral Agent*)
United States: Symmetrel
Canada: Symmetrel

☐ This medicine has many uses and the reason it was prescribed depends upon your condition. If you do not understand why you are taking it, check with your doctor.

HOW TO USE THIS MEDICINE

☐ Take the medicine with a glass of water.

☐ Do not take the medicine within 3 hours of bedtime because it may cause insomnia (difficulty in sleeping).

☐ Do not take any more of this medicine than your doctor has prescribed and do not stop taking this medicine without the approval of your doctor.

SPECIAL INSTRUCTIONS

☐ If you forget to take a dose, take it as soon as possible. However, if it is almost time for your next dose, do not take the missed dose. Instead, continue with your regular dosing schedule.

☐ Do not drink alcoholic beverages while taking this drug without the approval of your doctor.

☐ If your mouth becomes dry, suck a hard sour candy (sugarless) or ice chips, or chew gum. It is especially important to brush your teeth regularly if you develop a dry mouth.

☐ In some people, this drug may cause dizziness, drowsiness, or blurred vision. Do not drive a car or operate dangerous machinery or do jobs that require you to be alert until you know how you are going to react to this drug.

☐ If this medicine causes dizziness, you should be careful going up and down stairs and you should not change positions too rapidly. Get out of bed slowly

in the morning and dangle your feet over the edge of the bed for a few minutes before standing up. Sit down or lie down at the first sign of dizziness. Tell your doctor you have been dizzy. Avoid hot showers and baths because they could make you dizzy.

☐ If you become constipated, try increasing the amount of bulk in your diet (for example, bran and salads), exercising more often, or drinking more water.

☐ Most people experience few or no side effects from their drugs. However, any medicine can sometimes cause unwanted effects. Call your doctor if you develop a skin rash, fainting spells, swelling of the legs or ankles, shortness of breath, or if you become depressed.

* * * * *

Ambenonium (Oral Anticholinesterase)
United States: Mytelase

☐ This medicine is used to treat the fatigue and muscular weakness of myasthenia gravis.

HOW TO USE THIS MEDICINE
☐ This medicine may be taken with food or a glass of water.

SPECIAL INSTRUCTIONS
☐ If you forget to take a dose, take it as soon as possible. However, if it is almost time for your next dose, do not take the missed dose. Instead, continue with your regular dosing schedule.

☐ In some people, this drug may cause "double vision." Do not drive a car or operate dangerous machinery or do jobs that require you to be alert until you know how you are going to react to this drug.

☐ It is important that you obtain the advice of your doctor or pharmacist before taking pain relievers, nonprescription drugs, sleeping pills or tranquilizers or medicines for depression while you are taking this drug.

☐ It is a good idea to keep a diary of "peaks and valleys" of your muscle strength. This will help your doctor in designing your treatment.

☐ Most people experience few or no side effects from their drugs. However, any medicine can sometimes cause unwanted effects. Call your doctor if you develop slow or fast heart beats, changes in vision, muscle cramps, nausea, vomiting or diarrhea, difficulty in breathing, fainting spells or dizziness, convulsions, or unusual sweating or if you urinate ("pass your water") more frequently than usual.

* * * * *

Aminophylline (*Oral Antiasthmatic*)

United States: Aminodur Dura-Tabs, Lixaminol, Mini-Lix, Phyllo-contin, Somophyllin

Canada: Aminophyl, Corphyllin, Somophyllin

☐ This medicine is used to help open up the bronchioles (air passages in the lungs) to make breathing easier.

☐ IMPORTANT: If you have ever had an allergic reaction to caffeine or any medicine for lung conditions, tell your doctor or pharmacist before you take any of this medicine.

HOW TO USE THIS MEDICINE

☐ It is best to take this medicine on an empty stomach with a glass of water. However, if it upsets your stomach, it may be taken with a glass of milk or a snack. Call your doctor if the stomach upset continues.

☐ It is very important that you take this medicine exactly as your doctor has prescribed and that you do not miss any doses. Try to take this medicine at the same time every day. Do not take extra tablets without your doctor's approval.

☐ This medicine must be swallowed whole. Do not crush, chew, or break it into pieces. (**United States:** Aminodur Dura-Tabs, Phyllocontin)

SPECIAL INSTRUCTIONS

☐ Do not change the dose of any other asthma or bronchitis medicines except on the advice of your doctor.

☐ Women who are breast-feeding should tell their doctor before taking this medicine.

☐ If you forget to take a dose, take it as soon as possible. However, if it is almost time for your next dose, do not take the missed dose. Instead, continue with your regular dosing schedule.

☐ In some people, this drug may cause dizziness or drowsiness. Do not drive a car or operate dangerous machinery or do jobs that require you to be alert until you know how you are going to react to this drug.

☐ If you become dizzy, you should be careful going up and down stairs. Sit or lie down at the first sign of dizziness.

☐ It is important that you obtain the advice of your doctor or pharmacist before taking ANY other medicines including pain relievers, sleeping pills, tranquilizers or medicines for depression, cough/cold or allergy medicines, or weight-reducing medicines.

☐ Do not smoke while you are on this medicine because smoking can make the drug less effective.

- [ ] Avoid drinking large amounts of coffee, tea, cocoa, or cola drinks because you could be more sensitive to the caffeine in these beverages.

- [ ] Most people experience few or no side effects from their drugs. However, any medicine can sometimes cause unwanted effects. Call your doctor if you develop a skin rash, vomiting, stomach pain or red or black stools, fast heart beats, confusion, unusual tiredness, restlessness, or thirst or increased urination ("passing your water").

* * * * *

Aminophylline-Ephedrine-Amobarbital
United States: Amesec, Roamphed
Canada: Amesec, Chemphyl, Relasma

Aminophylline-Ephedrine-Phenobarbital
United States: Amodrine

- [ ] This medicine is used to help open up the bronchioles (air passages in the lungs) to make breathing easier.

- [ ] IMPORTANT: If you have ever had an allergic reaction to caffeine or any medicine for lung conditions or barbiturate medicine, tell your doctor or pharmacist before you take any of this medicine.

HOW TO USE THIS MEDICINE
- [ ] It is best to take this medicine on an empty stomach with a glass of water. However, if it upsets your stomach, it may be taken with a glass of milk or a snack. Call your doctor if the stomach upset continues.

- [ ] It is very important that you take this medicine exactly as your doctor has prescribed.

SPECIAL INSTRUCTIONS
- [ ] Do not change the dose of any other asthma or bronchitis medicines except on the advice of your doctor.

- [ ] Women who are pregnant, breast-feeding, or planning to become pregnant should tell their doctor before taking this medicine.

- [ ] If you forget to take a dose, take it as soon as possible. However, if it is almost time for your next dose, do not take the missed dose. Instead, continue with your regular dosing schedule.

- [ ] In some people, this drug may cause dizziness or drowsiness. Do not drive a car or operate dangerous machinery or do jobs that require you to be alert until you know how you are going to react to this drug.

☐ If you become dizzy, you should be careful going up and down stairs. Sit or lie down at the first sign of dizziness.

☐ It is important that you obtain the advice of your doctor or pharmacist before taking ANY other medicines including pain relievers, sleeping pills, tranquilizers or medicines for depression, cough/cold or allergy medicines, or weight-reducing medicines.

☐ Do not smoke while you are on this medicine because smoking can make the drug less effective.

☐ Avoid drinking large amounts of coffee, tea, cocoa, or cola drinks because you could be more sensitive to the caffeine in these beverages.

☐ Most people experience few or no side effects from their drugs. However, any medicine can sometimes cause unwanted effects. Call your doctor if you develop a skin rash, vomiting, stomach pain or red or black stools, fast heart beats, confusion, unusual tiredness, restlessness, or thirst, increased urination ("passing your water") or if your sputum turns yellow or green in color. Also call your doctor if you develop a yellow color to the skin or eyes, easy bruising, or nightmares.

*   *   *   *   *

Aminophylline (*Rectal Antiasthmatic*)
United States: Rectalad-Aminophylline
Canada: Amphylline, Corophyllin

☐ This medicine is used to help open up the bronchioles (air passages in the lungs) to make breathing easier.

☐ IMPORTANT: If you have ever had an allergic reaction to caffeine or any medicine for lung conditions, tell your doctor or pharmacist before you use any of this medicine.

HOW TO USE THIS MEDICINE
☐ Administration of suppositories:
- Remove the wrapper from the suppository.
- Lie on your side and raise your knee to your chest.
- Insert the suppository with the tapered (pointed) end first into the rectum.
- Remain lying down for a few minutes so that the suppository will dissolve in the rectum.
- Try to avoid having a bowel movement for at least one hour so that the drug will have time to work.

☐ It is very important that you use this medicine exactly as your doctor has prescribed and that you do not miss any doses. Do not use extra suppositories without your doctor's approval.

SPECIAL INSTRUCTIONS

- [ ] Do not change the dose of any other asthma or bronchitis medicines except on the advice of your doctor.

- [ ] Women who are breast-feeding should tell their doctor before taking this medicine.

- [ ] If you forget a dose, insert it as soon as possible. However, if it is almost time for your next dose, do not use the missed dose. Instead, continue with your regular dosing schedule.

- [ ] In some people, this drug may cause dizziness or drowsiness. Do not drive a car or operate dangerous machinery or do jobs that require you to be alert until you know how you are going to react to this drug.

- [ ] If you become dizzy, you should be careful going up and down stairs. Sit or lie down at the first sign of dizziness.

- [ ] It is important that you obtain the advice of your doctor or pharmacist before taking ANY other medicines including pain relievers, sleeping pills, tranquilizers or medicines for depression, cough/cold or allergy medicines, or weight-reducing medicines.

- [ ] Do not smoke while you are on this medicine because smoking can make the drug less effective.

- [ ] Avoid drinking large amounts of coffee, tea, cocoa, or cola drinks because you could be more sensitive to the caffeine in these beverages.

- [ ] Most people experience few or no side effects from their drugs. However, any medicine can sometimes cause unwanted effects. Call your doctor if you develop a skin rash, vomiting, stomach pain or red or black stools, fast heart beats, confusion, unusual tiredness, restlessness, or thirst, increased urination ("passing your water"), or sputum that turns yellow or green in color, or if you develop rectal burning or pain that was not present before you used the medicine.

* * * * *

Amitriptyline HCl (*Oral Antidepressant*)
United States: Amitril, Elavil, Endep, Rolavil
Canada: Amiline, Deprex, Elavil, Levate, Meravil, Novotriptyn

- [ ] This medicine is used to help relieve the symptoms of depression. It is important that you take the medicine regularly and that you do not miss any doses. The full effect of the medicine will not be noticed immediately, but may take from a few days to several weeks. Early signs of improvement are increased appetite, better sleep, increased energy, and later improved mood. DO NOT STOP TAKING the medicine when you first feel better or you may feel worse in 3 or 4 days.

☐ This medicine has also been used in children to treat bed-wetting.

HOW TO USE THIS MEDICINE

☐ This medicine may be taken with food unless otherwise directed.

☐ Shake the bottle of liquid medicine before using so that you can measure an accurate dose (**Canada:** Elavil Syrup)

SPECIAL INSTRUCTIONS

☐ If you forget to take a dose, take it as soon as possible. However, if it is almost time for your next dose, do not take the missed dose. Instead, continue with your regular dosing schedule.

☐ Any medicine has a few unwanted side effects. Because this medicine takes a few weeks to work, the side effects are the only thing that tell the doctor that the drug is being absorbed. Most of these side effects will go away as your body adjusts to the medicine.

☐ In some people, this drug may cause dizziness or drowsiness. Do not drive a car or operate dangerous machinery or do jobs that require you to be alert until you know how you are going to react to this drug.

☐ If this medicine causes dizziness, you should be careful going up and down stairs and you should not change positions too quickly. Get out of bed slowly in the morning and dangle your feet over the edge of the bed for a few minutes before standing up. Sit or lie down at the first sign of dizziness. Tell your doctor you have been dizzy and he may adjust your dose.

☐ Do not drink alcoholic beverages while taking this drug without the approval of your doctor.

☐ It is important that you obtain the advice of your doctor or pharmacist before taking any other medicines, including pain relievers, sleeping pills, tranquilizers, other medicines for depression, cough, cold, or allergy medicines, or weight-reducing medicine.

☐ If your mouth becomes dry, suck a hard sour candy (sugarless) or ice chips, or chew gum. It is especially important to brush your teeth regularly if you develop a dry mouth.

☐ If you become constipated, try increasing the amount of bulk in your diet (for example, bran, salads), exercising more often, or drinking water.

☐ Call your doctor if you develop a sore throat, fever, mouth sores, eye pain or blurred vision, difficulty in urinating ("passing your water"), fast heart beats, or a skin rash.

☐ Do not stop taking this medicine suddenly without your doctor's approval. When your doctor tells you to stop this medicine, you must follow these precautions for 1 week since some of the medicine will still be in your body.

☐ Carry an identification card indicating that you are taking this medicine. Always tell your dentist, pharmacist, and other doctors who are treating you that you are taking this medicine.

* * * * *

Amobarbital (*Oral Sedative-Hypnotic*)
United States: Amytal
Canada: Amytal

Amobarbital-Secobarbital
United States: Tuinal Pulvules
Canada: Bi-Secogen, Duo-Barb, Novamo-Secobarb, Tuo-Barb, Tuinal

☐ This medicine is used to cause sleep.

☐ IMPORTANT: If you have ever had an allergic reaction to a barbiturate medicine, tell your doctor or pharmacist before you take any of this medicine.

HOW TO USE THIS MEDICINE
☐ This medicine may be taken with food or a full glass of water.

SPECIAL INSTRUCTIONS
☐ Sleeping medicines are only useful for a short time. If used for too long, they lose their effectiveness. Do not take any more of this medicine than your doctor has prescribed and do not stop taking this medicine suddenly without the approval of your doctor.

☐ Women who are pregnant, breast-feeding, or planning to become pregnant should tell their doctor before taking this medicine.

☐ In some people, this drug may cause dizziness or drowsiness. Do not drive a car or operate dangerous machinery or do jobs that require you to be alert until you know how you are going to react to this drug.

☐ If you become dizzy, you should be careful going up and down stairs. Sit or lie down at the first sign of dizziness.

☐ Do not drink alcoholic beverages while taking this drug without the approval of your doctor.

☐ It is important that you obtain the advice of your doctor or pharmacist before taking ANY other medicines including pain relievers, sleeping pills, tranquilizers or medicines for depression, or cough/cold or allergy medicines.

- ☐ Since you are taking this medicine to help you sleep, take it about 20 minutes before you want to go to sleep. Go to bed after you have taken it. Do not smoke in bed after you have taken it.

- ☐ Do not store this medicine at the bedside and keep it out of the reach of children.

- ☐ Call your doctor immediately if you think you may be allergic to the medicine or if you develop a skin rash, hives, itching, swelling of the face, or difficulty in breathing. If you cannot reach your doctor, phone a hospital emergency department.

- ☐ Most people experience few or no side effects from their drugs. However, any medicine can sometimes cause unwanted effects. Call your doctor if you develop a sore throat, bothersome sleepiness or laziness during the day, nightmares, staggering walk, unusual nervousness, a yellow color to the skin or eyes, easy bruising, or slow heart beats.

* * * * *

Amodiaquine HCl (*Oral Antimalarial*)
United States: Camoquin HCl

- ☐ This medicine has many uses and the reason it was prescribed depends upon your condition. If you do not understand why you are taking it, check with your doctor.

HOW TO USE THIS MEDICINE
- ☐ Take this medicine immediately before or after meals or with food in order to help prevent stomach upset.

- ☐ It is very important that you take this medicine exactly as your doctor has prescribed and that you do not miss any doses. Try to take this medicine at the same time every day. Do not take extra tablets without your doctor's approval. Take the medicine for the full treatment.

SPECIAL INSTRUCTIONS
- ☐ If you forget to take a dose, take it as soon as possible. However, if it is almost time for your next dose, do not take the missed dose. Instead, continue with your regular dosing schedule.

- ☐ Women who are pregnant, breast-feeding, or planning to become pregnant should tell their doctor before taking this medicine.

- ☐ This medicine may cause the urine to turn rusty-yellow or brown in color. This is not unusual.

- ☐ If you find that your eyes become more sensitive to light, it may help to wear sunglasses.

□ Most people experience few or no side effects from their drugs. However, any medicine can sometimes cause unwanted effects. Call your doctor if you develop muscle weakness, blurred vision, night blindness or any changes in eyesight or hearing, a skin rash, sore throat, fever or mouth sores, blue-black color to skin or nails, numbness or tingling in the hands or feet, or unusual bruising or bleeding.

□ Keep this medicine well out of the reach of children.

* * * * *

Amoxicillin Trihydrate (*Oral Antibiotic*)

United States: Amoxil, Larotid, Polymox, Robamox, Sumox, Trimox, Utimox, Wymox

Canada: Amoxican, Amoxil, Novamoxin, Penamox, Polymox

□ This medicine is an antibiotic used to treat certain types of infections.

□ IMPORTANT: If you have ever had an allergic reaction to penicillin or any other antibiotic, tell your doctor or pharmacist before you take any of this medicine.

HOW TO USE THIS MEDICINE

□ This medicine may be taken with meals or on an empty stomach.

□ For LIQUID MEDICINE

• If you were prescribed a SUSPENSION, shake the bottle well before using so that you can measure an accurate dose. (**United States:** Amoxil, Larotid, Polymox, Robamox, Sumox, Trimox, Utimox, Wymox Suspensions; Amoxil, Larotid and Polymox Pediatric Drops; **Canada:** Amoxican, Amoxil, Penamox, Polymox Suspensions)

• If a dropper is used to measure the dose and you do not fully understand how to use it, check with your pharmacist. (**United States:** Amoxil, Larotid, Polymox Pediatric Drops; **Canada:** Amoxil, Penamox Pediatric Drops)

• Store the bottle of medicine in a refrigerator unless otherwise directed. Do not freeze. Do not use after the expiration date. (**United States:** Amoxil, Larocin, Polymox Suspensions; **Canada:** Amoxican, Amoxil, Penamox, Polymox Suspensions; Polymox Pediatric Drops)

SPECIAL INSTRUCTIONS

□ It is important to take **all** of this medicine plus any refills that your doctor told you to take. Do not stop taking this medicine earlier than your doctor has recommended in spite of the fact that you may feel better. Otherwise, the infection may return.

□ If you forget to take a dose, take it as soon as you remember and then continue with your regular schedule.

- [ ] Women who are breast-feeding should tell their doctor before taking this medicine.

- [ ] Most people experience few or no side effects from their drugs. However, any medicine may cause unwanted effects. Call your doctor if you develop a dark-colored tongue, yellow-green stools or, in women, a vaginal discharge that was not present before you started taking the medicine.

- [ ] This medicine sometimes causes diarrhea (loose bowel movements). Call your doctor if the diarrhea becomes severe or lasts for more than two days.

- [ ] Call your doctor immediately if you think you may be allergic to the medicine or if you develop a skin rash, hives, itching, swelling of the face, or difficulty in breathing. If you cannot reach your doctor, phone a hospital emergency department.

- [ ] If for some reason you cannot take all of the medicine, discard the unused portion by flushing it down the toilet. Do not take or save old medicine.

*   *   *   *   *

Amphetamine Sulfate (*Oral Sympathomimetic*)
United States: Benzedrine

- [ ] This medicine has many uses and the reason it was prescribed depends upon your condition. If you do not fully understand why you are taking it, check with your doctor.

- [ ] IMPORTANT: If you have ever had an allergic reaction to an amphetamine medicine or any other medicine, tell your doctor or pharmacist before you take any of this medicine.

HOW TO USE THIS MEDICINE
- [ ] This medicine may be taken with food or a glass of water.

- [ ] Do not take the medicine late in the day or it may cause insomnia (difficulty in sleeping).

- [ ] This medicine must be swallowed whole. Do not crush, chew, or break it into pieces. (**United States:** Benzedrine Spansules)

SPECIAL INSTRUCTIONS
- [ ] If you forget to take a dose, take it as soon as possible. However, if it is almost time for your next dose, do not take the missed dose. Instead, continue with your regular dosing schedule.

- [ ] Women who are pregnant, breast-feeding, or planning to become pregnant should tell their doctor before taking this medicine.

- [ ] Do not take any more of this medicine than your doctor has prescribed

89

and do not stop taking this medicine suddenly without the approval of your doctor.

☐ If your mouth becomes dry, suck a hard sour candy (sugarless) or ice chips, or chew gum. It is especially important to brush your teeth regularly if you develop a dry mouth.

☐ In some people, this drug may cause dizziness. Do not drive a car or operate dangerous machinery or do jobs that require you to be alert until you know how you are going to react to this drug. Therefore, you should be careful going up and down stairs. Sit or lie down at the first sign of dizziness.

☐ If this medicine is for a child, do not let him (her) ride a bike or climb trees until you can determine how he (she) is going to react to the medicine. They could hurt themselves if they participated in these activities if they were dizzy.

☐ Do not treat yourself with baking soda or antacids without the approval of your doctor.

☐ Most people experience few or no side effects from their drugs. However, any medicine can sometimes cause unwanted effects. Call your doctor if you develop a skin rash, chest pain or palpitations, unusual movements of the head, arms or legs, or unusual restlessness.

☐ Carry an identification card indicating that you are taking this medicine. Always tell your pharmacist, dentist, and other doctors who are treating you that you are taking this medicine.

*   *   *   *   *

Amphotericin B (*Topical Antifungal*)
United States: Fungizone

☐ This medicine is used to treat fungal infections of the skin.

HOW TO USE THIS MEDICINE

- Each time you apply the medicine, wash your hands and gently cleanse the skin area well with water unless otherwise directed by your doctor.
- Do not allow the skin to dry completely. Pat with a clean towel until almost dry.
- Apply a small amount of the drug to the affected area and spread lightly. Only the medicine that is actually touching the skin will work.
- A thick layer is not more effective than a thin layer. Do not bandage unless directed by your doctor.

☐ Do not use the drug more frequently or in larger quantities than prescribed by your doctor.

SPECIAL INSTRUCTIONS

- ☐ It is important to use **all** of this medicine, plus any refills that your doctor told you to use. Do not stop using it earlier than your doctor has recommended in spite of the fact that your symptoms seem to have improved. Otherwise, the infection may return.

- ☐ If you forget to apply the medicine, apply it as soon as possible. However, if it is almost time for your next dose, do not apply the missed dose, but continue with your regular schedule.

- ☐ Any staining of clothing from the cream or lotion can be removed by hand-washing the fabric with soap and warm water. Any staining from the ointment can be removed by applying a standard cleaning fluid or dry cleaning.

- ☐ Do not apply cosmetics or lotions on top of the drug unless your doctor approves.

- ☐ Keep this preparation away from the eyes. If you should accidentally get some in your eyes, wash it away with water immediately.

- ☐ Call your doctor if the condition for which this drug is being used persists or becomes worse or if you develop a constant irritation such as itching or burning that was not present before you started using this medicine.

- ☐ For external use only. Do not swallow.

*   *   *   *   *

Ampicillin (*Oral Antibiotic*)

United States: A-Cillin, Amcill, Ampico, Amplin, Omnipen, Pen A, Penbritin, Pensyn, Polycillin, Principen, SK-Ampicillin, Supen, Totacillin

Canada: Amcill, Ampicin, Ampilean, Biosan, Penbritin

- ☐ This medicine is an antibiotic used to treat certain types of infections.
- ☐ IMPORTANT: If you have ever had an allergic reaction to penicillin or any other antibiotic, tell your doctor or pharmacist before you take any of this medicine.

HOW TO USE THIS MEDICINE

- ☐ It is best to take this medicine on an empty stomach 1 hour before (or 2 hours after) meals or food unless otherwise directed by your doctor. Take it at the proper time even if you skip a meal.

- ☐ For TABLETS and CAPSULES
  - Take the tablets or capsules with a full glass of water.

- ☐ For LIQUID MEDICINE
  - If you were prescribed a suspension, shake the bottle well before using

so that you can measure an accurate dose. Store in the refrigerator but do not freeze. (*United States:* A-Cillin, Amcill, Ampico, Amplin, Omnipen, Pen A, Penbritin, Pensyn, Polycillin, Principen, SK-Ampicillin, Supen, Totacillin Suspensions; *Canada:* Amcill, Ampicin, Ampilean, Polycillin Suspensions)
- If a dropper is used to measure the dose and you do not fully understand how to use it, check with your pharmacist. (*United States:* Amcill, Omnipen, Penbritin, Polycillin, SK-Ampicillin Suspensions; *Canada:* Amcill, Ampicin, Ampilean, Polycillin Suspensions)
- If there is a discard date on the bottle, throw away any unused medicine after that date.

☐ For CHEWABLE TABLETS
- Chew or crush the tablets well before swallowing (*United States:* Amcill, SK-Ampicillin Chewable Tablets)

SPECIAL INSTRUCTIONS

☐ It is important to take **all** of this medicine plus any refills that your doctor told you to take. Do not stop taking this medicine earlier than your doctor has recommended in spite of the fact that you may feel better. Otherwise, the infection may return.

☐ If you forget to take a dose, take it as soon as you remember and then continue with your regular schedule.

☐ Women who are breast-feeding should tell their doctor before taking this medicine.

☐ Most people experience few or no side effects from their drugs. However, any medicine may sometimes cause unwanted effects. Call your doctor if you develop a dark-colored tongue, yellow-green stools or, in women, a vaginal discharge that was not present before you started taking the medicine.

☐ This medicine sometimes causes diarrhea (loose bowel movements). Call your doctor if the diarrhea becomes severe or lasts for more than two days.

☐ Call your doctor immediately if you think you may be allergic to the medicine or if you develop a skin rash, hives, itching, swelling of the face, or difficulty in breathing. If you cannot reach your doctor, phone a hospital emergency department.

*   *   *   *   *

Ampicillin-Probenecid (*Oral Gonorrhea Therapy*)
United States: Polycillin-PRB, Principen with Probenecid, Probampacin, Probenicillin
Canada: Ampicin-PRB, Pro-Biosan 500 Kit

☐ This medicine is used in the treatment of gonorrhea.

92

☐ IMPORTANT: If you have ever had an allergic reaction to penicillin or any other antibiotic or probenecid, tell your doctor or pharmacist before you take any of this medicine.

HOW TO USE THIS MEDICINE

☐ It is best to take this medicine on an empty stomach at least one hour before (or 2 hours after) eating food. Take it with a full glass of water.

☐ FOR LIQUID MEDICINE
  • Shake the bottle well before using so that you can measure an accurate dose. Store in the refrigerator before taking it.

SPECIAL INSTRUCTIONS

☐ It is important to take **all** of this medicine plus any refills that your doctor told you to take. Do not stop taking it earlier than your doctor has recommended in spite of the fact that you may feel better. Otherwise, the infection may return.

☐ Women who are breast-feeding should tell their doctor before taking this medicine.

☐ Call your doctor immediately if you think you may be allergic to the medicine or if you develop a skin rash, hives, itching, swelling of the face, or difficulty in breathing. If you cannot reach your doctor, phone a hospital emergency department.

☐ Most people experience few or no side effects from their drugs. However, any medicine can sometimes cause unwanted effects. Call your doctor if you develop a dark-colored tongue, yellow-green stools, a sore throat or fever, blood in the urine, difficulty in urinating ("passing your water"), or shortness of breath.

☐ This medicine sometimes causes diarrhea (loose bowel movements). Call your doctor if the diarrhea becomes severe or lasts for more than 2 days.

*   *   *   *   *

Amyl Nitrite *(Inhalation Vasodilator)*
United States: Amyl Nitrite
Canada: Amyl Nitrite

☐ This medicine is used to help relieve a type of heart pain called angina.

HOW TO USE THIS MEDICINE

☐ Instructions for use:
  • As soon as you feel an attack of angina coming, wrap the ampule in a handkerchief and crush it in the palm of your hand.
  • Sit down and inhale the vapor.

☐ It is important that all cigarettes are extinguished before using this medicine as it could be ignited.

SPECIAL INSTRUCTIONS

☐ This medicine should have a strong ether-like and fruity odor and will make a popping sound when the ampule is crushed.

☐ This medicine may produce flushing of the face, a headache, or dizziness. Sit down or lie down until these effects pass.

☐ It is recommended that patients avoid the use of alcoholic beverages while taking this medicine.

*   *   *   *   *

Anileridine (*Oral Analgesic*)
United States: Leritine
Canada: Leritine

☐ This medicine is used to help relieve pain.

HOW TO USE THIS MEDICINE

☐ This medicine may be taken with food or a glass of water.

☐ Do not take any more of this medicine than your doctor has prescribed. The drug could become habit-forming or you could take an overdose if you take it more often or longer than prescribed.

☐ Do not wait to take this medicine until the pain becomes severe. This medicine works best if you take it at the beginning of the pain. Call your doctor if you feel you need it more often than he prescribed.

SPECIAL INSTRUCTIONS

☐ Do not drink alcoholic beverages while taking this drug without the approval of your doctor.

☐ It is important that you obtain the advice of your doctor or pharmacist before taking ANY other medicines including other pain relievers, sleeping pills, tranquilizers or medicines for depression, cough/cold or allergy medicines, or weight-reducing medicines.

☐ In some people, this drug may cause dizziness or drowsiness. Do not drive a car or operate dangerous machinery or do jobs that require you to be alert until you know how you are going to react to this drug.

☐ If you become dizzy, you should be careful going up and down stairs. Sit or lie down at the first sign of dizziness. Get up slowly if you have been lying or sitting down.

- [ ] If you do feel nauseated when you first start taking the medicine, it may help if you lie down for a few minutes.

- [ ] If you become constipated, try increasing the amount of bulk in your diet (for example, bran and salads), exercising more often, or drinking more water. Call your doctor if the constipation continues.

- [ ] Most people experience few or no side effects from their drugs. However, any medicine can sometimes cause unwanted effects. Call your doctor if you develop shortness of breath, slow heart beat, unusual nervousness, stomach pain, or difficulty in urinating ("passing your water").

- [ ] Always tell your dentist, pharmacist, and other doctors who are treating you that you are taking this medicine.

*   *   *   *   *

Anisindione
United States: Miradon

- [ ] This medicine is used to help prevent harmful blood clots from forming. It is commonly called a "blood thinner."

HOW TO USE THIS MEDICINE
- [ ] Take this medicine **exactly** as your doctor has prescribed. Try to take the medicine at the same time every day and do not miss any doses. Do not take extra tablets without your doctor's approval because overtreatment will cause bleeding.

- [ ] Regular blood tests, called "prothrombin tests," are necessary in order for your doctor to prescribe the correct dose for you. Your dose may change from time to time depending on these tests.

- [ ] It is best to take this medicine with a glass of water. Do not take it with food or other drugs unless otherwise directed.

- [ ] If you forget to take a dose, take it as soon as possible. However, if it is almost time for your next dose, do not take the missed dose. Instead, continue with your regular dosing schedule. Record the date of the missed dose so that you can tell your doctor the next time you see him for a blood test. Call your doctor if you miss more than one dose.

SPECIAL INSTRUCTIONS
- [ ] Do not take any other drugs or stop taking any drugs you are presently taking without first consulting with your doctor. This even includes many products that you can buy without a prescription such as pain relievers and antacids. Always check with your pharmacist before you take or buy ANY nonprescription products.

- [ ] Do not take aspirin or medicines containing aspirin or salicylates. It is usually safe to take acetaminophen as a substitute for aspirin for occasional headaches and pain. Check with your pharmacist.

☐ It is best to avoid alcoholic beverages while you are taking this medicine because the combination may cause undesirable side effects. Ask your doctor if he feels it is safe for you to have an occasional drink.

☐ Do not eat unusually large amounts of leafy, green vegetables or change your diet without telling your doctor.

☐ If you have a tendency to cut yourself while shaving, you may wish to use an electric razor to avoid possible bleeding.

☐ Try to avoid contact sports or activities in which you could become injured because such injuries could result in internal bleeding.

☐ This medicine may cause your urine to turn orange in color. This is not an unusual effect, but tell your doctor so that he can check to make sure you do not have any blood in your urine.

☐ If your body gets more medicine than it needs, bleeding may occur. Call your doctor if you notice any of the following signs of bleeding which you cannot explain or are unusual for you: nosebleeds, bruising or heavy menstrual bleeding, bleeding from the gums after brushing the teeth, heavy bleeding from cuts, red or black stools, red or dark brown urine, or vomiting or coughing up blood. Your doctor will do some blood tests and adjust your dose.

☐ Women who are pregnant, breast-feeding, or planning to become pregnant should tell their doctor before taking this medicine.

☐ Most people experience few or no side effects from their drugs. However, any medicine can sometimes cause unwanted effects. Call your doctor if you develop stomach or back pain, unusual headaches, changes in eyesight, constipation or diarrhea, dizziness, a skin rash, sore throat, fever, mouth sores, a yellow color to the skin or eyes, or unusual tiredness.

☐ Carry an identification card indicating that you are taking this medicine. Always tell your pharmacist, dentist, and other doctors who are treating you that you are taking this medicine.

☐ Do not go without this medicine between prescription refills. Call your pharmacist 2 or 3 days before you will run out of the medicine.

☐ After you stop taking the medicine, it will take your body some time to return to normal. Your doctor or pharmacist will tell you how long you must follow these instructions AFTER you have stopped taking this medicine.

*   *   *   *   *

Anisotropine (*Oral Antispasmodic*)
United States: Valpin 50
Canada: Valpin

- ☐ This medicine is used to help relax muscles of the stomach and bowels as well as to decrease the amount of acid formed in the stomach.

- ☐ IMPORTANT: If you have ever had an allergic reaction to atropine or bromides or any other drug used to relax the stomach or bowels, tell your doctor or pharmacist before you take any of this medicine.

HOW TO USE THIS MEDICINE

- ☐ Take this medicine approximately 30 minutes before a meal unless otherwise directed.

- ☐ If you miss a dose of this medicine, do not take the missed dose and do not double the next dose.

SPECIAL INSTRUCTIONS

- ☐ Women who are pregnant, breast-feeding, or planning to become pregnant should tell their doctor before taking this medicine.

- ☐ If your mouth becomes dry, suck a hard sour candy (sugarless) or ice chips, or chew gum. It is especially important to brush your teeth regularly if you develop a dry mouth.

- ☐ In some people, this drug may cause dizziness or drowsiness. Do not drive a car or operate dangerous machinery or do jobs that require you to be alert until you know how you are going to react to this drug.

- ☐ If you become dizzy, you should be careful going up and down stairs. Sit or lie down at the first sign of dizziness. Tell your doctor you have been dizzy.

- ☐ A desire to urinate ("pass your water") with an inability to do so is not an uncommon effect with this drug. Urinating before taking the drug each time may help relieve this problem. Call your doctor if it continues.

- ☐ You may become more sensitive to heat because your body may perspire less while you are taking this drug. Be careful not to become overheated during exercise or in hot weather.

- ☐ Do not take antacids within 1 hour of taking this medicine as it could make this medicine less effective.

- ☐ If you become constipated, try increasing the amount of bulk in your diet (for example, bran and salads), exercising more often, or drinking more water. Call your doctor if the constipation continues.

- ☐ If your eyes become more sensitive to sunlight, it may help to wear sunglasses.

- ☐ Most people experience few or no side effects from their drugs. However, any medicine can sometimes cause unwanted effects. Call your doctor if you develop a skin rash, diarrhea, unusual restlessness, flushing, or eye pain.

* * * * *

Antazoline (Oral Antihistamine)
Canada: Antistine

☐ This medicine is used to help relieve the symptoms of certain types of allergic conditions.

HOW TO USE THIS MEDICINE
☐ This medicine may be taken with food or a glass of milk it it upsets your stomach.

SPECIAL INSTRUCTIONS
☐ If you forget to take a dose, take it as soon as possible. However, if it is almost time for your next dose, do not take the missed dose. Instead, continue with your regular dosing schedule.

☐ In some people, this drug may initially cause dizziness or drowsiness. Do not drive a car or operate dangerous machinery or do jobs that require you to be alert until you know how you are going to react to this drug. If you become dizzy, you should be careful going up and down stairs. Sit or lie down at the first sign of dizziness. Tell your doctor if it continues.

☐ Do not drink alcoholic beverages while taking this drug without the approval of your doctor.

☐ If your mouth becomes dry, suck a hard sour candy (sugarless) or ice chips, or chew gum. It is especially important to brush your teeth regularly if you develop a dry mouth.

☐ It is important that you obtain the advice of your doctor or pharmacist before taking pain relievers, nonprescription drugs, sleeping pills or tranquilizers, or other medicines for allergies.

☐ Do not take this medicine more often or longer than recommended by your doctor.

☐ Most people experience few or no side effects from their drugs. However, any medicine can sometimes cause unwanted effects. Call your doctor if you develop a skin rash, fast heart beats, blurred vision, stomach pain or difficulty in urinating ("passing your water").

* * * * *

Anthralin (*Topical Psoriasis Therapy*)

United States: Anthera, Anthra-Derm Ointment, Lasan
Canada: Anthra-Derm Oil, Lasan

☐ This medicine is used in the treatment of psoriasis.

HOW TO USE THIS MEDICINE

☐ Instructions for use: (**United States:** Anthera Ointment, Anthra-Derm Ointment, Lasan Unguent; **Canada:** Lasan Ointment)
   - Apply the ointment carefully to the plaque sites at bedtime.
   - In the morning remove with warm oil and follow with a bath.

☐ Instructions for use: (**United States** and **Canada:** Lasan Pomade)
   - Before applying pomade, apply a film of petrolatum on the normal skin areas of the scalp and ears. Be careful to avoid getting the pomade on the scalp behind the ears.
   - Apply carefully and massage medicine into scalp at bedtime. Remove the following morning with a shampoo.

☐ Instructions for use: (**Canada:** Anthra-Derm Oil)
   - Cleanse the skin area well with soap and water unless otherwise specified by your doctor.
   - Apply a thin film with gauze (not cotton), but do not rub in.

SPECIAL INSTRUCTIONS

☐ Do not apply this drug to normal skin. It must only be used on areas of active psoriasis.

☐ Do not use the drug more frequently or in larger quantities than prescribed by your doctor.

☐ If you forget to apply the medicine, apply it as soon as possible. However, if it is almost time for your next dose, do not apply the missed dose, but continue with your regular schedule.

☐ Do not allow any of this medicine to come into contact with the eyes. Wash hands thoroughly and carefully after using.

☐ This medicine may stain bed linen and clothing. Use old bed linen. Avoid getting any of the medicine on clothing.

☐ Plastic gloves may be used when applying the preparation in order to prevent staining of the hands.

☐ A plastic cap or shower cap may be worn at night in order to prevent staining of the pillow and sheets.

☐ Discontinue using this medicine if irritation develops or if normal skin becomes red.

☐ Wash hands thoroughly and carefully after applying this medicine.

- [ ] Cap bottle tightly after use. (**Canada:** Anthra-Derm Oil)
- [ ] For external use only. Do not swallow.

*   *   *   *   *

Antipyrine-Benzocaine (*Otic Analgesic-Antiphlogistic*)
United States: Auralgan, Aurasol, Eardro, Oto
Canada: Auralgan, Auricrine, Oto-Pediat

- [ ] This medicine is used to treat ear conditions.

HOW TO USE THIS MEDICINE
- [ ] For EAR DROPS

INSTILLATION OF EAR DROPS

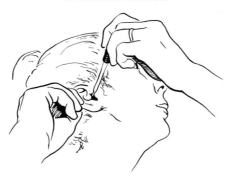

- Clean outer ear carefully and thoroughly with cotton.
- Warm the medicine to body temperature by holding it in your hands for a few minutes.
- Tilt head to the side or lie on side so that the ear to be treated is uppermost.
- Drop the prescribed amount of medicine into the ear canal.
- Remain in the same position for a short time (about 5 minutes) following administration.
- Dry the external ear thoroughly.
- Do not use the solution if it is discolored or if it appears to have changed in any way since you purchased it.
- If possible, have another person administer the ear drops for you.

- [ ] Place a cotton wick soaked in the solution into the ear **only** if your doctor directs you to do so.

- [ ] Do **not** rinse the dropper with water. Keep it dry. Wipe the end of the dropper off with a tissue.

SPECIAL INSTRUCTIONS
- [ ] If you forget to use the medicine, use it as soon as possible. However, if it

100

is almost time for your next dose, do not use the missed dose but continue with your regular schedule.

☐ Do not use this medicine at the same time as any other ear medicine without the approval of your doctor. Some medicines cannot be mixed.

☐ Call your doctor if the condition for which you are using this medicine persists or becomes worse or if the medicine causes itching or burning for more than a few minutes after instillation.

☐ Store in a cool dark place and keep the container tightly closed.

☐ For external use only. Do not swallow.

*　*　*　*　*

Aprobarbital (Oral Hypnotic)
United States: Alurate

☐ This medicine is used to cause sleep.

☐ IMPORTANT: If you have ever had an allergic reaction to a barbiturate medicine, tell your doctor or pharmacist before you take any of this medicine.

HOW TO USE THIS MEDICINE

☐ This medicine may be taken with food or a full glass of water.

SPECIAL INSTRUCTIONS

☐ Sleeping medicines are only useful for a short time. If used for too long, they lose their effectiveness. Do not take any more of this medicine than your doctor has prescribed and do not stop taking this medicine suddenly without the approval of your doctor.

☐ Women who are pregnant, breast-feeding, or planning to become pregnant should tell their doctor before taking this medicine.

☐ In some people, this drug may cause dizziness or drowsiness. Do not drive a car or operate dangerous machinery or do jobs that require you to be alert until you know how you are going to react to this drug.

☐ If you become dizzy, you should be careful going up and down stairs. Sit or lie down at the first sign of dizziness.

☐ Do not drink alcoholic beverages while taking this drug without the approval of your doctor.

☐ It is important that you obtain the advice of your doctor or pharmacist before taking ANY other medicines including pain relievers, sleeping pills, tranquilizers or medicines for depression, or cough/cold or allergy medicines.

☐ Since you are taking this medicine to help you sleep, take it about 20 minutes before you want to go to sleep. Go to bed after you have taken it. Do not smoke in bed after you have taken it.

- Do not store this medicine at the bedside and keep it out of the reach of children.

- Call your doctor immediately if you think you may be allergic to the medicine or if you develop a skin rash, hives, itching, swelling of the face, or difficulty in breathing. If you cannot reach your doctor, phone a hospital emergency department.

- Most people experience few or no side effects from their drugs. However, any medicine can sometimes cause unwanted effects. Call your doctor if you develop a sore throat, bothersome sleepiness or laziness during the day, nightmares, staggering walk, unusual nervousness, a yellow color to the skin or eyes, easy bruising, or slow heart beats.

*　*　*　*　*

Atropine Sulfate or Alkaloid (*Mydriatic-Cycloplegic*)

United States: Atropisol, Bufopto Atropine Solution, Isopto Atropine
Canada: Isopto Atropine, Optotropinal

- This medicine is used to treat conditions of the eye. The drug will cause the pupil of the eye to dilate (become larger in size). This is a normal effect of the drug.

HOW TO USE THIS MEDICINE
- For EYE DROPS

INSTILLATION OF EYE DROPS

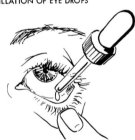

- The person administering the eye drops should wash his hands with soap and water.
- The eye drops must be kept clean. Do not touch the dropper against the face or anything else.
- Lie down or tilt your head backward and look at the ceiling.
- Gently pull down the lower lid of your eye to form a pouch.
- Hold the dropper in your other hand and approach the eye from the side. Place the dropper as close to the eye as possible without touching it.
- Place the prescribed number of drops into the pouch of the eye.

102

- Close your eyes. Do not rub them.
- Apply gentle pressure for a minute with your fingers to the bridge of the nose (inside corner of the eye) to prevent the eye drops from being drained from the eye.
- Blot excess solution around the eye with a tissue.

☐ If necessary, have someone else administer the eye drops for you.

☐ Do not use the eye drops if they change in color or change in any way since being purchased.

☐ Keep the eye drop bottle tightly closed when not in use.

☐ For EYE OINTMENT

INSTILLATION OF EYE OINTMENT

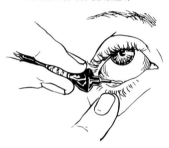

- The person administering the eye ointment should wash his hands with soap and water.
- The eye ointment must be kept clean. Do not touch the tube against the face or anything else.
- Lie down or tilt your head backward and look at the ceiling.
- Gently pull down the lower lid of your eye to form a pouch.
- Hold the tube in your other hand and place the tube as close as possible to the eye without touching it.
- Squeeze the prescribed amount of ointment (usually $\frac{1}{2}$ inch in adults) from the tube along the pouch.
- Close your eyes. Do not rub them.
- Wipe off any excess ointment around the eye with a tissue.
- Clean the tip of the ointment tube with a tissue.

☐ If necessary, have someone else administer the eye ointment for you.

☐ Keep the eye ointment tube tightly closed when not in use.

SPECIAL INSTRUCTIONS

☐ Vision may be blurred for a few minutes after using the eye medicine. Do not drive a car or operate dangerous machinery or do jobs that require you to be alert until your vision has cleared.

☐ If you forget to use the medicine, use it as soon as possible. However, if it is almost time for your next dose, do not use the missed dose but continue with your regular schedule.

- [ ] Do not use this medicine at the same time as any other eye medicine without the approval of your doctor. Some medicines cannot be mixed.

- [ ] If your eyes become more sensitive to light, it may help to wear sunglasses.

- [ ] Contact your doctor if the condition for which you are using this medicine does not improve or if the eye becomes irritated by it for more than a few minutes. Many eye medicines sting for a short time immediately after use. Also call your doctor if you develop eye pain, a skin rash, flushing, dryness of the skin, a fast pulse, or fever.

- [ ] Always tell any future doctors who are treating you that you have used this medicine.

- [ ] Keep the container tightly closed and store in a cool place.

- [ ] Do not use the drug more frequently or in larger quantities than prescribed by your doctor.

- [ ] For external use only. Do not swallow.

*　*　*　*　*

Atropine-Phenobarbital (Oral Antispasmodic-Sedative)
United States: Alised, Antrocol, Atrobarb
Canada: Atrobarbital, Atrosed

Atropine-Hyoscine-Hyoscyamine-Phenobarbital
United States: Barbidonna, Donnatal, Donphen, Hasp, Hybephen, Pylora, Sedralex, Setamine, Spalix, Spasmolin, Spasmorel
Canada: Donnatal

- [ ] This medicine is used to help relieve cramps or spasms of the stomach, bowels, or bladder.

- [ ] IMPORTANT: If you have ever had an allergic reaction to atropine, bromides, or barbiturates or any other drug used to relax the stomach or bowels, tell your doctor or pharmacist before you take any of this medicine.

HOW TO USE THIS MEDICINE
- [ ] Take this medicine approximately 30 minutes before a meal unless otherwise directed.

- [ ] If you miss a dose of this medicine, do not take the missed dose and do not double the next dose.

☐ This medicine must be swallowed whole. Do not crush, chew, or break it into pieces. (**United States:** Donnatal Extentabs, Spasmorel; **Canada:** Donnatal Extentabs)

SPECIAL INSTRUCTIONS

☐ Women who are pregnant, breast-feeding, or planning to become pregnant should tell their doctor before taking this medicine.

☐ If your mouth becomes dry, suck a hard sour candy (sugarless) or ice chips, or chew gum. It is especially important to brush your teeth regularly if you develop a dry mouth.

☐ In some people, this drug may cause dizziness or drowsiness. Do not drive a car or operate dangerous machinery or do jobs that require you to be alert until you know how you are going to react to this drug.

☐ If you become dizzy, you should be careful going up and down stairs. Sit or lie down at the first sign of dizziness. Tell your doctor you have been dizzy.

☐ Do not drink alcoholic beverages while taking this drug without the approval of your doctor.

☐ It is important that you obtain the advice of your doctor or pharmacist before taking pain relievers, nonprescription drugs, sleeping pills, tranquilizers, or medicine for depression while you are taking this drug.

☐ Do not take any more of this medicine than your doctor has prescribed and do not stop taking this medicine suddenly without the approval of your doctor.

☐ Call your doctor immediately if you think you may be allergic to the medicine or if you develop a skin rash, hives, itching, swelling of the face, or difficulty in breathing. If you cannot reach your doctor, phone a hospital emergency department.

☐ A desire to urinate ("pass your water") with an inability to do so is not an uncommon effect with this drug. Urinating before each time you take the drug may help relieve this problem. Call your doctor if it continues.

☐ You may become more sensitive to heat because your body may perspire less while you are taking this drug. Be careful not to become overheated during exercise or in hot weather.

☐ Do not take antacids within 1 hour of taking this medicine as it could make this medicine less effective.

☐ If you become constipated, try increasing the amount of bulk in your diet (for example, bran and salads), exercising more often, or drinking more water. Call your doctor if the constipation continues.

☐ If your eyes become more sensitive to sunlight, it may help to wear sunglasses.

- [ ] Most people experience few or no side effects from their drugs. However, any medicine can sometimes cause unwanted effects. Call your doctor if you develop a skin rash, diarrhea, unusual restlessness, flushing or eye pain, a sore throat, fever, a yellow color to the skin or eyes, easy bruising or bleeding, unusual tiredness, or slow heart beats.

* * * * *

Azathioprine (*Oral Immunosupressive Agent*)
United States: Imuran
Canada: Imuran

- [ ] This medicine is used in certain medical conditions to help reduce the body's natural immunity.

HOW TO USE THIS MEDICINE
- [ ] It is best to take this medicine 1 hour before breakfast or 2 hours after supper in order to help prevent nausea or vomiting.
- [ ] It is very important that you take this medicine exactly as your doctor has prescribed and that you do not miss any doses. Try to take this medicine at the same time every day.
- [ ] Even if you become nauseated or lose your appetite, do not stop taking the medicine but check with your doctor.
- [ ] If you miss a dose of this medicine, do not take the missed dose and do not double your next dose. Check with your doctor.

SPECIAL INSTRUCTIONS
- [ ] Always keep your doctor appointments so that your doctor can watch your progress.
- [ ] If your doctor has prescribed some other medicines for you, it is important that you take them in the right order and that you do not miss them.
- [ ] Men and women should take appropriate birth control measures to avoid pregnancy while taking this medicine and for at least 4 months after the medicine has been stopped.
- [ ] Always tell your pharmacist, dentist, and any other doctors who are treating you that you are taking this medicine. This is especially important if you plan to have surgery or any vaccinations.
- [ ] Call your doctor if you develop a sore throat, fever, a skin rash, easy bruising or bleeding, black tarry stools, severe stomach pain, a yellow color to the skin or eyes, dark-colored urine, or diarrhea (loose bowel movements), or if you develop an infection.

* * * * *

Azatadine Maleate *(Oral Antihistamine)*
United States: Optimine
Canada: Optimine

☐ This medicine is used to help relieve the symptoms of certain types of allergic conditions, coughs and colds, and certain skin conditions.

HOW TO USE THIS MEDICINE
☐ This medicine may be taken with food or a glass of milk if it upsets your stomach.

SPECIAL INSTRUCTIONS
☐ If you forget to take a dose, take it as soon as possible. However, if it is almost time for your next dose, do not take the missed dose. Instead, continue with your regular dosing schedule.

☐ In some people, this drug may initially cause dizziness or drowsiness. Do not drive a car or operate dangerous machinery or do jobs that require you to be alert until you know how you are going to react to this drug. If you become dizzy, you should be careful going up and down stairs. Sit or lie down at the first sign of dizziness. Tell your doctor if it continues.

☐ Do not drink alcoholic beverages while taking this drug without the approval of your doctor.

☐ If your mouth becomes dry, suck a hard sour candy (sugarless) or ice chips, or chew gum. It is especially important to brush your teeth regularly if you develop a dry mouth.

☐ It is important that you obtain the advice of your doctor or pharmacist before taking pain relievers, nonprescription drugs, sleeping pills or tranquilizers, or other medicines for allergies.

☐ Do not take this medicine more often or longer than recommended by your doctor.

☐ Most people experience few or no side effects from their drugs. However, any medicine can sometimes cause unwanted effects. Call your doctor if you develop a skin rash, fast heart beats, blurred vision, stomach pain, or difficulty in urinating ("passing your water").

*   *   *   *   *

Bacitracin *(Ophthalmic Antibiotic)*
United States: Baciguent
Canada: Baciguent

☐ This medicine is an antibiotic used to treat certain types of eye infections.

HOW TO USE THIS MEDICINE

☐ For EYE OINTMENT

INSTILLATION OF EYE OINTMENT

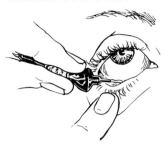

- The person administering the eye ointment should wash his hands with soap and water.
- The eye ointment must be kept clean. Do not touch the tube against the face or anything else.
- Lie down or tilt your head backward and look at the ceiling.
- Gently pull down the lower lid of your eye to form a pouch.
- Hold the tube in your other hand and place the tube as close as possible to the eye without touching it.
- Squeeze the prescribed amount of ointment (usually $\frac{1}{2}$ inch in adults), from the tube along the pouch.
- Close your eyes. Do not rub them.
- Wipe off any excess ointment around the eye with a tissue.
- Clean the tip of the ointment tube with a tissue.

☐ If necessary, have someone else administer the eye ointment for you.

☐ Keep the eye ointment tube tightly closed when not in use.

☐ Do not use the drug more frequently or in larger quantities than prescribed by your doctor.

SPECIAL INSTRUCTIONS

☐ Vision may be blurred for a few minutes after using the eye medicine. Do not drive a car or operate dangerous machinery or do jobs that require you to be alert until your vision has cleared.

☐ Eye medicines should be used as prescribed by your doctor. Often, eye infections clear rapidly after a few days of using the medicine, but not always completely. It is important to use **all** of this medicine, plus any refills that your doctor told you to use. Do not stop using it earlier than your doctor has recommended in spite of the fact that your symptoms seem to have improved. Otherwise, the infection may return.

☐ If you forget to use the medicine, use it as soon as possible. However, if it is almost time for your next dose, do not use the missed dose but continue with your regular schedule.

□ Do not use this medicine at the same time as any other eye medicine without the approval of your doctor. Some medicines cannot be mixed.

□ Contact your doctor if the condition for which you are using this medicine does not improve or if the eye becomes irritated by it for more than a few minutes. Many eye medicines sting for a short time immediately after use.

□ For external use only. Do not swallow.

*   *   *   *   *

Bacitracin (*Topical Antibiotic*)
United States: Baciguent
Canada: Baciguent, Bacitin

□ This medicine is an antibiotic used to treat infections of the skin.

HOW TO USE THIS MEDICINE
• Each time you apply the medicine, wash your hands and gently cleanse the skin area well with water unless otherwise directed by your doctor. Do not allow the skin to dry completely. Pat with a clean towel until almost dry.
• Apply a small amount of the drug to the affected area and spread lightly. Only the medicine that is actually touching the skin will work. A thick layer is not more effective than a thin layer. Do not bandage unless directed by your doctor.

□ Do not use the drug more frequently or in larger quantities than prescribed by your doctor.

SPECIAL INSTRUCTIONS
□ It is important to use **all** of this medicine, plus any refills that your doctor told you to use. Do not stop using it earlier than your doctor has recommended in spite of the fact that your symptoms seem to have improved. Otherwise, the infection may return.

□ If you forget to apply the medicine, apply it as soon as possible. However, if it is almost time for your next dose, do not apply the missed dose but continue with your regular schedule.

□ Do not apply cosmetics or lotions on top of the drug unless your doctor approves.

□ Keep this preparation away from the eyes. If you should accidentally get some in your eyes, wash it away with water immediately.

□ Call your doctor if the condition for which this drug is being used persists or becomes worse or if you develop a constant irritation such as itching or burning that was not present before you started using this medicine.

☐ For external use only. Do not swallow.

* * * * *

Baclofen (*Oral Skeletal Muscle Relaxant*)
United States: Lioresal
Canada: Lioresal

☐ This medicine is used to relax muscles and helps to relieve muscle pain and stiffness.

☐ IMPORTANT: If you have ever had an allergic reaction to any medicines, tell your doctor or pharmacist before you take any of this medicine.

HOW TO USE THIS MEDICINE

☐ This medicine may be taken with food or a glass of water.

☐ If you forget to take a dose, take it as soon as possible. However, if it is almost time for your next dose, do not take the missed dose. Instead, continue with your regular dosing schedule.

SPECIAL INSTRUCTIONS

☐ Women who are pregnant, breast-feeding, or planning to become pregnant should tell their doctor before taking this medicine.

☐ Do not drink alcoholic beverages while taking this drug without the approval of your doctor.

☐ It is important that you obtain the advice of your doctor or pharmacist before taking ANY other medicines including pain relievers, sleeping pills, tranquilizers or medicine for depression, or cough/cold or allergy medicines.

☐ In some people, this drug may cause dizziness or drowsiness. Do not drive a car or operate dangerous machinery or do jobs that require you to be alert until you know how you are going to react to this drug.

☐ If this medicine causes dizziness, you should be careful going up and down stairs and you should not change positions too rapidly. Get out of bed slowly in the morning and dangle your feet over the edge of the bed for a few minutes before standing up. Sit down or lie down at the first sign of dizziness. Tell your doctor you have been dizzy. Avoid hot showers and baths because they could make you dizzy.

☐ Do not take any more of this medicine than your doctor has prescribed and do not stop taking this medicine suddenly without the approval of your doctor.

110

☐ If you become constipated, try increasing the amount of bulk in your diet (for example, bran and salads), exercising more often, or drinking more water.

☐ Most people experience few or no side effects from their drugs. However, any medicine can sometimes cause unwanted effects. Call your doctor if you develop a skin rash, chest pain, frequent or painful urination ("passing your water"), blurred vision, severe constipation, fainting, or bothersome headaches or confusion, or if you become depressed.

*　*　*　*　*

Beclomethasone Dipropionate (*Inhalation Topical Steroid*)
United States: Beclovent Inhaler, Vanceril Inhaler
Canada: Beclovent Inhaler, Vanceril Oral Inhaler

☐ This medicine is used to help prevent asthmatic attacks.

HOW TO USE THIS MEDICINE
☐ Patients vary in the dose they require, and your doctor will determine the dosage that is best for you. Take the medicine regularly and do not take the medicine more often than directed by your doctor. If you develop difficulty in breathing, contact your doctor immediately.

☐ INSTRUCTIONS FOR USE
  • If troubled with sputum, try to clear your chest as completely as possible before inhalation of the drug. This will help get the drug more deeply into your lungs.
  • Hold the inhaler **upright** during use.
  • **Shake** the canister.

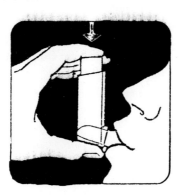

  • Breathe out fully and place lips tightly around mouthpiece and tilt head slightly back.
  • Start to breathe in slowly and press down on the valve firmly and fully at the middle of inspiration ("breathing in") to release a "puff."

111

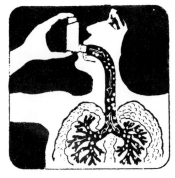

- Hold breath for a few seconds. Breathe out through the nose.
- Allow at least 30 seconds before shaking again to release a second "puff" if prescribed.
- Gargle and rinse your mouth with warm water after administering the medication.
- The mouthpiece of the inhaler should be cleaned after each use.
- Failure to follow these instructions carefully can result in inadequate treatment.

SPECIAL INSTRUCTIONS

☐ If you forget to take a dose, take it as soon as possible. However, if it is almost time for your next dose, do not take the missed dose. Instead, continue with your regular dosing schedule.

☐ It may take 1 to 4 weeks before you feel the full benefit of this medicine. If you are also using another inhaler that opens up the air passages (bronchodilator) in your lungs, use it several minutes before you use this inhaler.

☐ If an asthmatic attack should occur, continue the medicine and if no relief is obtained, you should notify your doctor.

☐ Do not take any more of this medicine than your doctor has prescribed and do not stop taking this medicine suddenly without the approval of your doctor. If you should suddenly stop taking it or reduce the dose, you may experience a worsening of your asthma.

☐ Carry an identification card indicating that you are taking this medicine. Always tell your pharmacist, dentist, and other doctors who are treating you that you are taking this medicine.

☐ Store the container in a cool place. Do not place the container in hot water or near radiators, stoves, or other sources of heat. Do not puncture, burn, or incinerate the container (even after it is empty).

☐ Most people experience few or no side effects from their drugs. However, any medicine can sometimes cause unwanted effects. Call your doctor if you develop a soreness in the mouth or throat, a bad taste in the mouth that will not go away, or if your asthma gets worse.

*　*　*　*　*

Beclomethasone Dipropionate Nasal Spray (*Nasal Allergic Rhinitis Therapy*)

Canada: Beconase, Vancenase

☐ This medicine is used in the treatment of hay fever to help relieve the symptoms of nasal stuffiness and "runny nose."

HOW TO USE THIS MEDICINE

☐ INSTRUCTIONS FOR USE

- Blow your nose gently.
- Sit upright with your head slightly back.
- Shake the canister.
- Insert the nozzle firmly into the nostril. The nozzle should be aimed upwards and outwards to obtain the best results. Close the other nostril by pressing your finger on the side of it.
- With the mouth closed, begin breathing in and press down on the value of the container.
- Hold your breath for a few seconds.
- Repeat for the other nostril if necessary.

☐ It is very important that you use this nasal spray regularly as your doctor has prescribed. It will not relieve your symptoms immediately. It is NOT like ordinary nasal decongestants that you take only when you feel it is necessary.

SPECIAL INSTRUCTIONS

☐ If you forget to take a dose, take it as soon as possible. However, if it is almost time for your next dose, do not take the missed dose. Instead, continue with your regular dosing schedule.

☐ Do not take any more of this medicine than your doctor has prescribed and do not stop taking this medicine suddenly without the approval of your doctor. It may be necessary for your doctor to slowly reduce your dose since your body becomes used to this medicine and it might be harmful if you suddenly did not receive this medicine.

☐ Carry an identification card indicating that you are taking this medicine. Always tell your pharmacist, dentist, and other doctors who are treating you that you are taking this medicine.

☐ Store the container in a cool place. Do not place the container in hot water or near radiators, stoves, or other sources of heat. Do not puncture, burn, or incinerate the container (even after it is empty).

☐ Most people experience few or no side effects from their drugs. However, any medicine can sometimes cause unwanted effects. Call your doctor if you develop soreness in your mouth or throat, a bad taste in your mouth that will not go away, burning or soreness of the nose, or nosebleeds.

*   *   *   *   *

Beclomethasone Dipropionate (*Topical Corticosteroid*)
Canada: Propaderm

Beclomethasone Dipropionate-Clioquinol
Canada: Propaderm C

☐ This medicine is used to help relieve redness, swelling and itching, and in-flammation of certain types of skin conditions.

HOW TO USE THIS MEDICINE

☐ For CREAM, OINTMENT, and LOTION
- Each time you apply the medicine, wash your hands and gently cleanse the skin area well with water unless otherwise directed by your doctor. Do not allow the skin to dry completely. Pat dry with a clean towel until slightly damp.
- Apply a small amount of the drug to the affected area and spread lightly. Only the medicine that is actually touching the skin will work. A thick layer is not more effective than a thin layer. Do not bandage unless directed by your doctor.

☐ Shake the liquid preparation well before using.

☐ The liquid preparation may cause a slight temporary stinging sensation after it is applied.

☐ Keep this medicine away from the hair, nails, and clothing because it could cause staining. (**Canada:** Propaderm C)

☐ Do not use the drug more frequently or in larger quantities than prescribed by your doctor. Overuse of this medicine may cause you to absorb too much of the drug and increase the risk of side effects.

☐ Keep the medicine away from the eyes, nose, and mouth.

SPECIAL INSTRUCTIONS

☐ If you forget to apply the medicine, apply it as soon as possible. However, if it is almost time for your next dose, do not apply the missed dose but continue with your regular schedule.

☐ Do not use this medicine for any other skin problems without checking with your doctor.

☐ Do not apply cosmetics or lotions on top of the drug unless your doctor approves.

☐ Call your doctor if the condition for which this drug is being used persists or becomes worse or if you have a constant irritation such as itching or burning that was not present before you started using this medicine. Also call your doctor if you develop abnormal lines or thinning of the skin especially under the arms or between the legs.

☐ Store in a cool place, but do not freeze.

☐ For external use only. Do not swallow.

☐ Tell future doctors that you have used this medicine.

*   *   *   *   *

Bendroflumethiazide (Oral Antihypertensive-Diuretic)
United States: Naturetin
Canada: Naturetin

☐ This medicine is used to help rid the body of excess water and to decrease swelling. It is also used to treat high blood pressure. It is commonly called a "water pill."

☐ IMPORTANT: If you have ever had an allergic reaction to sulfa drugs or thiazide diuretics, tell your doctor or pharmacist before taking any of this medicine.

HOW TO USE THIS MEDICINE
☐ Take the medicine with food, meals, or milk.

☐ Try to take it at the same time(s) every day so that you have a constant level of the medicine in your body. Do not miss any doses. Otherwise, you cannot expect the drug to work as well.

☐ When you first start taking this medicine, you will probably urinate ("pass your water") more often and in larger amounts than usual. Therefore, if you are to take one dose every day, take it in the morning after breakfast. If you are to take more than one dose every day, take the last dose 6 hours before bedtime so that you will not have to get up during the night to go to the bathroom. This effect will usually lessen after you have taken the drug for awhile.

SPECIAL INSTRUCTIONS
☐ If you forget to take a dose, take it as soon as possible. However, if it is almost time for your next dose, do not take the missed dose. Instead, continue with your regular dosing schedule.

☐ Women who are pregnant, breast-feeding, or planning to become pregnant should tell their doctor before taking this medicine.

☐ This medicine normally causes your body to lose potassium. The body has warning signs to let you know if too much potassium is being lost. Call your doctor if you become unusually thirsty or if you develop leg cramps, unusual weakness, fatigue, vomiting, confusion, or irregular pulse.

☐ If your doctor recommends that you eat foods that are high in potassium, one or more of the foods listed in Appendix A should be eaten daily. All of these foods are rich in potassium. Your goal should be to take in 1000 to 2000 mg. of potassium (approximately 25.6 to 51 mEq) each day. The calorie content and sodium content are included for your convenience in meal planning.
CHANGE YOUR DIET ONLY IF YOUR DOCTOR TELLS YOU TO.

☐ If this medicine causes dizziness, you should be careful going up and down stairs and you should not change positions too rapidly. Get out of bed slowly in the morning and dangle your feet over the edge of the bed for a few minutes before standing up. Sit down or lie down at the first sign of dizziness. Tell your doctor you have been dizzy. Be careful drinking alcoholic beverages while taking this medicine because it could make the dizziness worse. Do not drive a car or operate dangerous machinery or do jobs that require you to be alert if you are dizzy.

☐ In order to help prevent dizziness and fainting, your doctor may also recommend that you avoid strenuous exercises, standing for long periods of time (especially in hot weather), or hot showers or hot baths.

☐ This medicine may make some people more sensitive to sunlight and sunlamps. When you begin taking this medicine, try to avoid too much sun until you see how you are going to react. If your skin does become more sensitive to sunlight, tell your doctor and try to stay out of direct sunlight. While in the sun, wear protective clothing and sunglasses. You may wish to ask your pharmacist about suitable sunscreen products. Check with your doctor if you become sunburned.

☐ Call your doctor immediately if you think you may be allergic to the medicine or if you develop a skin rash, hives, itching, swelling of the face, or difficulty in breathing. If you cannot reach your doctor, phone a hospital emergency department.

☐ Most people experience few or no side effects from their drugs. However, any medicine can sometimes cause unwanted effects. Call your doctor if you develop a sore throat, fever, sharp stomach pain, chest pain, sharp joint pain, easy bruising or bleeding, a yellow color to the skin or eyes, or a sudden weight gain of 5 pounds or more.

* * * * *

Benzalkonium Chloride (*Topical Antiseptic Detergent*)
Canada: Dermo-sterol, Drapolex Cream

☐ This medicine is used to cleanse the skin and help prevent skin infections.

HOW TO USE THIS MEDICINE

☐ Instructions for use:
- Cleanse the skin area well.
- Remove **all** traces of soap by rinsing throughly.
- Apply the preparation and rub in lightly.

SPECIAL INSTRUCTIONS

☐ Consult your doctor if the condition for which this medicine is being used persists or becomes worse, or if the medicine causes an irritation such as itching or burning which was not present before you started using this medicine.

☐ For external use only.

* * * * *

Benzocaine (*Topical Anesthetic*)
United States: Americaine

☐ This medicine is used to help relieve pain and itching of the skin.

☐ IMPORTANT: If you have ever had an allergic reaction to benzocaine or any "caine" type of medicine, tell your doctor or pharmacist before you use any of this drug.

HOW TO USE THIS MEDICINE

☐ For OINTMENT
- Each time you apply the medicine, wash your hands and gently cleanse the skin area well with water unless otherwise directed by your doctor. Do not allow the skin to dry completely. Pat with a clean towel until almost dry.
- Apply a small amount of the drug to the affected area and spread lightly. Only the medicine that is actually touching the skin will work. A thick layer is not more effective than a thin layer. Do not bandage unless directed by your doctor.

☐ For AEROSOL
- Shake the container well each time before using.
- Cleanse the affected area well with water unless otherwise directed by your doctor.
- Hold the container straight up and about 6 to 8 inches away from the skin.
- Spray the affected area for 1 to 3 seconds.
- Shake the container well between sprays.
- Do not spray into the eyes, nose, or mouth and try to avoid inhaling the vapors.

117

- Do not smoke while using this spray or use near an open flame, fire, or heat. Do not use the spray near food.

☐ Do not place the aerosol container in hot water or near radiators, stoves, or other sources of heat. Do not puncture or incinerate the container (even when empty). Do not store at temperatures greater than 120°F (49°C).

☐ Do not use the drug more frequently, in larger quantities, or for a longer period of time than prescribed by your doctor.

SPECIAL INSTRUCTIONS
☐ Call your doctor if the condition for which this drug is being used persists or becomes worse or if you have a constant irritation such as itching or burning that was not present before you started using this medicine. Also call your doctor if you develop a slow heart beat, fainting, or tremors.

* * * * *

Benzonatate (*Oral Antitussive*)
United States: Tessalon
Canada: Tessalon

☐ This medicine is used to help relieve dry irritating coughs.

☐ IMPORTANT: If you have ever had an allergic reaction to a guaifenesin or cough medicine, tell your doctor or pharmacist before you take any of this medicine.

HOW TO USE THIS MEDICINE
☐ Swallow the capsule whole. Do not chew or break them.

SPECIAL INSTRUCTIONS
☐ In some people, this drug may cause drowsiness. Do not drive a car or operate dangerous machinery or do jobs that require you to be alert until you know how you are going to react to this drug.

☐ Call your doctor if the cough lasts longer than 1 week or if you develop a fever, skin rash, or persistent headache.

☐ Do not use this medicine for more than 1 week without the advice of your doctor.

* * * * *

Benzoyl Peroxide (*Topical Acne Therapy*)

United States: Benoxyl, Benzac, Benzagel, Desquam-X, Dry & Clear, Epi-Clear, Oxy, Panoxyl, Persadox, Persa-gel, Xerac BP

Canada: Acetoxyl, Benoxyl, Benzagel, Dermoxyl, Desquam-X, Oxy-derm, Panoxyl, Persa-Gel

Benzoyl Peroxide-Chlorhydroxyquinoline

United States: Loroxide, Vanoxide

Canada: Loroxide, Vanoxide

☐ This medicine is used in the treatment of acne.

HOW TO USE THIS MEDICINE
☐ For BENOXYL LOTION

- Cleanse the skin well with water unless otherwise specified by your physician.
- Apply medicine and spread lightly.
- Apply once daily for the first 4 days.
- Leave on for 2 hours and then remove with warm water.
- Apply once daily for the next 4 days, but leave on for 4 hours and then remove with warm water.
- Leave on overnight for the next 7 days.
- Finally apply after each washing.

☐ For LOTION, CREAM, and GEL

- Cleanse the affected areas well with water.
- Apply a thin film of medicine and blend well into the skin.
- Allow the medicine to dry.

GENERAL INSTRUCTIONS FOR ACNE PATIENTS
☐ Avoid greasy hair oils and creams.

☐ Try to keep your hands away from your hair and face.

☐ Shampoo your hair frequently—at least once or twice a week. Keep your hair brushed back off the face.

☐ Remember to keep your brush and comb clean with regular washing.

☐ Get plenty of exercise, fresh air, and sleep and eat a balanced diet.

☐ Do not squeeze or pick the blemishes.

SPECIAL INSTRUCTIONS
☐ Do not use the drug more frequently or in larger quantities than prescribed by your doctor.

- ☐ Call your doctor if the condition for which this drug is being used persists or becomes worse or if you develop a constant irritation such as itching or burning that was not present before you started using this medicine.

- ☐ IMPORTANT: If you have ever had an allergic reaction to an acne or skin medicine, tell your doctor or pharmacist before you use any of this drug.

- ☐ Avoid contact of the medicine with fabrics and clothing as it may cause bleaching.

- ☐ During the first few days, slight redness of the skin will occur. This is a desirable effect.

- ☐ During the first month of using this medicine, peeling of the skin may occur. This is not unusual. Stop using the medicine for 1 to 2 days and it should disappear. If it does not disappear, contact your doctor.

- ☐ Discontinue use of the medicine temporarily if *excessive* dryness or irritation of the skin should occur.

- ☐ Keep away from the eyes, nose, lips, or neck.

- ☐ For external use only.

* * * * *

Benzphetamine HCl (*Oral Anorexiant*)
United States: Didrex

- ☐ This medicine is used to help reduce the appetite in weight reduction programs. It can help you develop new eating habits and is only useful for a short time. Do not take any more of this medicine than your doctor has prescribed and do not stop taking this medicine suddenly without the approval of your doctor.

- ☐ IMPORTANT: If you have ever had an allergic reaction to an amphetamine medicine or any other medicine, tell your doctor or pharmacist before you take any of this medicine.

HOW TO USE THIS MEDICINE
- ☐ This medicine may be taken with a glass of water.

- ☐ Do not take the medicine late in the day or it may cause insomnia (difficulty in sleeping).

SPECIAL INSTRUCTIONS
- ☐ If you forget to take a dose, take it as soon as possible. However, if it is almost time for your next dose, do not take the missed dose. Instead, continue with your regular dosing schedule.

- ☐ Women who are pregnant, breast-feeding, or planning to become pregnant should tell their doctor before taking this medicine.

- [ ] It is very important that you follow the diet prescribed by your doctor.

- [ ] If your mouth becomes dry, suck a hard sour candy (sugarless) or ice chips, or chew gum. It is especially important to brush your teeth regularly if you develop a dry mouth.

- [ ] In some people, this drug may cause dizziness. Do not drive a car or operate dangerous machinery or do jobs that require you to be alert until you know how you are going to react to this drug. Therefore, you should be careful going up and down stairs. Sit or lie down at the first sign of dizziness.

- [ ] Do not treat yourself with baking soda or antacids without the approval of your doctor.

- [ ] Most people experience few or no side effects from their drugs. However, any medicine can sometimes cause unwanted effects. Call your doctor if you develop a skin rash, chest pain or palpitations, unusual movements of the head, arms or legs, or unusual restlessness.

- [ ] Carry an identification card indicating that you are taking this medicine. Always tell your pharmacist, dentist, and other doctors who are treating you that you are taking this medicine.

*   *   *   *   *

Benzthiazide (Oral Antihypertensive-Diuretic)

United States: Aquastat, Aquatag, ExNa, Hydrex, Marazide, Proaqua, Rola-Benz, S-Aqua, Urazide

Canada: ExNa

- [ ] This medicine is used to help rid the body of excess water and to decrease swelling. It is also used to treat high blood pressure. It is commonly called a "water pill."

- [ ] IMPORTANT: If you have ever had an allergic reaction to sulfa drugs or thiazide diuretics, tell your doctor or pharmacist before taking any of this medicine.

HOW TO USE THIS MEDICINE

- [ ] Take the medicine with food, meals, or milk.

- [ ] Try to take it at the same time(s) every day so that you have a constant level of the medicine in your body. Do not miss any doses. Otherwise, you cannot expect the drug to work as well.

- [ ] When you first start taking this medicine, you will probably urinate ("pass your water") more often and in larger amounts than usual. Therefore, if you are to take one dose every day, take it in the morning after breakfast. If you are to take more than one dose every day, take the last dose 6 hours before bedtime so that you will not have to get up during the night to go to the bathroom. This effect will usually lessen after you have taken the drug for awhile.

SPECIAL INSTRUCTIONS

☐ If you forget to take a dose, take it as soon as possible. However, if it is almost time for your next dose, do not take the missed dose. Instead, continue with your regular dosing schedule.

☐ Women who are pregnant, breast-feeding, or planning to become pregnant should tell their doctor before taking this medicine.

☐ This medicine normally causes your body to lose potassium. The body has warning signs to let you know if too much potassium is being lost. Call your doctor if you become unusually thirsty or if you develop leg cramps, unusual weakness, fatigue, vomiting, confusion, or irregular pulse.

☐ If your doctor recommends that you eat foods that are high in potassium, one or more of the foods listed in Appendix A should be eaten daily. All of these foods are rich in potassium. Your goal should be to take in 1000 to 2000 mg. of potassium (approximately 25.6 to 51 mEq) each day. The calorie content and sodium content are included for your convenience in meal planning.
CHANGE YOUR DIET ONLY IF YOUR DOCTOR TELLS YOU TO.

☐ If this medicine causes dizziness, you should be careful going up and down stairs and you should not change positions too rapidly. Get out of bed slowly in the morning and dangle your feet over the edge of the bed for a few minutes before standing up. Sit down or lie down at the first sign of dizziness. Tell your doctor you have been dizzy. Be careful drinking alcoholic beverages while taking this medicine because it could make the dizziness worse. Do not drive a car or operate dangerous machinery or do jobs that require you to be alert if you are dizzy.

☐ In order to help prevent dizziness and fainting, your doctor may also recommend that you avoid strenuous exercises, standing for long periods of time (especially in hot weather), or hot showers or hot baths.

☐ This medicine may make some people more sensitive to sunlight and sunlamps. When you begin taking this medicine, try to avoid too much sun until you see how you are going to react. If your skin does become more sensitive to sunlight, tell your doctor and try to stay out of direct sunlight. While in the sun, wear protective clothing and sunglasses. You may wish to ask your pharmacist about suitable sunscreen products. Check with your doctor if you become sunburned.

☐ Call your doctor immediately if you think you may be allergic to the medicine or if you develop a skin rash, hives, itching, swelling of the face, or difficulty in breathing. If you cannot reach your doctor, phone a hospital emergency department.

☐ Most people experience few or no side effects from their drugs. However, any medicine can sometimes cause unwanted effects. Call your doctor if you develop a sore throat, fever, sharp stomach pain, chest pain, sharp joint pain, easy bruising or bleeding, a yellow color to the skin or eyes, or a sudden weight gain of 5 pounds or more.

* * * * *

Benztropine Mesylate (*Oral Antiparkinsonian Agent*)
United States: Cogentin
Canada: Bensylate, Cogentin

☐ This medicine is used to improve muscle control and relieve muscle spasm in Parkinson's disease and certain other medical conditions.

HOW TO USE THIS MEDICINE
☐ Take this medicine with food or immediately after meals to help prevent stomach upset unless otherwise directed.

☐ If you forget to take a dose, take it as soon as possible. However, if your next dose is within 8 hours, do not take the missed dose but continue with your regular schedule.

SPECIAL INSTRUCTIONS
☐ If your mouth becomes dry, suck a hard sour candy (sugarless) or ice chips, or chew gum. It is especially important to brush your teeth regularly if you develop a dry mouth.

☐ In some people, this drug may cause dizziness, drowsiness, or blurred vision during the first 2 weeks of use. This will usually go away as your body adjusts to this medicine. Do not drive a car or operate dangerous machinery or do jobs that require you to be alert until you know how you are going to react to this drug.

☐ If you become dizzy, you should be careful going up and down stairs. Sit or lie down at the first sign of dizziness.

☐ If your eyes become more sensitive to sunlight, it may help to wear sunglasses.

☐ Do not take antacids or diarrhea medicines within 1 hour of taking this medicine as it could make this medicine less effective.

☐ A desire to urinate ("pass your water") with an inability to do so is not an uncommon effect with this drug. Urinating each time before the drug is taken may help relieve this problem. Call your doctor if it continues.

☐ Do not drink alcoholic beverages while taking this drug without the approval of your doctor.

- [ ] It is important that you obtain the advice of your doctor or pharmacist before taking pain relievers, nonprescription drugs, sleeping pills, tranquilizers, or medicine for depression while you are taking this drug.

- [ ] You may become more sensitive to heat because your body may perspire less while you are taking this medicine. Be careful not to become overheated during exercise or in hot weather.

- [ ] Most people experience few or no side effects from their drugs. However, any medicine can sometimes cause unwanted effects. Call your doctor if you develop a skin rash, eye pain, dizziness or fainting, fast heart beats, or constipation.

*　*　*　*　*

Benzyl Benzoate-Benzocaine (*Topical Scabicide*)
Canada: Scabanca, Scabide

- [ ] This medicine is used to treat scabies.

HOW TO USE THIS MEDICINE
- [ ] Instructions for use: (***Canada:*** Scabide Lotion, Scabanca Lotion)
    - Take a hot bath and scrub the body thoroughly with soap and water for 10 minutes.
    - Shake the bottle well before using in order to get an accurate dose.
    - While the body is still wet, brush the lotion from the neck downward on the entire body (except the head and scalp) with a stiff bristle brush for 5 minutes.
    - Allow to dry.
    - Reapply more lotion for a further 5 minutes.
    - Gently dry body with a towel.
    - Put on clean clothing and change bed linen.
    - Take a bath 24 hours later and clean body well with soap and water.

- [ ] Instructions for use: (***Canada:*** Scabanca Creme)
    - Take a hot bath, or sponge bath, and scrub the affected parts well with soap and water.
    - Gently dry body with a towel.
    - Apply the creme over the entire body except for the face and scalp.
    - Allow body to dry.
    - Apply the creme a second time and allow to dry.
    - Put on clean clothing and change the bed linen.
    - In 24 hours take another bath and cleanse body well.

SPECIAL INSTRUCTIONS
- [ ] IMPORTANT: If you have ever had an allergic reaction to benzocaine or any "caine" types of medicine, tell your doctor or pharmacist before you use any of this drug.

124

- [ ] Put on freshly laundered clean clothing after each application of the medicine. Use fresh towels and fresh bed sheets after each application. Launder or dry-clean contaminated clothing.

- [ ] Keep this medicine away from the eyes, mouth, or open wounds. If some does get in the eyes, flush it away with water immediately.

- [ ] Call your doctor if the condition for which this drug is being used persists or becomes worse or if you have a constant irritation such as itching or burning that was not present before you started using this medicine.

- [ ] Do not use this drug more frequently or for a longer period of time than prescribed by your doctor.

- [ ] For external use only. Do not swallow.

* * * * *

Betamethasone Disodium Phosphate (*Eye/Ear Corticosteroid*)
Canada: Betnesol

- [ ] This medicine is used to help relieve the pain, redness, and swelling of certain types of eye and ear conditions.

HOW TO USE THIS MEDICINE

- [ ] Do not use this drug more frequently or in larger quantities than prescribed by your doctor.

- [ ] For EAR DROPS

INSTILLATION OF EAR DROPS

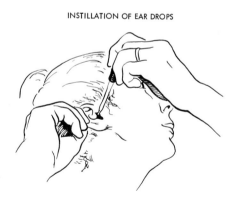

- Warm the ear drops to body temperature by holding the bottle in your hands for a few minutes. Do NOT heat the drops in hot water.
- The person administering the ear drops should wash his hands with soap and water.
- The ear drops must be kept clean. Do not touch the dropper against the ear or anything else.

125

- Tilt your head or lie on your side so that the ear to be treated is facing up.
- In ADULTS, hold the ear lobe up and back.
  In CHILDREN, hold the ear lobe down and back.
- Place the prescribed number of drops into the ear. Do not insert the dropper into the ear as it may cause injury.
- Remain in the same position for a short time (2 minutes) after you have administered the drops.
- Dry the ear lobe if there are any drops on it.
- If necessary, have someone else administer the ear drops for you.
- Do not use the ear drops if they change in color or change in any way since being purchased.
- Keep the bottle tightly closed when not in use.

☐ For EYE OINTMENT

INSTILLATION OF EYE OINTMENT

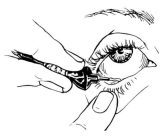

- The person administering the eye ointment should wash his hands with soap and water.
- The eye ointment must be kept clean. Do not touch the tube against the face or anything else.
- Lie down or tilt your head backward and look at the ceiling.
- Gently pull down the lower lid of your eye to form a pouch.
- Hold the tube in your other hand and place the tube as close as possible to the eye without touching it.
- Squeeze the prescribed amount of ointment (usually $\frac{1}{2}$ inch in adults) from the tube along the pouch.
- Close your eyes. Do not rub them.
- Wipe off any excess ointment around the eye with a tissue.
- Clean the tip of the ointment tube with a tissue.
- If necessary, have someone else administer the eye ointment for you.
- Keep the eye ointment tube tightly closed when not in use.

☐ For EYE DROPS

INSTILLATION OF EYE DROPS

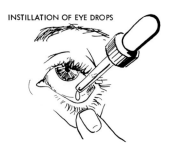

- The person administering the *eye* drops should wash his hands with soap and water.
- The *eye* drops must be kept clean. Do not touch the dropper against the face or anything else.
- Lie down or tilt your head backward and look at the ceiling.
- Gently pull down the lower lid of your *eye* to form a pouch.
- Hold the dropper in your other hand and approach the *eye* from the side. Place the dropper as close to the *eye* as possible without touching it.
- Place the prescribed number of drops into the pouch of the *eye*.
- Close your eyes. Do not rub them.
- Apply gentle pressure for a minute with your fingers to the bridge of the nose (inside corner of the *eye*) to prevent the *eye* drops from being drained from the *eye*.
  - Blot excess solution around the *eye* with a tissue.
- If necessary, have someone else administer the *eye* drops for you.
- Do not use the *eye* drops if they change in color or change in any way since being purchased.
- Keep the *eye* drop bottle tightly closed when not in use.

SPECIAL INSTRUCTIONS

☐ This medicine should be used as long as prescribed by your doctor. Do not stop using it earlier than your doctor has recommended in spite of the fact that your symptoms seem to have improved.

☐ If you forget to use the medicine, use it as soon as possible. However, if it is almost time for your next dose, do not use the missed dose, but continue with your regular schedule.

☐ Vision may be blurred for a few minutes after using the *eye* medicine. Do not drive a car or operate dangerous machinery or do jobs that require you to be alert until your vision has cleared.

☐ Do not use this medicine at the same time as any other *eye* or *ear* medicine without the approval of your doctor. Some medicines cannot be mixed.

☐ Call your doctor if the condition for which you are using this medicine persists or becomes worse or if the medicine causes itching or burning for more than a few minutes after instillation.

☐ Do not use the drug more frequently or in larger quantities than prescribed by your doctor.

☐ For external use only. Do not swallow.

* * * * *

Betamethasone (*Oral Corticosteroid*)
United States: Celestone
Canada: Betnelan, Betnesol, Celestone

☐ This medicine is similar to cortisone, which is a hormone normally produced by the body. This medicine is used to help decrease inflammation, which then relieves pain, redness, and swelling. It is used to treat certain kinds of arthritis and severe allergies or skin conditions.

HOW TO USE THIS MEDICINE

☐ Take this medicine with food or a glass of milk in order to help prevent stomach upset. Call your doctor if you develop stomach upset or stomach pain or heartburn (especially if it awakens you during the night). Do not try to treat yourself.

☐ If your doctor has prescribed only ONE dose of this medicine every day, it is best to take it before 9 A.M. or with breakfast.

☐ If you forget to take a dose, take it as soon as possible. However, if it is almost time for your next dose, do not take the missed dose. Instead, continue with your regular dosing schedule.

☐ Dissolve these tablets in a glass of water just before taking this medicine. (**Canada:** Betnesol Tablets)

☐ Place the pellet on the mouth sore and allow it to dissolve. (**Canada:** Betnesol Pellets)

☐ This medicine must be swallowed whole. Do not crush, chew, or break it into pieces. (**Canada:** Celestone Repetabs)

SPECIAL INSTRUCTIONS

☐ Women who are pregnant, breast-feeding, or planning to become pregnant should tell their doctor before taking this medicine.

☐ It is best not to drink alcoholic beverages while you are taking this medicine because the combination can cause stomach problems.

☐ Do not take any more of this medicine than your doctor has prescribed and do not stop taking this medicine suddenly without the approval of your doctor. It may be necessary for your doctor to slowly reduce your dose since your body becomes used to this medicine and it might be harmful if you suddenly did not receive this medicine.

☐ Do not take aspirin or medicines containing aspirin without the approval of your doctor.

☐ While you are taking this medicine you may gain some weight. This could be due to an increase in your appetite or increased water in your system. Your doctor may prescribe a special diet to decrease the number of calories you eat and/or to lower the amount of sodium or increase the amount of potassium in your diet. Follow any diet that your doctor may order.

☐ You may find that you bruise more easily. Try to protect yourself from all injuries to prevent bruising.

☐ Diabetic patients should regularly check the sugar in their urine and report any unusual levels to their doctor.

☐ Carry an identification card indicating that you are taking this medicine. Always tell your pharmacist, dentist, and other doctors who are treating you that you are taking this medicine. If you have an acute infection, an injury, an operation, or dental surgery within 1 year of taking this medicine, it is important to tell your doctor.

☐ Most people experience few or no side effects from their drugs. However, any medicine can sometimes cause unwanted effects. Call your doctor if you develop stomach pain, sore throat, fever, swelling of the legs or ankles, a wound which does not heal, eye pain or blurred vision, frequent urination ("passing your water"), nightmares or depression, muscle cramps, red or black stools, puffing of the face, or menstrual problems.

* * * * *

Betamethasone Benzoate (*Topical Corticosteroid*)
United States: Benisone, Flurobate, Uticort
Canada: Beben

☐ This medicine is used to help relieve redness, swelling, and itching and inflammation of certain types of skin conditions.

HOW TO USE THIS MEDICINE
☐ For CREAM, LOTION, and GEL
  • Each time you apply the medicine, wash your hands and gently cleanse the skin area well with water unless otherwise directed by your doctor. Do not allow the skin to dry completely. Pat with a clean towel until slightly damp.
  • Apply a small amount of the drug to the affected area and spread lightly. Only the medicine that is actually touching the skin will work. A thick layer is not more effective than a thin layer. Do not bandage unless directed by your doctor.

☐ Shake the liquid preparation well before using. (*United States:* Uticort Lotion)

☐ Do not use the drug more frequently or in larger quantities than prescribed by your doctor. Overuse of this medicine may cause you to absorb too much of the drug and increase the risk of side effects.

☐ Keep the medicine away from the eyes, nose, and mouth.

SPECIAL INSTRUCTIONS
☐ If you forget to apply the medicine, apply it as soon as possible. However, if it is almost time for your next dose, do not apply the missed dose, but continue with your regular schedule.

☐ Do not use this medicine for any other skin problems without checking with your doctor.

129

□ Do not apply cosmetics or lotions on top of the drug unless your doctor approves.

□ Call your doctor if the condition for which this drug is being used persists or becomes worse or if you have a constant irritation such as itching or burning that was not present before you started using this medicine. Also call your doctor if you develop abnormal lines or thinning of the skin especially under the arms or between the legs.

□ Store in a cool place but do not freeze.

□ For external use only. Do not swallow.

□ Tell future physicians that you have used this medicine.

* * * * *

Betamethasone Dipropionate (*Topical Corticosteroid*)
United States: Diprosone
Canada: Diprosone

□ This medicine is used to help relieve redness, swelling, itching, and inflammation of certain types of skin conditions.

HOW TO USE THIS MEDICINE
□ For CREAM, OINTMENT, and LOTION
  • Each time you apply the medicine, wash your hands and gently cleanse the skin area well with water unless otherwise directed by your doctor. Do not allow the skin to dry completely. Pat with a clean towel until almost dry.
  • Apply a small amount of the drug to the affected area and spread lightly. Only the medicine that is actually touching the skin will work. A thick layer is not more effective than a thin layer. Do not bandage unless directed by your doctor.

□ For AEROSOL
  • Shake the container well each time before using.
  • Cleanse the affected area well with water unless otherwise directed by your doctor.
  • Hold the container straight up and about 6 to 8 inches away from the skin.
  • Spray the affected area for 1 to 3 seconds.
  • Shake the container well between sprays.
  • Do not spray into the eyes, nose, or mouth, and try to avoid inhaling the vapors.
  • Do not smoke while using this spray or use near an open flame, fire, or heat. Do not use the spray near food.

- ☐ Shake the liquid preparation well before using. (**United States** and **Canada:** Diprosone Lotion)

- ☐ The liquid preparation may cause a slight temporary stinging sensation after it is applied.

- ☐ Do not use the drug more frequently or in larger quantities than prescribed by your doctor. Overuse of this medicine may cause you to absorb too much of the drug and increase the risk of side effects.

- ☐ Keep the medicine away from the eyes, nose, and mouth.

SPECIAL INSTRUCTIONS

- ☐ If you forget to apply the medicine, apply it as soon as possible. However, if it is almost time for your next dose, do not apply the missed dose, but continue with your regular schedule.

- ☐ Do not use this medicine for any other skin problems without checking with your doctor.

- ☐ Do not apply cosmetics or lotions on top of the drug unless your doctor approves.

- ☐ Call your doctor if the condition for which this drug is being used persists or becomes worse or if you have a constant irritation such as itching or burning that was not present before you started using this medicine. Also call your doctor if you develop abnormal lines or thinning of the skin, especially under the arms or between the legs.

- ☐ Store in a cool place but do not freeze.

- ☐ For external use only. Do not swallow.

- ☐ Do not place the aerosol container in hot water or near radiators, stoves, or other sources of heat. Do not puncture or incinerate the container (even when empty). Do not store at temperatures greater than 120°F (49°C).

- ☐ Tell future physicians that you have used this medicine.

*   *   *   *   *

Betamethasone Valerate (*Topical Corticosteroid*)
United States: Valisone
Canada: Betacort, Betnovate, Celestoderm-V, Celestoderm-V/2, Valisone Scalp Lotion

- ☐ This medicine is used to help relieve redness, swelling, itching, and inflammation of certain types of skin conditions.

HOW TO USE THIS MEDICINE

☐ For CREAM, OINTMENT, and LOTION

- Each time you apply the medicine, wash your hands and gently cleanse the skin area well with water unless otherwise directed by your doctor.
- Do not allow the skin to dry completely. Pat with a clean towel until almost dry.
- Apply a small amount of the drug to the affected area and spread lightly. Only the medicine that is actually touching the skin will work. A thick layer is not more effective than a thin layer. Do not bandage unless directed by your doctor.

☐ For AEROSOL

- Shake the container well each time before using.
- Cleanse the affected area well with water unless otherwise directed by your doctor.
- Hold the container straight up and about 6 to 8 inches away from the skin.
- Spray the affected area for 1 to 3 seconds.
- Shake the container well between sprays.
- Do not spray into the eyes, nose, or mouth and try to avoid inhaling the vapors.
- Do not smoke while using this spray or use near an open flame, fire, or heat. Do not use the spray near food.

☐ Shake the liquid preparation well before using. (**United States:** Valisone Lotion; **Canada:** Betnovate Lotion, Valisone Scalp Lotion)

☐ The liquid preparation may cause a slight temporary stinging sensation after it is applied.

☐ Do not use the drug more frequently or in larger quantities than prescribed by your doctor. Overuse of this medicine may cause you to absorb too much of the drug and increase the risk of side effects.

☐ Keep the medicine away from the eyes, nose, and mouth.

SPECIAL INSTRUCTIONS

☐ If you forget to apply the medicine, apply it as soon as possible. However, if it is almost time for your next dose, do not apply the missed dose but continue with your regular schedule.

☐ Do not use this medicine for any other skin problems without checking with your doctor.

☐ Do not apply cosmetics or lotions on top of the drug unless your doctor approves.

☐ Call your doctor if the condition for which this drug is being used persists or becomes worse or if you have a constant irritation such as itching or burning that was not present before you started using this medicine. Also call your doctor if you develop abnormal lines or thinning of the skin especially under the arms or between the legs.

☐ Store in a cool place but do not freeze.

☐ For external use only. Do not swallow.

☐ Do not place the aerosol container in hot water or near radiators, stoves, or other sources of heat. Do not puncture or incinerate the container (even when empty). Do not store at temperatures greater than 120°F (49°C).

☐ Tell future physicians that you have used this medicine.

*   *   *   *   *

Bethanechol (*Oral Parasympathomimetic Agent*)
United States: Myotonachol, Urecholine
Canada: Duvoid, Urecholine

☐ This medicine is used to help relax muscles in the bladder and intestines.

HOW TO USE THIS MEDICINE
☐ Take this medicine on an empty stomach to help prevent stomach upset.

SPECIAL INSTRUCTIONS
☐ If you forget to take a dose, take it as soon as possible. However, if it is almost time for your next dose, do not take the missed dose. Instead, continue with your regular dosing schedule.

☐ In some people, this drug may cause "double vision." Do not drive a car or operate dangerous machinery or do jobs that require you to be alert until you know how you are going to react to this drug.

☐ It is important that you obtain the advice of your doctor or pharmacist before taking pain relievers, nonprescription drugs, sleeping pills, or tranquilizers or medicines for depression while you are taking this drug.

☐ It is a good idea to keep a diary of "peaks and valleys" of your muscle strength. This will help your doctor in designing your treatment.

☐ Most people experience few or no side effects from their drugs. However, any medicine can sometimes cause unwanted effects. Call your doctor if you develop slow or fast heartbeats, changes in vision, muscle cramps, nausea, vomiting or diarrhea, difficulty in breathing, fainting spells or dizziness, convulsions, or unusual sweating, or if you urinate ("pass your water") more frequently than usual.

*   *   *   *   *

Bili-Labstix (*Diagnostic Acid*)
United States: Bili-Labstix
Canada: Bili-Labstix

☐ This preparation is used to test for various chemicals in the urine.

☐ Directions for use:
  - Dip test end of strip into the urine.
  - Tap strip against the edge of container to remove excess urine.
  - Compare color changes with the color chart at the correct times.

☐ For further information, refer to the package insert that accompanies this preparation.*

*   *   *   *   *

Biperiden HCl (*Oral Anticholinergic*)
United States: Akineton
Canada: Akineton

☐ This medicine is used to improve muscle control and relieve muscle spasm in Parkinson's disease and certain other medical conditions.

HOW TO USE THIS MEDICINE

☐ Take this medicine with food or immediately after meals to help prevent stomach upset unless otherwise directed.

☐ If you forget to take a dose, take it as soon as possible. However, if your next dose is within 2 hours, do not take the missed dose but continue with your regular schedule.

SPECIAL INSTRUCTIONS

☐ If your mouth becomes dry, suck a hard sour candy (sugarless) or ice chips, or chew gum. It is especially important to brush your teeth regularly if you develop a dry mouth.

☐ In some people, this drug may cause dizziness, drowsiness, or blurred vision during the first 2 weeks of using this drug. This will usually go away as your body adjusts to this medicine. Do not drive a car or operate dangerous machinery or do jobs that require you to be alert until you know how you are going to react to this drug.

☐ If you become dizzy, you should be careful going up and down stairs. Sit or lie down at the first sign of dizziness.

---

*Bili-Labstix (Package Insert), Ames Company Division, Miles Laboratories, Ltd., Rexdale, Ontario.

- [ ] If your eyes become more sensitive to sunlight, it may help to wear sunglasses.

- [ ] Do not take antacids or diarrhea medicines within 1 hour of taking this medicine as it could make this medicine less effective.

- [ ] A desire to urinate ("pass your water") with an inability to do so is not an uncommon effect with this drug. Urinating each time before the drug is taken may help relieve this problem. Call your doctor if it continues.

- [ ] Do not drink alcoholic beverages while taking this drug without the approval of your doctor.

- [ ] It is important that you obtain the advice of your doctor or pharmacist before taking pain relievers, nonprescription drugs, sleeping pills, tranquilizers, or medicine for depression while you are taking this drug.

- [ ] You may become more sensitive to heat because your body may perspire less while you are taking this medicine. Be careful not to become overheated during exercise or in hot weather.

- [ ] Most people experience few or no side effects from their drugs. However, any medicine can sometimes cause unwanted effects. Call your doctor if you develop a skin rash, eye pain, dizziness or fainting, fast heartbeats, or constipation, or if you become confused.

* * * * *

Bisacodyl (*Oral Laxative*)
United States: Bisco-Lax, Dulcolax, Fleet Bisacodyl, SK-Bisacodyl, Theralax
Canada: Bisacolax, Dulcolax, Laco

Bisacodyl-Dioctyl Sodium Sulfosuccinate (*Oral Laxative*)
Canada: Dulcodos

- [ ] This medicine is a laxative used to treat constipation or to empty the bowels before certain types of hospital procedures.

HOW TO USE THIS MEDICINE
- [ ] Take the medicine in the evening or before breakfast with a full glass of water.

- [ ] This medicine has a special coating and must be swallowed whole. Do not crush, chew, or break it into pieces. Do not take milk or antacids within 1 hour of taking this medicine.

☐ Do not take mineral oil while you are taking this medicine. (**Canada:** Dulcodos)

SPECIAL INSTRUCTIONS

☐ Do not take this medicine more often or longer than your doctor has prescribed as your bowels may become dependent upon it. If you feel you require this medicine every day and cannot have a bowel movement without it, call your doctor.

☐ Unless otherwise directed, you should also try increasing the amount of bulk foods in your diet (for example, bran, fresh fruits, and salads), exercising more often, and drinking 6 to 8 glasses of water every day.

☐ Do not take this medicine if you have any stomach pain, nausea, or vomiting.

☐ Call your doctor if your constipation is not relieved or if you develop rectal bleeding, muscle cramps, unusual weakness, or dizziness.

*   *   *   *   *

Bisacodyl (*Rectal Laxative*)

United States: Bisco-Lax, Dulcolax, Fleet Bisacodyl, Theralax
Canada: Bisacolax, Dulcolax, Erilax, Laco

☐ This medicine is a laxative used in the treatment of constipation or to empty the bowels before certain types of hospital procedures.

HOW TO USE THIS MEDICINE

☐ Administration of suppositories:
  • Remove the wrapper from the suppository.
  • Lie on your side and raise your knee to your chest.
  • Insert the suppository with the tapered end (pointed) first into the rectum.
  • Remain lying down for a few minutes so that the suppository will dissolve in the rectum.
  • Try to avoid having a bowel movement for at least 1 hour so that the drug will have time to work.

☐ Store the suppositories in a cool place.

SPECIAL INSTRUCTIONS

☐ Do not use this medicine more often or longer than your doctor has prescribed as your bowels may become dependent upon it. If you feel you require this medicine every day and cannot have a bowel movement without it, call your doctor.

☐ Unless otherwise directed, you should also try increasing the amount of bulk foods in your diet (for example, bran, fresh fruits, and salads), exercising more often, and drinking 6 to 8 glasses of water every day.

☐ Do not use this medicine if you have any stomach pain, nausea, or vomiting.

☐ Call your doctor if your constipation is not relieved or if you develop rectal bleeding, muscle cramps, unusual weakness, or dizziness.

* * * * *

Bromocriptine Mesylate (Oral Prolactin Inhibitor)
United States: Parlodel
Canada: Parlodel

☐ This medicine is used to help prevent lactation (milk production).

☐ IMPORTANT: If you have ever had an allergic reaction to an ergot medicine, tell your doctor or pharmacist before you take any of this medicine.

HOW TO USE THIS MEDICINE
☐ Take the medicine with food or at mealtime.

☐ If you forget to take a dose, take it as soon as possible. However, if it is almost time for your next dose, do not take the missed dose. Instead, continue with your regular dosing schedule.

SPECIAL INSTRUCTIONS
☐ If you are pregnant or plan to become pregnant, tell your doctor before taking this medicine.

☐ In some people, this drug may cause dizziness or drowsiness. Do not drive a car or operate dangerous machinery or do jobs that require you to be alert until you know how you are going to react to this drug.

☐ If this medicine causes dizziness, you should be careful going up and down stairs and you should not change positions too rapidly. Get out of bed slowly in the morning and dangle your feet over the edge of the bed for a few minutes before standing up. Sit down or lie down at the first sign of dizziness. Tell your doctor you have been dizzy. Avoid hot showers and baths because they could make you dizzy.

☐ Most people experience few or no side effects from their drugs. However, any medicine can sometimes cause unwanted effects. Call your doctor if you develop severe nausea, vomiting, headaches, severe stomach pain, fainting spells, confusion, or hallucinations.

* * * * *

Bromodiphenhydramine HCl *(Oral Antihistamine)*
United States: Ambodryl

☐ This medicine is used to help relieve the symptoms of certain types of allergic conditions, coughs and colds, and certain skin conditions.

HOW TO USE THIS MEDICINE
☐ This medicine may be taken with food or a glass of milk if it upsets your stomach.

SPECIAL INSTRUCTIONS
☐ If you forget to take a dose, take it as soon as possible. However, if it is almost time for your next dose, do not take the missed dose. Instead, continue with your regular dosing schedule.

☐ In some people, this drug may initially cause dizziness or drowsiness. Do not drive a car or operate dangerous machinery or do jobs that require you to be alert until you know how you are going to react to this drug. If you become dizzy, you should be careful going up and down stairs. Sit or lie down at the first sign of dizziness. Tell your doctor if it continues.

☐ Do not drink alcoholic beverages while taking this drug without the approval of your doctor.

☐ If your mouth becomes dry, suck a hard sour candy (sugarless) or ice chips, or chew gum. It is especially important to brush your teeth regularly if you develop a dry mouth.

☐ It is important that you obtain the advice of your doctor or pharmacist before taking pain relievers, nonprescription drugs, sleeping pills or tranquilizers, or other medicines for allergies.

☐ Do not take this medicine more often or longer than recommended by your doctor.

☐ Most people experience few or no side effects from their drugs. However, any medicine can sometimes cause unwanted effects. Call your doctor if you develop a skin rash, fast heartbeats, blurred vision, stomach pain, or difficulty in urinating ("passing your water").

* * * * *

Brompheniramine Maleate *(Oral Antihistamine)*
United States: Dimetane, Veltane
Canada: Dimetane

Brompheniramine Maleate-Guaifenesin-Phenylephrine-Phenylpropanolamine

United States: Dimetane Expectorant

Canada: Dimetane Expectorant

Brompheniramine Maleate-Guaifenesin-Phenylephrine-Phenylpropanolamine-Hydrocodone

Canada: Dimetane Expectorant-DC

Brompheniramine Maleate-Guaifenesin-Phenylephrine-Phenylpropanolamine-Codeine

United States: Dimetane Expectorant-DC

Brompheniramine Maleate-Phenylephrine-Phenylpropanolamine

United States: Dimetapp

Canada: Dimetapp

Brompheniramine Maleate-Phenylephrine-Dextromethorphan-Phenylpropanolamine

Canada: Dimetapp-DM

Brompheniramine Maleate-Phenylephrine-Phenylpropanolamine-Codeine Phosphate

Canada: Dimetapp with Codeine

□ This medicine is used to help relieve the symptoms of certain types of allergic conditions, coughs and colds, and certain skin conditions.

HOW TO USE THIS MEDICINE

☐ This medicine may be taken with food or a glass of milk if it upsets your stomach.

☐ These tablets must be swallowed whole. Do not crush, chew, or break them into pieces. (**United States** and **Canada:** Dimetane Extentabs, Dimetapp Extentabs)

SPECIAL INSTRUCTIONS

☐ If you forget to take a dose, take it as soon as possible. However, if it is almost time for your next dose, do not take the missed dose. Instead, continue with your regular dosing schedule.

☐ In some people, this drug may initially cause dizziness or drowsiness. Do not drive a car or operate dangerous machinery or do jobs that require you to be alert until you know how you are going to react to this drug. If you become dizzy, you should be careful going up and down stairs. Sit or lie down at the first sign of dizziness. Tell your doctor if it continues.

☐ Do not drink alcoholic beverages while taking this drug without the approval of your doctor.

☐ If your mouth becomes dry, suck a hard sour candy (sugarless) or ice chips, or chew gum. It is especially important to brush your teeth regularly if you develop a dry mouth.

☐ It is important that you obtain the advice of your doctor or pharmacist before taking pain relievers, nonprescription drugs, sleeping pills or tranquilizers, or other medicines for allergies.

☐ Do not take this medicine more often or longer than recommended by your doctor.

☐ Most people experience few or no side effects from their drugs. However, any medicine can sometimes cause unwanted effects. Call your doctor if you develop a skin rash, fast heartbeats, blurred vision, stomach pain, or difficulty in urinating ("passing your water").

☐ Prolonged use of this medicine should be avoided. Do not use more often than recommended by your physician. (**United States:** Dimetane Expectorant, Dimetane Expectorant-DC; **Canada:** Dimetane Expectorant, Dimetane Expectorant-DC, Dimetapp with Codeine)

*   *   *   *   *

Buclizine
United States: Bucladin-S Softabs

☐ This medicine is used to help control nausea, vomiting, dizziness, and motion sickness.

HOW TO USE THIS MEDICINE

☐ These tablets can be taken without water. Place the tablet in the mouth and either let it dissolve, chew it, or swallow it whole.

SPECIAL INSTRUCTIONS

☐ Women who are breast-feeding should tell their doctor before taking this medicine.

☐ In some people, this drug may cause drowsiness. Do not drive a car or operate dangerous machinery or do jobs that require you to be alert until you know how you are going to react to this drug.

☐ If your mouth becomes dry, suck a hard sour candy (sugarless) or ice chips, or chew gum. It is especially important to brush your teeth regularly if you develop a dry mouth.

☐ Do not drink alcoholic beverages while taking this drug without the approval of your doctor.

☐ It is important that you obtain the advice of your doctor or pharmacist before taking pain relievers, nonprescription drugs, sleeping pills, tranquilizers, or medicines for depression while you are taking this drug.

☐ Most people experience few or no side effects from their drugs. However, any medicine can sometimes cause unwanted effects. Call your doctor if you develop a skin rash, sore throat, fever, or mouth sores.

*   *   *   *   *

Burow's Solution (*Otitis Externa Therapy*)
United States: Domeboro Otic
Canada: Domeboro Otic

☐ This medicine is used to treat ear infections.

HOW TO USE THIS MEDICINE

☐ For EAR DROPS

INSTILLATION OF EAR DROPS

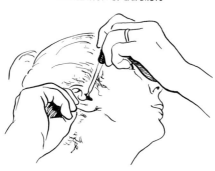

- Warm the ear drops to body temperature by holding the bottle in your hands for a few minutes. Do NOT heat the drops in hot water.
- The person administering the ear drops should wash his hands with soap and water.
- The ear drops must be kept clean. Do not touch the dropper against the ear or anything else.
- Tilt your head or lie on your side so that the ear to be treated is facing up.
- In ADULTS, hold the ear lobe up and back.
  In CHILDREN, hold the ear lobe down and back.
- Place the prescribed number of drops into the ear. Do not insert the dropper into the ear as it may cause injury.
- Remain in the same position for a short time (2 minutes) after you have administered the drops.
- Dry the ear lobe if any drops are on it.

☐ If necessary, have someone else administer the ear drops for you.

☐ Do not use the ear drops if they change in color or change in any way since being purchased.

☐ Keep the bottle tightly closed when not in use.

☐ EAR DROPS AFTER APPLICATION OF EAR WICK
- Warm the medicine to body temperature by holding it in your hands for a few minutes.
- Tilt your head to the side or lie on your side so that the ear to be treated is uppermost.
- Drop the prescribed amount of medicine into the ear canal on top of the ear wick.
- Do not use the solution if it is discolored or if it appears to have changed in any way since being purchased.

SPECIAL INSTRUCTIONS

☐ Consult your doctor if the condition for which this medicine is being used persists or becomes worse, or if the medicine causes an irritation such as itching or burning for more than just a few minutes after use.

☐ Store this medicine in a cool place, but do not freeze.

☐ For external use only. Do not swallow.

* * * * *

Busulfan (*Oral Antineoplastic*)
United States: Myleran
Canada: Myleran

☐ This medicine is used in certain medical conditions to help slow down the growth and reproduction of some of the body's cells.

HOW TO USE THIS MEDICINE

- ☐ It is best to take this medicine 1 hour before breakfast or 2 hours after supper in order to help prevent nausea or vomiting.

- ☐ It is very important that you take this medicine exactly as your doctor has prescribed and that you do not miss any doses. Try to take this medicine at the same time every day.

- ☐ Even if you become nauseated or lose your appetite, do not stop taking the medicine, but do check with your doctor.

- ☐ If you miss a dose of this medicine, do not take the missed dose and do not double your next dose. Check with your doctor.

SPECIAL INSTRUCTIONS

- ☐ Always keep your doctor appointments so that your doctor can watch your progress.

- ☐ If your doctor has prescribed some other medicines for you, it is important that you take them in the right order and that you do not miss them.

- ☐ Men and women should take appropriate birth control measures to avoid conception while taking this medicine.

- ☐ This medicine may cause a temporary loss of hair. Brush your hair gently and no more often than is necessary. After your treatment is finished, your hair should grow back in.

- ☐ Always tell your pharmacist, dentist, and any other doctors who are treating you that you are taking this medicine. This is especially important if you plan to have surgery or any vaccinations.

- ☐ This is a very strong medicine and, in addition to its beneficial effects, you may have some unwanted effects, even for a short time after you stop taking the medicine. Call your doctor if you develop unusual bruising or bleeding, sore throat, fever or mouth sores, a skin rash, swelling of the legs or ankles, shortness of breath, an unexplained cough, stomach pain, or difficulty in urinating ("passing your water").

* * * * *

Butabarbital (Oral Sedative-Hypnotic)
United States: Buticaps, Butisol Sodium
Canada: Buta-Barb, Butisol Sodium, Day-Barb, Neo-Barb

- ☐ This medicine is used to cause sleep and for certain types of nervous tension.

- ☐ IMPORTANT: If you have ever had an allergic reaction to a barbiturate medicine, tell your doctor or pharmacist before you take any of this medicine.

HOW TO USE THIS MEDICINE

☐ This medicine may be taken with food or a full glass of water.

SPECIAL INSTRUCTIONS

☐ Sleeping medicines are only useful for a short time. If used for too long, they lose their effectiveness. Do not take any more of this medicine than your doctor has prescribed, and do not stop taking this medicine suddenly without the approval of your doctor.

☐ Women who are pregnant, breast-feeding, or planning to become pregnant should tell their doctor before taking this medicine.

☐ In some people, this drug may cause dizziness or drowsiness. Do not drive a car or operate dangerous machinery or do jobs that require you to be alert until you know how you are going to react to this drug.

☐ If you become dizzy, you should be careful going up and down stairs. Sit or lie down at the first sign of dizziness.

☐ Do not drink alcoholic beverages while taking this drug without the approval of your doctor.

☐ It is important that you obtain the advice of your doctor or pharmacist before taking ANY other medicines including pain relievers, sleeping pills, tranquilizers or medicines for depression, cough/cold medicines, or allergy medicines.

☐ If you are taking this medicine to help you sleep, take it about 20 minutes before you want to go to sleep. Go to bed after you have taken it. Do not smoke in bed after you have taken it.

☐ Do not store this medicine at the bedside and keep it out of the reach of children.

☐ Call your doctor immediately if you think you may be allergic to the medicine or if you develop a skin rash, hives, itching, swelling of the face, or difficulty in breathing. If you cannot reach your doctor, phone a hospital emergency department.

☐ Most people experience few or no side effects from their drugs. However, any medicine can sometimes cause unwanted effects. Call your doctor if you develop a sore throat, bothersome sleepiness or laziness during the day, nightmares, staggering walk, unusual nervousness, a yellow color to the skin or eyes, easy bruising, or slow heartbeats.

*   *   *   *   *

144

Butaperazine Maleate (*Oral Antipsychotic-Antianxiety*)
United States: Repoise

☐ This medicine is used to help treat certain types of mental and emotional problems. Check with your doctor if you do not fully understand why you are taking it.

☐ IMPORTANT: If you have ever had an allergic reaction to a phenothiazine medicine, tell your doctor or pharmacist before you take any of this medicine.

HOW TO USE THIS MEDICINE

☐ This medicine may be taken with food or a full glass of water.

☐ Do not take this medicine at the same time as antacids or diarrhea medicine. Try to space them at least 1 hour apart.

☐ The effect of the medicine may not be noticed immediately, but may take from 2 to 4 weeks. Be patient. Take the medicine regularly and try not to miss any doses.

☐ Do not stop taking this medicine suddenly without the approval of your doctor.

SPECIAL INSTRUCTIONS

☐ If you forget to take a dose, take it as soon as possible. However, if it is almost time for your next dose, do not take the missed dose. Instead, continue with your regular dosing schedule.

☐ Any medicine has a few unwanted side effects. Because this medicine takes a few weeks to work, the side effects show the doctor that the drug is being absorbed. Many of these side effects will go away as your body adjusts to the medicine.

☐ Women who are pregnant, breast-feeding, or planning to become pregnant should tell their doctor before taking this medicine.

☐ In some people, this drug may cause dizziness or drowsiness. Do not drive a car or operate dangerous machinery or do jobs that require you to be alert until you know how you are going to react to this drug.

☐ If this medicine causes dizziness, you should be careful going up and down stairs and you should not change positions too rapidly. Get out of bed slowly in the morning and dangle your feet over the edge of the bed for a few minutes before standing up. Sit down or lie down at the first sign of dizziness. Tell your doctor you have been dizzy. Avoid hot showers and baths because they could make you dizzy.

☐ Do not drink alcoholic beverages while taking this drug without the approval of your doctor.

☐ This medicine may make some people more sensitive to sunlight and sun-lamps. When you begin taking this medicine, try to avoid getting too much sun until you see how you are going to react. If your skin does become more sensitive to sunlight, tell your doctor and try to stay out of direct sunlight. While in the sun, wear protective clothing and sunglasses. You may wish to ask your pharmacist about suitable sunscreen products. Check with your doctor if you become sunburned.

☐ If your mouth becomes dry, suck a hard sour candy (sugarless) or ice chips, or chew gum. It is especially important to brush your teeth regularly if you develop a dry mouth.

☐ It is important that you obtain the advice of your doctor or pharmacist before taking **any** other medicines including pain relievers, sleeping pills, other tranquilizers or medicines for depression, cough, cold or allergy medicines, weight-reducing medicines, or laxatives.

☐ This medicine may cause your urine to turn pink, red, or red-brown in color. This is not unusual.

☐ In hot weather or during exercise, be careful not to become overheated. You may be more sensitive to heat since this medicine may affect your body's ability to regulate temperature.

☐ If you become constipated, try increasing the amount of bulk in your diet (for example, bran and salads), exercising more often, or drinking more water. Call your doctor if the constipation continues.

☐ Call your doctor if you develop a sore throat, fever, mouth sores, skin rash, changes in eyesight, rapid heartrate, a yellow color in the eyes or skin, unusual weakness or unusual movements of the face, tongue, or hands, or difficulty in urinating ("passing your water"). Also call your doctor if you become restless or unable to sit still or sleep.

☐ Carry an identification card indicating that you are taking this medicine. Always tell your dentist, pharmacist, and other doctors who are treating you that you are taking this medicine.

* * * * *

Butobarbitone (Oral Sedative-Hypnotic)
Canada: Soneryl

☐ This medicine is used to cause sleep.

☐ IMPORTANT: If you have ever had an allergic reaction to a barbiturate medicine, tell your doctor or pharmacist before you take any of this medicine.

HOW TO USE THIS MEDICINE

☐ This medicine may be taken with food or a full glass of water.

☐ This medicine must be swallowed whole. Do not crush, chew, or break it into pieces.

SPECIAL INSTRUCTIONS

☐ Sleeping medicines are only useful for a short time. If used for too long, they lose their effectiveness. Do not take any more of this medicine than your doctor has prescribed and do not stop taking this medicine suddenly without the approval of your doctor.

☐ Women who are pregnant, breast-feeding, or planning to become pregnant should tell their doctor before taking this medicine.

☐ In some people, this drug may cause dizziness or drowsiness. Do not drive a car or operate dangerous machinery or do jobs that require you to be alert until you know how you are going to react to this drug.

☐ If you become dizzy, you should be careful going up and down stairs. Sit or lie down at the first sign of dizziness.

☐ Do not drink alcoholic beverages while taking this drug without the approval of your doctor.

☐ It is important that you obtain the advice of your doctor or pharmacist before taking ANY other medicines including pain relievers, sleeping pills, tranquilizers or medicines for depression, cough/cold medicines, or allergy medicines.

☐ Since you are taking this medicine to help you sleep, take it about 20 minutes before you want to go to sleep. Go to bed after you have taken it. Do not smoke in bed after you have taken it.

☐ Do not store this medicine at the bedside, and keep it out of the reach of children.

☐ Call your doctor immediately if you think you may be allergic to the medicine or if you develop a skin rash, hives, itching, swelling of the face, or difficulty in breathing. If you cannot reach your doctor, phone a hospital emergency department.

☐ Most people experience few or no side effects from their drugs. However, any medicine can sometimes cause unwanted effects. Call your doctor if you develop a sore throat, bothersome sleepiness or laziness during the day, nightmares, staggering walk, unusual nervousness, a yellow color to the skin or eyes, easy bruising, or slow heartbeats.

*   *   *   *   *

Calcitriol (*Oral Vitamin D₃ Metabolite*)

United States: Rocaltrol

Canada: Rocaltrol

☐ This medicine is used in the treatment of certain conditions to help restore to normal the calcium levels in the body.

☐ IMPORTANT: If you have ever had an allergic reaction to a vitamin D medicine, tell your doctor or pharmacist before you take any of this medicine.

HOW TO USE THIS MEDICINE

☐ It is very important that you take this medicine exactly as your doctor has prescribed and that you do not miss any doses. Try to take this medicine at the same time every day. Do not take extra tablets without your doctor's approval.

SPECIAL INSTRUCTIONS

☐ Do not take any nonprescription drugs while you are taking this medicine unless otherwise directed. This includes antacids containing magnesium and the prolonged use of mineral oil.

☐ Follow any diet that your doctor has prescribed, especially with respect to dairy products and calcium supplements.

☐ Do not take any other vitamin products containing vitamin D unless otherwise directed by your doctor.

☐ Most people experience few or no side effects from their drugs. However, any medicine can sometimes cause unwanted effects. Call your doctor if you develop unusual weakness, headache, irregular pulse, nausea, vomiting, dry mouth, muscle or bone pain, constipation, a metallic taste in the mouth, or excessive thirst.

*　*　*　*　*

Calcium Preparations (*Oral Calcium Supplement*)

United States: Calcium Chloride Powder, Calora, D.C.P., D.C.P. 340, Neo-Calglucon

Canada: Calcium-Eri, Calcium-Rougier, Calcium-Sandoz, Dicalgin, Gramacal

☐ This medicine is a calcium supplement. It has many uses and the reason it was prescribed depends upon your condition. Check with your doctor.

HOW TO USE THIS MEDICINE

☐ Take this medicine 1 hour to 1½ hours after a meal with a glass of water. (**Canada:** Calcium-Eri, Calcium-Rougier)

148

☐ The effervescent tablets should be dissolved in a glass of water before being swallowed. (**Canada:** Calcium-Sandoz, Gramacal)

SPECIAL INSTRUCTIONS

☐ Do not self-medicate with vitamin D preparations without the approval of your doctor.

☐ Do not eat unusually large amounts of bran, whole cereals, milk, or dairy products while you are taking this medicine.

☐ Most people experience few or no side effects from their drugs. However, any medicine can sometimes cause unwanted effects. Call your doctor if you develop troublesome diarrhea or constipation.

*　*　*　*　*

Calusterone (*Oral Androgen*)
United States: Methosarb

☐ This medicine is used in certain medical conditions to help slow down the growth and reproduction of some of the body's cells.

HOW TO USE THIS MEDICINE

☐ It is best to take this medicine on an empty stomach at least 1 hour before (or 2 hours after) eating food. Take it at the proper time even if you skip a meal.

☐ It is very important that you take this medicine exactly as your doctor has prescribed and that you do not miss any doses. Try to take this medicine at the same time every day. Do not take extra tablets without your doctor's approval.

☐ Even if you become nauseated, do not stop taking the medicine until you check with your doctor.

SPECIAL INSTRUCTIONS

☐ Always keep your doctor's appointments so that your doctor can watch your progress.

☐ Men and women should take appropriate birth control measures to avoid conception while taking this medicine.

☐ Always tell your pharmacist, dentist, and other doctors who are treating you that you are taking this medicine.

☐ Most people experience few or no side effects from their drugs. However, any medicine can sometimes cause unwanted effects. Call your doctor if you develop pain or swelling in the legs or ankles, sudden weight gain, dark-colored urine or a yellow color to the skin or eyes, severe vomiting, or increased facial hair. Also call your doctor if you become unusually thirsty, drowsy, or confused or if you urinate ("pass your water") more frequently than usual.

* * * * *

Carbachol (Ophthalmic Parasympathomimetic-Miotic)

United States: Carbacel Ophthalmic, Isopto Carbachol Ophthalmic
Canada: Isopto Carbachol

☐ This medicine is used in the treatment of glaucoma and other eye conditions.

HOW TO USE THIS MEDICINE

☐ For EYE DROPS

INSTILLATION OF EYE DROPS

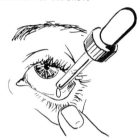

- The person administering the eye drops should wash his hands with soap and water.
- The eye drops must be kept clean. Do not touch the dropper against the face or anything else.
- Lie down or tilt your head backward and look at the ceiling.
- Gently pull down the lower lid of your eye to form a pouch.
- Hold the dropper in your other hand and approach the eye from the side. Place the dropper as close to the eye as possible without touching it.
- Place the prescribed number of drops into the pouch of the eye.
- Close your eyes. Do not rub them.
- Apply gentle pressure for a minute with your fingers to the bridge of the nose (inside corner of the eye) to prevent the eye drops from being drained from the eye.
- Blot excess solution around the eye with a tissue.

☐ If necessary, have someone else administer the eye drops for you.

☐ Do not use the eye drops if they change in color or change in any way since being purchased.

☐ Keep the eye drop bottle tightly closed when not in use.

☐ Wash your hands after you have instilled the drops.

150

□ Do not use the drug more frequently or in larger quantities than prescribed by your doctor.

SPECIAL INSTRUCTIONS

□ Vision may be blurred for a few minutes after using the eye medicine. Do not drive a car or operate dangerous machinery or do jobs that require you to be alert until your vision has cleared.

□ During the first few days of using the eye drops, you may experience aching in the eyes and head. This is not unusual and should disappear. Call your doctor if the pain persists.

□ If you forget to use the medicine, use it as soon as possible. However, if it is almost time for your next dose, do not use the missed dose, but continue with your regular schedule.

□ Do not use this medicine at the same time as any other eye medicine without the approval of your doctor. Some medicines cannot be mixed.

□ Contact your doctor if the condition for which you are using this medicine does not improve or if the eye becomes irritated by it for more than a few minutes. Many eye medicines sting for a short time immediately after use. Also call your doctor if you develop excessive sweating, flushing, stomach cramps, diarrhea (loose bowel movements), difficulty in breathing, or difficulty in urinating ("passing your water").

□ Always tell any future doctors who are treating you that you have used this medicine.

□ For external use only. Do not swallow.

*   *   *   *   *

Carbamazepine (Oral Trigeminal Neuralgia Therapy— Anticonvulsant)
United States: Tegretol
Canada: Tegretol

□ This medicine is used to help control convulsions and seizures. It is commonly used in the treatment of epilepsy and is also used to help relieve a certain type of face pain.

□ IMPORTANT: If you have ever had an allergic reaction to an anticonvulsant medicine or a medicine for depression, tell your doctor or pharmacist before you take any of this medicine.

HOW TO USE THIS MEDICINE

□ Take this medicine with food if it upsets your stomach. Call your doctor if you continue to have stomach upset.

151

☐ It is very important that you take this medicine regularly and that you do not miss any doses. Try to take the medicine at the same time(s) every day. This is the only way that you can receive the full benefit of the medicine.

SPECIAL INSTRUCTIONS

☐ If you forget to take a dose, take it as soon as possible. However, if it is almost time for your next dose, do not take the missed dose. Instead, continue with your regular dosing schedule. Do not double doses.

☐ Do not stop taking this medicine suddenly or change the amount you are taking without the approval of your doctor.

☐ Avoid swimming alone or participating in high-risk sports in which a sudden seizure could cause injury.

☐ In some people, this drug may cause dizziness or drowsiness. Do not drive a car or operate dangerous machinery or do jobs that require you to be alert until you know how you are going to react to this drug. If you become dizzy, you should be careful going up and down stairs. Sit or lie down at the first sign of dizziness.

☐ If this medicine is for a child, do not let him (her) ride a bike or climb trees until you can determine how he (she) is going to react to the medicine. They could hurt themselves if they participated in these activities if they were dizzy.

☐ Do not drink alcoholic beverages while taking this drug without the approval of your doctor.

☐ It is important that you obtain the advice of your doctor or pharmacist before taking pain relievers, nonprescription drugs, sleeping pills, tranquilizers or medicines for depression while you are taking this drug.

☐ If your mouth becomes dry, suck a hard sour candy (sugarless) or ice chips, or chew gum. It is especially important to brush your teeth regularly if you develop a dry mouth.

☐ This medicine may make some people more sensitive to sunlight and sunlamps. When you begin taking this medicine, try to avoid getting too much sun until you see how you are going to react. If your skin does become more sensitive to sunlight, tell your doctor and try to stay out of direct sunlight. While in the sun, wear protective clothing and sunglasses. You may wish to ask your pharmacist about suitable sunscreen products. Check with your doctor if you become sunburned.

☐ Women who are pregnant, breast-feeding, or planning to become pregnant should tell their doctor before taking this medicine.

☐ Most people experience few or no side effects from their drugs. However, any medicine can sometimes cause unwanted effects. Call your doctor if you develop a sore throat, fever or mouth sores, easy bruising or bleeding, dark-colored urine or a yellow color to the skin or eyes, fast eye movements, numbness or tingling of the hands or feet, nightmares or depression, palpitations, swelling of the legs or ankles, or if you urinate ("pass your water") in smaller amounts than usual.

- □ Do not go without this medicine between prescription refills. Call your pharmacist 2 or 3 days before you will run out of the medicine.
- □ Carry an identification card indicating that you are taking this medicine. Always tell your pharmacist, dentist, and other doctors who are treating you that you are taking this medicine.

*   *   *   *   *

Carbarsone (*Oral Amebicide*)
United States: Carbarsone

- □ This medicine is used in the treatment of certain types of bowel infections.

HOW TO USE THIS MEDICINE
- □ If you cannot swallow capsules, open the capsules and mix the contents with half a glass of milk or orange juice or in jelly or food.

SPECIAL INSTRUCTIONS
- □ It is important to follow any restrictions on diet or exercise that your doctor may prescribe.
- □ Do not take any more of this medicine than your doctor has prescribed, but it is important that you do not miss any doses. Otherwise, the infection will not be eliminated.
- □ Most people experience few or no side effects from their drugs. However, any medicine can sometimes cause unwanted effects. Call your doctor if you develop vomiting, stomach cramps, severe diarrhea, sore throat, fever or mouth sores, swelling of the legs or ankles, or a yellow color to the skin or eyes.

GENERAL INSTRUCTIONS
- □ Good personal hygiene is very important to prevent reinfection.
- □ It is recommended that you have a shower every morning in order to remove any eggs in the anal area that have appeared during the night.
- □ Wash your hands frequently, especially before handling food or anything that will be put into the mouth. Wash the hands after urination and bowel movements.
- □ Keep the nails short and clean and avoid biting them. Do not put your fingers in your mouth or nose.
- □ On the day of therapy, change the bed linen, underwear, and nightclothes. Wash or dry-clean immediately.
- □ Do not scratch the affected area.
- □ Disinfect the toilet seat and bathtub daily.

*   *   *   *   *

Carbenicillin Indanyl Sodium (*Oral Antibiotic*)

United States: Geocillin

Canada: Geopen Oral

☐ This medicine is an antibiotic used to treat certain types of infections of the urinary tract and prostate gland.

☐ IMPORTANT: If you have ever had an allergic reaction to penicillin or any other antibiotic, tell your doctor or pharmacist before you take any of this medicine.

HOW TO USE THIS MEDICINE

☐ It is best to take this medicine on an empty stomach 1 hour before (or 2 hours after) meals or food unless otherwise directed. Take it at the proper time even if you skip a meal.

☐ Take the medicine with a full glass of water.

SPECIAL INSTRUCTIONS

☐ It is important to take **all** of this medicine plus any refills that your doctor told you to take. Do not stop taking this medicine earlier than your doctor has recommended in spite of the fact that you may feel better. Otherwise, the infection may return.

☐ If you forget to take a dose, take it as soon as you remember and then continue with your regular schedule.

☐ Women who are breast-feeding should tell their doctor before taking this medicine.

☐ Most people experience few or no side effects from their drugs. However, any medicine can sometimes cause unwanted effects. Contact your doctor if you develop easy bruising or a dark-colored tongue, yellow-green stools or, in women, a vaginal discharge that was not present before you started taking the medicine.

☐ Check with your doctor if you develop diarrhea or a bitter taste in the mouth which does not go away as your body adjusts to the medicine.

☐ Call your doctor immediately if you think you may be allergic to the medicine or if you develop a skin rash, hives, itching, swelling of the face, or difficulty in breathing. If you cannot reach your doctor, phone a hospital emergency department.

☐ If for some reason you cannot take all of the medicine, throw away the unused portion by flushing it down the toilet. Do not take or save old medicine.

* * * * *

Carbenoxolone Sodium (*Oral Gastric Ulcer Therapy*)
Canada: Biogastrone, Duogastrone

☐ This medicine promotes healing of certain types of gastric and duodenal ulcers.

HOW TO USE THIS MEDICINE
☐ Take the tablets after meals. (*Canada:* Biogastrone)

☐ Take the capsules 30 minutes before eating. (*Canada:* Duogastrone)

☐ Swallow the medicine whole. Do not crush, chew, or break it into pieces.

SPECIAL INSTRUCTIONS
☐ Diabetic patients should regularly check the sugar in their urine and report any abnormal results to their doctor.

☐ In some people, this drug may cause dizziness. Do not drive a car or operate dangerous machinery or do jobs that require you to be alert until you know how you are going to react to this drug. If you become dizzy, you should be careful going up and down stairs. Sit or lie down at the first sign of dizziness.

☐ Most people experience few or no side effects from their drugs. However, any medicine can sometimes cause unwanted effects. Call your doctor if you develop a noticeable gain in weight, swelling of the hands, feet, or ankles, shortness of breath, nausea, unusual weakness and tiredness, or unusual headaches.

☐ You must follow any diet prescribed by your doctor and continue to take this medicine even if your pain fades. If you stop the medicine too soon, your ulcer may not be fully healed and could quickly return. Ulcer healing usually takes 4 to 6 weeks. It is best to avoid smoking as well as coffee, tea, alcohol, spiced food, and aspirin because these agents can irritate the stomach. Check with your pharmacist before you purchase any nonprescription drugs.

☐ Do not go without the medicine between prescription refills. Call your pharmacist 2 or 3 days before you will run out of the medicine.

*   *   *   *   *

Carbimazole (*Oral Antithyroid Agent*)
Canada: Neo-Mercazole

☐ This medicine is used to treat an overactive thyroid gland and is also used before thyroid surgery.

155

HOW TO USE THIS MEDICINE

☐ This medicine may be taken with meals or on an empty stomach. To make sure that you always get the same effect, always take it the same way.

☐ If you miss a dose of this medicine, take it as soon as you remember.

SPECIAL INSTRUCTIONS

☐ It is very important that you take this medicine exactly as your doctor has prescribed and that you do not miss any doses. Try to take this medicine at the same time every day. Do not take extra tablets without your doctor's approval. Do not stop taking this medicine without the approval of your doctor.

☐ Women who are breast-feeding should tell their doctor before taking this medicine.

☐ Check with your doctor or pharmacist before taking any nonprescription drugs that contain iodides (for example, some cough, cold, or asthma products).

☐ Call your doctor immediately if you become sick or develop a fever, sore throat, skin abscess, or other symptoms of an infection.

☐ Most people experience few or no side effects from their drugs. However, any medicine can sometimes cause unwanted effects. Call your doctor if you develop a sore throat, fever or mouth sores, a skin rash, easy bruising or bleeding, stomach upset, joint pain, or unusual tiredness.

* * * * *

Carbinoxamine Maleate (Oral Antihistamine)
United States: Clistin

☐ This medicine is used to help relieve the symptoms of certain types of allergic conditions, coughs and colds, and certain skin conditions.

HOW TO USE THIS MEDICINE

☐ This medicine may be taken with food or a glass of milk if it upsets your stomach.

☐ These tablets must be swallowed whole. Do not crush, chew, or break them into pieces. (**United States:** Clistin R-A Tablets).

SPECIAL INSTRUCTIONS

☐ If you forget to take a dose, take it as soon as possible. However, if it is almost time for your next dose, do not take the missed dose. Instead, continue with your regular dosing schedule.

156

- [ ] In some people, this drug may initially cause dizziness or drowsiness. Do not drive a car or operate dangerous machinery or do jobs that require you to be alert until you know how you are going to react to this drug. If you become dizzy, you should be careful going up and down stairs. Sit or lie down at the first sign of dizziness. Tell your doctor if it continues.

- [ ] Do not drink alcoholic beverages while taking this drug without the approval of your doctor.

- [ ] If your mouth becomes dry, suck a hard sour candy (sugarless) or ice chips, or chew gum. It is especially important to brush your teeth regularly if you develop a dry mouth.

- [ ] It is important that you obtain the advice of your doctor or pharmacist before taking pain relievers, nonprescription drugs, sleeping pills or tranquilizers, or other medicines for allergies.

- [ ] Do not take this medicine more often or longer than recommended by your doctor.

- [ ] Most people experience few or no side effects from their drugs. However, any medicine can sometimes cause unwanted effects. Call your doctor if you develop a skin rash, fast heartbeats, blurred vision, stomach pain, or difficulty in urinating ("passing your water").

* * * * *

Carisoprodol (Oral Skeletal Muscle Relaxant)
United States: Rela, Soma
Canada: Soma

- [ ] This medicine is used to relax muscles and helps to relieve muscle pain and stiffness.

- [ ] IMPORTANT: If you have ever had an allergic reaction to any medicines, tell your doctor or pharmacist before you take any of this medicine.

HOW TO USE THIS MEDICINE
- [ ] This medicine may be taken with food or a glass of water.

- [ ] If you forget to take a dose, take it as soon as possible. However, if it is almost time for your next dose, do not take the missed dose. Instead, continue with your regular dosing schedule.

SPECIAL INSTRUCTIONS
- [ ] Women who are breast-feeding should tell their doctor before taking this medicine.

- [ ] Do not drink alcoholic beverages while taking this drug without the approval of your doctor.

157

- [ ] It is important that you obtain the advice of your doctor or pharmacist before taking ANY other medicines including pain relievers, sleeping pills, tranquilizers or medicines for depression, cough/cold medicines, or allergy medicines.

- [ ] In some people, this drug may cause dizziness or drowsiness. Do not drive a car or operate dangerous machinery or do jobs that require you to be alert until you know how you are going to react to this drug.

- [ ] If this medicine causes dizziness, you should be careful going up and down stairs and you should not change positions too rapidly. Get out of bed slowly in the morning and dangle your feet over the edge of the bed for a few minutes before standing up. Sit down or lie down at the first sign of dizziness. Tell your doctor you have been dizzy. Avoid hot showers and baths because they could make you dizzy.

- [ ] Call your doctor immediately if you think you may be allergic to the medicine or if you develop a skin rash, hives, itching, swelling of the face, or difficulty in breathing. If you cannot reach your doctor, phone a hospital emergency department.

- [ ] Most people experience few or no side effects from their drugs. However, any medicine can sometimes cause unwanted effects. Call your doctor if you develop stomach pain, trembling, unusual nervousness, fast heartbeats, fainting spells, or if you become depressed.

*   *   *   *   *

Carphenazine Maleate (*Oral Antipsychotic-Antianxiety*)
United States: Proketazine

- [ ] This medicine is used to treat certain types of mental and emotional problems. Check with your doctor if you do not fully understand why you are taking it.

- [ ] IMPORTANT: If you have ever had an allergic reaction to a phenothiazine medicine, tell your doctor or pharmacist before you take any of this medicine.

HOW TO USE THIS MEDICINE
- [ ] This medicine may be taken with food or a full glass of water.

- [ ] Do not take this medicine at the same time as antacids or diarrhea medicine. Try to space them at least 1 hour apart.

- [ ] The effect of the medicine may not be noticed immediately, but may take from 2 to 4 weeks. Be patient. Take the medicine regularly and try not to miss any doses.

- [ ] Do not stop taking this medicine suddenly without the approval of your doctor.

158

SPECIAL INSTRUCTIONS

☐ If you forget to take a dose, take it as soon as possible. However, if it is almost time for your next dose, do not take the missed dose. Instead, continue with your regular dosing schedule.

☐ Any medicine has a few unwanted side effects. Because this medicine takes a few weeks to work, the side effects show the doctor that the drug is being absorbed. Many of these side effects will go away as your body adjusts to the medicine.

☐ Women who are pregnant, breast-feeding, or planning to become pregnant should tell their doctor before taking this medicine.

☐ In some people, this drug may cause dizziness or drowsiness. Do not drive a car or operate dangerous machinery or do jobs that require you to be alert until you know how you are going to react to this drug.

☐ If this medicine causes dizziness, you should be careful going up and down stairs and you should not change positions too rapidly. Get out of bed slowly in the morning and dangle your feet over the edge of the bed for a few minutes before standing up. Sit down or lie down at the first sign of dizziness. Tell your doctor you have been dizzy. Avoid hot showers and baths because they could make you dizzy.

☐ Do not drink alcoholic beverages while taking this drug without the approval of your doctor.

☐ This medicine may make some people more sensitive to sunlight and sunlamps. When you begin taking this medicine, try to avoid getting too much sun until you see how you are going to react. If your skin does become more sensitive to sunlight, tell your doctor and try to stay out of direct sunlight. While in the sun, wear protective clothing and sunglasses. You may wish to ask your pharmacist about suitable sunscreen products. Check with your doctor if you become sunburned.

☐ If your mouth becomes dry, suck a hard sour candy (sugarless) or ice chips, or chew gum. It is especially important to brush your teeth regularly if you develop a dry mouth.

☐ It is important that you obtain the advice of your doctor before taking **any** other medicines including pain relievers, sleeping pills, other tranquilizers or medicines for depression, cough, cold or allergy medicines, reducing medicines, or laxatives.

☐ This medicine may cause your urine to turn pink, red, or red-brown in color. This is not unusual.

☐ In hot weather or during exercise, be careful not to become overheated. You may be more sensitive to heat since this medicine may affect your body's ability to regulate temperature.

- [ ] If you become constipated, try increasing the amount of bulk in your diet (for example, bran and salads), exercising more often, or drinking more water. Call your doctor if the constipation continues.

- [ ] Call your doctor if you develop a sore throat, fever, mouth sores, skin rash, changes in eyesight, rapid heartrate, a yellow color in the eyes or skin, unusual weakness or unusual movements of the face, tongue, or hands, or difficulty in urinating ("passing your water"). Also call your doctor if you become restless or unable to sit still or sleep.

- [ ] Carry an identification card indicating that you are taking this medicine. Always tell your pharmacist, dentist, and other doctors who are treating you that you are taking this medicine.

*   *   *   *   *

Casanthranol-Docusate Sodium
United States: Afko-Lube Lax, Bu-Lax-Plus, Comfolax-Plus, Constiban, Disanthrol, D-S-S Plus, Molatoc-CST, Peri-Colace, Peri-Conate, Peri-Doss, Stimulax
Canada: Peri-Colace

Cascara Sagrada *(Oral Laxative)*
United States: Cas-Evac
Canada: Cas-Evac

- [ ] This medicine is a laxative used to help relieve constipation.

HOW TO USE THIS MEDICINE
- [ ] Take the medicine in the evening or before breakfast with a full glass of water.

- [ ] Do not take mineral oil while you are taking this medicine. (*United States:* Afko-Lube Lax, Bu-Lax-Plus, Comfolax-Plus, Constiban, Disanthrol, D-S-S Plus, Molatoc-CST, Peri-Colace, Peri-Conate, Peri-Doss, Stimulax; *Canada:* Peri-Colace)

SPECIAL INSTRUCTIONS
- [ ] Do not take this medicine more often or longer than your doctor has prescribed as your bowels may become dependent upon it. If you feel you require this medicine every day and cannot have a bowel movement without it, call your doctor.

- [ ] Women who are breast-feeding should tell their doctor before taking this medicine.

160

☐ Unless otherwise directed, you should also try increasing the amount of bulk foods in your diet (for example, bran, fresh fruits, and salads), exercising more often, and drinking 6 to 8 glasses of water every day.

☐ This medicine may cause your urine to turn yellow-brown or red in color. This is not unusual.

☐ Do not take this medicine if you have any stomach pain, nausea, or vomiting.

☐ Call your doctor if your constipation is not relieved or if you develop rectal bleeding, muscle cramps, unusual weakness, or dizziness.

* * * * *

Castor Oil (*Oral Laxative*)
United States: Alphamul, Neoloid
Canada: Neoloid, Unisoil

☐ This medicine is a laxative.

HOW TO USE THIS MEDICINE
☐ Mix this medicine with ½ to 1 glass of water, milk, fruit juice, or soft drinks. (**Canada:** Unisoil)

SPECIAL INSTRUCTIONS
☐ Avoid excessive and continual use of this medicine as your body may become dependent on it. If you feel you require this medicine every day, consult your doctor.

☐ Do not take this medicine if abdominal pain (stomach pain), nausea, or vomiting is present.

* * * * *

Cefaclor (*Oral Antibiotic*)
United States: Ceclor
Canada: Ceclor

☐ This medicine is used to treat certain types of infections.

☐ IMPORTANT: If you have ever had an allergic reaction to penicillin or any other antibiotic, tell your doctor or pharmacist before you take any of this medicine.

HOW TO USE THIS MEDICINE
☐ This medicine may be taken with meals or on an empty stomach. If it upsets your stomach, take it with some food. Call your doctor if you continue to have stomach upset.

□ For LIQUID MEDICINE (*United States* and *Canada:* Ceclor Suspensions)
- Shake the bottle well before using so that you can measure an accurate dose.
- Store in the refrigerator but do not freeze. Do not use after the expiration date.

SPECIAL INSTRUCTIONS

□ It is important to take *all* of this medicine plus any refills that your doctor told you to take. Do not stop taking this medicine earlier than your doctor has recommended in spite of the fact that you may feel better. Otherwise, the infection may return.

□ If you forget to take a dose, take it as soon as you remember, and then continue with your regular schedule.

□ Most people experience few or no side effects from their drugs. However, any medicine may cause unwanted effects. Call your doctor if you develop a dark-colored tongue, yellow-green stools, sore mouth or, in women, a vaginal discharge that was not present before you started taking the medicine.

□ Call your doctor immediately if you think you may be allergic to the medicine or if you develop a skin rash, hives, itching, swelling of the face, or difficulty in breathing. If you cannot reach your doctor, phone a hospital emergency department.

□ If for some reason you cannot take all of the medicine, discard the unused portion by flushing it down the toilet. Do not take or save old medicine.

*   *   *   *   *

Cefadroxil (*Oral Antibiotic*)
United States: Duricef

□ This medicine is used to treat certain types of infections.

□ IMPORTANT: If you have ever had an allergic reaction to penicillin or any other antibiotic, tell your doctor or pharmacist before you take any of this medicine.

HOW TO USE THIS MEDICINE

□ This medicine may be taken with meals or on an empty stomach. If it upsets your stomach, take it with some food. Call your doctor if you continue to have stomach upset.

SPECIAL INSTRUCTIONS

□ It is important to take *all* of this medicine plus any refills that your doctor told you to take. Do not stop taking this medicine earlier than your doctor has recommended in spite of the fact that you may feel better. Otherwise, the infection may return.

- If you forget to take a dose, take it as soon as you remember and then continue with your regular schedule.

- Most people experience few or no side effects from their drugs. However, any medicine may cause unwanted effects. Call your doctor if you develop a dark-colored tongue, yellow-green stools, sore mouth or, in women, a vaginal discharge that was not present before you started taking the medicine.

- Call your doctor immediately if you think you may be allergic to the medicine or if you develop a skin rash, hives, itching, swelling of the face, or difficulty in breathing. If you cannot reach your doctor, phone a hospital emergency department.

- If for some reason you cannot take all of the medicine, discard the unused portion by flushing it down the toilet. Do not take or save old medicine.

* * * * *

Cephalexin Monohydrate (*Oral Antibiotic*)
United States: Keflex
Canada: Ceporex, Keflex

- This medicine is used to treat certain types of infections.

- IMPORTANT: If you have ever had an allergic reaction to penicillin or any other antibiotic, tell your doctor or pharmacist before you take any of this medicine.

HOW TO USE THIS MEDICINE
- This medicine may be taken with meals or on an empty stomach. If it upsets your stomach, take it with some food. Call your doctor if you continue to have a stomach upset.

- For LIQUID MEDICINE

    - Shake the bottle well before using so that you can measure an accurate dose. Store in the refrigerator but do not freeze. Do not use after the discard date. (**United States:** Keflex Suspension; **Canada:** Ceporex, Keflex Suspensions)

    - If a dropper is used to measure a dose and you do not fully understand how to use it, check with your pharmacist. (**United States:** Keflex Pediatric Drops)

SPECIAL INSTRUCTIONS
- It is important to take **all** of this medicine plus any refills that your doctor told you to take. Do not stop taking this medicine earlier than your doctor has recommended in spite of the fact that you may feel better. Otherwise, the infection may return.

☐ If you forget to take a dose, take it as soon as you remember and then continue with your regular schedule.

☐ Most people experience few or no side effects from their drugs. However, any medicine may cause unwanted effects. Call your doctor if you develop a dark-colored tongue, yellow-green stools, sore mouth or, in women, a vaginal discharge that was not present before you started taking the medicine.

☐ Call your doctor immediately if you think you may be allergic to the medicine or if you develop a skin rash, hives, itching, swelling of the face, or difficulty in breathing. If you cannot reach your doctor, phone a hospital emergency department.

☐ If for some reason you cannot take all of the medicine, discard the unused portion by flushing it down the toilet. Do not take or save old medicine.

* * * * *

Cephaloglycin (*Oral Antibiotic*)
United States: Kafocin

☐ This medicine is used to treat certain types of infections of the urinary tract.

☐ IMPORTANT: If you have ever had an allergic reaction to penicillin or any other antibiotic, tell your doctor or pharmacist before you take any of this medicine.

HOW TO USE THIS MEDICINE
☐ This medicine may be taken with meals or on an empty stomach. If it upsets your stomach, take it with some food. Call your doctor if you continue to have stomach upset.

SPECIAL INSTRUCTIONS
☐ It is important to take **all** of this medicine plus any refills that your doctor told you to take. Do not stop taking this medicine earlier than your doctor has recommended in spite of the fact that you may feel better. Otherwise, the infection may return.

☐ If you forget to take a dose, take it as soon as you remember and then continue with your regular schedule.

☐ Most people experience few or no side effects from their drugs. However, any medicine may cause unwanted effects. Call your doctor if you develop a dark-colored tongue, yellow-green stools, sore mouth or, in women, a vaginal discharge that was not present before you started taking the medicine.

☐ Call your doctor if you develop severe diarrhea (loose bowel movements), severe stomach cramps, or bloody or black stools.

- [ ] Call your doctor immediately if you think you may be allergic to the medicine or if you develop a skin rash, hives, itching, swelling of the face, or difficulty in breathing. If you cannot reach your doctor, phone a hospital emergency department.

- [ ] If for some reason you cannot take all of the medicine, discard the unused portion by flushing it down the toilet. Do not take or save old medicine.

* * * * *

Cephradine (*Oral Antibiotic*)
United States: Anspor, Velosef
Canada: Velosef

- [ ] This medicine is an antibiotic used to treat certain types of infections.

- [ ] IMPORTANT: If you have ever had an allergic reaction to penicillin or any other antibiotic, tell your doctor or pharmacist before you take any of this medicine.

HOW TO USE THIS MEDICINE
- [ ] This medicine may be taken with meals or on an empty stomach. If it upsets your stomach, take it with some food. Call your doctor if you continue to have stomach upset.

- [ ] For LIQUID MEDICINE

- [ ] Shake the bottle well before using so that you can measure an accurate dose. Store it in the refrigerator but do not freeze. Do not use after the discard date. (*United States:* Anspor, Velosef Suspensions; *Canada:* Velosef Suspension)

SPECIAL INSTRUCTIONS
- [ ] It is important to take **all** of this medicine plus any refills that your doctor told you to take. Do not stop taking this medicine earlier than your doctor has recommended in spite of the fact that you may feel better. Otherwise, the infection may return.

- [ ] If you forget to take a dose, take it as soon as you remember and then continue with your regular schedule.

- [ ] Most people experience few or no side effects from their drugs. However, any medicine may cause unwanted effects. Call your doctor if you develop a dark-colored tongue, yellow-green stools, sore mouth or, in women, a vaginal discharge that was not present before you started taking the medicine.

- [ ] Call your doctor immediately if you think you may be allergic to the medicine or if you develop a skin rash, hives, itching, swelling of the face, or difficulty in breathing. If you cannot reach your doctor, phone a hospital emergency department.

165

☐ If for some reason you cannot take all of the medicine, discard the unused portion by flushing it down the toilet. Do not take or save old medicine.

* * * * *

Chlophedianol HCl (*Oral Antitussive*)
United States: Ulo
Canada: Ulone

☐ This medicine is used to help relieve dry, irritating coughs.

HOW TO USE THIS MEDICINE
☐ Do not dilute the syrup. The soothing effect of the syrup will be enhanced if you do not drink liquids immediately after taking the medicine.

SPECIAL INSTRUCTIONS
☐ In some people, this drug may cause drowsiness. Do not drive a car or operate dangerous machinery or do jobs that require you to be alert until you know how you are going to react to this drug.

☐ Most people experience few or no side effects from their drugs. However, any medicine can sometimes cause unwanted effects. Call your doctor if you develop nightmares, hallucinations, a skin rash, or vomiting.

☐ Call your doctor if the cough lasts longer than 1 week or if you develop a fever, skin rash, or persistent headache.

☐ Do not use this medicine for more than 1 week without the advice of your doctor.

* * * * *

Chloral Betaine
United States: Beta-Chlor

☐ This medicine is used to cause sleep and for certain types of nervous tension.

HOW TO USE THIS MEDICINE
☐ Take the tablets with a full glass of water, fruit juice, or ginger ale to help prevent stomach upset.

☐ This medicine must be swallowed whole. Do not crush, chew, or break it into pieces.

SPECIAL INSTRUCTIONS
☐ Sleeping medicines are only useful for a short time. If used for too long, they

lose their effectiveness. Do not take any more of this medicine than your doctor has prescribed and do not stop taking this medicine suddenly without the approval of your doctor.

☐ Women who are pregnant, breast-feeding, or planning to become pregnant should tell their doctor before taking this medicine.

☐ In some people, this drug may cause dizziness or drowsiness. Do not drive a car or operate dangerous machinery or do jobs that require you to be alert until you know how you are going to react to this drug.

☐ If you become dizzy, you should be careful going up and down stairs. Sit or lie down at the first sign of dizziness.

☐ Do not drink alcoholic beverages while taking this drug without the approval of your doctor.

☐ It is important that you obtain the advice of your doctor or pharmacist before taking ANY other medicines including pain relievers, sleeping pills, tranquilizers or medicines for depression, cough/cold medicines, or allergy medicines.

☐ If you are taking this medicine to help you sleep, take it about 20 minutes before you want to go to sleep. Go to bed after you have taken it. Do not smoke in bed after you have taken it.

☐ Call your doctor immediately if you think you may be allergic to the medicine or if you develop a skin rash, hives, itching, swelling of the face, or difficulty in breathing. If you cannot reach your doctor, phone a hospital emergency department.

☐ Most people experience few or no side effects from their drugs. However, any medicine can sometimes cause unwanted effects. Call your doctor if you develop slow heartbeats, bothersome sleepiness or laziness during the day, stomach pain, vomiting, or unusual nervousness.

* * * * *

Chloral Hydrate (*Oral Sedative-Hypnotic*)

United States: Cohidrate, Noctec, Oradrate, SK-Chloral Hydrate, Somnos

Canada: Chloralex, Chloralvan, Noctec, Novochlorhydrate

☐ This medicine is used to cause sleep and for certain types of nervous tension.

HOW TO USE THIS MEDICINE

☐ For CAPSULES AND TABLETS

☐ Take the medicine with a full glass of water, fruit juice, milk, or ginger ale to help prevent stomach upset. This medicine must be swallowed whole.

167

☐ Do not crush, chew, or break it into pieces. (**United States:** Cohidrate, Noctec, Oradrate, SK-Chloral Hydrate, Somnos; **Canada:** Noctec, Novochlorhydrate)

☐ For LIQUID MEDICINE

    ☐ Mix each dose with a half glass of water, fruit juice, milk, or ginger ale to help prevent stomach upset. (**United States:** Somnos; **Canada:** Noctec, Novochlorhydrate)

SPECIAL INSTRUCTIONS

☐ Sleeping medicines are only useful for a short time. If used for too long, they lose their effectiveness. Do not take any more of this medicine than your doctor has prescribed, and do not stop taking this medicine suddenly without the approval of your doctor.

☐ Women who are pregnant, breast-feeding, or planning to become pregnant should tell their doctor before taking this medicine.

☐ In some people, this drug may cause dizziness or drowsiness. Do not drive a car or operate dangerous machinery or do jobs that require you to be alert until you know how you are going to react to this drug.

☐ If you become dizzy, you should be careful going up and down stairs. Sit or lie down at the first sign of dizziness.

☐ Do not drink alcoholic beverages while taking this drug without the approval of your doctor.

☐ It is important that you obtain the advice of your doctor or pharmacist before taking ANY other medicines including pain relievers, sleeping pills, tranquilizers or medicines for depression, cough/cold medicines, or allergy medicines.

☐ If you are taking this medicine to help you sleep, take it about 20 minutes before you want to go to sleep. Go to bed after you have taken it. Do not smoke in bed after you have taken it.

☐ Call your doctor immediately if you think you may be allergic to the medicine or if you develop a skin rash, hives, itching, swelling of the face, or difficulty in breathing. If you cannot reach your doctor, phone a hospital emergency department.

☐ Most people experience few or no side effects from their drugs. However, any medicine can sometimes cause unwanted effects. Call your doctor if you develop slow heartbeats, bothersome sleepiness or laziness during the day, stomach pain, vomiting, or unusual nervousness.

*   *   *   *   *

Chloral Hydrate (*Rectal Sedative-Hypnotic*)
United States: Aquachloral, Rectules

☐ This medicine is used to cause sleep and for certain types of nervous tension.

HOW TO USE THIS MEDICINE

☐ Administration of suppositories:
- Remove the wrapper from the suppository.
- Lie on your side and raise your knee to your chest.
- Insert the suppository with the tapered (pointed) end first into the rectum.
- Remain lying down for a few minutes so that the suppository will dissolve in the rectum.
- Try to avoid having a bowel movement for at least one hour so that the drug will have time to work.

☐ Store the suppositories in a cool place.

SPECIAL INSTRUCTIONS

☐ Sleeping medicines are only useful for a short time. If used for too long, they lose their effectiveness. Do not use any more of this medicine than your doctor has prescribed and do not stop using this medicine suddenly without the approval of your doctor.

☐ Women who are pregnant, breast-feeding, or planning to become pregnant should tell their doctor before taking this medicine.

☐ In some people, this drug may cause dizziness or drowsiness. Do not drive a car or operate dangerous machinery or do jobs that require you to be alert until you know how you are going to react to this drug.

☐ If you become dizzy, you should be careful going up and down stairs. Sit or lie down at the first sign of dizziness.

☐ Do not drink alcoholic beverages while taking this drug without the approval of your doctor.

☐ It is important that you obtain the advice of your doctor or pharmacist before taking ANY other medicines including pain relievers, sleeping pills, tranquilizers or medicines for depression, cough/cold medicines, or allergy medicines.

☐ If you are using this medicine to help you sleep, use it about 20 minutes before you want to go to sleep. Go to bed after you have used it. Do not smoke in bed after you have used it.

☐ Call your doctor immediately if you think you may be allergic to the medicine or if you develop a skin rash, hives, itching, swelling of the face, or difficulty in breathing. If you cannot reach your doctor, phone a hospital emergency department.

☐ Most people experience few or no side effects from their drugs. However, any medicine can sometimes cause unwanted effects. Call your doctor if you develop slow heartbeats, bothersome sleepiness or laziness during the day, rectal pain, vomiting, or unusual nervousness.

* * * * *

Chlorambucil (*Oral Antineoplastic*)
United States: Leukeran
Canada: Leukeran

☐ This medicine is used in certain medical conditions to help slow down the growth and reproduction of some of the body's cells.

HOW TO USE THIS MEDICINE
☐ It is best to take this medicine 1 hour before breakfast or 2 hours after supper in order to help prevent nausea or vomiting.

☐ It is very important that you take this medicine exactly as your doctor has prescribed and that you do not miss any doses. Try to take this medicine at the same time every day.

☐ Even if you become nauseated or lose your appetite, do not stop taking the medicine, but do check with your doctor.

☐ If you miss a dose of this medicine, do not take the missed dose and do not double your next dose. Check with your doctor.

SPECIAL INSTRUCTIONS
☐ Always keep your doctor appointments so that your doctor can watch your progress.

☐ If your doctor has prescribed some other medicines for you, it is important that you take them in the right order and that you do not miss them.

☐ Men and women should take appropriate birth control measures to avoid conception while taking this medicine.

☐ Always tell your pharmacist, dentist, and any other doctors who are treating you that you are taking this medicine. This is especially important if you plan to have surgery or any vaccinations.

☐ This is a very strong medicine and, in addition to its benefits, it may cause some unwanted effects even for a short time after you stop taking the medicine. Call your doctor if you develop unusual bruising or bleeding, sore throat, fever or mouth sores, or a skin rash.

* * * * *

Chloramphenicol (*Oral Antibiotic*)

United States: Amphicol, Chloromycetin, Mychel

Canada: Chloromycetin, Novochlorocap

☐ This medicine is an antibiotic used to treat certain types of infections.

HOW TO USE THIS MEDICINE

☐ It is best to take this medicine on an empty stomach 1 hour before (or 2 hours after) eating food unless otherwise directed. Take it with a full glass of water.

☐ For LIQUID MEDICINE

    ☐ Shake the bottle well before using so that you can measure an accurate dose. (**United States** and **Canada:** Chloromycetin Palmitate Suspension)

SPECIAL INSTRUCTIONS

☐ It is important to take **all** of this medicine plus any refills that your doctor told you to take. Do not stop taking it earlier than your doctor has recommended in spite of the fact that you may feel better. Otherwise, the infection may return.

☐ If you forget to take a dose, take it as soon as you remember and then continue with your regular schedule.

☐ Women who are pregnant, breast-feeding, or planning to become pregnant should tell their doctor before taking this medicine.

☐ Most people experience few or no side effects from their drugs. However, any medicine may sometimes cause unwanted effects. Call your doctor if you develop easy bruising, eye pain, blurred vision, numbness, pain or weakness of the hands or feet, fever, or sore throat. These effects may occur weeks after you have stopped taking this medicine.

☐ If this medicine is for a newborn or premature infant, call your doctor immediately if the baby develops a grey skin color, bloated stomach, low body temperature, uneven breathing, or extreme sleepiness.

☐ If for some reason you cannot take all of the medicine, discard the unused portion by flushing it down the toilet. Do not take or save old medicine.

*   *   *   *   *

Chloramphenicol (*Eye-Ear Antibiotic*)

United States: Chloromycetin Ophthalmic, Chloroptic, Chloroptic S.O.P., Econochlor Ophthalmic, Ophthochlor

Canada: Chloromycetin Ophthalmic, Chloromycetin Otic, Chloroptic, Fenicol, Isopto Fenicol, Nova-Phenicol Ophthalmic, Pentamycetin Ophthalmic, Pentamycetin Otic, Sopamycetin Ophthalmic, Sopamycetin Otic

☐ This medicine is an antibiotic used to treat certain types of eye and ear infections.

HOW TO USE THIS MEDICINE

☐ For EYE DROPS

INSTILLATION OF EYE DROPS

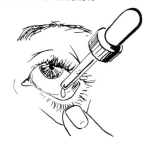

- The person administering the eye drops should wash his hands with soap and water.
- The eye drops must be kept clean. Do not touch the dropper against the face or anything else.
- Lie down or tilt your head backward and look at the ceiling.
- Gently pull down the lower lid of your eye to form a pouch.
- Hold the dropper in your other hand and approach the eye from the side. Place the dropper as close to the eye as possible without touching it.
- Place the prescribed number of drops into the pouch of the eye.
- Close your eyes. Do not rub them.
- Apply gentle pressure for a minute with your fingers to the bridge of the nose (inside corner of the eye) to prevent the eye drops from being drained from the eye.
- Blot excess solution around the eye with a tissue.
- If necessary, have someone else administer the eye drops for you.
- Do not use the eye drops if they change in color or change in any way since being purchased.
- Keep the eye drop bottle tightly closed when not in use.

☐ For EYE OINTMENT

INSTILLATION OF EYE OINTMENT

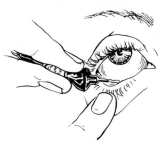

- The person administering the eye ointment should wash his hands with soap and water.
- The eye ointment must be kept clean. Do not touch the tube against the face or anything else.
- Lie down or tilt your head backward and look at the ceiling.
- Gently pull down the lower lid of your eye to form a pouch.
- Hold the tube in your other hand and place the tube as close as possible to the eye without touching it.
- Squeeze the prescribed amount of ointment (usually $\frac{1}{2}$ inch in adults) from the tube along the pouch.
- Close your eyes. Do not rub them.
- Wipe off any excess ointment around the eye with a tissue.
- Clean the tip of the ointment tube with a tissue.
- If necessary, have someone else administer the eye ointment for you.
- Keep the eye ointment tube tightly closed when not in use.

☐ For EAR DROPS

INSTILLATION OF EAR DROPS

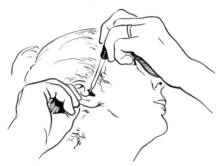

- Warm the ear drops to body temperature by holding the bottle in your hands for a few minutes. Do NOT heat the drops in hot water.
- The person administering the ear drops should wash his hands with soap and water.
- The ear drops must be kept clean. Do not touch the dropper against the ear or anything else.
- Tilt your head or lie on your side so that the ear to be treated is facing up.
- In ADULTS, hold the ear lobe up and back.
  In CHILDREN, hold the ear lobe down and back.
- Place the prescribed number of drops into the ear. Do not insert the dropper into the ear as it may cause injury.
- Remain in the same position for a short time (2 minutes) after you have administered the drops.
- Dry the ear lobe if there are any drops on it.
- If necessary, have someone else administer the ear drops for you.
- Do not use the ear drops if they change in color or change in any way since being purchased.
- Keep the bottle tightly closed when not in use.

☐ Do not use the drug more frequently or in larger quantities than prescribed by your doctor.

SPECIAL INSTRUCTIONS

☐ Vision may be blurred for a few minutes after using the eye medicine. Do not drive a car or operate dangerous machinery or do jobs that require you to be alert until your vision has cleared.

☐ It is important to use **all** of this medicine, plus any refills that your doctor told you to use. Do not stop using it earlier than your doctor has recommended in spite of the fact that your symptoms seem to have improved. Otherwise, the infection may return.

☐ If you forget to use the medicine, use it as soon as possible. However, if it is almost time for your next dose, do not use the missed dose but continue with your regular schedule.

☐ Do not use this medicine at the same time as any other eye or ear medicine without the approval of your doctor. Some medicines cannot be mixed.

☐ Call your doctor if the condition for which you are using this medicine persists or becomes worse or if the medicine causes itching or burning for more than a few minutes after instillation. Also call your doctor if you develop a sore throat, fever, mouth sores, or changes in vision.

☐ For external use only. Do not swallow.

* * * * *

Chloramphenicol (*Topical Antibiotic*)
United States: Chloromycetin Cream
Canada: Chloromycetin Cream

☐ This medicine is an antibiotic used to treat infections of the skin.

HOW TO USE THIS MEDICINE

☐ • Each time you apply the medicine, wash your hands and gently cleanse the skin area well with water unless otherwise directed by your doctor.
• Do not allow the skin to dry completely. Pat dry with a clean towel until almost dry.
• Apply a small amount of the drug to the affected area and spread lightly. Only the medicine that is actually touching the skin will work. A thick layer is not more effective than a thin layer. Do not bandage unless directed by your doctor.

☐ Do not use the drug more frequently or in larger quantities than prescribed by your doctor.

174

SPECIAL INSTRUCTIONS

☐ It is important to use *all* of this medicine, plus any refills that your doctor told you to use. Do not stop using it earlier than your doctor has recommended in spite of the fact that your symptoms seem to have improved. Otherwise, the infection may return.

☐ If you forget to apply the medicine, apply it as soon as possible. However, if it is almost time for your next dose, do not apply the missed dose but continue with your regular schedule.

☐ Do not apply cosmetics or lotions on top of the drug unless your doctor approves.

☐ Keep this preparation away from the eyes. If you should accidentally get some in your eyes, wash it away with water immediately.

☐ Call your doctor if the condition for which this drug is being used persists or becomes worse, or if you develop a constant irritation such as itching or burning that was not present before you started using this medicine. Also call your doctor if you develop a rash, redness, or swelling.

☐ For external use only. Do not swallow.

*   *   *   *   *

Chlordantoin (*Vaginal Candidiasis Therapy*)
United States: Sporostacin

☐ This medicine is used to treat infections of the vagina.

HOW TO USE THIS MEDICINE

☐ Use this medicine every morning and every evening for 2 weeks unless otherwise prescribed by your doctor.

☐ For VAGINAL CREAM
     • Remove the cap from the tube of medicine.
     • Screw the applicator to the tube.

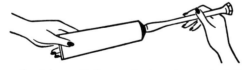

     • Squeeze the tube until the applicator plunger is fully extended. The applicator will now be filled with medicine.

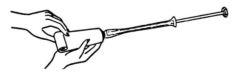

- Unscrew the applicator from the tube of medicine.
- Hold the applicator by the cylinder and gently insert it into the vaginal canal as far as it will comfortably go.
- While still holding the cylinder, gently press the plunger and deposit the medicine.

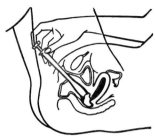

- While keeping the plunger depressed, remove the applicator from the vaginal canal.
- After each use, take the applicator apart and wash it thoroughly with warm water and soap. Reassemble the applicator.

SPECIAL INSTRUCTIONS

☐ It is important to use **all** of this medicine, plus any refills that your doctor told you to use. Do not stop using it earlier than your doctor has recommended in spite of the fact that your symptoms seem to have improved. Otherwise, the infection may return.

☐ If you forget to apply the medicine, apply it as soon as possible. However, if it is almost time for your next dose, do not apply the missed dose, but continue with your regular schedule.

☐ For external use only. Do not swallow.

☐ Consult your doctor if the condition for which this medicine is being used persists or becomes worse, or if the medicine causes an irritation such as itching or burning.

*   *   *   *   *

Chlordiazepoxide HCl (*Oral Antianxiety Agent*)

United States: Librium, Libritabs, SK-Lygen

Canada: Corax, C-Tran, Librium, Medilium, Nack, Novopoxide, Relaxil, Solium, Trilium

☐ This medicine is used to help relieve anxiety and tension. It is also used to help relax muscles as well as to treat some other conditions. Check with your doctor if you do not fully understand why you are taking it.

☐ IMPORTANT: If you have ever had an allergic reaction to a benzodiazepine medicine, tell your doctor or pharmacist before you take any of this medicine.

176

HOW TO USE THIS MEDICINE

□ This medicine may be taken with food or a full glass of water.

SPECIAL INSTRUCTIONS

□ If you forget to take a dose, take it as soon as possible. However, if it is almost time for your next dose, do not take the missed dose. Instead, continue with your regular dosing schedule.

□ Women who are pregnant, breast-feeding, or planning to become pregnant should tell their doctor before taking this medicine.

□ In some people, this drug may cause dizziness or drowsiness. Do not drive a car or operate dangerous machinery or do jobs that require you to be alert until you know how you are going to react to this drug.

□ If you become dizzy, you should be careful going up and down stairs. Sit or lie down at the first sign of dizziness.

□ Do not drink alcoholic beverages while taking this drug without the approval of your doctor.

□ It is important that you obtain the advice of your doctor or pharmacist before taking ANY other medicines including pain relievers, sleeping pills, tranquilizers or medicines for depression, cough/cold or allergy medicines, or weight-reducing medicines.

□ Do not take any more of this medicine than your doctor has prescribed. The drug could become habit-forming. Do not stop taking this medicine suddenly without the approval of your doctor.

□ Most people experience few or no side effects from their drugs. However, any medicine can sometimes cause unwanted effects. Call your doctor if you develop a sore throat, fever, mouth sores, a staggering walk, a yellow color to the skin or eyes, slow heartbeats or shortness of breath, unusual tiredness or nervousness, or stomach pain.

*　*　*　*　*

Chlordiazepoxide-Clidinium (*Oral Anticholinergic-Anxiolytic*)
United States: Clipoxide, Librax, Lidinium
Canada: Librax

□ This medicine is used to treat stomach and bowel conditions.

□ IMPORTANT: If you have ever had an allergic reaction to a benzodiazepine medicine, tell your doctor or pharmacist before you take any of this medicine.

177

HOW TO USE THIS MEDICINE

☐ This medicine may be taken with food or a full glass of water $\frac{1}{2}$ hour to 1 hour before meals unless otherwise directed.

SPECIAL INSTRUCTIONS

☐ If you forget to take a dose of this medicine and do not remember to take it right away, do not take the missed dose but continue with your regular schedule.

☐ Women who are pregnant, breast-feeding, or planning to become pregnant should tell their doctor before taking this medicine.

☐ In some people, this drug may cause dizziness or drowsiness. Do not drive a car or operate dangerous machinery or do jobs that require you to be alert until you know how you are going to react to this drug.

☐ If you become dizzy, you should be careful going up and down stairs. Sit or lie down at the first sign of dizziness.

☐ Do not drink alcoholic beverages while taking this drug without the approval of your doctor.

☐ It is important that you obtain the advice of your doctor or pharmacist before taking ANY other medicines including pain relievers, sleeping pills, tranquilizers or medicines for depression, cough/cold or allergy medicines, or weight-reducing medicines.

☐ If your mouth becomes dry, suck a hard sour candy (sugarless) or ice chips, or chew gum. It is especially important to brush your teeth regularly if you develop a dry mouth.

☐ Do not take any more of this medicine than your doctor has prescribed and do not stop taking this medicine suddenly without the approval of your doctor.

☐ Most people experience few or no side effects from their drugs. However, any medicine can sometimes cause unwanted effects. Call your doctor if you develop a sore throat, fever, mouth sores, a staggering walk, a yellow color to the skin or eyes, slow heartbeats or shortness of breath, unusual tiredness or nervousness or stomach pain, difficulty in urinating ("passing your water"), or constipation.

*   *   *   *   *

Chlormezanone (*Oral Antianxiety-Muscle Relaxant*)
United States: Trancopal
Canada: Trancopal

☐ This medicine is used to help relieve anxiety and tension as well as to treat some other conditions. Check with your doctor if you do not fully understand why you are taking it.

178

☐ IMPORTANT: If you have ever had an allergic reaction to meprobamate medicines, tell your doctor or pharmacist before you take any of this medicine.

HOW TO USE THIS MEDICINE

☐ This medicine may be taken with food or a full glass of water.

SPECIAL INSTRUCTIONS

☐ If you forget to take a dose, take it as soon as possible. However, if it is almost time for your next dose, do not take the missed dose. Instead, continue with your regular dosing schedule.

☐ In some people, this drug may cause dizziness or drowsiness. Do not drive a car or operate dangerous machinery or do jobs that require you to be alert until you know how you are going to react to this drug.

☐ If you become dizzy, you should be careful going up and down stairs. Sit or lie down at the first sign of dizziness.

☐ Do not drink alcoholic beverages while taking this drug without the approval of your doctor.

☐ It is important that you obtain the advice of your doctor or pharmacist before taking ANY other medicines including pain relievers, sleeping pills, tranquilizers or medicines for depression, cough/cold or allergy medicines, or weight-reducing medicines.

☐ Do not take any more of this medicine than your doctor has prescribed and do not stop taking this medicine suddenly without the approval of your doctor.

☐ Most people experience few or no side effects from their drugs. However, any medicine can sometimes cause unwanted effects. Call your doctor if you develop a skin rash, sore throat, fever, dark-colored urine or a yellow color to the skin or eyes, difficulty in urinating ("passing your water"), or unusual tiredness.

*   *   *   *   *

Chlorophenoxamine HCl (*Oral Parkinsonism Therapy*)
United States: Phenoxene
Canada: Phenoxene

☐ This medicine is used to improve muscle control and relieve muscle spasm in Parkinson's disease and certain other medical conditions

HOW TO USE THIS MEDICINE

☐ Take this medicine with food or immediately after meals to help prevent stomach upset unless otherwise directed.

179

☐ If you forget to take a dose, take it as soon as possible. However, if it is almost time for your next dose, do not take the missed dose. Instead, continue with your regular dosing schedule.

SPECIAL INSTRUCTIONS

☐ If your mouth becomes dry, suck a hard sour candy (sugarless) or ice chips, or chew gum. It is especially important to brush your teeth regularly if you develop a dry mouth.

☐ In some people, this drug may cause dizziness, drowsiness, or blurred vision during the first 2 weeks of using this drug. This will usually go away as your body adjusts to this medicine. Do not drive a car or operate dangerous machinery or do jobs that require you to be alert until you know how you are going to react to this drug.

☐ If you become dizzy, you should be careful going up and down stairs. Sit or lie down at the first sign of dizziness.

☐ A desire to urinate ("pass your water") with an inability to do so is not an uncommon effect with this drug. Urinating each time before the drug is taken may help relieve this problem. Call your doctor if it continues.

☐ Do not drink alcoholic beverages while taking this drug without the approval of your doctor.

☐ If you become constipated, try increasing the amount of bulk in your diet (for example, bran and salads), exercising more often, or drinking more water. Call your doctor if the constipation continues.

☐ It is important that you obtain the advice of your doctor or pharmacist before taking pain relievers, nonprescription drugs, sleeping pills, tranquilizers, or medicine for depression while you are taking this drug.

☐ Most people experience few or no side effects from their drugs. However, any medicine can sometimes cause unwanted effects. Call your doctor if you develop a skin rash, eye pain, dizziness or fainting, or fast heartbeats, or if you become confused.

*　*　*　*　*

Chloroquine Phosphate (*Oral Antimalarial-Antiparasitic*)
United States: Aralen
Canada: Aralen

☐ This medicine has many uses and the reason it was prescribed depends upon your condition. If you do not understand why you are taking it, check with your doctor.

HOW TO USE THIS MEDICINE

☐ Take this medicine immediately before or after meals or with food in order to help prevent stomach upset.

☐ It is very important that you take this medicine exactly as your doctor has prescribed and that you do not miss any doses. Try to take this medicine at the same time every day. Do not take extra tablets without your doctor's approval. Take the medicine for the full treatment.

SPECIAL INSTRUCTIONS

☐ If you forget to take a dose, take it as soon as possible. However, if it is almost time for your next dose, do not take the missed dose. Instead, continue with your regular dosing schedule.

☐ Women who are pregnant, breast-feeding, or planning to become pregnant should tell their doctor before taking this medicine.

☐ This medicine may cause the urine to turn rusty-yellow or brown in color. This is not unusual.

☐ If you find that your eyes become more sensitive to light, it may help to wear sunglasses.

☐ Most people experience few or no side effects from their drugs. However, any medicine can sometimes cause unwanted effects. Call your doctor if you develop muscle weakness, blurred vision, night blindness or any changes in eyesight or hearing, a skin rash, sore throat, fever or mouth sores, blue-black color to skin or nails, numbness or tingling in the hands or feet, or unusual bruising or bleeding.

☐ Keep this medicine well out of the reach of children.

* * * * *

Chlorothiazide (*Oral Diuretic*)
United States: Diuril, Ro-Chlorozide
Canada: Diuril

☐ This medicine is used to help rid the body of excess water and to decrease swelling. It is also used to treat high blood pressure. It is commonly called a "water pill."

☐ IMPORTANT: If you have ever had an allergic reaction to sulfa drugs or thiazide diuretics, tell your doctor or pharmacist before taking any of this medicine.

HOW TO USE THIS MEDICINE

☐ Take the medicine with food, meals, or milk.

□ Try to take it at the same time(s) every day so that you have a constant level of the medicine in your body. Do not miss any doses. Otherwise, you cannot expect the drug to work as well.

□ When you first start taking this medicine, you will probably urinate ("pass your water") more often and in larger amounts than usual. Therefore, if you are to take one dose every day, take it in the morning after breakfast. If you are to take more than one dose every day, take the last dose 6 hours before bedtime so that you will not have to get up during the night to go to the bathroom. This effect will usually lessen after you have taken the drug for awhile.

□ Shake the bottle well before using in order to measure an accurate dose. (**United States:** Diuril Suspension)

SPECIAL INSTRUCTIONS

□ If you forget to take a dose, take it as soon as possible. However, if it is almost time for your next dose, do not take the missed dose. Instead, continue with your regular dosing schedule.

□ Women who are pregnant, breast-feeding, or planning to become pregnant should tell their doctor before taking this medicine.

□ This medicine normally causes your body to lose potassium. The body has warning signs to let you know if too much potassium is being lost. Call your doctor if you become unusually thirsty or if you develop leg cramps, unusual weakness, fatigue, vomiting, confusion, or irregular pulse.

□ If your doctor recommends that you eat foods that are high in potassium, one or more of the foods listed in Appendix A should be eaten daily. All of these foods are rich in potassium. Your goal should be to take in 1000 to 2000 mg. of potassium (approximately 25.6 to 51 mEq) each day. The calorie content and sodium content are included for your convenience in meal planning. CHANGE YOUR DIET ONLY IF YOUR DOCTOR TELLS YOU TO.

□ If this medicine causes dizziness, you should be careful going up and down stairs and you should not change positions too rapidly. Get out of bed slowly in the morning and dangle your feet over the edge of the bed for a few minutes before standing up. Sit down or lie down at the first sign of dizziness. Tell your doctor you have been dizzy. Be careful drinking alcoholic beverages while taking this medicine because it could make the dizziness worse. Do not drive a car or operate dangerous machinery or do jobs that require you to be alert if you are dizzy.

□ In order to help prevent dizziness and fainting, your doctor may also recommend that you avoid strenuous exercises, standing for long periods of time (especially in hot weather), or hot showers or hot baths.

□ This medicine may make some people more sensitive to sunlight and sunlamps. When you begin taking this medicine, try to avoid too much sun until you see how you are going to react. If your skin does become more sensitive to sunlight, tell your doctor and try to stay out of direct sunlight. While in the sun, wear protective clothing and sunglasses. You may wish to ask your pharmacist about suitable sunscreen products. Check with your doctor if you become sunburned.

☐ Call your doctor immediately if you think you may be allergic to the medicine or if you develop a skin rash, hives, itching, swelling of the face, or difficulty in breathing. If you cannot reach your doctor, phone a hospital emergency department.

☐ Most people experience few or no side effects from their drugs. However, any medicine can sometimes cause unwanted effects. Call your doctor if you develop a sore throat, fever, sharp stomach pain, chest pain, sharp joint pain, easy bruising or bleeding, a yellow color to the skin or eyes, or a sudden weight gain of 5 pounds or more.

*   *   *   *   *

Chlorotrianisene (Oral Estrogen)
United States: Tace
Canada: Tace

☐ This medicine is a hormone. It has many uses and the reason it was prescribed depends on your condition. If you do not understand why you are taking it, check with your doctor.

HOW TO USE THIS MEDICINE
☐ The tablets may be taken after meals or with a snack if they upset your stomach.

SPECIAL INSTRUCTIONS
☐ Women who are pregnant, breast-feeding, or planning to become pregnant should tell their doctor before taking this medicine.

☐ It is recommended that you do not smoke while you are taking this medicine because smoking may increase the incidence of heart attacks.

☐ Diabetic patients should regularly check the sugar in their urine while they are taking this medicine.

☐ Contact your doctor if any of the following side effects occur:
  • Severe or persistent headaches
  • Vomiting, dizziness, or fainting
  • Blurred vision or slurred speech
  • Pain in the calves of the legs or numbness in an arm or leg
  • Chest pain, shortness of breath, or coughing of blood
  • Lumps in the breast

- Severe depression
- A yellow color to the skin or eyes or dark-colored urine
- Severe abdominal pain
- Breakthrough vaginal bleeding

☐ Carry an identification card indicating that you are taking this medicine. Always tell your pharmacist, dentist, and other doctors who are treating you that you are taking this medicine.

* * * * *

Chlorphenesin Carbamate (*Oral Skeletal Muscle Relaxant*)
United States: Maolate

☐ This medicine is used to relax muscles and helps to relieve muscle pain and stiffness.

☐ IMPORTANT: If you have ever had an allergic reaction to any medicines, tell your doctor or pharmacist before you take any of this medicine.

HOW TO USE THIS MEDICINE
☐ This medicine may be taken with food or a glass of water.

☐ If you forget to take a dose, take it as soon as possible. However, if it is almost time for your next dose, do not take the missed dose. Instead, continue with your regular dosing schedule.

SPECIAL INSTRUCTIONS
☐ Do not drink alcoholic beverages while taking this drug without the approval of your doctor.

☐ It is important that you obtain the advice of your doctor or pharmacist before taking ANY other medicines including pain relievers, sleeping pills, tranquilizers or medicine for depression, cough/cold medicines, or allergy medicines.

☐ In some people, this drug may cause dizziness or drowsiness. Do not drive a car or operate dangerous machinery or do jobs that require you to be alert until you know how you are going to react to this drug.

☐ If you become dizzy, you should be careful going up and down stairs. Sit or lie down at the first sign of dizziness.

☐ Call your doctor immediately if you think you may be allergic to the medicine or if you develop a skin rash, hives, itching, swelling of the face, or difficulty in breathing. If you cannot reach your doctor, phone a hospital emergency department.

☐ Most people experience few or no side effects from their drugs. However, any medicine can sometimes cause unwanted effects. Call your doctor if you develop a sore throat, fever or mouth sores, easy bruising or bleeding, unusual tiredness, stomach pain, or unusual nervousness.

* * * * *

Chlorphenesin (*Topical Fungicide*)
Canada: Mycil

☐ This medicine is used to treat fungal infections of the feet and skin.

HOW TO USE THIS MEDICINE
☐ For CREAM
   • Clean affected area well with soap and water and dry thoroughly. Apply cream to affected areas.
☐ For POWDER
   • Dust the powder into socks and shoes or on body as required.

SPECIAL INSTRUCTIONS
☐ It is important to use **all** of this medicine, plus any refills that your doctor told you to use. Do not stop using it earlier than your doctor has recommended in spite of the fact that your symptoms seem to have improved. Otherwise, the infection may return.

☐ If you forget to apply the medicine, apply it as soon as possible. However, if it is almost time for your next dose, do not apply the missed dose but continue with your regular schedule.

☐ If you have a fungal infection of the feet, it is important to dry the feet (especially between the toes) well after washing.

☐ Do not apply cosmetics or lotions on top of the drug unless your doctor approves.

☐ Keep this preparation away from the eyes. If you should accidentally get some in your eyes, wash it away with water immediately.

☐ Call your doctor if the condition for which this drug is being used persists or becomes worse or if you develop a constant irritation such as itching or burning that was not present before you started using this medicine.

☐ For external use only. Do not swallow.

* * * * *

Chlorpheniramine Maleate (*Oral Antihistamine*)

United States: Allerbid, Tymcaps, Chlor-Trimeton, Histaspan, Teldrin

Canada: Chlor-Tripolon, Histalon, Novopheniram

Chlorpheniramine Maleate-Phenylephrine

United States: Demazin Repetabs, Histaspan-Plus, Novahistine LP

Canada: Histaspan-P

☐ This medicine is used to help relieve the symptoms of certain types of allergic conditions, coughs and colds, and certain skin conditions.

HOW TO USE THIS MEDICINE

☐ This medicine may be taken with food or a glass of milk if it upsets your stomach.

☐ This medicine must be swallowed whole. It must not be chewed, crushed, or broken into pieces. (**United States:** Allerbid Tymcaps, Chlor-Trimeton Repetabs, Histaspan, Teldrin Spansules; **Canada:** Chlor-Tripolon Repetabs, Histaspan-P)

SPECIAL INSTRUCTIONS

☐ If you forget to take a dose, take it as soon as possible. However, if it is almost time for your next dose, do not take the missed dose. Instead, continue with your regular dosing schedule.

☐ In some people, this drug may initially cause dizziness or drowsiness. Do not drive a car or operate dangerous machinery or do jobs that require you to be alert until you know how you are going to react to this drug. If you become dizzy, you should be careful going up and down stairs. Sit or lie down at the first sign of dizziness. Tell your doctor if it continues.

☐ Do not drink alcoholic beverages while taking this drug without the approval of your doctor.

☐ If your mouth becomes dry, suck a hard sour candy (sugarless) or ice chips, or chew gum. It is especially important to brush your teeth regularly if you develop a dry mouth.

☐ It is important that you obtain the advice of your doctor or pharmacist before taking pain relievers, nonprescription drugs, sleeping pills or tranquilizers, or other medicines for allergies.

☐ Do not take this medicine more often or longer than recommended by your doctor.

☐ Most people exerience few or no side effects from their drugs. However, any medicine can sometimes cause unwanted effects. Call your doctor if you develop a skin rash, fast heartbeats, blurred vision, stomach pain, or difficulty in urinating ("passing your water").

* * * * *

Chlorpheniramine-Phenylpropanolamine-Isopropamide *(Oral Nasal Decongestant)*
United States: Ornade

Chlorpheniramine-Phenylpropanolamine
Canada: Ornade

☐ This medicine is used to help relieve nasal stuffiness and to treat allergies.

HOW TO USE THIS MEDICINE
☐ This medicine may be taken with food if it upsets your stomach.

☐ These capsules must be swallowed whole. Do not crush, chew, or break them into pieces.

SPECIAL INSTRUCTIONS
☐ Women who are pregnant, breast-feeding, or planning to become pregnant should tell their doctor before taking this medicine.

☐ If you forget to take a dose, take it as soon as possible. However, if it is almost time for your next dose, do not take the missed dose. Instead, continue with your regular dosing schedule.

☐ In some people, this drug may initially cause dizziness or drowsiness. Do not drive a car or operate dangerous machinery or do jobs that require you to be alert until you know how you are going to react to this drug. If you become dizzy, you should be careful going up and down stairs. Sit or lie down at the first sign of dizziness. Tell your doctor if it continues.

☐ Do not drink alcoholic beverages while taking this drug without the approval of your doctor.

☐ If your mouth becomes dry, suck a hard sour candy (sugarless) or ice chips, or chew gum. It is especially important to brush your teeth regularly if you develop a dry mouth.

☐ It is important that you obtain the advice of your doctor or pharmacist before taking pain relievers, nonprescription drugs, sleeping pills or tranquilizers, or other medicines for allergies.

☐ Do not take this medication more often or longer than recommended by your doctor.

☐ Do not use this medicine for longer than 7 days without the approval of your doctor.

☐ Most people experience few or no side effects from their drugs. However, any medicine can sometimes cause unwanted effects. Call your doctor if you develop a skin rash, fast heartbeats, blurred vision, stomach pain, or difficulty in urinating ("passing your water").

*   *   *   *   *

Chlorphentermine HCl (*Oral Anorexiant*)

United States: Chlorophen, Pre-Sate, Teramine
Canada: Pre-Sate

☐ This medicine is used to help reduce the appetite in weight reduction programs. It can help you develop new eating habits and is only useful for a short time. Do not take any more of this medicine than your doctor has prescribed, and do not stop taking this medicine suddenly without the approval of your doctor.

HOW TO USE THIS MEDICINE

☐ This medicine may be taken with a glass of water.

☐ Do not take the medicine late in the day or it may cause insomnia (difficulty in sleeping).

SPECIAL INSTRUCTIONS

☐ If you forget to take a dose, take it as soon as possible. However, if it is almost time for your next dose, do not take the missed dose. Instead, continue with your regular dosing schedule.

☐ It is very important that you follow the diet prescribed by your doctor.

☐ If your mouth becomes dry, suck a hard sour candy (sugarless) or ice chips, or chew gum. It is especially important to brush your teeth regularly if you develop a dry mouth.

☐ In some people, this drug may cause dizziness. Do not drive a car or operate dangerous machinery or do jobs that require you to be alert until you know how you are going to react to this drug. Therefore, you should be careful going up and down stairs. Sit or lie down at the first sign of dizziness.

☐ Most people experience few or no side effects from their drugs. However, any medicine can sometimes cause unwanted effects. Call your doctor if you develop a skin rash, sore throat, fever, mouth sores, unusual nervousness, difficulty in urinating ("passing your water"), or palpitations, or if you become depressed.

☐ Carry an identification card indicating that you are taking this medicine. Always tell your pharmacist, dentist, and other doctors who are treating you that you are taking this medicine.

* * * * *

Chlorpromazine HCl (*Oral Antipsychotic-Antiemetic-Antianxiety*)

United States: Chlor-PZ, Promachel, Promapar, Sonazine, Thorazine
Canada: Chlorprom, Chlor-Promanyl, Largactil

- This medicine is used to help relieve the symptoms of certain types of emotional problems. This drug has several other uses and the reason it was prescribed depends upon your condition. Check with your doctor if you do not fully understand why you are taking it.

- IMPORTANT: If you have ever had an allergic reaction to a phenothiazine medicine, tell your doctor or pharmacist before you take any of this medicine.

HOW TO USE THIS MEDICINE

- This medicine may be taken with food or a full glass of water.

- Do not take this medicine at the same time as antacids or diarrhea medicine. Try to space them at least 1 hour apart.

- If a dropper is used to measure the dose and you do not fully understand how to use it, check with your pharmacist. (**Canada:** Largactil Oral Drops)

- Store the liquid medicines in a cool, dark place and do not get the liquid on your skin or clothing.

- These capsules must be swallowed whole. Do not open the capsules. (**United States:** Thorazine Spansules; **Canada:** Largactil Spansules)

- Do not stop taking this medicine suddenly without the approval of your doctor.

SPECIAL INSTRUCTIONS

- If your forget to take a dose, take it as soon as possible. However, if it is almost time for your next dose, do not take the missed dose. Instead, continue with your regular dosing schedule.

- Any medicine has a few unwanted side effects. Because this medicine takes a few weeks to work, the side effects show the doctor that the drug is being absorbed. Many of these side effects will go away as your body adjusts to the medicine.

- Women who are pregnant, breast-feeding, or planning to become pregnant should tell their doctor before taking this medicine.

- In some people, this drug may cause dizziness or drowsiness. Do not drive a car or operate dangerous machinery or do jobs that require you to be alert until you know how you are going to react to this drug.

- If this medicine causes dizziness, you should be careful going up and down stairs and you should not change positions too rapidly. Get out of bed slowly in the morning and dangle your feet over the edge of the bed for a few minutes before standing up. Sit down or lie down at the first sign of dizziness. Tell your doctor you have been dizzy. Avoid hot showers and baths because they could make you dizzy.

- Do not drink alcoholic beverages while taking this drug without the approval of your doctor.

- [ ] This medicine may make some people more sensitive to sunlight and sunlamps. When you begin taking this medicine, try to avoid getting too much sun until you see how you are going to react. If your skin does become more sensitive to sunlight, tell your doctor and try to stay out of direct sunlight. While in the sun, wear protective clothing and sunglasses. You may wish to ask your pharmacist about suitable sunscreen products. Check with your doctor if you become sunburned.

- [ ] If your mouth becomes dry, suck a hard sour candy (sugarless) or ice chips, or chew gum. It is especially important to brush your teeth regularly if you develop a dry mouth.

- [ ] It is important that you obtain the advice of your doctor or pharmacist before taking *any* other medicines including pain relievers, sleeping pills, other tranquilizers or medicines for depression, cough, cold or allergy medicines, weight-reducing medicines, or laxatives.

- [ ] This medicine may cause your urine to turn pink, red, or red-brown in color. This is not unusual.

- [ ] In hot weather or during exercise, be careful not to become overheated. You may be more sensitive to heat since this medicine may affect your body's ability to regulate temperature.

- [ ] If you become constipated, try increasing the amount of bulk in your diet (for example, bran and salads), exercising more often, or drinking more water. Call your doctor if the constipation continues.

- [ ] Call your doctor if you develop a sore throat, fever, mouth sores, skin rash, changes in eyesight, rapid heartrate, a yellow color in the eyes or skin, unusual weakness or unusual movements of the face, tongue, or hands, or difficulty in urinating ("passing your water"). Also call your doctor if you become restless or unable to sit still or sleep.

- [ ] Carry an identification card indicating that you are taking this medicine. Always tell your pharmacist, dentist, and other doctors who are treating you that you are taking this medicine.

* * * * *

Chlorpromazine HCl (*Rectal Antipsychotic-Antiemetic-Antianxiety*)

United States: Thorazine
Canada: Largactil

- [ ] This medicine is used to help relieve the symptoms of certain types of emotional problems. This drug has several other uses and the reason it was prescribed depends upon your condition. Check with your doctor if you do not fully understand why you are taking it.

190

☐ IMPORTANT: If you have ever had an allergic reaction to a phenothiazine medicine, tell your doctor or pharmacist before you take any of this medicine.

HOW TO USE THIS MEDICINE

☐ Administration of SUPPOSITORIES
- Remove the wrapper from the suppository.
- Lie on your side and raise your knee to your chest.
- Insert the suppository with the tapered (pointed) end first into the rectum.
- Remain lying down for a few minutes so that the suppository will dissolve in the rectum.
- Try to avoid having a bowel movement for at least one hour so that the drug will have time to work.

☐ Store the suppositories in a cool place.

☐ Do not stop using this medicine suddenly without the approval of your doctor.

SPECIAL INSTRUCTIONS

☐ If you forget to use a dose, use it as soon as possible. However, if it is almost time for your next dose, do not use the missed dose. Instead, continue with your regular dosing schedule.

☐ Any medicine has a few unwanted side effects. Because this medicine takes a few weeks to work, the side effects show the doctor that the drug is being absorbed. Many of these side effects will go away as your body adjusts to the medicine.

☐ Women who are pregnant, breast-feeding, or planning to become pregnant should tell their doctor before taking this medicine.

☐ In some people, this drug may cause dizziness or drowsiness. Do not drive a car or operate dangerous machinery or do jobs that require you to be alert until you know how you are going to react to this drug.

☐ If this medicine causes dizziness, you should be careful going up and down stairs and you should not change positions too rapidly. Get out of bed slowly in the morning and dangle your feet over the edge of the bed for a few minutes before standing up. Sit down or lie down at the first sign of dizziness. Tell your doctor you have been dizzy. Avoid hot showers and baths because they could make you dizzy.

☐ Do not drink alcoholic beverages while taking this drug without the approval of your doctor.

☐ This medicine may make some people more sensitive to sunlight and sun-lamps. When you begin taking this medicine, try to avoid getting too much sun until you see how you are going to react. If your skin does become more sensitive to sunlight, tell your doctor and try to stay out of direct sunlight.

191

While in the sun, wear protective clothing and sunglasses. You may wish to ask your pharmacist about suitable sunscreen products. Check with your doctor if you become sunburned.

□ If your mouth becomes dry, suck a hard sour candy (sugarless) or ice chips, or chew gum. It is especially important to brush your teeth regularly if you develop a dry mouth.

□ It is important that you obtain the advice of your doctor or pharmacist before taking **any** other medicines including pain relievers, sleeping pills, other tranquilizers or medicines for depression, cough, cold, or allergy medicines, weight-reducing medicines, or laxatives.

□ This medicine may cause your urine to turn pink, red, or red-brown in color. This is not unusual.

□ In hot weather or during exercise, be careful not to become overheated. You may be more sensitive to heat since this medicine may affect your body's ability to regulate temperature.

□ Call your doctor if you develop a sore throat, fever, mouth sores, skin rash, changes in eyesight, rapid heartrate, a yellow color in the eyes or skin, unusual weakness or unusual movements of the face, tongue, or hands, or difficulty in urinating ("passing your water"). Also call your doctor if you become restless or unable to sit still or sleep.

□ Carry an identification card indicating that you are using this medicine. Always tell your pharmacist, dentist, and other doctors who are treating you that you are using this medicine.

*   *   *   *   *

Chlorpropamide (*Oral Hypoglycemic*)

United States: Diabinese

Canada: Chloromide, Chloronase, Diabinese, Novopropamide, Stabinol

□ This medicine is used in the treatment of diabetes. When you have diabetes, the body either is not producing enough insulin or is not able to use what is produced. Insulin is needed for the body's proper use of food, especially sugar. In a diabetic person, the sugar in the blood can build up to dangerous levels and is passed out in the urine. Your doctor has prescribed this medicine to help keep your blood sugar at nearly normal levels.

HOW TO USE THIS MEDICINE

□ This medicine may be taken with food to help prevent stomach upset.

□ It is very important that you take this medicine exactly as your doctor has prescribed. Do not miss any doses. Try to take this medicine at the same time every day. Do not take extra tablets without your doctor's approval.

☐ Do not take this medicine at bedtime unless your doctor tells you to.

☐ If you forget to take a dose, take it as soon as possible. However, if it is almost time for your next dose, do not take the missed dose. Instead, continue with your regular dosing schedule.

SPECIAL INSTRUCTIONS

☐ Women who are pregnant, breast-feeding, or planning to become pregnant should tell their doctor before taking this medicine.

☐ This medicine may make some people more sensitive to sunlight and sunlamps. When you begin taking this medicine try to avoid getting too much sun until you see how you are going to react. If your skin does become more sensitive to sunlight, tell your doctor and try to stay out of direct sunlight. While in the sun, wear protective clothing and sunglasses. You may wish to ask your pharmacist about suitable sunscreen products. Check with your doctor if you become sunburned.

☐ Most people experience few or no side effects from their drugs. However, any medicine can sometimes cause unwanted effects. Call your doctor if you develop a skin rash, sore throat, fever, mouth sores, dark-colored urine, a yellow color to the skin or eyes, easy bruising or bleeding, unusual tiredness, diarrhea or light-colored stools, swelling of the face, hands, or legs, muscle cramps, or seizures.

GENERAL INSTRUCTIONS FOR DIABETIC PATIENTS

☐ Keep a regular schedule of daily activities. Eat, exercise, and take your insulin at approximately the same time every day.

☐ The diet that your doctor has prescribed has been carefully planned especially for you. It is to your advantage to follow it very closely.

☐ Test your urine regularly for sugar and if your doctor recommends, test it for acetone.

☐ Learn the signs of hypoglycemia (low blood sugar). When this happens, your urine sugar will be negative. Hypoglycemia may occur if you delay or skip a meal, exercise too much, become sick or emotionally upset, take too much insulin, drink alcohol, or take certain drugs. If you develop sweating, drowsiness, headache, unusual hunger, dizziness, nausea, nervousness, blurred vision, weakness, or shaking or trembling, eat or drink any of the following:

  • 2 sugar cubes or 2 teaspoons of sugar in water
  • 4 ounces orange juice
  • 4 ounces regular ginger ale, cola beverage, or any other sweetened carbonated beverage. Do NOT use low-calorie or diet beverages.
  • 2 to 3 teaspoons honey or corn syrup
  • 4 Lifesaver candies

☐ Artificial sweeteners are of no use. Call your doctor if this does not relieve your symptoms in about 15 minutes.

☐ Always carry sugar cubes or hard candy in case you have a hypoglycemic (low blood sugar) reaction.

☐ Before you purchase any nonprescription medicine (for example, cough and cold medicines), ask your pharmacist if the medicine is safe for diabetic patients to use. Some nonprescription medicines have very high sugar contents which could interfere with the control of your diabetes. Aspirin and medicines containing salicylates or vitamin C could affect your urine test results. Check with your pharmacist.

☐ Ask your doctor if it is safe for you to drink alcoholic beverages because the combination may cause low blood sugar as well as a pounding headache, flushing, upset stomach, dizziness, or sweating.

☐ Take special care of your feet.
  • Wash your feet daily and dry them well.
  • Check your feet daily for minor injuries. Bring these to the attention of your doctor immediately.
  • Wear clean shoes and stockings and choose shoes that fit well.
  • If you develop corns or calluses, soak your feet in lukewarm water for about 10 minutes. Then rub them off gently with a pumice stone. Never use a knife to cut corns or calluses on your feet. Do NOT use commercial corn removers, or commercial arch supports.
  • Soften dry skin by rubbing with oil or lotion.
  • Trim your toenails straight across with a file or a nail cutter. Do not cut your own toenails if your eyesight is poor.
  • Do not wear garters or socks with tight elastic tops. Do NOT sit with your knees crossed.
  • Do not warm your feet with a hot water bottle or a heating pad. Use loose bed socks instead. If your feet are cold under normal conditions, tell your doctor. Your circulation may be poor and your doctor can offer advice.
  • Call your doctor if you injure your toes or feet. Cuts and scratches in the diabetic person can become infected easily and take longer to heal. Do not apply iodine or strong antiseptics to the feet at any time.

☐ Call your doctor immediately if you develop any of the following symptoms of hyperglycemia (high blood sugar): high urine sugar, acetone in urine, drowsiness, hunger, unusual thirst, fast breathing, nausea, confusion, a flushed dry skin, increase in urination ("passing your water"), or a fruity odor to the breath. These symptoms may occur if you are taking too little insulin, miss a dose, overeat, or if you have a fever or infection.

☐ Call your doctor if you become sick and have a fever, an infection, nausea, or vomiting.

☐ Carry an identification card or wear a bracelet indicating that you are a diabetic and that you are taking this medicine. Always tell your pharmacist, dentist, and other doctors who are treating you that you are taking this medicine.

*   *   *   *   *

Chlorprothixene (*Oral Antipsychotic-Antiemetic-Antianxiety*)
United States: Taractan
Canada: Tarasan

☐ This medicine is used to help relieve the symptoms of certain types of emotional conditions.

☐ IMPORTANT: If you have ever had an allergic reaction to a medicine that you took for the same reason, tell your doctor or pharmacist before you take any of this medicine.

HOW TO USE THIS MEDICINE

☐ This medicine may be taken with food or a full glass of water.

☐ Do not take this medicine at the same time as antacids or diarrhea medicine. Try to space them at least 1 hour apart.

☐ The effect of the medicine may not be noticed immediately, but may take from 2 to 4 weeks. Be patient. Take the medicine regularly and try not to miss any doses.

☐ Do not stop taking this medicine suddenly without the approval of your doctor.

SPECIAL INSTRUCTIONS

☐ If you forget to take a dose, take it as soon as possible. However, if it is almost time for your next dose, do not take the missed dose. Instead, continue with your regular dosing schedule.

☐ Any medicine has a few unwanted side effects. Because this medicine takes a few weeks to work, the side effects show the doctor that the drug is being absorbed. Many of these side effects will go away as your body adjusts to the medicine.

☐ In some people, this drug may cause dizziness or drowsiness. Do not drive a car or operate dangerous machinery or do jobs that require you to be alert until you know how you are going to react to this drug.

☐ If this medicine causes dizziness, you should be careful going up and down stairs and you should not change positions too rapidly. Get out of bed slowly in the morning and dangle your feet over the edge of the bed for a few minutes before standing up. Sit down or lie down at the first sign of dizziness. Tell your doctor you have been dizzy. Avoid hot showers and baths because they could make you dizzy.

☐ Do not drink alcoholic beverages while taking this drug without the approval of your doctor.

☐ This medicine may make some people more sensitive to sunlight and sunlamps. When you begin taking this medicine, try to avoid getting too much sun until you see how you are going to react. If your skin does become more sensitive to sunlight, tell your doctor and try to stay out of direct sunlight. While in the sun, wear protective clothing and sunglasses.

You may wish to ask your pharmacist about suitable sunscreen products. Check with your doctor if you become sunburned.

☐ If your mouth becomes dry, suck a hard sour candy (sugarless) or ice chips, or chew gum. It is especially important to brush your teeth regularly if you develop a dry mouth.

☐ It is important that you obtain the advice of your doctor or pharmacist before taking **any** other medicines including pain relievers, sleeping pills, other tranquilizers or medicines for depression, cough, cold, or allergy medicines, weight-reducing medicines, or laxatives.

☐ In hot weather or during exercise, be careful not to become overheated. You may be more sensitive to heat since this medicine may affect the body's ability to regulate temperature.

☐ Call your doctor if you develop a sore throat, fever, mouth sores, skin rash, changes in eyesight, rapid heartrate, dark-colored urine or a yellow color in the eyes or skin, unusual weakness or unusual movements of the face, tongue, or hands, or difficulty in urinating ("passing your water"). Also call your doctor if you become restless or unable to sit still or sleep.

☐ Carry an identification card indicating that you are taking this medicine. Always tell your pharmacist, dentist, and other doctors who are treating you that you are taking this medicine.

* * * * *

Chlortetracycline (*Ophthalmic Antibiotic*)
United States: Aureomycin
Canada: Aureomycin

☐ This medicine is an antibiotic used to treat certain types of eye infections.

☐ IMPORTANT: If you have ever had an allergic reaction to tetracycline or any antibiotic medicine, tell your doctor or pharmacist before you use any of this drug.

HOW TO USE THIS MEDICINE
☐ For EYE OINTMENT

INSTILLATION OF EYE OINTMENT

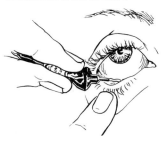

- The person administering the eye ointment should wash his hands with soap and water.
- The eye ointment must be kept clean. Do not touch the tube against the face or anything else.
- Lie down or tilt your head backward and look at the ceiling.
- Gently pull down the lower lid of your eye to form a pouch.
- Hold the tube in your other hand and place the tube as close as possible to the eye without touching it.
- Squeeze the prescribed amount of ointment (usually $\frac{1}{2}$ inch in adults) from the tube along the pouch.
- Close your eyes. Do not rub them.
- Wipe off any excess ointment around the eye with a tissue.
- Clean the tip of the ointment tube with a tissue.

☐ If necessary, have someone else administer the eye ointment for you.

☐ Keep the eye ointment tube tightly closed when not in use.

SPECIAL INSTRUCTIONS

☐ Vision may be blurred for a few minutes after using the eye medicine. Do not drive a car or operate dangerous machinery or do jobs that require you to be alert until your vision has cleared.

☐ Eye medicines should be used as prescribed by your doctor. Often eye infections clear rapidly after a few days of use of the medicine, but do not always clear completely. It is important to use *all* of this medicine, plus any refills that your doctor told you to use. Do not stop using it earlier than your doctor has recommended in spite of the fact that your symptoms seem to have improved. Otherwise, the infection may return.

☐ If you forget to use the medicine, use it as soon as possible. However, if it is almost time for your next dose, do not use the missed dose but continue with your regular schedule.

☐ Do not use this medicine at the same time as any other eye medicine without the approval of your doctor. Some medicines cannot be mixed.

☐ Contact your doctor if the condition for which you are using this medicine does not improve or if the eye becomes irritated by it for more than a few minutes. Many eye medicines sting for a short time immediately after use.

☐ For external use only. Do not swallow.

*   *   *   *   *

Chlortetracycline (*Oral Antibiotic*)
United States: Aureomycin

☐ This medicine is used to treat certain types of infections and to help control acne.

☐ IMPORTANT: If you have ever had an allergic reaction to tetracycline or any other antibiotic, tell your doctor or pharmacist before you take any of this medicine.

HOW TO USE THIS MEDICINE

☐ It is best to take this medicine on an empty stomach 1 hour before eating food or 2 hours after eating food. Take it at the proper time even if you skip a meal. If this medicine upsets your stomach, take it with some crackers (not with dairy products). Call your doctor if you continue to have stomach upset.

☐ Take this medicine with a full glass of water.

☐ Do not drink milk or eat cheese, cottage cheese, ice cream, or other dairy products 1 hour before or 2 hours after you have taken a dose of this medicine.

SPECIAL INSTRUCTIONS

☐ It is important that you take **all** of this medicine plus any refills that your doctor told you to take. Do not stop taking this medicine earlier than your doctor has recommended in spite of the fact that you may feel better. Otherwise, the infection may return.

☐ If you forget to take a dose, take it as soon as you remember and then continue with your regular schedule.

☐ Women who are pregnant, breast-feeding, or planning to become pregnant should tell their doctor before taking this medicine.

☐ Some antacids and some laxatives can make this medicine less effective if they are taken at the same time. If you must take them, they should be taken at least 2 to 3 hours after this medicine. If you have any questions, ask your pharmacist.

☐ If you must take iron products or vitamins containing iron, take them 2 hours before (or 3 hours after) this medicine.

☐ This medicine may make some people more sensitive to sunlight or sunlamps. When you begin taking this medicine, try to avoid getting too much sun until you see how you are going to react. If your skin does become more sensitive, try to stay out of direct sunlight. While in the sun, wear protective clothing and sunglasses. You may wish to ask your pharmacist about suitable sunscreen products. You may remain sensitive to sunlight and sunlamps for several weeks after you have stopped taking the drug. Check with your doctor if you become sunburned.

☐ Most people experience few or no side effects from their drugs. However, any medicine can sometimes cause unwanted effects. Call your doctor if you develop a dark-colored tongue, sore mouth, yellow-green stools or, in women, a vaginal discharge that was not present before you started taking this medicine.

- [ ] Store the medicine in a cool, dark place and keep tightly closed.

- [ ] If for some reason you cannot take all of the medicine, discard the unused portion by flushing it down the toilet. Do not save this medicine for future use. Outdated chlortetracycline can be harmful.

* * * * *

Chlortetracycline HCl (*Topical Antibiotic*)
United States: Aureomycin
Canada: Aureomycin

- [ ] This medicine is an antibiotic used to treat infections of the skin.

- [ ] IMPORTANT: If you have ever had an allergic reaction to chlortetracycline, tetracycline, or any antibiotic medicine, tell your doctor or pharmacist before you use any of this drug.

HOW TO USE THIS MEDICINE
- [ ]
  - Each time you apply the medicine, wash your hands and gently cleanse the skin area well with water unless otherwise directed by your doctor. Do not allow the skin to dry completely. Pat with a clean towel until almost dry.
  - Apply a small amount of the drug to the affected area and spread lightly. Only the medicine that is actually touching the skin will work. A thick layer is not more effective than a thin layer. Do not bandage unless directed by your doctor.

- [ ] Do not use the drug more frequently or in larger quantities than prescribed by your doctor.

SPECIAL INSTRUCTIONS
- [ ] It is important to use **all** of this medicine, plus any refills that your doctor told you to use. Do not stop using it earlier than your doctor has recommended in spite of the fact that your symptoms seem to have improved. Otherwise, the infection may return.

- [ ] If you forget to apply the medicine, apply it as soon as possible. However, if it is almost time for your next dose, do not apply the missed dose but continue with your regular schedule.

- [ ] Do not apply cosmetics or lotions on top of the drug unless your doctor approves.

- [ ] Keep this preparation away from the eyes. If you should accidentally get some in your eyes, wash it away with water immediately.

- [ ] Call your doctor if the condition for which this drug is being used persists or becomes worse, or if you develop a constant irritation such as itching or burning that was not present before you started using this medicine. Also call your doctor if you develop pain, redness, swelling, or become more sensitive to sunlight.

☐ For external use only. Do not swallow.

* * * * *

Chlorthalidone (*Oral Diuretic-Antihypertensive*)
United States: Hygroton
Canada: Hygroton, Novothalidone, Uridon

☐ This medicine is used to help rid the body of excess water and to decrease swelling. It is also used to treat high blood pressure. It is commonly called a "water pill."

☐ IMPORTANT: If you have ever had an allergic reaction to sulfa drugs or thiazide diuretics, tell your doctor or pharmacist before taking any of this medicine.

HOW TO USE THIS MEDICINE
☐ Take the medicine with food, meals, or milk.

☐ Try to take it at the same time(s) every day so that you have a constant level of the medicine in your body. Do not miss any doses. Otherwise, you cannot expect the drug to work as well.

☐ When you first start taking this medicine, you will probably urinate ("pass your water") more often and in larger amounts than usual. Therefore, if you are to take one dose every day, take it in the morning after breakfast. If you are to take more than one dose every day, take the last dose 6 hours before bedtime so that you will not have to get up during the night to go to the bathroom. This effect will usually lessen after you have taken the drug for awhile.

SPECIAL INSTRUCTIONS
☐ If you forget to take a dose, take it as soon as possible. However, if it is almost time for your next dose, do not take the missed dose. Instead, continue with your regular dosing schedule.

☐ Women who are pregnant, breast-feeding, or planning to become pregnant should tell their doctor before taking this medicine.

☐ This medicine normally causes your body to lose potassium. The body has warning signs to let you know if too much potassium is being lost. Call your doctor if you become unusually thirsty or if you develop leg cramps, unusual weakness, fatigue, vomiting, confusion, or irregular pulse.

☐ If your doctor recommends that you eat foods which are high in potassium,

200

one or more of the foods listed in Appendix A should be eaten daily. All of these foods are rich in potassium. Your goal should be to take in 1000 to 2000 mg. of potassium (approximately 25.6 to 51 mEq) each day. The calorie content and sodium content are included for your convenience in meal planning.
CHANGE YOUR DIET ONLY IF YOUR DOCTOR TELLS YOU TO.

☐ If this medicine causes dizziness, you should be careful going up and down stairs and you should not change positions too rapidly. Get out of bed slowly in the morning and dangle your feet over the edge of the bed for a few minutes before standing up. Sit down or lie down at the first sign of dizziness. Tell your doctor you have been dizzy. Be careful drinking alcoholic beverages while taking this medicine because it could make the dizziness worse. Do not drive a car or operate dangerous machinery or do jobs that require you to be alert if you are dizzy.

☐ In order to help prevent dizziness and fainting, your doctor may also recommend that you avoid strenuous exercises, standing for long periods of time (especially in hot weather), or hot showers or hot baths.

☐ This medicine may make some people more sensitive to sunlight and sunlamps. When you begin taking this medicine, try to avoid getting too much sun until you see how you are going to react. If your skin does become more sensitive to sunlight, tell your doctor and try to stay out of direct sunlight. While in the sun, wear protective clothing and sunglasses. You may wish to ask your pharmacist about suitable sunscreen products. Check with your doctor if you become sunburned.

☐ Call your doctor immediately if you think you may be allergic to the medicine or if you develop a skin rash, hives, itching, swelling of the face, or difficulty in breathing. If you cannot reach your doctor, phone a hospital emergency department.

☐ Most people experience few or no side effects from their drugs. However, any medicine can sometimes cause unwanted effects. Call your doctor if you develop a sore throat, fever, sharp stomach pain, sharp joint pain, easy bruising or bleeding, a yellow color to the skin or eyes, or a sudden weight gain of 5 pounds or more.

*   *   *   *   *

Chlorzoxazone (*Oral Skeletal Muscle Relaxant*)
United States: Paraflex

☐ This medicine is used to relax muscles and helps to relieve muscle pain and stiffness.

☐ IMPORTANT: If you have ever had an allergic reaction to any medicines, tell your doctor or pharmacist before you take any of this medicine.

HOW TO USE THIS MEDICINE

☐ This medicine may be taken with food or a glass of water.

☐ If you forget to take a dose, take it as soon as possible. However, if it is almost time for your next dose, do not take the missed dose. Instead, continue with your regular dosing schedule.

SPECIAL INSTRUCTIONS

☐ Do not drink alcoholic beverages while taking this drug without the approval of your doctor.

☐ It is important that you obtain the advice of your doctor or pharmacist before taking ANY other medicines including pain relievers, sleeping pills, tranquilizers or medicine for depression, cough/cold medicines, or allergy medicines.

☐ In some people, this drug may cause dizziness or drowsiness. Do not drive a car or operate dangerous machinery or do jobs that require you to be alert until you know how you are going to react to this drug.

☐ If you become dizzy, you should be careful going up and down staris. Sit or lie down at the first sign of dizziness.

☐ Call your doctor immediately if you think you may be allergic to the medicine or if you develop a skin rash, hives, itching, swelling of the face, or difficulty in breathing. If you cannot reach your doctor, phone a hospital emergency department.

☐ This medicine may cause the urine to turn orange or purple-red in color.

☐ Most people experience few or no side effects from their drugs. However, any medicine can sometimes cause unwanted effects. Call your doctor if you develop a skin rash or itching, stomach pain, red or black stools, a yellow color to the skin or eyes, unusual tiredness, or easy bruising.

*   *   *   *   *

Cholestyramine Resin (*Oral Bile Acid Adsorbent*)
United States: Questran
Canada: Questran

☐ This drug has many uses and the reason it was prescribed depends on your condition. Check with your doctor.

HOW TO USE THIS MEDICINE

☐ It is best to take this medicine before meals unless otherwise directed.

☐ This drug must not be taken in the dry form and must be mixed with fruit juice, water, milk, applesauce, soups, or puréed fruit. Just before taking the medicine, place the drug on the top of 4 to 6 oz. of the preferred beverage or food and allow to stand for approximately 2 minutes. Then stir slowly and take immediately. Rinse the glass to make sure you have taken the full dose.

SPECIAL INSTRUCTIONS

☐ Do not take any other medicines at the same time as this drug. If you must take other medicines, take them 1 hour before or 4 hours after this drug.

☐ It is very important to follow any diet that your doctor may also prescribe for you.

☐ If you forget to take a dose, take it as soon as possible. However, if it is almost time for your next dose, do not take the missed dose. Instead, continue with your regular dosing schedule.

☐ Do not take any more of this medicine than your doctor has prescribed and do not stop taking this medicine suddenly without the approval of your doctor.

☐ Most people experience few or no side effects from their drugs. However, any medicine can sometimes cause unwanted effects. Call your doctor if you develop severe constipation, easy bruising, bleeding from the mouth, gums and/or nose, black stools or blood in the urine, sharp stomach pain, numbness or coldness in the hands or feet, chest pain, or shortness of breath.

$$* \quad * \quad * \quad * \quad *$$

Choline Salicylate (*Oral Analgesic-Anti-inflammatory*)
United States: Arthropan
Canada: Arthropan

☐ This medicine is used to help relieve pain, reduce fever, and relieve redness and swelling in certain kinds of arthritis.

☐ IMPORTANT: If you have a stomach ulcer or if you have ever had an allergic reaction to aspirin, tell your doctor or pharmacist before you take any of this medicine.

HOW TO USE THIS MEDICINE

☐ This medicine may be mixed with water, fruit juice, or ginger ale.

☐ Do not take this medicine if it smells strongly like vinegar since this means the medicine is not fresh.

☐ Do not take this medicine regularly for more than 10 days without consulting your doctor, and do not administer it to children under 12 years of age for more than 5 days without your doctor's approval.

SPECIAL INSTRUCTIONS

☐ Do not take any other medicines containing aspirin while you are taking this medicine because it could result in too high a dose.

☐ Women who are pregnant, breast-feeding, or planning to become pregnant should tell their doctor before taking this medicine.

☐ If you are taking this medicine for arthritis, it is very important that you take it regularly and that you DO NOT MISS ANY DOSES. If you miss a dose, the level of the medicine in your body will fall and the drug will not be as effective. Only if the level of drug is high enough will the inflammation in your joints be decreased and help prevent further damage. If you forget a dose, take it as soon as possible. However, if it is almost time for your next dose, do not take the missed dose. Instead, continue with your regular dosing schedule.

☐ It is best not to drink alcoholic beverages while you are taking this medicine since the combination can cause stomach problems.

☐ Most people experience few or no side effects from their drugs. However, any medicine can sometimes cause unwanted effects. Call your doctor if you develop "ringing" or "buzzing" in the ears, skin rash, stomach pain, red or black stools, dizziness, fever, sweating, wheezing, or shortness of breath.

☐ Call your doctor if the medicine does not relieve your symptoms.

* * * * *

Chymotrypsin (*Oral Anti-inflammatory Agent*)
United States: Avazyme

Chymotrypsin-Trypsin
United States: Chymoral, Orenzyme
Canada: Orenzyme

☐ The medicine is used to help reduce inflammation and/or swelling.

☐ These tablets have a special coating; they must be swallowed whole. Do *not* crush, chew, or break them into pieces. Do not take milk or antacids within 1 hour of taking these tablets. Do not take chipped tablets.

* * * * *

Cimetidine
United States: Tagamet
Canada: Tagamet

☐ This medicine is used in the treatment of certain types of stomach ulcers and in conditions in which the stomach is producing too much acid.

HOW TO USE THIS MEDICINE
☐ Take this medicine with food or immediately after meals unless otherwise directed.

- [ ] If you develop stomach pain between doses of this medicine, ask your doctor if you may take an antacid between doses.

SPECIAL INSTRUCTIONS

- [ ] If you miss a dose of this medicine, do not take the missed dose and do not double your next dose.

- [ ] It is very important to follow the diet your doctor has prescribed for you. People with peptic ulcers should generally avoid the following: alcoholic beverages, aspirin medicines, coffee, tea, colas, spices (including mustard, ketchup and meat sauce), corn, popcorn, nuts, citrus fruits and juices (especially pineapple and tomato), soda water, and carbonated beverages. Smoking may delay healing of an ulcer. People with an ulcer can usually eat lean meat, dairy products, eggs, and cooked and creamed vegetables.

- [ ] It is very important that you take this medicine for the full length of treatment as your doctor has prescribed. Try not to miss any doses because the medicine will not be as effective. It may take several days or a few weeks before you feel the full benefit of this medicine.

- [ ] In some people, this drug may cause dizziness. Do not drive a car or operate dangerous machinery or do jobs that require you to be alert until you know how you are going to react to this drug.

- [ ] If you become dizzy, you should be careful going up and down stairs. Sit or lie down at the first sign of dizziness.

- [ ] Some men taking this medicine may notice a slight increase in the size of their breasts or some breast soreness. This is temporary and will go away after the treatment has ended.

- [ ] Call your doctor immediately if you are being treated for an ulcer and you develop faintness, weakness, thirst, dizziness, sweating, vomiting of blood, or red or black stools.

- [ ] Most people experience few or no side effects from their drugs. However, any medicine can sometimes cause unwanted effects. Call your doctor if you develop a skin rash, muscle cramps, severe diarrhea, or if you become confused.

* * * * *

Clemastine (*Oral Antihistamine*)
United States: Tavist
Canada: Tavist

- [ ] This medicine is used to help relieve the symptoms of certain types of allergic conditions, coughs and colds, and certain skin conditions.

205

HOW TO USE THIS MEDICINE

☐ This medicine may be taken with food or a glass of milk if it upsets your stomach.

☐ This medicine must be swallowed whole. Do not crush, chew, or break it into pieces. (*United States:* Tavist-1)

SPECIAL INSTRUCTIONS

☐ If you forget to take a dose, take it as soon as possible. However, if it is almost time for your next dose, do not take the missed dose. Instead, continue with your regular dosing schedule.

☐ In some people, this drug may initially cause dizziness or drowsiness. Do not drive a car or operate dangerous machinery or do jobs that require you to be alert until you know how you are going to react to this drug. If you become dizzy, you should be careful going up and down stairs. Sit or lie down at the first sign of dizziness. Tell your doctor if it continues.

☐ Do not drink alcoholic beverages while taking this drug without the approval of your doctor.

☐ If your mouth becomes dry, suck a hard sour candy (sugarless) or ice chips or chew gum. It is especially important to brush your teeth regularly if you develop a dry mouth.

☐ It is important that you obtain the advice of your doctor or pharmacist before taking pain relievers, nonprescription drugs, sleeping pills or tranquilizers, or other medicines for allergies.

☐ Do not take this medicine more often or longer than recommended by your doctor.

☐ Most people experience few or no side effects from their drugs. However, any medicine can sometimes cause unwanted effects. Call your doctor if you develop a skin rash, fast heartbeats, stomach pain, or difficulty in urinating ("passing your water").

* * * * *

Clindamycin (*Oral Antibiotic*)
United States: Cleocin
Canada: Dalacin C

☐ This medicine is an antibiotic used to treat certain types of infections.

☐ IMPORTANT: If you have ever had an allergic reaction to any antibiotics, tell your doctor or pharmacist before you take any of this medicine.

206

HOW TO USE THIS MEDICINE

☐ Take the capsules with a full glass of water. They may be taken with meals or on an empty stomach.

☐ For LIQUID MEDICINE

  • Do not refrigerate the liquid form of this medicine because it may thicken and become difficult to pour. Store the medicine at room temperature. (*United States:* Cleocin Pediatric; *Canada:* Dalacin C Solution)

SPECIAL INSTRUCTIONS

☐ It is important to take **all** of this medicine plus any refills that your doctor told you to take. Do not stop taking it earlier than your doctor has recommended in spite of the fact that you may feel better. Otherwise, the infection may return.

☐ If you forget to take a dose, take it as soon as you remember and then continue with your regular schedule.

☐ Most people experience few or no side effects from their drugs. However, any medicine can sometimes cause unwanted effects. Call your doctor if you develop a skin rash, fever, severe stomach cramps, or severe diarrhea (loose bowel movements) that may be accompanied by blood or mucus.

☐ Do not self-treat any diarrhea (loose bowel movements) without first checking with your doctor or pharmacist because some antidiarrheal products can cancel the effect of this antibiotic and may make your diarrhea worse or last longer.

☐ If for some reason you cannot take all of the medicine, throw away the unused portion by flushing it down the toilet. Do not take or save old medicine.

*   *   *   *   *

Clioquinol (*Topical Dermatitis Therapy*)
United States: Mycoquin, Vioform
Canada: Vioform

Clioquinol-Hydrocortisone
United States: Caquin Cream, Domeform-HC, Formtone-HC Cream, HCV Creme, Hexaderm I.Q. Modified Cream, Hydroquin, Hysone Ointment, Iodocort Cream, Mity-Quin Cream, Racet Cream, Vioform-Hydrocortisone
Canada: Vioform-Hydrocortisone

☐ This medicine is used to treat skin infections.

☐ IMPORTANT: If you have ever had an allergic reaction to iodine medicine, tell your doctor or pharmacist before you use any of this drug.

HOW TO USE THIS MEDICINE

☐ For CREAM and OINTMENT

- Each time you apply the medicine, wash your hands and gently cleanse the skin area well with water unless otherwise directed by your doctor. Do not allow the skin to dry completely. Pat with a clean towel until almost dry.
- Apply a small amount of the drug to the affected area and spread lightly. Only the medicine that is actually touching the skin will work. A thick layer is not more effective than a thin layer. Do not bandage unless directed by your doctor.

☐ Do not use the drug more frequently or in larger quantities than prescribed by your doctor.

SPECIAL INSTRUCTIONS

☐ It is important to use **all** of this medicine, plus any refills that your doctor told you to use. Do not stop using it earlier than your doctor has recommended in spite of the fact that your symptoms seem to have improved. Otherwise, the infection may return.

☐ If you forget to apply the medicine, apply it as soon as possible. However, if it is almost time for your next dose, do not apply the missed dose but continue with your regular schedule.

☐ Do not apply cosmetics or lotions on top of the drug unless your doctor approves.

☐ Keep this preparation away from the eyes. If you should accidentally get some in your eyes, wash it away with water immediately.

☐ Avoid getting this medication on your clothing as it may cause staining.

☐ Call your doctor if the condition for which this drug is being used persists or becomes worse or if you develop a constant irritation such as itching or burning that was not present before you started using this medicine.

☐ For external use only. Do not swallow.

* * * * *

Clobetasol Propionate (*Topical Corticosteroid*)
Canada: Dermovate

☐ This medicine is used to help relieve redness, swelling, itching, and inflammation of certain types of skin conditions.

208

HOW TO USE THIS MEDICINE

☐ For CREAM and OINTMENT
- Each time you apply the medicine, wash your hands and gently cleanse the skin area well with water unless otherwise directed by your doctor.
- Do not allow the skin to dry completely. Pat with a clean towel until almost dry.
- Apply a small amount of the drug to the affected area and spread lightly. Only the medicine that is actually touching the skin will work. A thick layer is not more effective than a thin layer. Do not bandage unless directed by your doctor.

☐ Do not use the drug more frequently or in larger quantities than prescribed by your doctor. Overuse of this medicine may cause you to absorb too much of the drug and increase the risk of side effects.

☐ Keep the medicine away from the eyes, nose, and mouth.

SPECIAL INSTRUCTIONS

☐ If you forget to apply the medicine, apply it as soon as possible. However, if it is almost time for your next dose, do not apply the missed dose but continue with your regular schedule.

☐ Do not use this medicine for any other skin problems without checking with your doctor.

☐ Do not apply cosmetics or lotions on top of the drug unless your doctor approves.

☐ Call your doctor if the condition for which this drug is being used persists or becomes worse or if you have a constant irritation such as itching or burning that was not present before you started using this medicine. Also call your doctor if you develop abnormal lines or thinning of the skin, especially under the arms or between the legs.

☐ Store in a cool place but do not freeze.

☐ For external use only. Do not swallow.

☐ Tell future doctors that you have used this medicine.

*   *   *   *   *

Clobetasone Butyrate (*Topical Corticosteroid*)
Canada: Eumovate

☐ This medicine is used to help relieve redness, swelling, itching, and inflammation of certain types of skin conditions.

HOW TO USE THIS MEDICINE

☐ For CREAM and OINTMENT

- Each time you apply the medicine, wash your hands and gently cleanse the skin area well with water unless otherwise directed by your doctor. Do not allow the skin to dry completely. Pat with a clean towel until almost dry.
- Apply a small amount of the drug to the affected area and spread lightly. Only the medicine that is actually touching the skin will work. A thick layer is not more effective than a thin layer. Do not bandage unless directed by your doctor.

☐ Do not use the drug more frequently or in larger quantities than prescribed by your doctor. Overuse of this medicine may cause you to absorb too much of the drug and increase the risk of side effects.

☐ Keep the medicine away from the eyes, nose, and mouth.

SPECIAL INSTRUCTIONS

☐ If you forget to apply the medicine, apply it as soon as possible. However, if it is almost time for your next dose, do not apply the missed dose but continue with your regular schedule.

☐ Do not use this medicine for any other skin problems without checking with your doctor.

☐ Do not apply cosmetics or lotions on top of the drug unless your doctor approves.

☐ Call your doctor if the condition for which this drug is being used persists or becomes worse or if you have a constant irritation such as itching or burning that was not present before you started using this medicine. Also call your doctor if you develop abnormal lines or thinning of the skin, especially under the arms or between the legs.

☐ Store in a cool place but do not freeze.

☐ For external use only. Do not swallow.

☐ Tell future doctors you have used this medicine.

*   *   *   *   *

Clofibrate (Oral Antihyperlipidemic Agent)

United States: Atromid-S

Canada: Atromid-S, Claripex, Liprinal, Novofibrate

☐ This medicine is used in certain types of conditions to lower the amount of cholesterol and triglycerides (fatty substances) in the blood.

HOW TO USE THIS MEDICINE

□ Take this medicine with food or after meals to help prevent stomach upset.

SPECIAL INSTRUCTIONS

□ If you forget to take a dose, take it as soon as possible. However, if it is almost time for your next dose, do not take the missed dose. Instead, continue with your regular dosing schedule.

□ Women who are pregnant, breast-feeding, or planning to become pregnant should tell their doctor before taking this medicine.

□ It is very important to follow any diet that your doctor may also prescribe for you. The cholesterol content of some common foods is listed in Appendix B.

□ In some people, this drug may cause dizziness or drowsiness. Do not drive a car or operate dangerous machinery or do jobs that require you to be alert until you know how you are going to react to this drug. If you become dizzy, you should be careful going up and down stairs. Sit or lie down at the first sign of dizziness.

□ Do not take any more of this medicine than your doctor has prescribed and do not stop taking this medicine suddenly without the approval of your doctor.

□ Call your doctor immediately if you develop chest pain, sharp stomach pain, shortness of breath, or irregular pulse.

□ Most people experience few or no side effects from their drugs. However, any medicine can sometimes cause unwanted effects. Call your doctor if you develop a skin rash, sore throat, fever, chills, nausea or vomiting, sudden weight gain, swelling of the legs or ankles, muscle cramps, or if you urinate ("pass your water") less frequently or in smaller amounts than usual.

* * * * *

Clomiphene (*Oral Ovulatory Agent*)
United States: Clomid
Canada: Clomid

□ This medicine is used to regulate the ovaries and to increase fertility in women who want to become pregnant.

HOW TO USE THIS MEDICINE

□ Take this medicine exactly as your doctor has directed. It is important not to miss any doses.

□ If you do miss a dose, call your doctor or pharmacist.

211

- ☐ Women who are pregnant, breast-feeding, or planning to become pregnant should tell their doctor before taking this medicine.

- ☐ In some people, this drug may cause dizziness, drowsiness, or blurred vision. Do not drive a car or operate dangerous machinery or do jobs that require you to be alert until you know how you are going to react to this drug.

- ☐ Check with your doctor if you develop hot flushes which do not go away as your body adjusts to the medicine.

- ☐ Most people experience few or no side effects from their drugs. However, any medicine can sometimes cause unwanted effects. Call your doctor if you develop blurred vision or spots before the eyes, abnormal vaginal bleeding, sensitivity of eyes to light, a skin rash or a yellow color to the skin or eyes, stomach pain, or pelvic pain.

- ☐ Always keep your doctor appointments so that your treatment can be evaluated.

* * * * *

Clomipramine HCl (*Oral Antidepressant*)
Canada: Anafranil

- ☐ This medicine is used to help relieve the symptoms of depression. It is important that you take the medicine regularly and that you do not miss any doses. The full effect of the medicine may not be noticed immediately but may take from a few days to 4 weeks. Early signs of improvement are increased appetite, better sleep, increased energy and, later, improved mood. DO NOT STOP TAKING the medicine when you first feel better or you will feel worse in 3 or 4 days.

- ☐ This medicine has also been used in children to treat bed-wetting.

HOW TO USE THIS MEDICINE
- ☐ This medicine may be taken with food unless otherwise directed.

SPECIAL INSTRUCTIONS
- ☐ If you forget to take a dose, take it as soon as possible. However, if it is almost time for your next dose, do not take the missed dose. Instead, continue with your regular dosing schedule.

- ☐ Any medicine has a few unwanted side effects. Because this medicine takes a few weeks to work, the side effects are the only things that tell the doctor that the drug is being absorbed. Most of these side effects will go away as your body adjusts to the medicine.

- [ ] Women who are pregnant, breast-feeding, or planning to become pregnant should tell their doctor before taking this medicine.

- [ ] In some people, this drug may cause dizziness or drowsiness. Do not drive a car or operate dangerous machinery or do jobs that require you to be alert until you know how you are going to react to this drug.

- [ ] If this medicine causes dizziness, you should be careful going up and down stairs and you should not change positions too quickly. Get out of bed slowly in the morning and dangle your feet over the edge of the bed for a few minutes before standing up. Sit or lie down at the first sign of dizziness. Tell your doctor you have been dizzy.

- [ ] Do not drink alcoholic beverages while taking this drug without the approval of your doctor.

- [ ] It is important that you obtain the advice of your doctor or pharmacist before taking any other medicines, including pain relievers, sleeping pills, tranquilizers, other medicines for depression, cough, cold or allergy medicines, or weight-reducing medicine.

- [ ] If your mouth becomes dry, suck a hard sour candy (sugarless) or ice chips, or chew gum. It is especially important to brush your teeth regularly if you develop a dry mouth.

- [ ] This medicine may make some people more sensitive to sunlight and sunlamps. When you begin taking this medicine, try to avoid getting too much sun until you see how you are going to react. If your skin does become more sensitive to sunlight, tell your doctor and try to stay out of direct sunlight. While in the sun, wear protective clothing and sunglasses. You may wish to ask your pharmacist about suitable sunscreen products. Check with your doctor if you become sunburned.

- [ ] If you become constipated, try increasing the amount of bulk in your diet (for example, bran and salads), exercising more often, or drinking water.

- [ ] Call your doctor if you develop a sore throat, fever, mouth sores, eye pain or blurred vision, difficulty in urinating ("passing your water"), fast heartbeats, dark-colored urine or a yellow color to the skin or eyes, a skin rash, nightmares, or tingling of the hands or feet.

- [ ] Do not stop taking this medicine suddenly without your doctor's approval. When your doctor tells you to stop this medicine, you must follow these precautions for 2 weeks since some of the medicine may still be in your body.

- [ ] Carry an identification card indicating that you are taking this medicine. Always tell your pharmacist, dentist, and other doctors who are treating you that you are taking this medicine.

* * * * *

Clonazepam (*Oral Sedative-Anticonvulsant*)
United States: Clonopin
Canada: Rivotril

- ☐ This medicine is used to help control convulsions and seizures. It is commonly used in the treatment of epilepsy.

- ☐ IMPORTANT: If you have ever had an allergic reaction to a benzodiazepine or tranquilizer medicine, tell your doctor or pharmacist before you take any of this medicine.

HOW TO USE THIS MEDICINE
- ☐ Take this medicine with food or a full glass of water.

- ☐ It is very important that you take this medicine regularly and that you do not miss any doses. Try to take the medicine at the same time(s) every day. This is the only way that you can receive the full benefit of the medicine. If you forget to take this medicine, the amount of medicine in your blood will go down and you may have seizures.

SPECIAL INSTRUCTIONS
- ☐ If you forget to take a dose and remember it within 1 hour of the missed dose, take it and continue with your regular dosing schedule. Otherwise, do not take the missed dose at all.

- ☐ In some people, this drug may cause dizziness or drowsiness. Do not drive a car or operate dangerous machinery or do jobs that require you to be alert until you know how you are going to react to this drug.

- ☐ If you become dizzy, you should be careful going up and down stairs. Sit or lie down at the first sign of dizziness.

- ☐ If this medicine is for a child, do not let him (her) ride a bike or climb trees until you can determine how he (she) is going to react to the medicine. They could hurt themselves if they participated in these activities if they were dizzy.

- ☐ Do not drink alcoholic beverages while taking this drug without the approval of your doctor.

- ☐ It is important that you obtain the advice of your doctor or pharmacist before taking ANY other medicines including pain relievers, sleeping pills, tranquilizers or medicines for depression, cough/cold medicines, or allergy medicines.

- ☐ Avoid swimming alone or participating in high-risk sports in which a sudden seizure could cause injury.

- ☐ Women who are pregnant, breast-feeding, or planning to become pregnant should tell their doctor before taking this medicine.

- ☐ Call your doctor immediately if you think you may be allergic to the medicine or if you develop a skin rash, hives, itching, swelling of the face, or difficulty

in breathing. If you cannot reach your doctor, phone a hospital emergency department.

☐ Most people experience few or no side effects from their drugs. However, any medicine can sometimes cause unwanted effects. Call your doctor if you develop a sore throat, fever, mouth sores, dark-colored urine or a yellow color to the skin or eyes, fast heartbeats, fast eye movements, unusual nervousness, or nightmares, or if you become depressed or confused.

☐ Do not stop taking this medicine suddenly without the approval of your doctor.

☐ Do not go without this medicine between prescription refills. Call your pharmacist 2 or 3 days before you will run out of the medicine.

☐ Carry an identification card indicating that you are taking this medicine. Always tell your pharmacist, dentist, and other doctors who are treating you that you are taking this medicine.

* * * * *

Clonidine HCl (*Oral Antihypertensive*)
United States: Catapres
Canada: Catapres

☐ This medicine is used to help lower the blood pressure.

☐ Hypertension (high blood pressure) is a long-term condition, and it will probably be necessary for you to take the drug for a long time in spite of the fact that you feel better. It is very important that you take this medicine as your doctor has directed and that you do not miss any doses. Otherwise, you cannot expect the drug to keep your blood pressure down.

HOW TO USE THIS MEDICINE
☐ Try to take the medicine at the same time(s) every day.

☐ Unless otherwise directed, the last dose of the day should be given at bedtime to control the blood pressure during sleep.

SPECIAL INSTRUCTIONS
☐ If you forget to take a dose, take it as soon as possible. However, if it is almost time for your next dose, do not take the missed dose. Instead, continue with your regular dosing schedule.

☐ In some people, this drug may initially cause dizziness or drowsiness. Do not drive a car or operate dangerous machinery or do jobs that require you to be alert until you know how you are going to react to this drug. If you do become dizzy, lie or sit down. Always get up slowly from lying or sitting positions. Call your doctor if the dizziness does not go away.

215

☐ If your mouth becomes dry, suck a hard sour candy (sugarless) or ice chips, or chew gum. It is especially important to brush your teeth regularly if you develop a dry mouth.

☐ Do not drink alcoholic beverages while taking this drug without the approval of your doctor.

☐ It is important that you obtain the advice of your doctor or pharmacist before you take pain relievers, sleeping pills, medicines for seizures, tranquilizers, medicines for depression, or nonprescription drugs such as cough/cold or sinus products, asthma or allergy products, or diet or weight-reducing medicines.

☐ Follow any special diet your doctor may have ordered. He may want you to limit the amount of salt in your food.

☐ If you become constipated, try increasing the amount of bulk in your diet (for example, bran and salads), exercising more often, or drinking more water.

☐ Most people experience few or no side effects from their drugs. However, any medicine can sometimes cause unwanted effects. Call your doctor if you develop swelling of the legs or ankles, sudden weight gain of 5 pounds or more, chest pains, difficulty in breathing, dry eyes, nightmares, skin rash, or if you urinate ("pass your water") less frequently or in smaller amounts than usual.

☐ Carry an identification card indicating that you are taking this medicine. Always tell your pharmacist, dentist, and other doctors who are treating you that you are taking this medicine.

☐ Do not stop taking this medicine without your doctor's approval and do not go without medication between prescription refills. Call your pharmacist two or three days before you will run out of the medicine.

* * * * *

Clorazepate Dipotassium (*Oral Anxiolytic-Sedative*)
United States: Tranxene
Canada: Tranxene

Clorazepate Monopotassium
United States: Azene

☐ This medicine is used to help relieve anxiety as well as to treat some other conditions. Check with your doctor if you do not fully understand why you are taking it.

☐ IMPORTANT: If you have ever had an allergic reaction to a benzodiazepine medicine, tell your doctor or pharmacist before you take any of this medicine.

216

HOW TO USE THIS MEDICINE

- ☐ This medicine may be taken with food or a full glass of water.
- ☐ Swallow the tablets whole. Do not crush, chew, or break them into pieces. (**United States:** Tranxene-SD, Tranxene-SD Half Strength)

SPECIAL INSTRUCTIONS

- ☐ If you forget to take a dose, take it as soon as possible. However, if it is almost time for your next dose, do not take the missed dose. Instead, continue with your regular dosing schedule.
- ☐ Women who are pregnant, breast-feeding, or planning to become pregnant should tell their doctor before taking this medicine.
- ☐ In some people, this drug may cause dizziness or drowsiness. Do not drive a car or operate dangerous machinery or do jobs that require you to be alert until you know how you are going to react to this drug.
- ☐ If you become dizzy, you should be careful going up and down stairs. Sit or lie down at the first sign of dizziness.
- ☐ If your mouth becomes dry, suck a hard sour candy (sugarless) or ice chips, or chew gum. It is especially important to brush your teeth regularly if you develop a dry mouth.
- ☐ Do not drink alcoholic beverages while taking this drug without the approval of your doctor.
- ☐ It is important that you obtain the advice of your doctor or pharmacist before taking ANY other medicines including pain relievers, sleeping pills, tranquilizers or medicines for depression, cough/cold or allergy medicines, or weight-reducing medicines.
- ☐ Do not take any more of this medicine than your doctor has prescribed because the drug could become habit-forming. Do not stop taking this medicine suddenly without the approval of your doctor.
- ☐ Most people experience few or no side effects from their drugs. However, any medicine can sometimes cause unwanted effects. Call your doctor if you develop a sore throat, fever, mouth sores, a staggering walk, a yellow color to the skin or eyes, slow heartbeats or shortness of breath, unusual tiredness or nervousness, or stomach pain.

*   *   *   *   *

Clortermine HCl (*Oral Anorexiant*)
United States: Voranil

- ☐ This medicine is used to help reduce the appetite in weight reduction programs. It can help you develop new eating habits and is only useful for a short time. Do not take any more of this medicine than your doctor has prescribed and do not stop taking this medicine suddenly without the approval of your doctor.

HOW TO USE THIS MEDICINE

☐ This medicine may be taken with a glass of water.

☐ Do not take the medicine late in the day or it may cause insomnia (difficulty in sleeping).

SPECIAL INSTRUCTIONS

☐ If you forget to take a dose, take it as soon as possible. However, if it is almost time for your next dose, do not take the missed one. Instead, continue with your regular dosing schedule.

☐ It is very important that you follow the diet prescribed by your doctor.

☐ If your mouth becomes dry, suck a hard sour candy (sugarless) or ice chips, or chew gum. It is especially important to brush your teeth regularly if you develop a dry mouth.

☐ In some people, this drug may cause dizziness. Do not drive a car or operate dangerous machinery or do jobs that require you to be alert until you know how you are going to react to this drug. Therefore, you should be careful going up and down stairs. Sit or lie down at the first sign of dizziness.

☐ Most people experience few or no side effects from their drugs. However, any medicine can sometimes cause unwanted effects. Call your doctor if you develop a skin rash, sore throat, fever, mouth sores, unusual nervousness, difficulty in urinating ("passing your water"), or palpitations, or if you become depressed.

☐ Carry an identification card indicating that you are taking this medicine. Always tell your pharmacist, dentist, and other doctors who are treating you that you are taking this medicine.

* * * * *

Clotrimazole (*Topical Antifungal*)
United States: Lotrimin
Canada: Canesten

☐ This medicine is used to treat fungal infections of the skin.

HOW TO USE THIS MEDICINE
☐ INSTRUCTIONS FOR USE

• Cleanse the affected area well with soap and water unless otherwise directed by your doctor. Pat the skin with a clean towel until almost dry.

- Apply a small amount of drug to the affected and surrounding areas and massage gently until it disappears.

SPECIAL INSTRUCTIONS

☐ If you have a fungal infection of the feet, it is important to dry the feet (especially between the toes) well after washing.

☐ Consult your doctor if the condition for which this medicine is being used persists or becomes worse, or if the medicine causes an irritation.

☐ For external use only.

*   *   *   *   *

Cloxacillin (Oral Antibiotic)

United States: Cloxapen, Tegopen

Canada: Bactopen, Cloxapen, Cloxilean, Novocloxin, Orbenin, Tegopen

☐ This medicine is an antibiotic used to treat certain types of infections.

☐ IMPORTANT: If you have ever had an allergic reaction to penicillin or any other antibiotic, tell your doctor or pharmacist before you take any of this medicine.

HOW TO USE THIS MEDICINE

☐ It is best to take this medicine on an empty stomach 1 hour before (or 2 hours after) meals or food unless otherwise directed by your doctor. Take it at the proper time even if you skip a meal.

☐ Take this medicine with a full glass of water.

☐ For LIQUID MEDICINE (**United States:** Tegopen; **Canada:** Cloxilean, Orbenin, Tegopen)
  - Store the liquid medicine in the refrigerator. Do not freeze.
  - If there is a discard date on the bottle, throw away any unused medicine after that date.

SPECIAL INSTRUCTIONS

☐ It is important to take **all** of this medicine plus any refills that your doctor told you to take. Do not stop taking this medicine earlier than your doctor has recommended in spite of the fact that you may feel better. Otherwise, the infection may return.

☐ If you forget to take a dose, take it as soon as you remember and then continue with your regular schedule.

☐ Most people experience few or no side effects from their drugs. However, any medicine can sometimes cause unwanted effects. Call your doctor if you

develop a dark-colored tongue, yellow-green stools or, in women, a vaginal discharge that was not present before you started taking this medicine.

☐ This medicine sometimes causes diarrhea (loose bowel movements). Call your doctor if the diarrhea becomes severe or lasts for more than 2 days.

☐ Call your doctor immediately if you think you may be allergic to the medicine or if you develop a skin rash, hives, itching, swelling of the face, or difficulty in breathing. If you cannot reach your doctor, phone a hospital emergency department.

☐ If for some reason you cannot take all of the medicine, throw away the unused portion by flushing it down the toilet. Do not take or save old medicine.

*   *   *   *   *

Coal Tar (*Topical Antipsoriatic*)
United States: Estar, L.C.D., Zetar
Canada: Zetar

Coal Tar-Allantoin
United States: Alphonsyl
Canada: Alphonsyl, A.T.S.

Tar Distillate
United States: Balnetar, Cutar Bath Oil Emulsion, Doak Oil, Doak Oil Forte, Lavatar, Tar Doak
Canada: Doak Oil, Doak Oil Forte, Tar Doak Lotion, Tersa Tar

☐ This medicine is used to treat psoriasis, eczema, dandruff, and other skin conditions.

HOW TO USE THIS MEDICINE
☐ Follow the instructions appearing on the package.

☐ Do not use the drug more frequently or in larger quantities than prescribed by your doctor.

☐ Keep this preparation away from the eyes. If you should accidentally get some in your eyes, wash it away with water immediately.

☐ If you forget to apply the medicine, apply it as soon as possible. However, if it is almost time for your next dose, do not apply the missed dose but continue with your regular schedule.

SPECIAL INSTRUCTIONS
☐ Do not apply this medicine to open or oozing wounds or infected areas of the skin.

- [ ] Care must be taken when the skin is exposed to direct sunlight for 24 hours because you may be more sensitive to sunlight.

- [ ] This medicine may stain bed linen and clothing. Use old bed linen and avoid getting this medicine on your clothing.

- [ ] The gel or solution may cause a mild stinging sensation when you apply it. This is not unusual and is temporary.

- [ ] If you are using the shampoo and if you have blond, bleached, or tinted hair or hair that has a permanent, it may cause temporary discoloration.

- [ ] Call your doctor if the condition for which this drug is being used persists or becomes worse or if you develop a constant irritation such as itching or burning that was not present before you started using this medicine.

- [ ] For external use only. Do not swallow.

*   *   *   *   *

Codeine Phosphate (*Oral Analgesic-Antitussive*)
Canada: Paveral

- [ ] This medicine is used to help relieve pain and certain types of coughs.

HOW TO USE THIS MEDICINE
- [ ] This medicine may be taken with food or a glass of water.

- [ ] Do not take any more of this medicine than your doctor has prescribed. The drug could become habit-forming, or you could take an overdose if you take it more often or longer than prescribed.

- [ ] If you are taking this medicine to help relieve pain, do not wait until the pain becomes severe. This medicine works best if you take it at the beginning of the pain. Call your doctor if you feel you need it more often than he prescribed.

- [ ] For LIQUID MEDICINE
  - Do not dilute the syrup. The soothing effect of the syrup is better if you do not drink liquids immediately after taking the medicine. (**Canada:** Paveral)

SPECIAL INSTRUCTIONS
- [ ] Do not drink alcoholic beverages while taking this drug without the approval of your doctor.

- [ ] It is important that you obtain the advice of your doctor or pharmacist before taking ANY other medicines including other pain relievers, sleeping pills, tranquilizers or medicines for depression, cough/cold or allergy medicines, or weight-reducing medicines.

☐ In some people, this drug may cause dizziness or drowsiness. Do not drive a car or operate dangerous machinery or do jobs that require you to be alert until you know how you are going to react to this drug.

☐ If you become dizzy, you should be careful going up and down stairs. Sit or lie down at the first sign of dizziness. Get up slowly if you have been lying or sitting down.

☐ If you do feel nauseated when you first start taking the medicine, it may help if you lie down for a few minutes.

☐ If you become constipated, try increasing the amount of bulk in your diet (for example, bran and salads), exercising more often, or drinking more water. Call your doctor if the constipation continues.

☐ Most people experience few or no side effects from their drugs. However, any medicine can sometimes cause unwanted effects. Call your doctor if you develop shortness of breath, slow heartbeats, unusual nervousness, stomach pain, or difficulty in urinating ("passing your water").

☐ Always tell your dentist, pharmacist, and other doctors who are treating you that you are taking this medicine.

* * * * *

Colchicine (Oral Gout Therapy)
United States: Colchicine, Colsalide
Canada: Novocolchine

☐ This medicine is used to prevent and treat gout and gouty arthritis. It helps relieve the pain, redness, and swelling of these conditions.

HOW TO USE THIS MEDICINE
☐ Take the medicine with food to help prevent stomach upset.

☐ If you are taking this medicine to TREAT a gout attack, take it at the beginning of the attack. Stop taking the medicine as soon as the pain is relieved or if you develop nausea, vomiting, diarrhea, or stomach pain.

☐ If you are taking this medicine to PREVENT a gout attack, take it regularly as your doctor has prescribed. If you develop a gout attack, increase your dose at the beginning of the attack as your doctor has directed. Stop taking the medicine as soon as the pain is relieved or if you develop nausea, vomiting, diarrhea, or stomach pain. After the attack is over, resume your regular schedule.

☐ This medicine has a special coating and must be swallowed whole. Do not crush, chew, or break it into pieces. (**United States:** Colsalide)

☐ If you forget to take a dose, take it as soon as possible. However, if it is

222

almost time for your next dose, do not take the missed dose. Instead, continue with your regular dosing schedule.

SPECIAL INSTRUCTIONS

- ☐ Try to drink at least 8 to 10 glasses of water or other liquids every day while you are taking this medicine unless otherwise directed.

- ☐ Do not drink alcoholic beverages while taking this drug without the approval of your doctor. Fermented beverages (beer, ale, wine) may cause a gout attack.

- ☐ Most people experience few or no side effects from their drugs. However, any medicine can sometimes cause unwanted effects. Call your doctor if you develop a sore throat, fever or mouth sores, numbness or tingling in the hands or feet, easy bruising or bleeding, or unusual tiredness. Also call your doctor if any nausea, vomiting, diarrhea, or stomach pain from the medicine do not disappear.

- ☐ It is important to carry this medicine with you at all times so that you will be able to take it at the first sign of an attack.

*   *   *   *   *

Colestipol (*Oral Bile Acid Absorbent*)
United States: Colestid

- ☐ This medicine is used in certain types of conditions to lower the amount of cholesterol and triglycerides (fatty substances) in the blood.

HOW TO USE THIS MEDICINE

- ☐ This medicine must NOT be taken in the dry form and must be mixed with a liquid such as fruit juice, water, or milk, or with a food such as soups, applesauce, or cereals. Add the drug to at least 3 ounces of the liquid or food and stir until it is completely mixed. Rinse the glass to make sure you have taken the full dose.

SPECIAL INSTRUCTIONS

- ☐ Do not take any other medicines at the same time as this drug. If you must take other medicines, take them 1 hour before or 4 hours after this drug.

- ☐ It is very important to follow any diet that your doctor may also prescribe for you. The cholesterol content of some common foods is listed in Appendix B.

- ☐ If you forget to take a dose, take it as soon as possible. However, if it is almost time for your next dose, do not take the missed dose. Instead, continue with your regular dosing schedule.

- ☐ Do not take any more of this medicine than your doctor has prescribed and do not stop taking this medicine suddenly without the approval of your doctor.

☐ Most people experience few or no side effects from their drugs. However, any medicine can sometimes cause unwanted effects. Call your doctor if you develop severe constipation, easy bruising, bleeding from the mouth, gums, or nose, black stools or blood in the urine, sharp stomach pain, numbness or coldness in the hands or feet, chest pain, or shortness of breath.

*　*　*　*　*

Colistin-Neomycin-Hydrocortisone (*Otic Antibiotic-Corticosteroid*)
United States: Coly-Mycin S Otic
Canada: Coly-Mycin Otic

☐ This medicine is an antibiotic used to treat certain types of ear infections.

☐ IMPORTANT: If you have ever had an allergic reaction to a neomycin or any antibiotic medicine, tell your doctor or pharmacist before you use any of this drug.

HOW TO USE THIS MEDICINE
☐ For EAR DROPS

INSTILLATION OF EAR DROPS

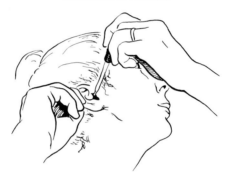

- Warm the ear drops to body temperature by holding the bottle in your hands for a few minutes. Do NOT heat the drops in hot water.
- The person administering the ear drops should wash his hands with soap and water.
- The ear drops must be kept clean. Do not touch the dropper against the ear or anything else.
- Shake the bottle well before using.
- Tilt your head or lie on your side so that the ear to be treated is facing up.
- In ADULTS, hold the ear lobe up and back.
  In CHILDREN, hold the ear lobe down and back.
- Place the prescribed number of drops into the ear. Do not insert the dropper into the ear as it may cause injury.

224

- Remain in the same position for a short time (2 minutes) after you have administered the drops.
- Dry the ear lobe if there are any drops on it.

☐ For EAR DROPS AFTER APPLICATION OF EAR WICK
- Warm the medication to body temperature by holding in your hands for a few minutes.
- Tilt head to the side or lie on side so that the ear to be treated is uppermost.
- Drop the prescribed amount of medication into the ear canal.
- Do not use the solution if it is discolored or if it appears to have changed in any way since you purchased it.

☐ If necessary, have someone else administer the ear drops for you.

☐ Do not use the ear drops if they change in color or change in any way after being purchased.

SPECIAL INSTRUCTIONS

☐ If you forget to use the medicine, use it as soon as possible. However, if it is almost time for your next dose, do not use the missed dose but continue with your regular schedule.

☐ Do not use this medicine at the same time as any other ear medicine without the approval of your doctor. Some medicines cannot be mixed.

☐ Call your doctor if the condition for which you are using this medicine persists or becomes worse or if the medicine causes itching or burning for more than a few minutes after instillation.

☐ Store in a cool dark place and keep the container tightly closed.

☐ For external use only. Do not swallow.

*   *   *   *   *

Combistix *Diagnostic Aid*
United States: Combistix
Canada: Combistix

☐ This preparation is used to test for various chemicals in the urine.

☐ Directions for use:
- Moisten test end of strip in urine by dipping and removing immediately.
- Tap tip of strip against edge of container to remove excess urine.
- Compare the middle part of the strip with the glucose chart 10 seconds after dipping.
- Compare tip of strip with protein color chart.
- Compare third portion of strip with pH color chart.

225

☐ For further information, refer to the package insert which accompanies the medicine.*

* * * * *

Cortisone Acetate (*Oral Corticosteroid*)
United States: Cortisone Acetate
Canada: Cortone

☐ This medicine is cortisone, which is a hormone normally produced by the body. This medicine is used to help decrease inflammation, which then relieves pain, redness, and swelling. It is used in the treatment of certain kinds of arthritis as well as for severe allergies or skin conditions.

HOW TO USE THIS MEDICINE

☐ Take this medicine with food or a glass of milk in order to help prevent stomach upset. Call your doctor if you develop stomach upset, stomach pain, or heartburn (especially if it awakens you during the night). Do not try to treat this yourself.

☐ If your doctor has prescribed only ONE dose of this medicine every day, it is best to take it before 9 A.M. or with breakfast.

☐ If you forget to take a dose, take it as soon as possible. However, if it is almost time for your next dose, do not take the missed dose. Instead, continue with your regular dosing schedule.

SPECIAL INSTRUCTIONS

☐ Women who are pregnant, breast-feeding, or planning to become pregnant should tell their doctor before taking this medicine.

☐ It is best not to drink alcoholic beverages while you are taking this medicine because the combination can cause stomach problems.

☐ Do not take any more of this medicine than your doctor has prescribed and do not stop taking this medicine suddenly without the approval of your doctor. It may be necessary for your doctor to slowly reduce your dose since your body becomes used to this medicine and it might be harmful if you suddenly did not receive this medicine.

☐ Do not take aspirin or medicines containing aspirin without the approval of your doctor.

☐ While you are taking this medicine you may gain some weight. This could be due to an increase in your appetite or increased water in your system. Your doctor may prescribe a special diet to decrease the number of calories you eat and/or to lower the amount of sodium or increase the amount of potassium in your diet. Follow any diet that your doctor may order.

☐ You may find that you bruise more easily. Try to protect yourself from all injuries to prevent bruising.

*Combistix (Package Insert), Ames Company Division, Miles Laboratories Ltd., Rexdale, Ontario.

226

- [ ] Diabetic patients should regularly check the sugar in their urine and report any unusual levels to their doctor.

- [ ] Carry an identification card indicating that you are taking this medicine. Always tell your pharmacist, dentist, and other doctors who are treating you that you are taking this medicine. If you have an acute infection, injury or operation, or dental surgery within 1 year of taking this medicine, it is important to tell your doctor.

- [ ] Most people experience few or no side effects from their drugs. However, any medicine can sometimes cause unwanted effects. Call your doctor if you develop stomach pain, sore throat, fever, swelling of the legs or ankles, a wound which does not heal, eye pain or blurred vision, frequent urination ("passing your water"), nightmares or depression, muscle cramps, red or black stools, puffing of the face, or menstrual problems.

*   *   *   *   *

Co-Trimoxazole (*See Sulfonamide Preparations*)

*   *   *   *   *

Cromoglycate Sodium (*Ophthalmic Anti-Allergic*)
Canada: Opticrom

- [ ] This medicine is used to help relieve the redness and swelling of certain types of eye conditions.

HOW TO USE THIS MEDICINE
- [ ] For EYE DROPS

INSTILLATION OF EYE DROPS

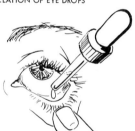

- The person administering the eye drops should wash his hands with soap and water.
- The eye drops must be kept clean. Do not touch the dropper against the face or anything else.
- Lie down or tilt your head backward and look at the ceiling.
- Gently pull down the lower lid of your eye to form a pouch.
- Hold the dropper in your other hand and approach the eye from the side. Place the dropper as close to the eye as possible without touching it.
- Place the prescribed number of drops into the pouch of the eye.
- Close your eyes. Do not rub them.

- Apply gentle pressure for a minute with your fingers to the bridge of the nose (inside corner of the eye) to prevent the eye drops from being drained from the eye.
- Blot excess solution around the eye with a tissue.

☐ If necessary, have someone else administer the eye drops for you.

☐ Do not use the eye drops if they have changed in color or have changed in any way since you purchased them.

☐ Keep the eye drop bottle tightly closed when not in use.

☐ Do not use the drug more frequently or in larger quantities than prescribed by your doctor.

SPECIAL INSTRUCTIONS

☐ If you forget to use the medicine, use it as soon as possible. However, if it is almost time for your next dose, do not use the missed dose but continue with your regular schedule.

☐ Do not use this medicine at the same time as any other eye medicine without the approval of your doctor. Some medicines cannot be mixed.

☐ Contact your doctor if the condition for which you are using this medicine does not improve or if the eye becomes irritated by it for more than a few minutes. Many eye medicines sting for a short time immediately after use.

☐ Always tell any future doctors who are treating you that you have used this medicine.

☐ Throw away any unused medicine 4 weeks after the bottle has been opened.

☐ For external use only. Do not swallow.

* * * * *

Cromolyn Sodium (*Inhalation Asthma Prophylaxis*)
United States: Intal
Canada: Intal

☐ This medicine is used to help prevent asthmatic attacks. It will not help an asthmatic attack that has already begun.

☐ IMPORTANT: If you have ever had an allergic reaction to lactose (milk sugar), milk, or milk products, tell your doctor or pharmacist before you take any of this medicine. There is a preparation which is free of lactose that your doctor can prescribe.

HOW TO USE THIS MEDICINE

☐ These capsules must be used in the inhaler. DO NOT SWALLOW the capsules.

☐ INSTRUCTIONS FOR USE: (Fig. 4).

228

How to use your Spinhaler®

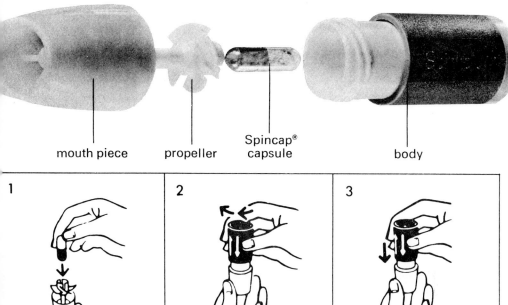

mouth piece	propeller	Spincap® capsule
		body

1	**2**	**3**
LOAD Unscrew grey body of the Spinhaler then with mouthpiece downwards and propeller on spindle, insert colored end of capsule firmly into cup.	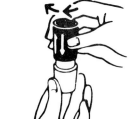 **TURN** Screw back the body by turning to right. Hold Spinhaler with mouthpiece down at all times.	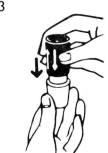 **PIERCE** To pierce the capsule, move grey sleeve down once and return to original position.
4	**5**	**6**
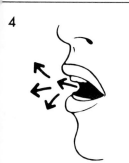 **EXHALE** Breathe out to empty as much air from the lungs as possible. Tilt head back. Place mouthpiece between lips and teeth, with air inlet slightly upwards.	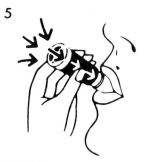 **INHALE** Draw in a deep breath through the Spinhaler as rapidly as possible. Hold for a few seconds then breathe out. **Repeat this procedure until capsule is empty.**	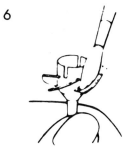 **WASH** Wash all parts of the Spinhaler once-a-week and allow to dry thoroughly before assembling. It is recommended that the Spinhaler be replaced after six months of use.

INTAL, Fissons (Canada) Limited, Don Mills, Ontario.

Figure 4. *Instructions for use of cromolyn sodium.*

SPECIAL INSTRUCTIONS

☐ If you forget to take a dose, take it as soon as possible. However, if it is almost time for your next dose, do not take the missed dose. Instead, continue with your regular dosing schedule.

☐ It may take 1 to 4 weeks before you feel the full benefit of this medicine. If you are also using another inhaler that opens up the air passages in your lungs (bronchodilator), use it several minutes before you use this inhaler.

☐ Do not take any more of this medicine than your doctor has prescribed and do not stop taking this medicine suddenly without the approval of your doctor. If you should suddenly stop taking it or reduce your dose, you may experience a worsening of your asthma.

☐ Carry an identification card indicating that you are taking this medicine. Always tell your pharmacist, dentist, and other doctors who are treating you that you are taking this medicine.

☐ Call your doctor immediately if you think you may be allergic to the medicine or if you develop a skin rash, hives, itching, swelling of the face, or difficulty in breathing. If you cannot reach your doctor, phone a hospital emergency department.

☐ Most people experience few or no side effects from their drugs. However, any medicine can sometimes cause unwanted effects. Call your doctor if you develop fever or coughing, difficulty in urinating ("passing your water"), dizziness or severe headaches, joint or muscle pain, nausea or vomiting, trouble in swallowing, or swollen glands.

* * * * *

Crotamiton (*Topical Scabicide*)
United States: Eurax
Canada: Eurax

☐ This medicine is used to treat skin conditions.

HOW TO USE THIS MEDICINE
☐ For SCABIES
- Apply the ointment over the skin of the entire body, except the face and scalp, and massage into the skin until dry.
- Wait 24 hours between applications.
- All bed linen and clothing should be changed the next morning.
- A cleansing bath may be taken 24 hours after the last application of ointment.

☐ For ITCHING SKIN
- Each time you apply the medicine, wash your hands and gently cleanse the skin area well with water unless otherwise directed by your doctor.

- Do not allow the skin to dry completely. Pat with a clean towel until almost dry.
- Apply a small amount of the drug to the affected area and spread lightly until almost dry. Only the medicine that is actually touching the skin will work. A thick layer is not more effective than a thin layer. Do not bandage unless directed by your doctor.

SPECIAL INSTRUCTIONS

☐ Put on freshly laundered clean clothing after each application of the medicine. Use fresh towels and fresh bed sheets after each application. Launder or dry-clean contaminated clothing.

☐ Keep this medicine away from the eyes, mouth or open wounds. If some does get in the eyes, flush it away with water immediately.

☐ Call your doctor if the condition for which this drug is being used persists or becomes worse or if you develop a constant irritation such as itching or burning that was not present before you started using this medicine.

☐ For external use only. Do not swallow.

*   *   *   *   *

Cryptenamine Tannate (*Oral Antihypertensive*)
United States: Unitensen

☐ This medicine is used to lower blood pressure.

☐ Hypertension (high blood pressure) is a long-term condition, and it will probably be necessary for you to take the drug for a long time in spite of the fact that you feel better. It is very important that you take this medicine as your doctor has directed and that you do not miss any doses. Otherwise, you cannot expect the drug to keep your blood pressure down.

HOW TO USE THIS MEDICINE

☐ Try to take the medicine at the same time(s) every day.

☐ If possible, avoid eating anything for 4 hours after you have taken the medicine. This will help prevent stomach upset.

SPECIAL INSTRUCTIONS

☐ If you forget to take a dose, take it as soon as possible. However, if it is almost time for your next dose, do not take the missed dose. Instead, continue with your regular dosing schedule.

☐ In some people, this drug may cause dizziness or blurred vision. Do not drive a car or operate dangerous machinery or do jobs that require you to be alert until you know how you are going to react to the drug.

☐ If this medicine causes dizziness, you should be careful going up and down stairs and you should not change positions too rapidly. Sit or lie down at the first sign of dizziness. Tell your doctor you have been dizzy.

☐ Follow any special diet that your doctor may have ordered. He may want you to limit the amount of salt in your food.

☐ Some nonprescription drugs can aggravate your condition. Do not take any of the following without the approval of your doctor or pharmacist: cough, cold or sinus products; asthma or allergy products; or diet or weight-reducing medicines.

☐ Most people experience few or no side effects from their drugs. However, any medicine can sometimes cause unwanted effects. Call your doctor if you develop swelling of the legs or ankles, sudden weight gain of 5 pounds or more, chest pains or difficulty in breathing, nausea, or a slow pulse rate.

☐ Carry an identification card indicating that you are taking this medicine. Always tell your pharmacist, dentist, and other doctors who are treating you that you are taking this medicine.

☐ Do not stop taking this medicine without your doctor's approval and do not go without medicine between prescription refills. Call your pharmacist 2 or 3 days before you will run out of the medicine.

*   *   *   *   *

Cupric Sulfate Reagent (*Glycosuria Diagnostic Aid*)
United States: Clinitest
Canada: Clinitest

☐ This preparation is used to test the amount of sugar (glucose) in the urine.

☐ Care and Handling of Clinitest Reagent Tablets:
   1. Keep tablets away from direct heat and sunlight. Keep in a cool, dry place but not in the refrigerator.
   2. Bottled tablets: Replace the bottle cap immediately after removing the tablet and before starting the test. Tablets absorb moisture and spoil (turn dark blue in color) if the bottle is not kept tightly closed.
   3. Tablets in foil: Use the tablet immediately after removing the foil. Avoid breaking the seal on the adjoining tablet. Clinitest Reagent Tablets normally have a spotted bluish-white color. Never use tablets that are dark blue. Handle tablets cautiously because they contain caustic soda.

☐ Directions for use:
   1. Collect urine in a clean receptable. With the dropper in an upright position, place 5 drops of urine in a test tube. Rinse the dropper and add 10 drops of water in the test tube.
   2. Drop 1 tablet into the test tube. Watch while the complete reaction takes place. Do not shake the test tube during the reaction or for 15 seconds after the boiling has stopped.

3. After the 15-second waiting period, shake the test tube gently and compare with the color chart supplied. Record the results on the Analysis Record Sheet.

☐ Interpretation of test:
    1. *Negative*—No sugar (glucose)
        —The fluid will be blue at the end of the waiting period of 15 seconds. The whitish sediment that may form has no bearing on the test.
    2. *Positive*—Sugar present
        —The fluid will change color. The more sugar, the greater the change and the more rapidly it occurs.
        —The amount of sugar is determined by comparing the color of the solution in the test tube with the color chart after the 15-second waiting period. Color changes developing later than 15 seconds should be disregarded.
    Important: Careful observation of the solution in the test tube while the reaction takes place during the 15-second waiting period is necessary to detect rapid "pass through" color changes caused by amounts of sugar over 2%. Should the color rapidly "pass through" green, tan, and orange to a dark greenish-brown, record the results as over 2% sugar without comparing final color development with the color chart.

☐ Clinitest Reagent Tablets, if swallowed, may cause chemical injury. Keep out of the reach of children. If the tablets are accidentally swallowed, do *not* induce vomiting. Call your physician immediately.

☐ For further information, refer to the package insert which accompanies this chemical.*

*   *   *   *   *

Cyclacillin (*Oral Antibiotic*)
United States: Cyclapen

☐ This medicine is an antibiotic used to treat certain types of infections.

☐ IMPORTANT: If you have ever had an allergic reaction to penicillin or any other antibiotic, tell your doctor or pharmacist before you take any of this medicine.

HOW TO USE THIS MEDICINE

☐ It is best to take this medicine on an empty stomach 1 hour before (or 2 hours after) meals or food unless otherwise directed by your doctor. Take it at the proper time even if you skip a meal.

*Clinitest Reagent Tablets (Package Insert), Ames Company Division, Miles Laboratories, Ltd., Rexdale, Ontario.

☐ Take the tablets or capsules with a full glass of water.

☐ For LIQUID MEDICINE

- If you were prescribed a suspension, shake the bottle well before using so that you can measure an accurate dose. Store in the refrigerator but do not freeze.

- If there is a discard date on the bottle, throw away any unused medicine after that date.

SPECIAL INSTRUCTIONS

☐ It is important to take *all* of this medicine plus any refills that your doctor told you to take. Do not stop taking this medicine earlier than your doctor has recommended in spite of the fact that you may feel better. Otherwise, the infection may return.

☐ If you forget to take a dose, take it as soon as you remember and then continue with your regular schedule.

☐ Most people experience few or no side effects from their drugs. However, any medicine may sometimes cause unwanted effects. Call your doctor if you develop a dark-colored tongue, yellow-green stools or, in women, a vaginal discharge that was not present before you started taking this medicine.

☐ This medicine sometimes causes diarrhea (loose bowel movements). Call your doctor if the diarrhea becomes severe or lasts for more than two days.

☐ Call your doctor immediately if you think you may be allergic to the medicine or if you develop a skin rash, hives, itching, swelling of the face, or difficulty in breathing. If you cannot reach your doctor, phone a hospital emergency department.

* * * * *

Cyclandelate (*Oral Vasodilator*)

United States: Cyclanfour, Cyclospasmol, Cydel

Canada: Cyclospasmol

☐ This medicine is used to help improve the circulation of blood in the body and to help relax muscles.

HOW TO USE THIS MEDICINE

☐ Take the medicine on an empty stomach; however, if stomach upset occurs, take it with meals or with antacids as recommended by your doctor.

☐ If you forget to take a dose, take it as soon as possible. However, if it is almost time for your next dose, do not take the missed dose. Instead, continue with your regular schedule.

SPECIAL INSTRUCTIONS

☐ Women who are pregnant, breast-feeding, or planning to become pregnant should tell their doctor before taking this medicine.

☐ In some people, this drug may cause dizziness or drowsiness. Do not drive a car or operate dangerous machinery or do jobs that require you to be alert until you know how you are going to react to this drug.

☐ This medicine may cause a warm sensation, flushing of the face, or headache. Sit or lie down until these effects pass.

☐ Some nonprescription drugs can aggravate your condition. Do not take any of the following without the approval of your doctor or pharmacist: cough, cold, or sinus products; asthma or allergy products; or diet or weight-reducing medicines.

☐ Do not drink alcoholic beverages while taking this drug without the approval of your doctor.

☐ The activity of this drug is improved if you keep warm. Avoid getting cold or exposing yourself to a cold environment.

☐ Most people experience few or no side effects from their drugs. However, any medicine can sometimes cause unwanted effects. Call your doctor if you develop a skin rash, nausea or vomiting, severe stomach pain, a rapid pulse, or fainting spells.

* * * * *

Cyclizine (*Oral Antinauseant*)
United States: Marezine
Canada: Marzine

☐ This medicine is used to help control nausea, vomiting, dizziness, and motion sickness.

HOW TO USE THIS MEDICINE
☐ Take the tablets with a little water.

SPECIAL INSTRUCTIONS
☐ Women who are breast-feeding should tell their doctor before taking this medicine.

☐ In some people, this drug may cause dizziness or drowsiness. Do not drive a car or operate dangerous machinery or do jobs that require you to be alert until you know how you are going to react to this drug.

☐ If you become dizzy, you should be careful going up and down stairs. Sit or lie down at the first sign of dizziness.

☐ If you become constipated, try increasing the amount of bulk in your diet (for example, bran and salads), exercising more often, or drinking more water.

- [ ] If your mouth becomes dry, suck a hard sour candy (sugarless) or ice chips, or chew gum. It is especially important to brush your teeth regularly if you develop a dry mouth.

- [ ] Do not drink alcoholic beverages while taking this drug without the approval of your doctor.

- [ ] It is important that you obtain the advice of your doctor or pharmacist before taking pain relievers, nonprescription drugs, sleeping pills, tranquilizers, or medicines for depression while you are taking this drug.

- [ ] Most people experience few or no side effects from their drugs. However, any medicine can sometimes cause unwanted effects. Call your doctor if you develop a skin rash, sore throat, fever or mouth sores, changes in vision or eye pain, fast heartbeats or chest pain, difficulty in urinating ("passing your water"), dark-colored urine or a yellow color to the skin or eyes.

*   *   *   *   *

Cyclobenzaprine (*Oral Skeletal Muscle Relaxant*)
United States: Flexeril
Canada: Flexeril

- [ ] This medicine is used to relax muscles and helps to relieve muscle pain and stiffness.

- [ ] IMPORTANT: If you have ever had an allergic reaction to any medicines, tell your doctor or pharmacist before you take any of this medicine.

HOW TO USE THIS MEDICINE
- [ ] This medicine may be taken with food or a glass of water.

- [ ] If you forget to take a dose, take it as soon as possible. However, if it is almost time for your next dose, do not take the missed dose. Instead, continue with your regular dosing schedule.

SPECIAL INSTRUCTIONS
- [ ] Do not drink alcoholic beverages while taking this drug without the approval of your doctor.

- [ ] It is important that you obtain the advice of your doctor or pharmacist before taking ANY other medicines including pain relievers, sleeping pills, tranquilizers or medicine for depression, cough/cold medicines, or allergy medicines.

- [ ] In some people, this drug may cause dizziness or drowsiness. Do not drive a car or operate dangerous machinery or do jobs that require you to be alert until you know how you are going to react to this drug.

- [ ] If you become dizzy, you should be careful going up and down stairs. Sit or lie down at the first sign of dizziness.

236

☐ Call your doctor immediately if you think you may be allergic to the medicine or if you develop a skin rash, hives, itching, swelling of the face, or difficulty in breathing. If you cannot reach your doctor, phone a hospital emergency department.

☐ If your mouth becomes dry, suck a hard sour candy (sugarless) or ice chips, or chew gum. It is especially important to brush your teeth regularly if you develop a dry mouth.

☐ Most people experience few or no side effects from their drugs. However, any medicine can sometimes cause unwanted effects. Call your doctor if you develop fast heartbeats, numbness of the hands or feet, stomach pain or constipation, trembling, difficulty in urinating ("passing your water"), or if you become confused or depressed.

* * * * *

Cyclopentolate HCl (*Ophthalmic—Cycloplegic-Mydriatic*)
United States: Cyclogyl
Canada: Cyclogyl, Mydplegic, Optopentolate

Cyclopentolate HCl-Phenylephrine
United States: Cyclomydril

☐ This medicine is used to treat conditions of the eye. The drug will cause the pupil of the eye to dilate (become larger in size). This is a normal effect of the drug.

HOW TO USE THIS MEDICINE
☐ For EYE DROPS

INSTILLATION OF EYE DROPS

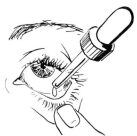

- The person administering the eye drops should wash his hands with soap and water.
- The eye drops must be kept clean. Do not touch the dropper against the face or anything else.
- Lie down or tilt your head backward and look at the ceiling.
- Gently pull down the lower lid of your eye to form a pouch.
- Hold the dropper in your other hand and approach the eye from the

237

side. Place the dropper as close to the eye as possible without touching it.
- Place the prescribed number of drops into the pouch of the eye.
- Close your eyes. Do not rub them.
- Apply gentle pressure for a minute with your fingers to the bridge of the nose (inside corner of the eye) to prevent the eye drops from being drained from the eye.
- Blot excess solution around the eye with a tissue.

☐ If necessary, have someone else administer the eye drops for you.

☐ Do not use the eye drops if they change in color or have changed in any way since you purchased them.

☐ Keep the eye drop bottle tightly closed when not in use.

SPECIAL INSTRUCTIONS

☐ Vision may be blurred for a few minutes after using the eye medicine. Do not drive a car or operate dangerous machinery or do jobs that require you to be alert until your vision has cleared.

☐ If you forget to use the medicine, use it as soon as possible. However, if it is almost time for your next dose, do not use the missed dose but continue with your regular schedule.

☐ Do not use this medicine at the same time as any other eye medicine without the approval of your doctor. Some medicines cannot be mixed.

☐ If your eyes become more sensitive to light, it may help to wear sunglasses.

☐ Contact your doctor if the condition for which you are using this medicine does not improve or if the eye becomes irritated by it for more than a few minutes. Many eye medicines sting for a short time immediately after use. Also call your doctor if you develop eye pain, a skin rash, flushing, dryness of the skin, a fast pulse, or fever.

☐ Always tell any future doctors who are treating you that you have used this medicine.

☐ Keep the container tightly closed and store in a cool place.

☐ For external use only. Do not swallow.

* * * * *

Cyclophosphamide (*Oral Antineoplastic*)
United States: Cytoxan
Canada: Cytoxan, Procytox

☐ This medicine is used in certain medical conditions to help slow down the growth and reproduction of some of the body's cells.

238

HOW TO USE THIS MEDICINE

☐ It is very important that you take this medicine exactly as your doctor has prescribed and that you do not miss any doses. Try to take this medicine at the same time every day.

☐ If you miss a dose of this medicine, do not take the missed dose and do not double your next dose.

☐ It is best to take this medicine 1 hour before breakfast in order to help prevent nausea or vomiting.

☐ Even if you become nauseated or lose your appetite, do not stop taking the medicine but check with your doctor.

SPECIAL INSTRUCTIONS

☐ Always keep your doctor appointments so that your doctor can watch your progress.

☐ If your doctor has prescribed some other medicines for you, it is important that you take them in the right order and that you do not miss them.

☐ Unless otherwise directed, drink plenty of fluids (2 to 3 quarts daily) while you are taking this medicine. This will help your kidneys handle the medicine and help prevent bladder problems. Smaller children should drink 1 to 2 quarts of fluids a day depending on their weight.

☐ This medicine may cause a temporary loss of hair. Brush your hair gently and no more often than necessary. After your treatment is finished, your hair should grow back in.

☐ Always tell your pharmacist, dentist, and any other doctors who are treating you that you are taking this medicine. This is especially important if you plan to have surgery or any vaccinations.

☐ Men and women should take appropriate birth control measures while taking this medicine to avoid conception.

☐ This is a very strong medicine. In addition to its benefits, there may be some unwanted effects even for a short time after you stop taking the medicine. Call your doctor if you develop unusual bruising or bleeding, sore throat, fever or mouth sores, a skin rash, swelling of the legs or ankles, shortness of breath, dark-colored urine, a yellow color to the skin or eyes, stomach or joint pain, difficulty or pain in urinating ("passing your water"), blood in the urine, black tarry stools, or fast heartbeats.

* * * * *

Cycloserine (Oral Tuberculosis Therapy)
United States: Seromycin

☐ This medicine is used to prevent or help the body overcome tuberculosis. Because tuberculosis (TB) heals very slowly, it may be necessary for you to take this medicine for a long time.

□ It is very important that you keep taking this medicine for the full length of time that your doctor has prescribed. Do not stop taking the medicine earlier than your doctor has recommended in spite of the fact that you may feel better. DO NOT MISS ANY DOSES and DO NOT RUN OUT OF THIS MEDICINE.

□ The most important thing you can do to protect others from catching your TB is to take your medicine regularly and to cover your coughs and sneezes with a double-ply tissue. This will reduce the spray of germs into the air. Covering your mouth with the bare hand does no good.

HOW TO USE THIS MEDICINE

□ This medicine may be taken with food if it upsets your stomach.

SPECIAL INSTRUCTIONS

□ If you forget to take a dose, take it as soon as you can remember and then continue with your regular schedule. However, if it is almost time for your next dose, omit the dose you forgot.

□ It is recommended that you avoid the use of alcoholic beverages while you are taking this medicine.

□ In some people, this drug may cause drowsiness. Do not drive a car or operate dangerous machinery or do jobs that require you to be alert until you know how you are going to react to this drug.

□ Most people experience few or no side effects from their drugs. However, any medicine can sometimes cause unwanted effects. Call you doctor if you develop numbness or tingling in the hands or feet, a skin rash, unusual tiredness or weakness, drowsiness, confusion, headache, or tremor.

* * * * *

Cyclothiazide (*Oral Diuretic*)
United States: Anhydron

□ This medicine is used to help rid the body of excess water and to decrease swelling. It is also used to treat high blood pressure. It is commonly called a "water pill."

□ IMPORTANT: If you have ever had an allergic reaction to sulfa drugs or thiazide diuretics, tell your doctor or pharmacist before taking any of this medicine.

HOW TO USE THIS MEDICINE

□ Take the medicine with food, meals, or milk.

□ Try to take it at the same time(s) every day so that you have a constant level of the medicine in your body. Do not miss any doses. Otherwise, you cannot expect the drug to work as well.

□ When you first start taking this medicine, you will probably urinate ("pass your water") more often and in larger amounts than usual. Therefore, if you are to take one dose every day, take it in the morning after breakfast. If you are to take more than one dose every day, take the last dose 6 hours before bedtime so that you will not have to get up during the night to go to the bathroom. This effect will usually lessen after you have taken the drug for awhile.

SPECIAL INSTRUCTIONS

□ If you forget to take a dose, take it as soon as possible. However, if it is almost time for your next dose, do not take the missed dose. Instead, continue with your regular dosing schedule.

□ Women who are pregnant, breast-feeding, or planning to become pregnant should tell their doctor before taking this medicine.

□ This medicine normally causes your body to lose potassium. The body has warning signs to let you know if too much potassium is being lost. Call your doctor if you become unusually thirsty or if you develop leg cramps, unusual weakness, fatigue, vomiting, confusion, or irregular pulse.

□ If your doctor recommends that you eat foods that are high in potassium, one or more of the foods listed in Appendix A should be eaten daily. All of these foods are rich in potassium. Your goal should be to take in 1000 to 2000 mg. of potassium (approximately 25.6 to 51 mEq) each day. The calorie content and sodium content are included for your convenience in meal planning.
CHANGE YOUR DIET ONLY IF YOUR DOCTOR TELLS YOU TO.

□ If this medicine causes dizziness, you should be careful going up and down stairs and you should not change positions too rapidly. Get out of bed slowly in the morning and dangle your feet over the edge of the bed for a few minutes before standing up. Sit down or lie down at the first sign of dizziness. Tell your doctor you have been dizzy. Be careful drinking alcoholic beverages while taking this medicine because it could make the dizziness worse. Do not drive a car or operate dangerous machinery or do jobs that require you to be alert if you are dizzy.

□ In order to help prevent dizziness and fainting, your doctor may also recommend that you avoid strenuous exercises, standing for long periods of time (especially in hot weather), or hot showers or hot baths.

□ This medicine may make some people more sensitive to sunlight and sunlamps. When you begin taking this medicine, try to avoid getting too much sun until you see how you are going to react. If your skin does become more sensitive to sunlight, tell your doctor and try to stay out of direct sunlight. While in the sun, wear protective clothing and sunglasses. You may wish to ask your pharmacist about suitable sunscreen products. Check with your doctor if you become sunburned.

□ Call your doctor immediately if you think you may be allergic to the medicine

241

or if you develop a skin rash, hives, itching, swelling of the face, or difficulty in breathing. If you cannot reach your doctor, phone a hospital emergency department.

☐ Most people experience few or no side effects from their drugs. However, any medicine can sometimes cause unwanted effects. Call your doctor if you develop a sore throat, fever, sharp stomach pain, chest pain, sharp joint pain, easy bruising or bleeding, a yellow color to the skin or eyes, or a sudden weight gain of 5 pounds or more.

*   *   *   *   *

Cycrimine HCl (*Oral Antispasmodic*)
United States: Pagitane HCl

☐ This medicine is used to improve muscle control and relieve muscle spasm in Parkinson's disease and certain other medical conditions.

HOW TO USE THIS MEDICINE
☐ Take this medicine with food or immediately after meals to help prevent stomach upset unless otherwise directed.

☐ If you forget to take a dose, take it as soon as possible. However, if your next dose is within 2 hours, do not take the missed dose but continue with your regular schedule.

SPECIAL INSTRUCTIONS
☐ If your mouth becomes dry, suck a hard sour candy (sugarless) or ice chips, or chew gum. It is especially important to brush your teeth regularly if you develop a dry mouth.

☐ In some people, this drug may cause dizziness, drowsiness, or blurred vision during the first 2 weeks of using this drug. This will usually go away as your body adjusts to this medicine. Do not drive a car or operate dangerous machinery or do jobs that require you to be alert until you know how you are going to react to this drug.

☐ If you become dizzy, you should be careful going up and down stairs. Sit or lie down at the first sign of dizziness.

☐ If your eyes become more sensitive to sunlight, it may help to wear sunglasses.

☐ Do not take antacids or diarrhea medicines within 1 hour of taking this medicine as it could make this medicine less effective.

☐ A desire to urinate ("pass your water") with an inability to do so is not an uncommon effect with this drug. Urinating each time before the drug is taken may help relieve this problem. Call your doctor if it continues.

☐ Do not drink alcoholic beverages while taking this drug without the approval of your doctor.

☐ It is important that you obtain the advice of your doctor or pharmacist before taking pain relievers, nonprescription drugs, sleeping pills, tranquilizers, or medicine for depression while you are taking this drug.

☐ You may become more sensitive to heat because your body may perspire less while you are taking this medicine. Be careful not to become overheated during exercise or in hot weather.

☐ Most people experience few or no side effects from their drugs. However, any medicine can sometimes cause unwanted effects. Call your doctor if you develop a skin rash, eye pain, dizziness or fainting, fast heartbeats, or constipation, or if you become confused.

*   *   *   *   *

Cyproheptadine HCl (*Oral Antihistamine*)
United States: Periactin
Canada: Periactin, Vimicon

☐ This medicine is used to help relieve symptoms (such as itching) of certain types of allergic conditions. This drug has several other uses and the reason it was prescribed depends upon your condition. Check with your doctor if you do not understand why you are taking it.

HOW TO USE THIS MEDICINE
☐ This medicine may be taken with food or a glass of milk if it upsets your stomach.

☐ For LIQUID MEDICINE
    • Do not freeze the liquid medicine (**United States:** Periactin Syrup; **Canada:** Periactin Syrup, Vimicon Syrup)

SPECIAL INSTRUCTIONS
☐ If you forget to take a dose, take it as soon as possible. However, if it is almost time for your next dose, do not take the missed dose. Instead, continue with your regular dosing schedule.

☐ Women who are breast-feeding should tell their doctor before taking this medicine.

☐ In some people, this drug may initially cause dizziness or drowsiness. Do not drive a car or operate dangerous machinery or do jobs that require you to be alert until you know how you are going to react to this drug. If you become dizzy, you should be careful going up and down stairs. Sit or lie down at the first sign of dizziness. Tell your doctor if it continues.

☐ Do not drink alcoholic beverages while taking this drug without the approval of your doctor.

☐ If your mouth becomes dry, suck a hard sour candy (sugarless) or ice chips, or chew gum. It is especially important to brush your teeth regularly if you develop a dry mouth.

243

- [ ] It is important that you obtain the advice of your doctor or pharmacist before taking pain relievers, nonprescription drugs, sleeping pills or tranquilizers, or other medicines for allergies.

- [ ] Do not take this medicine more often or longer than recommended by your doctor.

- [ ] Most people experience few or no side effects from their drugs. However, any medicine can sometimes cause unwanted effects. Call your doctor if you develop a sore throat, fever, mouth sores, fast heartbeats, blurred vision, stomach pain or difficulty in urinating ("passing your water").

* * * * *

Danazol (*Oral Pituitary Gonadotropin Inhibitor*)
United States: Danocrine
Canada: Cyclomen

- [ ] This medicine is similar to a hormone which is normally produced by the body. It is used in the treatment of endometriosis.

HOW TO USE THIS MEDICINE
- [ ] Take the drug after meals or with a snack if it upsets your stomach.

- [ ] It is very important that you take this drug as your doctor has prescribed.

SPECIAL INSTRUCTIONS
- [ ] Women who are pregnant, breast-feeding, or planning to become pregnant should tell their doctor before taking this medicine.

- [ ] Carry an identification card indicating that you are taking this medicine. Always tell your pharmacist, dentist, and other doctors who are treating you that you are taking this medicine.

- [ ] Most people experience few or no side effects from their drugs. However, any medicine can sometimes cause unwanted effects. Call your doctor if you develop swelling of the hands, legs, or ankles; acne; blood in the urine; blurred vision; hoarseness or a deepening of the voice; baldness or increased facial hair; or vaginal itching, dryness, burning, or bleeding.

* * * * *

Danthron (*Oral Laxative*)
United States: Dorbane, Modane, Modane Mild
Canada: Dorbane, Modane

Danthron-Docusate Sodium
United States: Danthross, Doctate-P, Dorbantyl, Dorbantyl Forte, Doxan, Doxidan
Canada: Doss, Doxidan, Regulex-D

Danthron-Docusate Calcium
United States: Doxidan
Canada: Doxidan

- [ ] This medicine is a laxative used to help relieve constipation.

HOW TO USE THIS MEDICINE

- [ ] Take the medicine in the evening or before breakfast with a full glass of water.

- [ ] Do not take mineral oil while you are taking this medicine. (***United States:*** Danthross, Doctate-P, Dorbantyl, Dorbantyl Forte, Doxan, Doxidan; ***Canada:*** Doss, Doxidan, Regulex-D)

SPECIAL INSTRUCTIONS

- [ ] Do not take this medicine more often or longer than your doctor has prescribed as your bowels may become dependent upon it. If you feel you require this medicine every day and cannot have a bowel movement without it, call your doctor.

- [ ] Women who are breast-feeding should tell their doctor before taking this medicine.

- [ ] Unless otherwise directed, you should also try to increase the amount of bulk foods in your diet (for example, bran, fresh fruits, and salads), exercising more often, and drinking 6 to 8 glasses of water every day.

- [ ] This medicine may cause your urine to turn pink or orange in color. This is not unusual.

- [ ] Do not take this medicine if you have any stomach pain, nausea, or vomiting.

- [ ] Call your doctor if your constipation is not relieved or if you develop rectal bleeding, muscle cramps, unusual weakness, or dizziness.

* * * * *

Dantrolene Sodium (*Oral Skeletal Muscle Relaxant*)
United States: Dantrium
Canada: Dantrium

- [ ] This medicine is used to relax muscles and helps to relieve muscle pain and stiffness.

- [ ] IMPORTANT: If you have ever had an allergic reaction to any medicines, tell your doctor or pharmacist before you take any of this medicine.

HOW TO USE THIS MEDICINE

- [ ] This medicine may be taken with food or a glass of water.

- [ ] If you forget to take a dose, take it as soon as possible. However, if it is almost time for your next dose, do not take the missed dose. Instead, continue with your regular dosing schedule.

245

☐ Shake the bottle well before using so that you can measure an accurate dose. (**United States:** Dantrium)

SPECIAL INSTRUCTIONS

☐ Do not drink alcoholic beverages while taking this drug without the approval of your doctor.

☐ It is important that you obtain the advice of your doctor or pharmacist before taking ANY other medicines including pain relievers, sleeping pills, tranquilizers or medicines for depression, cough/cold medicines, or allergy medicines.

☐ In some people, this drug may cause dizziness or drowsiness. Do not drive a car or operate dangerous machinery or do jobs that require you to be alert until you know how you are going to react to this drug.

☐ If you become dizzy, you should be careful going up and down stairs. Sit or lie down at the first sign of dizziness.

☐ This medicine may make some people more sensitive to sunlight and sunlamps. When you begin taking this medicine, try to avoid getting too much sun until you see how you are going to react. If your skin does become more sensitive to sunlight, tell your doctor and try to stay out of direct sunlight. While in the sun, wear protective clothing and sunglasses. You may wish to ask your pharmacist about suitable sunscreen products. Check with your doctor if you become sunburned.

☐ Most people experience few or no side effects from their drugs. However, any medicine can sometimes cause unwanted effects. Call your doctor if you develop a skin rash, itching, chest pain, red or black stools, severe diarrhea, blood in the urine, unusual weakness, a yellow color to the skin or eyes, or difficulty in urinating ("passing your water"), or if you become depressed.

* * * * *

Dapsone (*Oral Antibacterial Sulfone*)
United States: Avlosulfon
Canada: Avlosulfon

☐ This medicine is used in the treatment of certain types of skin conditions.

HOW TO USE THIS MEDICINE

☐ Take the medicine with food or a glass of water.

☐ It is very important that you take this medicine exactly as your doctor has prescribed and that you do not miss any doses. Try to take this medicine at the same time every day. Do not take extra tablets without your doctor's approval.

SPECIAL INSTRUCTIONS

□ If you forget to take a dose, take it as soon as possible. However, if it is almost time for your next dose, do not take the missed dose. Instead, continue with your regular dosing schedule.

□ Most people experience few or no side effects from their drugs. However, any medicine can sometimes cause unwanted effects. Call your doctor if you develop a sore throat, fever or mouth sores, numbness, swelling or pain in the hands or feet, muscle weakness, joint pain, a yellow color to the skin or eyes, unusual tiredness, or blood in the urine.

* * * * *

Deanol (*Oral CNS Stimulant*)
United States: Deaner
Canada: Deaner-100

□ This medicine has many uses and the reason it was prescribed depends upon your condition. Check with your doctor if you do not fully understand why you are taking it.

HOW TO USE THIS MEDICINE

□ This medicine may be taken with food or a glass of water.

SPECIAL INSTRUCTIONS

□ If you forget to take a dose, take it as soon as possible. However, if it is almost time for your next dose, do not take the missed dose. Instead, continue with your regular dosing schedule.

□ If this medicine causes dizziness, you should be careful going up and down stairs and you should not change positions too rapidly. Get out of bed slowly in the morning and dangle your feet over the edge of the bed for a few minutes before standing up. Sit down or lie down at the first sign of dizziness. Tell your doctor you have been dizzy. Do not drive a car or operate dangerous machinery if you are dizzy. Avoid hot showers and baths because they could make you dizzy.

□ Check with your doctor if you develop a headache which does not go away as your body adjusts to the medicine.

□ Most people experience few or no side effects from their drugs. However, any medicine can sometimes cause unwanted effects. Call your doctor if you develop a skin rash, insomnia (difficulty in sleeping), or muscle stiffness.

* * * * *

Demecarium Bromide (*Ophthalmic Miotic*)
United States: Humorsol Ophthalmic

□ This medicine is used in the treatment of glaucoma and other eye conditions.

□ IMPORTANT: If you have ever had an allergic reaction to bromides, tell your doctor or pharmacist before you use any of this drug.

HOW TO USE THIS MEDICINE

□ For EYE DROPS

INSTILLATION OF EYE DROPS

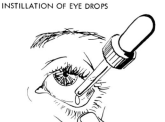

- The person administering the eye drops should wash his hands with soap and water.
- The eye drops must be kept clean. Do not touch the dropper against the face or anything else.
- Lie down or tilt your head backward and look at the ceiling.
- Gently pull down the lower lid of your eye to form a pouch.
- Hold the dropper in your other hand and approach the eye from the side. Place the dropper as close to the eye as possible without touching it.
- Place the prescribed number of drops into the pouch of the eye.
- Close your eyes. Do not rub them.
- Apply gentle pressure for a minute with your fingers to the bridge of the nose (inside corner of the eye) to prevent the eye drops from being drained from the eye.
- Blot excess solution around the eye with a tissue.

□ If necessary, have someone else administer the eye drops for you.

□ Do not use the eye drops if they change in color or have changed in any way since you purchased them.

□ Wash your hands after you have instilled the drops.

SPECIAL INSTRUCTIONS

□ If you are routinely exposed to organophosphorus insecticides or pesticides (for example, farmers, lawn service workers, aerial sprayers, or home users) you may be more sensitive to this medicine. It is advisable to wear a face mask when you are exposed to the insecticides and pesticides (for example, parathion and malathion), and to wash and change your clothes after exposure.

□ Vision may be blurred for a few minutes after using the eye medicine. Do not drive a car or operate dangerous machinery or do jobs that require you to be alert until your vision has cleared.

□ During the first few days of using the eye drops, you may experience aching in the eyes and head. This is not unusual and should disappear. Call your doctor if the pain persists.

☐ If you forget to use the medicine, use it as soon as possible. However, if it is almost time for your next dose, do not use the missed dose but continue with your regular schedule.

☐ Do not use this medicine at the same time as any other eye medicine without the approval of your doctor. Some medicines cannot be mixed.

☐ Contact your doctor if the condition for which you are using this medicine does not improve or if the eye becomes irritated by it for more than a few minutes. Many eye medicines sting for a short time immediately after use. Also call your doctor if you develop excessive sweating, flushing, stomach cramps, diarrhea (loose bowel movements), difficulty in breathing, difficulty in urinating ("passing your water"), or muscle weakness.

☐ Always tell any future doctors who are treating you that you have used this medicine.

☐ Store the eye drops in a cool place and кeep tightly capped.

☐ For external use only. Do not swallow.

* * * * *

Demeclocycline (Oral Antibiotic)
United States: Declomycin
Canada: Declomycin

☐ This medicine is an antibiotic used to treat certain types of infections.

☐ IMPORTANT: If you have ever had an allergic reaction to tetracycline or any other antibiotic, tell your doctor or pharmacist before you take any of this medicine.

HOW TO USE THIS MEDICINE

☐ It is best to take this medicine on an empty stomach 1 hour before eating food or 2 hours after eating food. Take it at the proper time even if you skip a meal. If this medicine upsets your stomach, take it with some crackers (not with dairy products). Call your doctor if you continue to have stomach upset.

☐ Take this medicine with a full glass of water.

☐ Do not drink milk or eat cheese, cottage cheese, ice cream, or other dairy products 1 hour before or 2 hours after you have taken a dose of this medicine.

SPECIAL INSTRUCTIONS

☐ It is important that you take **all** of this medicine plus any refills that your doctor told you to take. Do not stop taking this medicine earlier than your doctor has recommended in spite of the fact that you may feel better. Otherwise, the infection may return.

☐ If you forget to take a dose, take it as soon as you remember and then continue with your regular schedule.

☐ Women who are pregnant, breast-feeding, or planning to become pregnant should tell their doctor before taking this medicine.

☐ Some antacids and some laxatives can make this medicine less effective if they are taken at the same time. If you must take them, they should be taken at least 2 to 3 hours after this medicine. If you have any questions, ask your pharmacist.

☐ If you must take iron products or vitamins containing iron, take them 2 hours before (or 3 hours after) this medicine.

☐ This medicine may make some people more sensitive to sunlight or sun-lamps. When you begin taking this medicine, try to avoid getting too much sun until you see how you are going to react. If your skin does become more sensitive, try to stay out of direct sunlight. While in the sun, wear protective clothing and sunglasses. You may wish to ask your pharmacist about suitable sunscreen products. You may remain sensitive to sunlight and sunlamps for several weeks after you have stopped taking the drug. Check with your doctor if you become sunburned.

☐ Most people experience few or no side effects from their drugs. However, any medicine can sometimes cause unwanted effects. Call your doctor if you develop a dark-colored tongue, sore mouth, yellow-green stools or, in women, a vaginal discharge that was not present before you started taking this medicine.

☐ Store the medicine in a cool, dark place and keep tightly closed.

☐ If for some reason you cannot take all of the medicine, discard the unused portion by flushing it down the toilet. Do not save this medicine for future use. Outdated demeclocycline can be harmful.

* * * * *

Deserpidine (Oral Antihypertensive)
United States: Harmonyl

☐ This medicine is used to lower the blood pressure.

☐ Hypertension (high blood pressure) is a long-term condition and it will prob-ably be necessary for you to take the drug for a long time in spite of the fact that you feel better. It is very important that you take this medicine as your doctor has directed and that you do not miss any doses. Otherwise, you cannot expect the drug to keep your blood pressure down.

☐ IMPORTANT: If you have allergies, tell your doctor or pharmacist before you take any of this medicine.

HOW TO USE THIS MEDICINE
☐ Take this medicine with food, meals, or milk.

250

☐ Try to take the medicine at the same time(s) every day.

SPECIAL INSTRUCTIONS

☐ If you forget to take a dose, take it as soon as possible. However, if it is almost time for your next dose, do not take the missed dose. Instead, continue with your regular dosing schedule.

☐ In some people, this drug may cause dizziness or drowsiness. Do not drive a car or operate dangerous machinery or do jobs that require you to be alert until you know how you are going to react to this drug.

☐ In a few people, this medicine may cause dizziness or fainting if you get up quickly from a lying or sitting position. Get up slowly, especially in the morning. It is advisable to dangle your feet over the edge of the bed for a few minutes before standing up. Sit or lie down at the first sign of dizziness. Tell your doctor that you have been dizzy.

☐ In order to help prevent dizziness and fainting, it is also recommended that you avoid strenuous exercise, standing for long periods of time (especially in hot weather), and hot showers or hot baths.

☐ If you develop a stuffy nose, tell your doctor.

☐ Some nonprescription drugs can aggravate your condition. Do not take any of the following without the approval of your doctor or pharmacist: cough, cold, or sinus products; asthma or allergy products; or diet or weight-reducing medicines.

☐ Most people experience few or no side effects from their drugs. However, any medicine can sometimes cause unwanted effects. Call your doctor if you develop severe diarrhea (loose bowel movements), stomach pain, a skin rash, nightmares, loss of appetite or depression, swelling of the legs or ankles, sudden weight gain of 5 pounds or more, chest pains, or difficulty in breathing.

☐ Carry an identification card indicating that you are taking this medicine. Always tell your pharmacist, dentist, and other doctors who are treating you that you are taking this medicine.

☐ Do not stop taking this medicine without your doctor's approval and do not go without medicine between prescription refills. Call your pharmacist 2 or 3 days before you will run out of the medicine.

* * * * *

Desipramine HCl (Oral Antidepressant)
United States: Norpramin, Pertofrane
Canada: Norpramin, Pertofrane

☐ This medicine is used to help relieve the symptoms of depression. It is important that you take the medicine regularly and that you do not miss any

251

doses. The full effect of the medicine will not be noticed immediatley, but may take from a few days to several weeks. Early signs of improvement are increased appetite, better sleep, increased energy and, later, improved mood. DO NOT STOP TAKING the medicine when you first feel better or you may feel worse in 3 or 4 days.

HOW TO USE THIS MEDICINE

☐ This medicine may be taken with food unless otherwise directed.

SPECIAL INSTRUCTIONS

☐ If you forget to take a dose, take it as soon as possible. However, if it is almost time for your next dose, do not take the missed dose. Instead, continue with your regular dosing schedule.

☐ Any medicine has a few unwanted side effects. Because this medicine takes a few weeks to work, the side effects are the only thing that tell the doctor that the drug is being absorbed. Most of these side effects will go away as your body adjusts to the medicine.

☐ In some people, this drug may cause dizziness or drowsiness. Do not drive a car or operate dangerous machinery or do jobs that require you to be alert until you know how you are going to react to this drug.

☐ If this medicine causes dizziness, you should be careful going up and down stairs and you should not change positions too quickly. Get out of bed slowly in the morning and dangle your feet over the edge of the bed for a few minutes before standing up. Sit or lie down at the first sign of dizziness. Tell your doctor you have been dizzy and he may adjust your dose.

☐ Do not drink alcoholic beverages while taking this drug without the approval of your doctor.

☐ It is important that you obtain the advice of your doctor or pharmacist before taking any other medicines, including pain relievers; sleeping pills; tranquilizers; other medicines for depression; cough, cold, or allergy medicines; or weight-reducing medicine.

☐ If your mouth becomes dry, suck a hard sour candy (sugarless) or ice chips, or chew gum. It is especially important to brush your teeth regularly if you develop a dry mouth.

☐ If you become constipated, try increasing the amount of bulk in your diet (for example, bran and salads), exercising more often, or drinking water.

☐ Call your doctor if you develop a sore throat, fever, mouth sores, eye pain or blurred vision, difficulty in urinating ("passing your water"), fast heartbeats, or a skin rash.

☐ Do not stop taking this medicine suddenly without your doctor's approval. When your doctor tells you to stop this medicine, you must follow these precautions for 1 week since some of the medicine will still be in your body.

☐ Carry an identification card indicating that you are taking this medicine.

Always tell your dentist, pharmacist, and other doctors who are treating you
that you are taking this medicine.

* * * * *

Desmopressin (*Nasal Antidiuretic Hormone Analogue*)
United States: DDAVP
Canada: DDAVP

☐ This medicine is used in certain conditions to help decrease the amount of
water excreted in the urine and to decrease thirst.

HOW TO USE THIS MEDICINE (Fig. 5):

☐ INTRANASAL APPLICATION OF DDAVP WITH THE RHINYLE

1. Pull the plastic tag on the neck of the bottle and tear off the security
seal.
2. Remove the plastic cap and **retain it for reclosure.**
3. Twist off the inner seal at the tip of the plastic teat and **retain for
reclosure.**

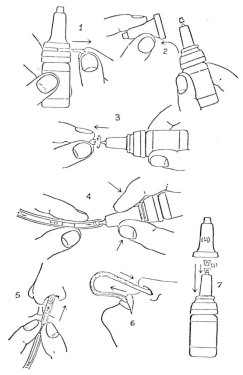

Figure 5. *Instructions for use of desmopressin Reproduced by permission of
Ferring Pharmaceuticals Limited, Canada.*

4. Take the arrow-marked end of the rhinyle in one hand and place the finger and thumb of the other hand around the plastic teat.
   Insert the tip of the plastic teat in a downward position into the arrow-marked end of the rhinyle and gently squeeze the teat until the solution has reached the desired graduation mark.
   Note: In order to prevent air bubbles from forming in the rhinyle, maintain steady pressure on the plastic teat.
      If it is difficult to fill the rhinyle, a diabetic or tuberculin syringe may be used to draw up the dose and load the rhinyle tube.
5. Hold the rhinyle with the tips of finger and thumb $1\frac{1}{2}$ to 2 cm from the arrow-marked end and insert it into a nostril until the finger tips touch the nostril.
6. Place the other end of the rhinyle in your mouth. Hold your breath, tilt back your head, and then blow with a short strong puff through the rhinyle so that the solution reaches the right place in the nasal cavity. Through this procedure, medicine is limited to the nasal cavity and the solution does not pass down into the pharynx.
7. After use, close the bottle using both the inner plastic tip seal (i) and the outer plastic cap (ii). **The use of both seals prevents wasteful loss by evaporation during refrigeration storage.**
   Rinse the rhinyle under running water and shake thoroughly until no more water is left. The rhinyle can then be used for the next application.

☐ Do not use this medicine more often than prescribed.

SPECIAL INSTRUCTIONS

☐ Your doctor may limit the amount of liquids you should drink.

☐ Call your doctor immediately if you think you may be allergic to the medicine or if you develop a skin rash, hives, itching, swelling of the face, or difficulty in breathing. If you cannot reach your doctor, phone a hospital emergency department.

☐ Most people experience few or no side effects form their drugs. However, any medicine can sometimes cause unwanted effects. Call your doctor if you develop nausea, unusual headaches, or stomach cramps.

☐ Store the medicine in a refrigerator but do not freeze. Do not use after the discard date.

*   *   *   *   *

Desonide (*Topical Corticosteroid*)
United States: Tridesilon
Canada: Tridesilon

☐ This medicine is used to help relieve redness, swelling, itching, and inflammation of certain types of skin conditions.

HOW TO USE THIS MEDICINE

☐ For CREAM and OINTMENT

- Each time you apply the medicine, wash your hands and gently cleanse the skin area well with water unless otherwise directed by your doctor. Do not allow the skin to dry completely. Pat with a clean towel until slightly damp.
- Apply a small amount of the drug to the affected area and spread lightly. Only the medicine that is actually touching the skin will work. A thick layer is not more effective than a thin layer. Do not bandage unless directed by your doctor.

☐ Do not use the drug more frequently or in larger quantities than prescribed by your doctor. Overuse of this medicine may cause you to absorb too much of the drug and increase the risk of side effects.

☐ Keep the medicine away from the eyes, nose, and mouth.

SPECIAL INSTRUCTIONS

☐ If you forget to apply the medicine, apply it as soon as possible. However, if it is almost time for your next dose, do not apply the missed dose but continue with your regular schedule.

☐ Do not use this medicine for any other skin problems without checking with your doctor.

☐ Do not apply cosmetics or lotions on top of the drug unless your doctor approves.

☐ Call your doctor if the condition for which this drug is being used persists or becomes worse or if you have a constant irritation such as itching or burning that was not present before you started using this medicine. Also call your doctor if you develop abnormal lines or thinning of the skin, especially under the arms or between the legs.

☐ Store in a cool place but do not freeze.

☐ For external use only. Do not swallow.

☐ Tell future doctors that you have used this medicine.

* * * * *

Desoximetasone (*Topical Corticosteroid*)
United States: Topicort
Canada: Topicort

☐ This medicine is used to help relieve redness, swelling, itching, and inflammation of certain types of skin conditions.

255

HOW TO USE THIS MEDICINE

☐ For CREAM

- Each time you apply the medicine, wash your hands and gently cleanse the skin area well with water unless otherwise directed by your doctor. Do not allow the skin to dry completely. Pat with a clean towel until almost dry.
- Apply a small amount of the drug to the affected area and spread lightly. Only the medicine that is actually touching the skin will work. A thick layer is not more effective than a thin layer. Do not bandage unless directed by your doctor.

☐ Do not use the drug more frequently or in larger quantities than prescribed by your doctor. Overuse of this medicine may cause you to absorb too much of the drug and increase the risk of side effects.

☐ Keep the medicine away from the eyes, nose, and mouth.

SPECIAL INSTRUCTIONS

☐ If you forget to apply the medicine, apply it as soon as possible. However, if it is almost time for your next dose, do not apply the missed dose but continue with your regular schedule.

☐ Do not use this medicine for any other skin problems without checking with your doctor.

☐ Do not apply cosmetics or lotions on top of the drug unless your doctor approves.

☐ Call your doctor if the condition for which this drug is being used persists or becomes worse or if you have a constant irritation such as itching or burning that was not present before you started using this medicine. Also call your doctor if you develop abnormal lines or thinning of the skin, especially under the arms or between the legs.

☐ Store in a cool place but do not freeze.

☐ For external use only. Do not swallow.

☐ Tell future doctors that you have used this medicine.

* * * * *

Dexamethasone (Eye/Ear Corticosteroid)

United States: Decadron, Maxidex Ophthalmic, Phosphate Ophthalmic

Canada: Decadron Eye-Ear Solution, Maxidex, Novadex, Optomethasone

☐ This medicine is used to help relieve the pain, redness and swelling of certain types of eye and ear conditions.

HOW TO USE THIS MEDICINE

☐ Shake this medicine well before using. (**United States** and **Canada:** Maxidex Ophthalmic Suspension)

☐ For EAR DROPS

INSTILLATION OF EAR DROPS

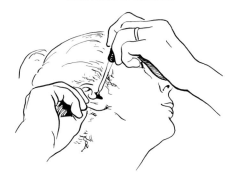

- Warm the ear drops to body temperature by holding the bottle in your hands for a few minutes. Do NOT heat the drops in hot water.
- The person administering the ear drops should wash his hands with soap and water.
- The ear drops must be kept clean. Do not touch the dropper against the ear or anything else.
- Tilt your head or lie on your side so that the ear to be treated is facing up.
- In ADULTS, hold the ear lobe up and back.
  In CHILDREN, hold the ear lobe down and back.
- Place the prescribed number of drops into the ear. Do not insert the dropper into the ear as it may cause injury.
- Remain in the same position for a short time (2 minutes) after you have administered the drops.
- Dry the ear lobe if there are any drops on it.
- If necessary, have someone else administer the ear drops for you.
- Do not use the ear drops if they change in color or have changed in any way since you purchased them.
- Keep the bottle tightly closed when not in use.

☐ For EAR DROPS AFTER APPLICATION OF EAR WICK
- Warm the medicine to body temperature by holding it in your hands for a few minutes.
- Tilt the head to the side or lie on your side so that the ear to be treated is uppermost.
- Drop the prescribed amount of medicine into the ear canal.

257

- Do not use the solution if it is discolored or if it appears to have changed in any way since you purchased it.
- Keep the wick moist and replace with a clean wick as directed by your doctor.

☐ For EAR OINTMENT
- Clean the ear thoroughly and apply a small amount of ointment to the affected area using a cotton-tipped swab.

☐ For EYE DROPS

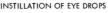

INSTILLATION OF EYE DROPS

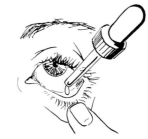

- The person administering the eye drops should wash his hands with soap and water.
- The eye drops must be kept clean. Do not touch the dropper against the face or anything else.
- Lie down or tilt your head backward and look at the ceiling.
- Gently pull down the lower lid of your eye to form a pouch.
- Hold the dropper in your other hand and approach the eye from the side. Place the dropper as close to the eye as possible without touching it.
- Place the prescribed number of drops into the pouch of the eye.
- Close your eyes. Do not rub them.
- Apply gentle pressure for a minute with your fingers to the bridge of the nose (inside corner of the eye) to prevent the eye drops from being drained from the eye.
- Blot excess solution around the eye with a tissue.
- If necessary, have someone else administer the eye drops for you.
- Do not use the eye drops if they change in color or have changed in any way since being purchased.
- Keep the eye drop bottle tightly closed when not in use.

☐ For EYE OINTMENT

INSTILLATION OF EYE OINTMENT

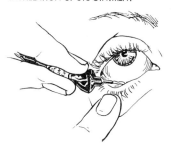

- The person administering the eye ointment should wash his hands with soap and water.
- The eye ointment must be kept clean. Do not touch the tube against the face or anything else.
- Lie down or tilt your head backward and look at the ceiling.
- Gently pull down the lower lid of your eye to form a pouch.
- Hold the tube in your other hand and place the tube as close as possible to the eye without touching it.
- Squeeze the prescribed amount of ointment (usually $\frac{1}{2}$ inch in adults) from the tube along the pouch.
- Close your eyes. Do not rub them.
- Wipe off any excess ointment around the eye with a tissue.
- Clean the tip of the ointment tube with a tissue.
- If necessary, have someone else administer the eye ointment for you.
- Keep the eye ointment tube tightly closed when not in use.

☐ Do not use this drug more frequently or in larger quantities than prescribed by your doctor.

SPECIAL INSTRUCTIONS

☐ This medicine should be used as long as prescribed by your doctor. Do not stop using it earlier than your doctor has recommended in spite of the fact that your symptoms seem to have improved.

☐ If you forget to use the medicine, use it as soon as possible. However, if it is almost time for your next dose, do not use the missed dose but continue with your regular schedule.

☐ Vision may be blurred for a few minutes after using the eye medicine. Do not drive a car or operate dangerous machinery or do jobs that require you to be alert until your vision has cleared.

☐ Do not use this medicine at the same time as any other eye or ear medicine without the approval of your doctor. Some medicines cannot be mixed.

☐ Call your doctor if the condition for which you are using this medicine persists or becomes worse or if the medicine causes itching or burning for more than a few minutes after instillation.

☐ For external use only. Do not swallow.

*　*　*　*　*

Dexamethasone (*Topical Corticosteroid*)
United States: Aeroseb-Dex, Decaderm, Decaspray, Hexadrol

☐ This medicine is used to help relieve redness, swelling and itching, and inflammation of certain types of skin conditions.

HOW TO USE THIS MEDICINE
☐ For CREAM and OINTMENT
- Each time you apply the medicine, wash your hands and gently cleanse the skin area well with water unless otherwise directed by your doctor. Do not allow the skin to dry completely. Pat with a clean towel until almost dry.
- Apply a small amount of the drug to the affected area and spread lightly. Only the medicine that is actually touching the skin will work. A thick layer is not more effective than a thin layer. Do not bandage unless directed by your doctor.

☐ For AEROSOL
- Shake the container well each time before using.
- Cleanse the affected area well with water unless otherwise directed by your doctor.
- Hold the container straight up and about 6 to 8 inches away from the skin.
- Spray the affected area for 1 to 3 seconds.
- Shake the container well between sprays.
- Do not spray into the eyes, nose, or mouth and try to avoid inhaling the vapors.
- Do not smoke while using this spray or use it near an open flame, fire, or heat. Do not use the spray near food.

☐ Do not use the drug more frequently or in larger quantities than prescribed by your doctor. Overuse of this medicine may cause you to absorb too much of the drug and increase the risk of side effects.

☐ Keep the medicine away from the eyes, nose, and mouth.

SPECIAL INSTRUCTIONS
☐ If you forget to apply the medicine, apply it as soon as possible. However, if it is almost time for your next dose, do not apply the missed dose but continue with your regular schedule.

260

- ☐ Do not use this medicine for any other skin problems without checking with your doctor.

- ☐ Do not apply cosmetics or lotions on top of the drug unless your doctor approves.

- ☐ Call your doctor if the condition for which this drug is being used persists or becomes worse or if you have a constant irritation such as itching or burning that was not present before you started using this medicine. Also call your doctor if you develop abnormal lines or thinning of the skin, especially under the arms or between the legs.

- ☐ Do not place the aerosol container in hot water or near radiators, stoves, or other sources of heat. Do not puncture or incinerate the container (even when empty). Do not store it at temperatures greater than 120°F (49°C).

- ☐ Store in a cool place, but do not freeze.

- ☐ For external use only. Do not swallow.

- ☐ Tell future doctors that you have used this medicine.

* * * * *

Dexamethasone (*Oral Corticosteroid*)

United States: Decadron, Dexone, Hexadrol, SK-Dexamethasone
Canada: Decadron, Dexasone, Hexadrol

- ☐ This medicine is similar to cortisone which is a hormone normally produced by the body. This medicine is used to help decrease inflammation which then relieves pain, redness, and swelling. It is used in the treatment of certain kinds of arthritis as well as severe allergies or skin conditions.

HOW TO USE THIS MEDICINE
- ☐ Take this medicine with food or a glass of milk in order to help prevent stomach upset. Call your doctor if you develop stomach upset or stomach pain or heartburn (especially if it awakens you during the night). Do not try to treat this yourself.

- ☐ If your doctor has prescribed only ONE dose of this medicine every day, it is best to take it before 9 A.M. or with breakfast.

- ☐ If you forget to take a dose, take it as soon as possible. However, if it is almost time for your next dose, do not take the missed dose. Instead, continue with your regular dosing schedule.

SPECIAL INSTRUCTIONS
- ☐ Women who are pregnant, breast-feeding, or planning to become pregnant should tell their doctor before taking this medicine.

261

☐ It is best not to drink alcoholic beverages while you are taking this medicine because the combination can cause stomach problems.

☐ Do not take any more of this medicine than your doctor has prescribed and do not stop taking this medicine suddenly without the approval of your doctor. It may be necessary for your doctor to slowly reduce your dose since your body becomes used to this medicine and it might be harmful if you suddenly did not receive this medicine.

☐ Do not take aspirin or medicines containing aspirin without the approval of your doctor.

☐ While you are taking this medicine you may gain some weight. This could be due to an increase in your appetite or increased water in your system. Your doctor may prescribe a special diet to decrease the number of calories you eat and/or to lower the amount of sodium or increase the amount of potassium in your diet. Follow any diet that your doctor may order.

☐ You may find that you bruise more easily. Try to protect yourself from all injuries to prevent bruising.

☐ Diabetic patients should regularly check the sugar in their urine and report any unusual levels to their doctor.

☐ Carry an identification card indicating that you are taking this medicine. Always tell your pharmacist, dentist, and other doctors who are treating you that you are taking this medicine. If you have an acute infection, injury, or operation or dental surgery within 1 year of taking this medicine, it is important to tell your doctor.

☐ Most people experience few or no side effects from their drugs. However, any medicine can sometimes cause unwanted effects. Call your doctor if you develop stomach pain, sore throat, fever, swelling of the legs or ankles, a wound that does not heal, eye pain or blurred vision, frequent urination ("passing your water"), nightmares or depression, muscle cramps, red or black stools, puffing of the face, or menstrual problems.

*   *   *   *   *

Dexamethasone Sodium Phosphate (*Inhalation Asthma Prophylaxis*)

United States: Decadron Phosphate Respihaler

☐ This medicine is used to help prevent asthmatic attacks.

HOW TO USE THIS MEDICINE

☐ INSTRUCTIONS FOR USE

    1. If troubled with sputum, try to clear your chest as completely as possible before inhaling the drug. This will help get the drug more deeply into your lungs.

2. Hold the inhaler UPRIGHT during use.
3. SHAKE the canister.
4. Breathe out fully and place your lips tightly around the mouthpiece and tilt your head slightly back.

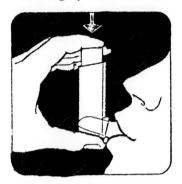

5. Start to breathe in slowly and press down on the valve firmly and fully at the middle of inspiration ("breathing in") to release a "puff."

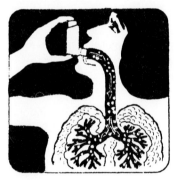

6. Hold your breath for a few seconds. Breathe out through the nose.
7. Allow at least 30 seconds before shaking again to release a second "puff" if prescribed.
8. Gargle and rinse your mouth with warm water after administering the medicine.
9. The mouthpiece of the inhaler should be cleaned after each use.
10. Failure to follow these instructions carefully can result in inadequate treatment.

SPECIAL INSTRUCTIONS

☐ If you forget to take a dose, take it as soon as possible. However, if it is almost time for your next dose, do not take the missed dose. Instead, continue with your regular dosing schedule.

☐ It may take 1 to 4 weeks before you feel the full benefit of this medicine. If you are also using another inhaler that opens up the air passages in your lungs (bronchodilator), use it several minutes before you use this inhaler.

263

- [ ] If an asthmatic attack should occur continue the medicine and if no relief is obtained, you should notify your doctor.

- [ ] Do not take any more of this medicine than your doctor has prescribed and do not stop taking this medicine suddenly without the approval of your doctor. If you should suddenly stop taking it or reduce your dose, you may experience a worsening of your asthma and it might be harmful if you suddenly did not receive this medicine.

- [ ] Carry an identification card indicating that you are taking this medicine. Always tell your pharmacist, dentist, and other doctors who are treating you that you are taking this medicine.

- [ ] Store the container in a cool place. Do not place the container in hot water or near radiators, stoves, or other sources of heat. Do not puncture, burn, or incinerate the container (even after it is empty).

- [ ] Most people experience few or no side effects from their drugs. However, any medicine can sometimes cause unwanted effects. Call your doctor if you develop a soreness in the mouth or throat, a bad taste in the mouth that will not go away, or a worsening of your asthma.

* * * * *

Dexchlorpheniramine Maleate (*Oral Antihistamine*)
United States: Polaramine
Canada: Polaramine

- [ ] This medicine is used to help relieve the symptoms of certain types of allergic conditions, coughs and colds, and certain skin conditions.

HOW TO USE THIS MEDICINE
- [ ] This medicine may be taken with food or a glass of milk if it upsets your stomach.

- [ ] Swallow these tablets whole. Do not crush, chew, or break them into pieces. (**United States** and **Canada:** Polaramine Repetabs)

SPECIAL INSTRUCTIONS
- [ ] If you forget to take a dose, take it as soon as possible. However, if it is almost time for your next dose, do not take the missed dose. Instead, continue with your regular dosing schedule.

- [ ] In some people, this drug may initially cause dizziness or drowsiness. Do not drive a car or operate dangerous machinery or do jobs that require you to be alert until you know how you are going to react to this drug. If you become dizzy, you should be careful going up and down stairs. Sit or lie down at the first sign of dizziness. Tell your doctor if it continues.

- [ ] Do not drink alcoholic beverages while taking this drug without the approval of your doctor.

264

- [ ] If your mouth becomes dry, suck a hard sour candy (sugarless) or ice chips, or chew gum. It is especially important to brush your teeth regularly if you develop a dry mouth.

- [ ] It is important that you obtain the advice of your doctor or pharmacist before taking pain relievers, nonprescription drugs, sleeping pills or tranquilizers, or other medicines for allergies.

- [ ] Do not take this medicine more often or longer than recommended by your doctor.

- [ ] Most people experience few or no side effects from their drugs. However, any medicine can sometimes cause unwanted effects. Call your doctor if you develop a skin rash, fast heartbeats, blurred vision, stomach pain, or difficulty in urinating ("passing your water").

* * * * *

Dextroamphetamine Sulfate (*Oral Sympathomimetic*)
United States: Dexampex, Dexedrine, Ferndex
Canada: Dexedrine

Dextroamphetamine Tannate
United States: Obotan

- [ ] This medicine has many uses and the reason it was prescribed depends upon your condition. If you do not fully understand why you are taking it, check with your doctor.

- [ ] IMPORTANT: If you have ever had an allergic reaction to an amphetamine medicine or any other medicine, tell your doctor or pharmacist before you take any of this medicine.

HOW TO USE THIS MEDICINE
- [ ] This medicine may be taken with food or a glass of water.

- [ ] Do not take the medicine late in the day or it may cause insomnia (difficulty in sleeping).

- [ ] This medicine must be swallowed whole. Do not crush, chew, or break it into pieces. (**United States** and **Canada:** Dexedrine Spansules)

SPECIAL INSTRUCTIONS
- [ ] If you forget to take a dose, take it as soon as possible. However, if it is almost time for your next dose, do not take the missed dose. Instead, continue with your regular dosing schedule.

- [ ] Women who are pregnant, breast-feeding, or planning to become pregnant should tell their doctor before taking this medicine.

- [ ] Do not take any more of this medicine than your doctor has prescribed and do not stop taking this medicine suddenly without the approval of your doctor.

☐ If your mouth becomes dry, suck a hard sour candy (sugarless) or ice chips, or chew gum. It is especially important to brush your teeth regularly if you develop a dry mouth.

☐ In some people, this drug may cause dizziness. Do not drive a car or operate dangerous machinery or do jobs that require you to be alert until you know how you are going to react to this drug. Therefore, you should be careful going up and down stairs. Sit or lie down at the first sign of dizziness.

☐ If this medicine is for a child, do not let him (her) ride a bike or climb trees until you can determine how he (she) is going to react to the medicine. They could hurt themselves if they participated in these activities when they were dizzy.

☐ Do not treat yourself with baking soda or antacids without the approval of your doctor.

☐ Most people experience few or no side effects from their drugs. However, any medicine can sometimes cause unwanted effects. Call your doctor if you develop a skin rash, chest pain or palpitations, unusual movements of the head, arms or legs, or unusual restlessness.

☐ Carry an identification card indicating that you are taking this medicine. Always tell your pharmacist, dentist, and other doctors who are treating you that you are taking this medicine.

*　*　*　*　*

Dextroamphetamine Sulfate-Amobarbital (*Oral Sympathomimetic-Sedative*)

United States: Dexamyl

Canada: Dexamyl

☐ This medicine has many uses and the reason it was prescribed depends upon your condition. If you do not fully understand why you are taking it, check with your doctor.

☐ IMPORTANT: If you have ever had an allergic reaction to an amphetamine medicine or barbiturate medicine or any other medicine, tell your doctor or pharmacist before you take any of this medicine.

HOW TO USE THIS MEDICINE

☐ This medicine may be taken with food or a glass of water.

☐ Do not take the medicine late in the day or it may cause insomnia (difficulty in sleeping).

☐ This medicine must be swallowed whole. Do not crush, chew, or break it into pieces. (**Canada:** Dexamyl Spansules)

266

SPECIAL INSTRUCTIONS

☐ If you forget to take a dose, take it as soon as possible. However, if it is almost time for your next dose, do not take the missed dose. Instead, continue with your regular dosing schedule.

☐ Women who are pregnant, breast-feeding, or planning to become pregnant should tell their doctor before taking this medicine.

☐ Do not take any more of this medicine than your doctor has prescribed and do not stop taking this medicine suddenly without the approval of your doctor.

☐ If your mouth becomes dry, suck a hard sour candy (sugarless) or ice chips, or chew gum. It is especially important to brush your teeth regularly if you develop a dry mouth.

☐ In some people, this drug may cause dizziness. Do not drive a car or operate dangerous machinery or do jobs that require you to be alert until you know how you are going to react to this drug. Therefore, you should be careful going up and down stairs. Sit or lie down at the first sign of dizziness.

☐ Do not drink alcoholic beverages while taking this drug without the approval of your doctor.

☐ It is important that you obtain the advice of your doctor or pharmacist before taking pain relievers, nonprescription drugs, sleeping pills, tranquilizers, or medicines for depression while you are taking this drug.

☐ Call your doctor immediately if you think you may be allergic to the medicine or if you develop a skin rash, hives, itching, swelling of the face, or difficulty in breathing. If you cannot reach your doctor, phone a hospital emergency department.

☐ Most people experience few or no side effects from their drugs. However, any medicine can sometimes cause unwanted effects. Call your doctor if you develop a sore throat, nightmares, staggering walk or unusual restlessness, a yellow color to the skin or eyes, easy bruising, or unusual movements of the head, arms or legs.

☐ Carry an identification card indicating that you are taking this medicine. Always tell your pharmacist, dentist, and other doctors who are treating you that you are taking this medicine.

* * * * *

Dextromethorphan HBr (*Oral Antitussive*)
United States: Benylin DM Cough, Romilar
Canada: Balminil D.M. Syrup, DM Syrup, Robidex, Sedatuss,

☐ This medicine is used to help relieve dry, irritating coughs.

☐ IMPORTANT: If you have ever had an allergic reaction to a bromide medicine, tell your doctor or pharmacist before you take any of this medicine.

267

HOW TO USE THIS MEDICINE

☐ Do not dilute the syrup. The soothing effect of the syrup will be enhanced if you do not drink liquids immediately after taking the medicine.

SPECIAL INSTRUCTIONS

☐ In some people, this drug may cause dizziness or drowsiness. Do not drive a car or operate dangerous machinery or do jobs that require you to be alert until you know how you are going to react to this drug.

☐ If you become dizzy, you should be careful going up and down stairs. Sit or lie down at the first sign of dizziness.

☐ Do not drink alcoholic beverages while taking this drug without the approval of your doctor.

☐ It is important that you obtain the advice of your doctor or pharmacist before taking pain relievers, nonprescription drugs, sleeping pills, tranquilizers, or medicines for depression while you are taking this drug.

☐ Call your doctor if the cough lasts longer than 1 week or if you develop a fever, skin rash, or persistent headache.

☐ Do not use this medicine for more than 1 week without the advice of your doctor.

* * * * *

Dextrothyroxine (*Oral Hypercholesterolemia Therapy*)
United States: Choloxin
Canada: Choloxin

☐ This medicine is used in certain types of conditions to lower the amount of cholesterol and triglycerides (fatty substances) in the blood.

HOW TO USE THIS MEDICINE

☐ This medicine may be taken with food or on an empty stomach.

SPECIAL INSTRUCTIONS

☐ It is very important to follow any diet that your doctor may also prescribe for you. The cholesterol content of some common foods is listed in Appendix B.

☐ If you forget to take a dose, take it as soon as possible. However, if it is almost time for your next dose, do not take the missed dose. Instead, continue with your regular dosing schedule.

☐ In some people, this drug may cause dizziness or blurred vision. Do not drive a car or operate dangerous machinery or do jobs that require you to be alert until you know how you are going to react to this drug.

☐ If you become dizzy, you should be careful going up and down stairs. Sit or lie down at the first sign of dizziness.

268

☐ Do not take any more of this medicine than your doctor has prescribed and do not stop taking this medicine suddenly without the approval of your doctor.

☐ Most people experience few or no side effects from their drugs. However, any medicine can sometimes cause unwanted effects. Call your doctor if you develop a skin rash, chest pain, rapid pulse, swelling of the legs or ankles, sudden weight gain, or shortness of breath.

☐ Carry an identification card indicating that you are taking this medicine. Always tell your pharmacist, dentist, and other doctors who are treating you that you are taking this medicine.

* * * * *

Diazepam (Oral Anxiolytic-Sedative)
United States: Valium
Canada: D-Tran, E-Pam, Meval, Neo-Calme, Novodiapam, Paxel, Serenack, Stress-Pam, Valium, Vivol

☐ This medicine is used to help relieve anxiety and tension. It is also used to help relax muscles as well as to treat some other conditions. Check with your doctor if you do not fully understand why you are taking it.

☐ IMPORTANT: If you have ever had an allergic reaction to a benzodiazepine medicine, tell your doctor or pharmacist before you take any of this medicine.

HOW TO USE THIS MEDICINE
☐ This medicine may be taken with food or a full glass of water.

☐ For LIQUID MEDICINE
  • Shake the bottle well before using so that you can measure an accurate dose. (Canada: Valium Suspension)

SPECIAL INSTRUCTIONS
☐ If you forget to take a dose, take it as soon as possible. However, if it is almost time for your next dose, do not take the missed dose. Instead, continue with your regular dosing schedule.

☐ Women who are pregnant, breast-feeding, or planning to become pregnant should tell their doctor before taking this medicine.

☐ In some people, this drug may cause dizziness or drowsiness. Do not drive a car or operate dangerous machinery or do jobs that require you to be alert until you know how you are going to react to this drug.

☐ If you become dizzy, you should be careful going up and down stairs. Sit or lie down at the first sign of dizziness.

269

- [ ] Do not drink alcoholic beverages while taking this drug without the approval of your doctor.

- [ ] It is important that you obtain the advice of your doctor or pharmacist before taking ANY other medicines including pain relievers, sleeping pills, tranquilizers or medicines for depression, cough/cold or allergy medicines, or weight-reducing medicines.

- [ ] Do not take any more of this medicine than your doctor has prescribed because the drug could become habit-forming. Do not stop taking this medicine suddenly without the approval of your doctor.

- [ ] Most people experience few or no side effects from their drugs. However, any medicine can sometimes cause unwanted effects. Call your doctor if you develop a sore throat, fever, mouth sores, a staggering walk, a yellow color to the skin or eyes, slow heartbeats or shortness of breath, unusual tiredness or nervousness, or stomach pain.

* * * * *

Dibucaine (*Rectal Topical Anesthetic*)
United States: Nupercainal Suppositories
Canada: Nupercainal Suppositories

- [ ] This medicine is used to help relieve pain and itching.

- [ ] IMPORTANT: If you have ever had an allergic reaction to dibucaine or any "caine" type of medicine, tell your doctor or pharmacist before you use any of this drug.

HOW TO USE THIS MEDICINE
- [ ] ADMINISTRATION OF SUPPOSITORIES
    - Remove the wrapper from the suppository.
    - Lie on your side and raise your knee to your chest.
    - Insert the suppository with the tapered (pointed) end first into the rectum.
    - Remain lying down for a few minutes so that the suppository will dissolve in the rectum.
    - Try to avoid having a bowel movement for at least one hour so that the drug will have time to work.

SPECIAL INSTRUCTIONS
- [ ] Call your doctor if the condition for which this drug is being used persists or becomes worse or if you have a constant irritation such as itching or burning that was not present before you started using this medicine. Also call your doctor if you develop any new rectal bleeding.

- [ ] For external use only. Do not swallow.

* * * * *

270

Dibucaine (*Topical Anesthetic*)
United States: Nupercainal
Canada: Nupercainal

☐ This medicine is used to help relieve pain and itching of the skin.

☐ IMPORTANT: If you have ever had an allergic reaction to dibucaine or any "caine" type of medicine, tell your doctor or pharmacist before you use any of this drug.

HOW TO USE THIS MEDICINE
☐ For CREAM and OINTMENT

- Each time you apply the medicine, wash your hands and gently cleanse the skin area well with water unless otherwise directed by your doctor. Do not allow the skin to dry completely. Pat with a clean towel until almost dry.
- Apply a small amount of the drug to the affected area and spread lightly. Only the medicine that is actually touching the skin will work. A thick layer is not more effective than a thin layer. Do not bandage unless directed by your doctor.

☐ Do not use the drug more frequently or in larger quantities than prescribed by your doctor.

☐ **Adults:** Do not use more than 2 tubes of cream or 1 tube of ointment on the skin in any 24-hour period.

☐ **Children:** Do not use more than $\frac{1}{2}$ tube of cream or $\frac{1}{4}$ tube of ointment on the skin in any 24-hour period.

SPECIAL INSTRUCTIONS
☐ If you have a severe sunburn, you should consult your doctor before using this medicine.

☐ Call your doctor if the condition for which this drug is being used persists or becomes worse or if you have a constant irritation such as itching or burning that was not present before you started using this medicine. Also call your doctor if you develop a slow heartbeat, fainting, or tremors.

☐ For external use only. Do not swallow.

*　*　*　*　*

Dichlorphenamide (*Oral Carbonic Anhydrase Inhibitor*)
United States: Daranide, Oratrol
Canada: Daranide

☐ This drug has many uses and the reason it was prescribed depends on your condition. Check with your doctor.

☐ If you forget to take a dose, take it as soon as possible. However, if it is almost time for your next dose, do not take the missed dose. Instead, continue with your regular dosing schedule.

☐ Most people experience few or no side effects from their drugs. However, any medicine can sometimes cause unwanted effects. Call your doctor if you develop a skin rash, sore throat, fever, blurred vision, easy bruising, numbness of the hands or feet, drowsiness, unusual weakness, stomach pain, or vomiting.

*   *   *   *   *

Dicloxacillin (*Oral Antibiotic*)

United States: Dycill, Dynapen, Pathocil, Veracillin
Canada: Dynapen

☐ This medicine is an antibiotic used to treat certain types of infections.

☐ IMPORTANT: If you have ever had an allergic reaction to penicillin or any other antibiotic, tell your doctor or pharmacist before you take any of this medicine.

HOW TO USE THIS MEDICINE

☐ It is best to take this medicine on an empty stomach 1 hour before (or 2 hours after) meals or food unless otherwise directed by your doctor. Take it at the proper time even if you skip a meal.

☐ Take this medicine with a full glass of water.

☐ For LIQUID MEDICINE (***United States:*** Dynapen and Pathocil Suspensions, ***Canada:*** Dynapen Suspension)
   • If you were prescribed a SUSPENSION, shake the bottle well before using so that you can measure an accurate dose.
   • Store the bottle of medicine in the refrigerator but do not freeze.
   • If there is a discard date on the bottle, throw away any unused medicine after that date.

SPECIAL INSTRUCTIONS

☐ It is important to take ***all*** of this medicine plus any refills that your doctor told you to take. Do not stop taking this medicine earlier than your doctor has recommended in spite of the fact that you may feel better. Otherwise, the infection may return.

☐ If you forget to take a dose, take it as soon as you remember and then continue with your regular schedule.

☐ Most people experience few or no side effects from their drugs. However, any medicine can sometimes cause unwanted effects. Call your doctor if you

develop a dark-colored tongue, yellow-green stools or, in women, a vaginal discharge that was not present before you started taking this medicine.

☐ This medicine sometimes causes diarrhea (loose bowel movements). Call your doctor if the diarrhea becomes severe or lasts for more than two days.

☐ Call your doctor immediately if you think you may be allergic to the medicine or if you develop a skin rash, hives, itching, swelling of the face, or difficulty in breathing. If you cannot reach your doctor, phone a hospital emergency department.

☐ If for some reason you cannot take all of the medicine, throw away the unused portion by flushing it down the toilet. Do not take or save old medicine.

*   *   *   *   *

Dicumarol (*Oral Anticoagulant*)
United States: Dicumarol
Canada: Dufalone

☐ This medicine is used to help prevent harmful blood clots from forming. It is commonly called a "blood thinner."

HOW TO USE THIS MEDICINE

☐ Take this medicine **exactly** as your doctor has prescribed. Try to take the medicine at the same time every day and do not miss any doses. Do not take extra tablets without your doctor's approval because overtreatment will cause bleeding.

☐ Regular blood tests, called "prothrombin times," are necessary in order for your doctor to prescribe the correct dose for you. Your dose may change from time to time depending on these tests.

☐ It is best to take this medicine with a glass of water. Do not take it with food or other drugs unless otherwise directed.

☐ If you forget to take a dose, take it as soon as possible. However, if it is almost time for your next dose, do not take the missed dose. Instead, continue with your regular dosing schedule. Record the date of the missed dose so that you can tell your doctor the next time you see him for a blood test. Call your doctor if you miss more than 1 dose.

SPECIAL INSTRUCTIONS

☐ Do not take any other drugs or stop taking any drugs you are currently taking without first consulting with your doctor. This even includes many products that you can buy without a prescription such as pain relievers and antacids. Always check with your pharmacist before you take or buy ANY nonprescription products.

☐ Do not take aspirin or medicines containing aspirin or salicylates. It is usually safe to take acetaminophen as a substitute for aspirin for occasional headaches and pain. Check with your pharmacist.

☐ It is best to avoid alcoholic beverages while you are taking this medicine because the combination may cause undesirable side effects. Ask your doctor if he feels it is safe for you to have the occasional drink.

☐ Do not eat unusually large amounts of leafy, green vegetables or change your diet without telling your doctor.

☐ If you have a tendency to cut yourself while shaving, you may wish to use an electric razor to avoid possible bleeding.

☐ Try to avoid contact sports or activities in which you could become injured because injuries could result in internal bleeding.

☐ If your body gets more medicine than it needs, bleeding may occur. Call your doctor if you notice any of the following signs of bleeding which you cannot explain or are unusual for you: nosebleeds, bruising or heavy menstrual bleeding; bleeding from the gums after brushing the teeth, heavy bleeding from cuts, red or black stools, red or dark brown urine, or vomiting or coughing up blood. Your doctor will do some blood tests and adjust your dose.

☐ Women who are pregnant, breast-feeding, or planning to become pregnant should tell their doctor before taking this medicine.

☐ Most people experience few or no side effects from their drugs. However, any medicine can sometimes cause unwanted effects. Call your doctor if you develop stomach or back pain, unusual headaches, changes in eyesight, constipation or diarrhea, dizziness, a skin rash, sore throat, fever, mouth sores, a yellow color to the skin or eyes, or unusual tiredness.

☐ Carry an identification card indicating that you are taking this medicine. Always tell your pharmacist, dentist, and other doctors who are treating you that you are taking this medicine.

☐ Do not go without this medicine between prescription refills. Call your pharmacist 2 or 3 days before you will run out of the medicine.

☐ After you stop taking the medicine, it will take your body some time to return to normal. Your doctor or pharmacist will tell you how long you must follow these instructions AFTER you have stopped taking this medicine.

*   *   *   *   *

Dicyclomine HCl (*Oral Antispasmodic*)

United States: Bentyl HCl, Dyspas, Rocyclo-10, Rocyclo-20
Canada: Bentylol, Cyclobec, Formulex, Spasmoban, Viscerol

☐ This medicine is used to help relieve cramps or spasms of the stomach, bowels, or bladder.

274

☐ IMPORTANT: If you have ever had an allergic reaction to atropine or any other drug used to relax the stomach or bowels, tell your doctor or pharmacist before you take any of this medicine.

HOW TO USE THIS MEDICINE

☐ Take this medicine approximately 30 minutes before a meal unless otherwise directed.

☐ This medicine must be swallowed whole. Do not crush, chew, or break it into pieces. (**Canada:** Bentylol Dospans)

☐ If you miss a dose of this medicine, do not take the missed dose and do not double the next dose.

SPECIAL INSTRUCTIONS

☐ If your mouth becomes dry, suck a hard sour candy (sugarless) or ice chips, or chew gum. It is especially important to brush your teeth regularly if you develop a dry mouth.

☐ In some people, this drug may cause dizziness or drowsiness. Do not drive a car or operate dangerous machinery or do jobs that require you to be alert until you know how you are going to react to this drug.

☐ If you become dizzy, you should be careful going up and down stairs. Sit or lie down at the first sign of dizziness. Tell your doctor you have been dizzy.

☐ Do not drink alcoholic beverages while taking this drug without the approval of your doctor.

☐ It is important that you obtain the advice of your doctor or pharmacist before taking pain relievers, nonprescription drugs, sleeping pills, tranquilizers or medicine for depression while you are taking this drug.

☐ A desire to urinate ("pass your water") with an inability to do so is not an uncommon effect with this drug. Urinating each time before taking the drug may help relieve this problem. Call your doctor if it continues.

☐ You may become more sensitive to heat because your body may perspire less while you are taking this drug. Be careful not to become overheated during exercise or in hot weather.

☐ Do not take antacids within 1 hour of taking this medicine as it could make this medicine less effective.

☐ If you become constipated, try increasing the amount of bulk in your diet (for example, bran and salads), exercising more often, or drinking more water. Call your doctor if the constipation continues.

☐ If your eyes become more sensitive to sunlight, it may help to wear sunglasses.

☐ Most people experience few or no side effects from their drugs. However, any medicine can sometimes cause unwanted effects. Call your doctor if you develop a skin rash, diarrhea, unusual restlessness, flushing, or eye pain.

*   *   *   *   *

Dicyclomine HCl-Phenobarbital (*Oral Antispasmodic-Sedative*)

United States: Bentyl with Phenobarb, Dibent-PB, Spastyl with Phenobarbital

Canada: Bentylol with Phenobarb, Spasmoban-PH, Viscephen

☐ This medicine is used to help relieve cramps or spasms of the stomach, bowels, or bladder.

☐ IMPORTANT: If you have ever had an allergic reaction to atropine or barbiturates or any other drug used to relax the stomach or bowels, tell your doctor or pharmacist before you take any of this medicine.

HOW TO USE THIS MEDICINE

☐ Take this medicine approximately 30 minutes before a meal unless otherwise directed.

☐ This medicine must be swallowed whole. Do not crush, chew, or break it into pieces. (***Canada:*** Bentylol Dospans with Phenobarb)

☐ If the syrup form has been prescribed for a child, it may be mixed with an equal amount of water.

☐ If you miss a dose of this medicine, do not take the missed dose and do not double the next dose.

SPECIAL INSTRUCTIONS

☐ Women who are pregnant, breast-feeding, or planning to become pregnant should tell their doctor before taking this medicine.

☐ If your mouth becomes dry, suck a hard sour candy (sugarless) or ice chips, or chew gum. It is especially important to brush your teeth regularly if you develop a dry mouth.

☐ In some people, this drug may cause dizziness or drowsiness. Do not drive a car or operate dangerous machinery or do jobs that require you to be alert until you know how you are going to react to this drug.

☐ If you become dizzy, you should be careful going up and down stairs. Sit or lie down at the first sign of dizziness. Tell your doctor you have been dizzy.

☐ Do not drink alcoholic beverages while taking this drug without the approval of your doctor.

☐ It is important that you obtain the advice of your doctor or pharmacist before taking pain relievers, nonprescription drugs, sleeping pills, tranquilizers, or medicine for depression while you are taking this drug.

☐ Do not take any more of this medicine than your doctor has prescribed and do not stop taking this medicine suddenly without the approval of your doctor.

☐ Call your doctor immediately if you think you may be allergic to the medicine or if you develop a skin rash, hives, itching, swelling of the face, or difficulty in breathing. If you cannot reach your doctor, phone a hospital emergency department.

☐ A desire to urinate ("pass your water") with an inability to do so is not an uncommon effect with this drug. Urinating each time before taking the drug may help relieve this problem. Call your doctor if it continues.

☐ You may become more sensitive to heat because your body may perspire less while you are taking this drug. Be careful not to become overheated during exercise or in hot weather.

☐ Do not take antacids within 1 hour of taking this medicine as it could make this medicine less effective.

☐ If you become constipated, try increasing the amount of bulk in your diet (for example, bran and salads), exercising more often, or drinking more water. Call your doctor if the constipation continues.

☐ If your eyes become more sensitive to sunlight, it may help to wear sunglasses.

☐ Most people experience few or no side effects from their drugs. However, any medicine can sometimes cause unwanted effects. Call your doctor if you develop a skin rash, diarrhea, unusual restlessness, flushing or eye pain, a sore throat, fever, a yellow color to the skin or eyes, easy bruising or bleeding, unusual tiredness, or slow heartbeats.

* * * * *

Dienestrol (*Vaginal Estrogen*)
United States: Dienestrol Cream, DV Cream, DV Suppositories, Estraguard
Canada: Dienestrol Cream

Dienestrol-Sulfanilamide (*Vaginal Estrogen-Antimicrobial*)
United States: AVC w/Dienestrol
Canada: AVC/Dienestrol

☐ This medicine is used to treat conditions of the vagina.

HOW TO USE THIS MEDICINE
☐ For VAGINAL CREAM
• Remove the cap from the tube.
• Screw the applicator to the tube of cream.

- Squeeze the tube until the plunger of the applicator is fully extended.
- Unscrew the applicator from the tube. Apply a small amount of cream to the outside of the applicator.
- Hold the filled applicator by the cylinder and gently insert it into the vaginal canal as far as it will go comfortably.
- Press the plunger and deposit the cream into the vagina.
- Keep the plunger depressed and remove the applicator from the vagina.
- After each use, it is important to take the applicator apart and clean it thoroughtly with soap and warm water. Rinse well. To take it apart, hold the cylinder of the plunger and turn the cap counterclockwise. To put it back together, drop the plunger into the cylinder as far as it will go. Place the cap on the end and turn it clockwise until the cap is tight.

☐ For VAGINAL SUPPOSITORIES
- Remove the wrapper from the suppository.
- Dip the suppository quickly into water just to moisten it.
- Insert the wide end of the suppository into the vaginal canal.

☐ Do not stop using this medicine suddenly without first consulting you physician. (**United States:** and **Canada:** AVC/Dienestrol)

☐ It is recommended that a pad or tampon be worn to protect underclothing. (**United States:** AVC/w/Dienestrol Cream; **Canada:** AVC/Dienestrol)

SPECIAL INSTRUCTIONS

☐ Women who are pregnant, breast-feeding, or planning to become pregnant should tell their doctor before taking this medicine.

☐ Do not use this medicine more often or longer than recommended by your doctor.

☐ It is recommmended that you do not smoke while you are on this medicine.

☐ Most people experience few or no side effects from their drugs. However, any medicine can sometimes cause unwanted effects. Call your doctor if you develop severe or persistent headaches, vomiting, dizziness or fainting, blurred vision or slurred speech, pain in the calves of the legs or numbness in an arm or leg, lumps in the breast, severe depression, a yellow color to the skin or eyes or dark-colored urine, severe abdominal pain, or an irritation caused by the medicine.

*   *   *   *   *

Diethylpropion (Oral Anorexiant)

United States: Tenuate, Tenuate Dospan, Tepanil, Tepanil Ten-Tab
Canada: Dietec, D.I.P., Nobesine-75, Regibon, Tenuate

☐ This medicine is used to help reduce the appetite in weight reduction programs. It can help you develop new eating habits and is only useful for a short time. Do not take any more of this medicine than your doctor has prescribed and do not stop taking this medicine suddenly without the approval of your doctor.

HOW TO USE THIS MEDICINE

- ☐ This medicine may be taken with food or a glass of water.

- ☐ Do not take the medicine late in the day or it may cause insomnia (difficulty in sleeping).

- ☐ This medicine must be swallowed whole. Do not crush, chew, or break it into pieces. (**United States:** Tenuate Dospan, Tepanil Ten-Tab; **Canada:** Nobesine-75, Tenuate Dospan)

SPECIAL INSTRUCTIONS

- ☐ If you forget to take a dose, take it as soon as possible. However, if it is almost time for your next dose, do not take the missed dose. Instead, continue with your regular dosing schedule.

- ☐ Women who are pregnant, breast-feeding, or planning to become pregnant should tell their doctor before taking this medicine.

- ☐ It is very important that you follow the diet prescribed by your doctor.

- ☐ If your mouth becomes dry, suck a hard sour candy (sugarless) or ice chips, or chew gum. It is especially important to brush your teeth regularly if you develop a dry mouth.

- ☐ In some people, this drug may cause dizziness. Do not drive a car or operate dangerous machinery or do jobs that require you to be alert until you know how you are going to react to this drug. Therefore, you should be careful going up and down stairs. Sit or lie down at the first sign of dizziness.

- ☐ Most people experience few or no side effects from their drugs. However, any medicine can sometimes cause unwanted effects. Call your doctor if you develop a skin rash, sore throat, fever, mouth sores, unusual nervousness, difficulty in urinating ("passing your water"), or palpitations, or if you become depressed.

- ☐ Carry an identification card indicating that you are taking this medicine. Always tell your pharmacist, dentist, and other doctors who are treating you that you are taking this medicine.

* * * * *

Diethylstilbestrol (*Oral Estrogen*)
United States: Stilbestrol
Canada: Honvol, Stibilium, Stilbestrol

- ☐ This medicine is a hormone and has many uses. The reason it was prescribed depends on your condition.

279

HOW TO USE THIS MEDICINE

☐ The tablets may be taken after meals or with a snack if they upset your stomach.

☐ This medicine has a special coating and must be swallowed whole. Do not crush, chew, or break it into pieces. (**United States:** Stilbestrol E.C.T.)

SPECIAL INSTRUCTIONS

☐ Women who are pregnant, breast-feeding, or planning to become pregnant should tell their doctor before taking this medicine.

☐ It is recommended that you do not smoke while you are taking this medicine because smoking may increase the incidence of heart attacks.

☐ Contact your doctor if any of the following side effects occur:
- Severe or persistent headaches
- Vomiting, dizziness, or fainting
- Blurred vision or slurred speech
- Pain in the calves of the legs or numbness in an arm or leg
- Chest pain, shortness of breath, or coughing of blood
- Lumps in the breast
- Severe depression
- A yellow color to the skin or eyes or dark-colored urine
- Severe abdominal pain
- Breakthrough vaginal bleeding which persists after the third month of therapy. During the first 3 months of therapy, breakthrough bleeding may be expected, but you should keep taking the tablets and it will usually clear up in a day or two.
- If you miss 2 consecutive menstrual periods or if you think you are pregnant.

☐ Carry an identification card indicating that you are taking this medicine. Always tell your pharmacist, dentist, and other doctors who are treating you that you are taking this medicine.

* * * * *

Diethylstilbestrol (*Vaginal Estrogen*)
United States: A.T.V., Prin V/S, DV, Test-Estrin

☐ This medicine is used to treat certain types of vaginal conditions.

HOW TO USE THIS MEDICINE

☐ For VAGINAL SUPPOSITORIES
- Remove the wrapper from the suppository.
- Insert the wide end of the suppository into the vaginal canal.

280

SPECIAL INSTRUCTIONS

- ☐ Women who are pregnant, breast-feeding, or planning to become pregnant should tell their doctor before taking this medicine.

- ☐ Do not use this medicine more often or longer than recommended by your doctor.

- ☐ It is recommended that you do not smoke while you are on this medicine.

- ☐ Most people experience few or no side effects from their drugs. However, any medicine can sometimes cause unwanted effects. Call your doctor if you develop severe or persistent headaches, vomiting, dizziness or fainting, blurred vision or slurred speech, pain in the calves of the legs or numbness in an arm or leg, lumps in the breast, severe depression, a yellow color to the skin or eyes or dark-colored urine, severe abdominal pain, or an irritation caused by the medicine.

- ☐ Store the suppositories in a cool place.

* * * * *

Diflorasone Diacetate (*Topical corticosteroid*)
United States: Florone
Canada: Florone

- ☐ This medicine is used to help relieve redness, swelling and itching, and inflammmation of certain types of skin conditions.

HOW TO USE THIS MEDICINE

- ☐ For CREAM and OINTMENT
    - • Each time you apply the medicine, wash your hands and gently cleanse the skin area well with water unless otherwise directed by your doctor.
    - • Do not allow the skin to dry completely. Pat with a clean towel until slightly damp.
    - • Apply a small amount of the drug to the affected area and spread lightly. Only the medicine that is actually touching the skin will work. A thick layer is not more effective than a thin layer. Do not bandage unless directed by your doctor.

- ☐ Do not use the drug more frequently or in larger quantities than prescribed by your doctor. Overuse of this medicine may cause you to absorb too much of the drug and increase the risk of side effects.

- ☐ Keep the medicine away from the eyes, nose, and mouth.

SPECIAL INSTRUCTIONS

- ☐ If you forget to apply the medicine, apply it as soon as possible. However, if it is almost time for your next dose, do not apply the missed dose but continue with your regular schedule.

281

- ☐ Do not use this medicine for any other skin problems without checking with your doctor.

- ☐ Do not apply cosmetics or lotions on top of the drug unless your doctor approves.

- ☐ Call your doctor if the condition for which this drug is being used persists or becomes worse or if you have a constant irritation such as itching or burning that was not present before you started using this medicine. Also call your doctor if you develop abnormal lines or thinning of the skin, especially under the arms or between the legs.

- ☐ Store in a cool place but do not freeze.

- ☐ For external use only. Do not swallow.

- ☐ Tell future doctors that you have used this medicine.

* * * * *

Digitoxin (*Oral Cardiotonic*)
United States: Crystodigin, Purodigin

Digoxin
United States: Lanoxin, SK-Digoxin
Canada: Lanoxin

Gitalin
United States: Gitaligin

Lanatoside C
United States: Cedilanid

- ☐ This medicine is used to help make the heartbeat strong and steady.

HOW TO USE THIS MEDICINE
- ☐ If this medicine causes stomach upset, take it with some food.

- ☐ For LIQUID MEDICINE
    - A specially marked dropper is used to measure the dose of the medicine. Check with your pharmacist if you do not fully understand how to use it. (**United States:** Lanoxin; **Canada:** Cedilanid, Lanoxin)

SPECIAL INSTRUCTIONS
- ☐ It is very important that you take this medicine exactly as your doctor has prescribed and that you do not miss any doses. Try to take this medicine at the same time every day. Do not take extra tablets without your doctor's approval.

282

- [ ] Do not stop taking this medicine without your doctor's approval and do not go without medicine between prescription refills.

- [ ] Some nonprescription drugs can interfere with this medicine or aggravate your heart condition. Do not take any of the following without the approval of your doctor or pharmacist: antacids; cough, cold, or sinus products; diarrhea products; asthma and allergy products; or diet or weight-reducing medicines.

- [ ] It is recommended that you learn how to check your pulse rate. If it becomes slow or irregular, check with your doctor and he may adjust your dose of the medicine.

- [ ] Most people experience few or no side effects from their drugs. However, any medicine can sometimes cause unwanted effects. Call your doctor if you develop nausea, vomiting, diarrhea, unusual tiredness or weakness, blurred vision or "yellow" or "green" vision, or loss of appetite.

- [ ] Carry an identification card indicating that you are taking this medicine. Always tell your pharmacist, dentist, and other doctors who are treating you that you are taking this medicine.

*   *   *   *   *

Dihydrotachysterol (*Oral Vitamin D Analogue*)
United States: Hytakerol
Canada: Hytakerol

- [ ] This medicine is used in the treatment of certain conditions to help restore to normal the calcium levels in the body.

HOW TO USE THIS MEDICINE
- [ ] Take the medicine with some water.

- [ ] If you forget to take a dose, take it as soon as possible. However, if it is almost time for your next dose, do not take the missed dose. Instead, continue with your regular dosing schedule.

SPECIAL INSTRUCTIONS
- [ ] Do not take any vitamin preparations containing calcium or vitamin D without the approval of your doctor.

- [ ] Do not take mineral oil while you are taking this medicine.

- [ ] Follow any special diet that your doctor may recommend, especially with respect to dairy products and calcium supplements.

- [ ] Most people experience few or no side effects from their drugs. However any medicine can sometimes cause unwanted effects. Call your doctor if you develop nausea, vomiting, weakness, excessive thirst, unusual constipation, or stomach cramps, or if you urinate ("pass your water") more often than usual. Your doctor may have to adjust your dose.

☐ Do not store the capsules in the refrigerator because they may crack.

* * * * *

Dihydroxyaluminum Aminoacetate (*Oral Antacid-Demulcent*)
United States: Robalate
Canada: Robalate

☐ This medicine is an antacid which is used to reduce the acidity of the stomach contents. It is used to help relieve the symptoms of heartburn and to treat peptic ulcer, "reflux," or hiatus hernia.

HOW TO USE THIS MEDICINE
☐ For CHEWABLE TABLETS

   • The tablets may be chewed or dissolved slowly in the mouth. Follow with a glass of water. Do not swallow the tablets.

SPECIAL INSTRUCTIONS
☐ Do not take this medicine more often than recommended by your doctor.

☐ If you are taking this medicine because you have an ULCER, you will have to have this antacid very often. This is because your stomach must not be without food or this medicine for usually more than 2 hours at a time. You must follow any diet prescribed by your doctor and continue to take this medicine even if your pain fades. If you stop the antacid too early, your ulcer may not be fully healed and could quickly return. It is best to avoid smoking as well as coffee, tea, alcohol, spices, and aspirin because all of these agents can irritate the stomach. Check with your pharmacist before you take any nonprescription drugs.

☐ If you are taking this medicine because you have REFLUX or HIATUS HERNIA, it is usually best to avoid overeating, to limit the amount of fluids you drink during a meal, to reduce the amount of fats you eat, and to keep your shoulders elevated about 30° in bed.

☐ Most people experience few or no side effects from their drugs. However, any medicine can sometimes cause unwanted effects. Call your doctor if you develop stomach pain which lasts more than 3 days, loss of appetite, tremors, weakness, or bone pain.

* * * * *

p-Diisobutylphenoxy-Polyethoxyethanol Compounds (*Vaginal Contraceptive*)
United States: Ortho-Gynol, Preceptin Gel
Canada: Ortho-Gynol Jelly

284

☐ This preparation is to be used with the diaphragm as a birth control measure.

HOW TO USE THIS MEDICINE

☐ Instructions for use: (**United States:** Ortho-Gynol; **Canada:** Ortho-Gynol Jelly)

(a) *Preparing Diaphragm*—Always insert your diaphragm with the jelly or cream before intercourse (sex). Do not depend upon the diaphragm alone for contraceptive protection. First, empty the bladder (urinate) and wash your hands thoroughly. Approximately one teaspoonful of spermicidal jelly or cream then is applied to the side of the diaphragm which will contact the cervix (entrance to the womb). Spread jelly or cream over this surface and on the rim of the diaphragm; this eases insertion and ensures a more perfect seal over the cervix (Figure a).

(b) *Inserting Diaphragm*—Hold the diaphragm firmly between thumb, index, and third fingers. Compress each side of the rim at midpoints opposite each other, while keeping the index finger securely in place inside the compressed diaphragm (Figure b). Separate the labia (lips) and insert the diaphragm into the vaginal canal, directing it backwards as far as it will go (Figure b). The diaphragm may be inserted while you are in a standing, squatting, or reclining position.

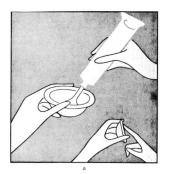 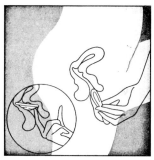

a   b

(c) *Placing Diaphragm*—Always insert the diaphragm as far back as it will go behind the mouth of the cervix. Then push the near part of the rim up behind the pubic bone. Test for correct position by running the index or middle finger over the diaphragm's dome to be sure it covers the cervix. The cervix will feel like the end of your nose. It also is normal to feel folds in the diaphragm when it is in place.

The diaphragm may be inserted into the vagina before retiring or just before intercourse. If intercourse is repeated, insert more jelly or cream into the vagina with the aid of an ORTHO applicator, but do not remove the diaphragm (Figure c). It should remain in position for at least 6 to 8 hours after intercourse. Do not douche until the diaphragm is removed.

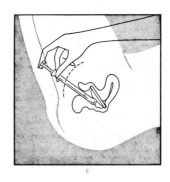

c

Bodily movements or changes in position will not dislodge a correctly inserted diaphragm. While it is in the vagina, you may urinate or move the bowels and your diaphragm will stay in place. Any discomfort or pain, while the diaphragm is in place, may be due to incorret diaphragm insertion, an abnormal pelvic condition, constipation, or incorrect diaphragm size. In such case, be sure to consult your doctor.

(d) *Inserting the Diaphragm with an Introducer*

1. *Preparing Diaphragm*—Another way to insert the diaphragm is with an introducer (handle). The diaphragm is placed on the introducer by fitting the rim into the end groove, then hooking the opposite rim over the notch corresponding to the diaphragm size.

2. *Inserting Diaphragm*—After applying the equivalent of one teaspoonful of Ortho-Gynol or Ortho-Creme* into the "pockets" formed in the diaphragm, then direct it by means of the introducer along the floor of the vagina to make sure it passes the cervix. To remove the introducer, after the diaphragm is in place, give it a quarter turn left or right which disengages it from the diaphragm. Then, gently withdraw the introducer. The near rim of the diaphragm is then pushed up behind the pubic bone. Check to make sure the dome is covering the cervix.

   To cleanse the introducer, wash with soap and warm water, rinse, and dry. To remove the diaphragm, place the forefinger (or if you prefer, the hook of the introducer) behind the front portion of the rim and pull the diaphragm down and out. Straining down as with a bowel movement helps push the rim down so that the index finger or introducer can reach the rim more easily. If suction is holding the diaphragm, the suction may be broken by placing a finger between the vaginal wall and the rim. If the menstrual period begins while the diaphragm is in place and blood is found in the cup of the diaphragm when it is removed, do not be concerned as this is not harmful.

(e) *Care of the Diaphragm*—After removal of the diaphragm, it should be cleansed thoroughly with mild soap and water, rinsed, and dried carefully. Never boil the diaphragm or use antiseptic solutions in

*Ortho-Creme (Package Insert), Ortho Pharmaceutical (Canada) Ltd., Don Mills, Ontario.

286

cleaning it. Dust lightly with talcum powder or corn starch and immediately return it to the original container. Do not allow the diaphragm to dry in the open as exposure to light or heat will deteriorate the rubber rapidly. The container provides the best storage protection. Examine the diaphragm carefully before each use by holding it in front of a light to make sure that no damage has occurred in handling. Never stretch or puncture the diaphragm with sharp fingernails.

☐ Instructions for use: (**United States:** Preceptin Vaginal Gel*)

   (a) This preparation should be used just before intercourse (sex), and an additional applicator full of gel should be used each time you have intercourse afterwards.
   (b) Remove the cap from the tube and attach the applicator in its place.

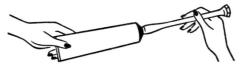

   (c) Squeeze the tube from the bottom slowly to force the contents into the transparent cylinder. Squeeze slowly until the plunger is pushed out as far as it will go.

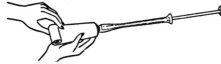

   (d) After filling the applicator and before detaching it, roll the tube from the bottom as shown. This will reduce wastage of the contents of the tube.
   (e) After each use replace the cap on the tube. Avoid keeping the tube in a cold place.
   (f) After detaching the applicator from the tube, hold the filled applicator by the cylinder, gently insert it well into the vaginal canal, so the gel is deposited near the cervix, press the plunger, and then, with the plunger still depressed, remove the applicator from the vaginal canal. The best method for insertion of the applicator is when lying on the back with the knees bent.

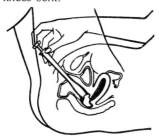

*Preceptin Vaginal Gel (Package Insert), Ortho Pharmaceutical (Canada) Ltd., Don Mills, Ontario.

(g) The applicator should be taken apart after each use and cleaned thoroughly. Grasp the plunger with one hand and turn the cap counterclockwise with the other. When the cap is removed, the plunger will then drop out of the cylinder.

(h) Wash the parts with warm water and soap, but do *not* boil. Rinse thoroughly and reassemble the applicator.

(i) If a vaginal douche is required, you must wait at least 6 to 8 hours after intercourse before douching.

* * * * *

Dimenhydrinate (*Oral Antiemetic*)

United States: Dramamine, Vertiban

Canada: Dramamine, Gravol, Nauseal, Novodimenate, Travamine

☐ This medicine is used to help prevent and treat the nausea and vomiting of motion sickness. It may also be used to help relieve the symptoms of certain types of allergic conditions, coughs and colds, and certain skin conditions.

HOW TO USE THIS MEDICINE

☐ This medicine may be taken with food or a glass of milk if it upsets your stomach.

☐ Swallow these capsules. Do not break them open. (***Canada:*** Gravol L/A)

SPECIAL INSTRUCTIONS

☐ If you forget to take a dose, take it as soon as possible. However, if it is almost time for your next dose, do not take the missed dose. Instead, continue with your regular dosing schedule.

☐ Women who are breast-feeding should tell their doctor before taking this medicine.

☐ In some people, this drug may initially cause dizziness or drowsiness. Do not drive a car or operate dangerous machinery or do jobs that require you to be alert until you know how you are going to react to this drug. If you become dizzy, you should be careful going up and down stairs. Sit or lie down at the first sign of dizziness. Tell your doctor if it continues.

☐ Do not drink alcoholic beverages while taking this drug without the approval of your doctor.

☐ If your mouth becomes dry, suck a hard candy (sugarless) or ice chips, or chew gum. It is especially important to brush your teeth regularly if you develop a dry mouth.

☐ It is important that you obtain the advice of your doctor or pharmacist before taking pain relievers, nonprescription drugs, sleeping pills or tranquilizers, or other medicines for allergies.

☐ Do not take this medicine more often or longer than recommended by your doctor.

288

- Most people experience few or no side effects from their drugs. However, any medicine can sometimes cause unwanted effects. Call your doctor if you develop a skin rash, fast heartbeats, blurred vision, stomach pain, or difficulty in urinating ("passing your water").

* * * * *

Dimenhydrinate (*Rectal Antiemetic*)
United States: Dramamine
Canada: Dramamine, Gravol, Nauseal, Nauseatol

- This medicine is used to help prevent and treat the nausea and vomiting of motion sickness. It is also used to help relieve the symptoms of certain types of allergic conditions, coughs and colds, and certain skin conditions.

HOW TO USE THIS MEDICINE
- ADMINISTRATION OF SUPPOSITORIES:
  - Remove the wrapper from the suppository.
  - Lie on your side and raise your knee to your chest.
  - Insert the suppository with the tapered (pointed) end first into the rectum.
  - Remain lying down for a few minutes so that the suppository will dissolve in the rectum.
  - Try to avoid having a bowel movement for at least 1 hour so that the drug will have time to work.

SPECIAL INSTRUCTIONS
- If you forget to use a dose, use it as soon as possible. However, if it is almost time for your next dose, do not use the missed dose. Instead, continue with your regular dosing schedule.

- Women who are breast-feeding should tell their doctor before taking this medicine.

- In some people, this drug may initially cause dizziness or drowsiness. Do not drive a car or operate dangerous machinery or do jobs that require you to be alert until you know how you are going to react to the drug. If you become dizzy, you should be careful going up and down stairs. Sit or lie down at the first sign of dizziness. Tell your doctor if it continues.

- Do not drink alcoholic beverages while taking this drug without the approval of your doctor.

- If your mouth becomes dry, suck a hard candy (sugarless) or ice chips, or chew gum. It is especially important to brush your teeth regularly if you develop a dry mouth.

- It is important that you obtain the advice of your doctor or pharmacist before taking pain relievers, nonprescription drugs, sleeping pills or tranquilizers, or other medicines for allergies.

289

□ Do not use this medicine more often or longer than recommended by your doctor.

□ Most people experience few or no side effects from their drugs. However, any medicine can sometimes cause unwanted effects. Call your doctor if you develop a skin rash, fast heartbeats, blurred vision, stomach pain, or difficulty in urinating ("passing your water").

*   *   *   *   *

Dimethindene Maleate (Oral Antihistamine)
United States: Forhistal, Triten
Canada: Forhistal

□ This medicine is used to help relieve the symptoms of certain types of allergic conditions, coughs and colds, and certain skin conditions.

HOW TO USE THIS MEDICINE
□ This medicine may be taken with food or a glass of milk if it upsets your stomach.

□ Swallow these tablets whole. Do not crush, chew, or break them into pieces. (**United States:** Forhistal Lontabs, Triten Tab-In)

SPECIAL INSTRUCTIONS
□ If you forget to take a dose, take it as soon as possible. However, if it is almost time for your next dose, do not take the missed dose. Instead, continue with your regular dosing schedule.

□ In some people, this drug may initially cause dizziness or drowsiness. Do not drive a car or operate dangerous machinery or do jobs that require you to be alert until you know how you are going to react to the drug. If you become dizzy, you should be careful going up and down stairs. Sit or lie down at the first sign of dizziness. Tell your doctor if it continues.

□ Do not drink alcoholic beverages while taking this drug without the approval of your doctor.

□ If your mouth becomes dry, suck a hard candy (sugarless) or ice chips, or chew gum. It is especially important to brush your teeth regularly if you develop a dry mouth.

□ It is important that you obtain the advice of your doctor or pharmacist before taking pain relievers, nonprescription drugs, sleeping pills or tranquilizers, or other medicines for allergies.

□ Do not take this medicine more often or longer than recommended by your doctor.

□ Most people experience few or no side effects from their drugs. However, any medicine can sometimes cause unwanted effects. Call your doctor if you develop a skin rash, fast heartbeats, blurred vision, stomach pain, or difficulty in urinating ("passing your water").

* * * * *

Dimethothiazine Mesylate (Oral Antihistamine)
Canada: Promaquid

☐ This medicine is used to help relieve the symptoms of certain types of allergic conditions, coughs and colds, certain skin conditions, and some types of headaches.

HOW TO USE THIS MEDICINE
☐ This medicine may be taken with food or a glass of milk if it upsets your stomach.

SPECIAL INSTRUCTIONS
☐ If you forget to take a dose, take it as soon as possible. However, if it is almost time for your next dose, do not take the missed dose. Instead, continue with your regular dosing schedule.

☐ Women who are pregnant, breast-feeding, or planning to become pregnant should tell their doctor before taking this medicine.

☐ In some people, this drug may initially cause dizziness or drowsiness. Do not drive a car or operate dangerous machinery or do jobs that require you to be alert until you know how you are going to react to this drug. If you become dizzy, you should be careful going up and down stairs. Sit or lie down at the first sign of dizziness. Tell your doctor if it continues.

☐ Do not drink alcoholic beverages while taking this drug without the approval of your doctor.

☐ If your mouth becomes dry, suck a hard candy (sugarless) or ice chips, or chew gum. It is especially important to brush your teeth regularly if you develop a dry mouth.

☐ It is important that you obtain the advice of your doctor or pharmacist before taking pain relievers, nonprescription drugs, sleeping pills or tranquilizers, or other medicines for allergies.

☐ Do not take this medicine more often or longer than recommended by your doctor.

☐ Most people experience few or no side effects from their drugs. However, any medicine can sometimes cause unwanted effects. Call your doctor if you develop a skin rash, sore throat, fever, or mouth sores.

* * * * *

Dioctyl Calcium Sulfosuccinate (See Docusate Calcium)

* * * * *

Dioctyl Sodium Sulfosuccinate (*See Docusate Sodium*)

*   *   *   *   *

Dioxyline Phosphate (*Oral Antispasmodic*)
United States: Paveril

- ☐ This medicine is used to help improve the circulation of blood in the body and to relax muscles.

HOW TO USE THIS MEDICINE

- ☐ This medicine may be taken with food or on an empty stomach.

- ☐ If you forget to take a dose, take it as soon as possible. However, if it is almost time for your next dose, do not take the missed dose. Instead, continue with your regular dosing schedule.

SPECIAL INSTRUCTIONS

- ☐ In some people, this drug may cause dizziness or drowsiness. Do not drive a car or operate dangerous machinery or do jobs that require you to be alert until you know how you are going to react to this drug.

- ☐ Some nonprescription drugs can aggravate your condition. Do not take any of the following without the approval of your doctor or pharmacist: cough, cold, or sinus products; asthma or allergy products; or diet or weight-reducing medicines.

- ☐ Do not drink alcoholic beverages while taking this drug without the approval of your doctor.

- ☐ The activity of this drug is improved if you keep warm. Avoid getting cold or exposing yourself to a cold environment.

- ☐ Most people experience few or no side effects from their drugs. However, any medicine can sometimes cause unwanted effects. Call your doctor if you develop a skin rash, nausea or vomiting, severe stomach pain, a rapid pulse, or fainting spells.

*   *   *   *   *

Diphemanil Methylsulfate (*Oral Antispasmodic*)
United States: Prantal

- ☐ This medicine is used to help relax muscles of the stomach and bowels as well as to decrease the amount of acid formed in the stomach.

- ☐ IMPORTANT: If you have ever had an allergic reaction to atropine or any other drug used to relax the stomach or bowels, tell your doctor or pharmacist before you take any of this medicine.

HOW TO USE THIS MEDICINE

- ☐ Take this medicine approximately 30 minutes before a meal unless otherwise directed.

- [ ] If you miss a dose of this medicine, do not take the missed dose and do not double the next dose.

SPECIAL INSTRUCTIONS

- [ ] If your mouth becomes dry, suck a hard sour candy (sugarless) or ice chips, or chew gum. It is especially important to brush your teeth regularly if you develop a dry mouth.

- [ ] In some people, this drug may cause dizziness or drowsiness. Do not drive a car or operate dangerous machinery or do jobs that require you to be alert until you know how you are going to react to this drug.

- [ ] If you become dizzy, you should be careful going up and down stairs. Sit or lie down at the first sign of dizziness. Tell your doctor you have been dizzy.

- [ ] A desire to urinate ("pass your water") with an inability to do so is not an uncommon effect with this drug. Urinating each time before taking the drug may help relieve this problem. Call your doctor if it continues.

- [ ] You may become more sensitive to heat because your body may perspire less while you are taking this drug. Be careful not to become overheated during exercise or in hot weather.

- [ ] Do not take antacids within 1 hour of taking this medicine as it could make this medicine less effective.

- [ ] If you become constipated, try increasing the amount of bulk in your diet (for example, bran and salads), exercising more often, or drinking more water. Call your doctor if the constipation continues.

- [ ] If your eyes become more sensitive to sunlight, it may help to wear sunglasses.

- [ ] Most people experience few or no side effects from their drugs. However, any medicine can sometimes cause unwanted effects. Call your doctor if you develop a skin rash, diarrhea, unusual restlessness, flushing, or eye pain.

* * * * *

Diphenoxylate HCl (*Oral Antidiarrheal*)
Canada: Lomotil

Diphenoxylate HCl-Atropine
United States: Lofene, Loflo, Lomotil, Lonox, Lo-Trol

- [ ] This medicine is used to treat diarrhea.

HOW TO USE THIS MEDICINE

- [ ] This medicine may be taken with food if it upsets your stomach.

- [ ] If a dropper or a dispensing spoon is used to measure the dose and you do not fully understand how to use it, check with your pharmacist. (***United States:*** Lomotil Liquid)

☐ Do not take any more of this medicine than your doctor has prescribed. The drug could become habit-forming or you could take an overdose if you take it more often or longer than prescribed. A doctor should be called if you develop any of these signs of an overdose: shallow breathing, pinpoint pupils, loss of consciousness, or unusual restlessness.

☐ If you miss a dose of this medicine, do not take the missed dose and do not double your next dose.

SPECIAL INSTRUCTIONS

☐ Women who are pregnant, breast-feeding, or planning to become pregnant should tell their doctor before taking this medicine.

☐ Call your doctor if you develop a fever or if the diarrhea continues.

☐ Do not drink alcoholic beverages while taking this drug without the approval of your doctor.

☐ It is important that you obtain the advice of your doctor or pharmacist before taking pain relievers, nonprescription drugs, sleeping pills, tranquilizers, or medicines for depression while you are taking this drug.

☐ In some people, this drug may cause dizziness or drowsiness. Do not drive a car or operate dangerous machinery or do jobs that require you to be alert until you know how you are going to react to this drug.

☐ If you become dizzy, you should be careful going up and down stairs. Sit or lie down at the first sign of dizziness.

☐ Most people experience few or no side effects from their drugs. However, any medicine can sometimes cause unwanted effects. Call your doctor if you develop bloating, constipation, nausea or vomiting, loss of appetite, or stomach pain.

☐ Also call your doctor if you develop a dry mouth, flushing, fast heartbeats, or difficulty in urinating ("passing your water"). (**United States:** Lofene, Loflo, Lomotil, Lonox, Lo-Trol)

☐ Carry an identification card indicating that you are taking this medicine. Always tell your pharmacist, dentist, and other doctors who are treating you that you are taking this medicine.

* * * * *

Diphenhydramine HCl (*Oral Antihistamine*)
United States: Benylin, Benadryl, SK-Diphenhydramine Rohydra
Canada: Benadryl

Diphenhydramine HCl-Ephedrine Sulfate
United States: Benadryl with Ephedrine

Diphenhydramine HCl-Ammonium Chloride
Canada: Benylin

☐ This medicine is an antihistamine which has many uses. The reason it was prescribed depends on your condition. If you do not fully understand why you are taking it, check with your doctor.

HOW TO USE THIS MEDICINE

☐ Take this medicine with food if it upsets your stomach.

SPECIAL INSTRUCTIONS

☐ If you forget to take a dose, take it as soon as possible. However, if it is almost time for your next dose, do not take the missed dose. Instead, continue with your regular dosing schedule.

☐ Women who are breast-feeding should tell their doctor before taking this medicine.

☐ In some people, this drug may initially cause dizziness or drowsiness. Do not drive a car or operate dangerous machinery or do jobs that require you to be alert until you know how you are going to react to this drug. If you become dizzy, you should be careful going up and down stairs. Sit or lie down at the first sign of dizziness. Tell your doctor if it continues.

☐ Do not drink alcoholic beverages while taking this drug without the approval of your doctor.

☐ If your mouth becomes dry, suck a hard sour candy (sugarless) or ice chips, or chew gum. It is especially important to brush your teeth regularly if you develop a dry mouth.

☐ It is important that you obtain the advice of your doctor or pharmacist before taking pain relievers, nonprescription drugs, sleeping pills or tranquilizers, or other medicines for allergies.

☐ Do not take this medicine more often or longer than recommended by your doctor.

☐ Most people experience few or no side effects from their drugs. However, any medicine can sometimes cause unwanted effects. Call your doctor if you develop a skin rash, fast heartbeats, blurred vision, stomach pain, or difficulty in urinating ("passing your water").

*　*　*　*　*

Diphenylpyraline (*Oral Antihistamine*)
United States: Diafen, Hispril

☐ This medicine is used to help relieve the symptoms of certain types of allergic conditions, coughs and colds, and certain skin conditions.

HOW TO USE THIS MEDICINE

☐ This medicine may be taken with food or a glass of milk if it upsets your stomach.

295

☐ The following capsules must be swallowed whole. Do not crush or break the capsules open. (**United States:** Hispril Spansules)

SPECIAL INSTRUCTIONS

☐ If you forget to take a dose, take it as soon as possible. However, if it is almost time for your next dose, do not take the missed dose. Instead, continue with your regular dosing schedule.

☐ In some people, this drug may initially cause dizziness or drowsiness. Do not drive a car or operate dangerous machinery or do jobs that require you to be alert until you know how you are going to react to this drug. If you become dizzy, you should be careful going up and down stairs. Sit or lie down at the first sign of dizziness. Tell your doctor if it continues.

☐ Do not drink alcoholic beverages while taking this drug without the approval of your doctor.

☐ If your mouth becomes dry, suck a hard sour candy (sugarless) or ice chips, or chew gum. It is especially important to brush your teeth regularly if you develop a dry mouth.

☐ It is important that you obtain the advice of your doctor or pharmacist before taking pain relievers, nonprescription drugs, sleeping pills or tranquilizers, or other medicines for allergies.

☐ Do not take this medicine more often or longer than recommended by your doctor.

☐ Most people experience few or no side effects from their drugs. However, any medicine can sometimes cause unwanted effects. Call your doctor if you develop a skin rash, fast heartbeats, blurred vision, stomach pain, or difficulty in urinating ("passing your water").

* * * * *

Diphenylpyraline-Phenylephrine (*Oral Antitussive-Decongestant*)
Canada: Novahistex

☐ This medicine is used to help relieve the symptoms of certain types of allergic conditions, coughs and colds, and certain skin conditions.

HOW TO USE THIS MEDICINE

☐ This medicine may be taken with food or a glass of milk if it upsets your stomach.

☐ This medicine must be swallowed whole. Do not crush, chew, or break it into pieces.

SPECIAL INSTRUCTIONS

☐ If you forget to take a dose, take it as soon as possible. However, if it is almost time for your next dose, do not take the missed dose. Instead, continue with your regular dosing schedule.

☐ In some people, this drug may initially cause dizziness or drowsiness. Do not drive a car or operate dangerous machinery or do jobs that require you to be alert until you know how you are going to react to this drug. If you become dizzy, you should be careful going up and down stairs. Sit or lie down at the first sign of dizziness. Tell your doctor if it continues.

☐ Do not drink alcoholic beverages while taking this drug without the approval of your doctor.

☐ If your mouth becomes dry, suck a hard sour candy (sugarless) or ice chips, or chew gum. It is especially important to brush your teeth regularly if you develop a dry mouth.

☐ It is important that you obtain the advice of your doctor or pharmacist before taking pain relievers, nonprescription drugs, sleeping pills or tranquilizers, or other medicines for allergies.

☐ Do not take this medicine more often or longer than recommended by your doctor.

☐ Most people experience few or no side effects from their drugs. However, any medicine can sometimes cause unwanted effects. Call your doctor if you develop a skin rash, fast heartbeats, blurred vision, stomach pain, or difficulty in urinating ("passing your water").

* * * * *

Diprophylline (See Dyphylline)

* * * * *

Dipyridamole (Oral Coronary Vasodilator)
United States: Persantine
Canada: Persantine

☐ This medicine is used to help prevent angina attacks and must be taken regularly as your doctor has prescribed. It may be necessary to take this medicine for 2 to 3 months before you feel its full benefit. Do not miss any doses. It will not relieve an angina attack that has already started because it works too slowly.

☐ This medicine also helps prevent harmful blood clots from forming in certain medical conditions.

HOW TO USE THIS MEDICINE

☐ It is best to take this medicine on an empty stomach 1 hour before (or 2 hours after) eating food. The drug may be taken with a light snack or a glass of milk if it upsets your stomach.

☐ If you do forget to take a dose, take it as soon as possible. However, if your next dose is within 4 hours, do not take the missed dose but continue with your regular schedule.

SPECIAL INSTRUCTIONS

- ☐ If you become dizzy or feel faint, breathe deeply and bend forward with your head between your knees. Always get up slowly after you have been sitting or lying down. Get out of bed slowly in the morning and dangle your feet over the edge of the bed for a few minutes before standing up. Do not drive a car or operate dangerous machinery or do jobs that require you to be alert if you are dizzy or drowsy.

- ☐ Do not drink alcoholic beverages while you are taking this medicine as it may make the dizziness and fainting worse.

- ☐ Some nonprescription drugs can aggravate your heart condition. Do not take any of the following without the approval of your doctor or pharmacist: cough, cold, or sinus products; asthma or allergy products; or diet or weight-reducing medicines.

- ☐ When you first start taking this medicine, you may get a headache or flushing. These are common side effects and will usually disappear within a few days. Call your doctor if they continue.

- ☐ Cigarette smoking can aggravate angina and is a special risk for people who have angina.

- ☐ Most people experience few or no side effects from their drugs. However, any medicine can sometimes cause unwanted effects. Call your doctor if you develop a skin rash, fainting spells, nausea or vomiting, severe headache, persistent stomach cramps, or if your chest pain is not relieved.

- ☐ Do not stop taking the medicine suddenly or it could cause an angina attack.

- ☐ Carry an identification card indicating that you are taking this medicine. Always tell your pharmacist, dentist, and other doctors who are treating you that you are taking this medicine.

* * * * *

Disopyramide
Canada: Rythmodan

Disopyramide Phosphate
United States: Norpace
Canada: Norpace

- ☐ This medicine is used to help make your heart beat at a regular and normal rate.

HOW TO USE THIS MEDICINE

- ☐ It is best to take this medicine on an empty stomach 1 hour before (or 2 hours after) eating food. However, if it upsets your stomach, take the medicine with some food or milk.

SPECIAL INSTRUCTIONS

☐ It is very important that you take this medicine exactly as your doctor has prescribed and that you do not miss any doses. Try to take this medicine at the same time every day. Do not take extra tablets without your doctor's approval. Do not go without this medicine between prescription refills.

☐ If you forget to take a dose and remember it within 2 hours of the missed dose, take it as soon as possible. Otherwise, do not take the missed dose and continue with your regular schedule.

☐ Some nonprescription drugs can aggravate your heart condition. Do not take any of the following without the approval of your doctor or pharmacist: cough, cold, or sinus products; asthma or allergy products; or diet or weight-reducing medicines.

☐ Tell your doctor if you become dizzy or feel faint. Sit or lie down at the first sign of dizziness and do not drive a car, operate dangerous machinery, or do jobs that require you to be alert.

☐ If your mouth becomes dry, suck a hard sour candy (sugarless) or ice chips, or chew gum. It is especially important to brush your teeth regularly if you develop a dry mouth.

☐ Most people experience few or no side effects from their drugs. However, any medicine can sometimes cause unwanted effects. Call your doctor if you develop difficulty in urinating ("passing your water"), shortness of breath, chest pain, or a skin rash.

☐ Carry an identification card indicating that you are taking this medicine. Always tell your pharmacist, dentist, and other doctors who are treating you that you are taking this medicine.

*　　*　　*　　*　　*

Disulfiram (*Oral Alcoholism Therapy*)
United States: Antabuse, Ro-Sulfiram
Canada: Antabuse

☐ This medicine is used in the treatment of alcoholism to help keep you from drinking. You must **not** drink alcohol while you are taking this drug. If you drink even a small amount of alcohol, you may experience these sensations: flushing, dizziness, sweating, shortness of breath, throbbing headache, and nausea. The more you drink, the more severe this reaction will be. Knowing that just one drink will make you sick can strengthen your determination not to drink.

☐ IMPORTANT: If you have ever had an allergic reaction to rubber, pesticides, or fungicides, tell your doctor or pharmacist before you take any of this medicine.

HOW TO USE THIS MEDICINE

☐ It is important that you take this medicine regularly and that you do not miss any doses. It is usually taken at breakfast. If you develop drowsiness, it may be taken at bedtime.

☐ If you forget to take a dose, take it as soon as possible. However, if it is almost time for your next dose, do not take the missed dose. Instead, continue with your regular dosing schedule.

SPECIAL INSTRUCTIONS

☐ Women who are pregnant, breast-feeding, or planning to become pregnant should tell their doctor before taking this medicine.

☐ Do not use or drink alcohol in any form because it may make you very sick. This includes rubbing alcohol and certain types of back rub solutions, after-shave lotions, cologne, toilet waters, vinegars and sauces, mouth washes, and gargles. You should make sure that any medicine you get from your doctor or pharmacist does not contain alcohol. Many cough medicines and tonics contain enough alcohol to cause a serious reaction. Do not eat any foods prepared with alcohol. This includes chocolates containing alcohol liqueurs.

☐ In some people, this drug may cause drowsiness. Do not drive a car or operate dangerous machinery or do jobs that require you to be alert until you know how you are going to react to this drug. The drowsiness will usually disappear in a few days.

☐ During the first 2 weeks of treatment, you may have a metallic or garlic taste in your mouth. This is a normal effect of the medicine and should disappear.

☐ You should not stop taking this drug without discussing it with your doctor. There may still be enough drug in your system to cause a reaction as long as 2 weeks after you have stopped taking it.

☐ Most people experience few or no side effects from their drugs. However, any medicine can sometimes cause unwanted effects. Call your doctor if you develop skin problems, numbness or tingling in the hands or feet, eye pain or changes in eyesight, a yellow color to the skin or eyes, fast heartbeats, or difficulty in breathing.

☐ Carry an identification card indicating that you are taking this medicine. Always tell your pharmacist, dentist, and other doctors who are treating you that you are taking this medicine.

☐ If you have a severe reaction, phone your doctor or go to the nearest hospital emergency department.

*   *   *   *   *

Docusate Calcium (*Oral Stool Softener*)
United States: Surfak
Canada: Surfak

☐ This medicine is used to help relieve constipation.

HOW TO USE THIS MEDICINE
☐ Take the capsules with a glass of water.

☐ It may take 2 or 3 days before you notice the full effect of this medicine.

SPECIAL INSTRUCTIONS
☐ Do not take this medicine longer than your doctor has prescribed. If you feel you need this medicine every day and cannot have a bowel movement without it, call your doctor.

☐ Unless otherwise directed, you should also try increasing the amount of bulk food in your diet (for example, bran, fresh fruits, and salads), exercising more often, and drinking 6 to 8 glasses of water every day.

☐ Do not take this medicine if you have any stomach pain, nausea, or vomiting.

☐ Do not take mineral oil while taking this medicine.

☐ Call your doctor if your constipation is not relieved or if you develop rectal bleeding.

* * * * *

Docusate Sodium (*Oral Stool Softener*)
United States: Bu-Lax, Colace, Comfolax, Dilax, DioMedicone, Diosuccin, Disonate, Doxinate, D-S-S, Laxinate, Modane Soft
Canada: Colace, Constiban, Regulex

☐ This medicine is used to help relieve constipation.

HOW TO USE THIS MEDICINE
☐ Take the capsules or tablets with a glass of water.

☐ It may take 2 or 3 days before you notice the full effect of this medicine.

☐ The syrup can be mixed with one-half glass of milk or fruit juice. (**United States** and **Canada:** Colace)

SPECIAL INSTRUCTIONS
☐ Do not take this medicine longer than your doctor has prescribed. If you feel you need this medicine every day and cannot have a bowel movement without it, call your doctor.

□ Unless otherwise directed, you should also try increasing the amount of bulk food in your diet (for example, bran, fresh fruits, and salads), exercising more often, and drinking 6 to 8 glasses of water every day.

□ Do not take this medicine if you have any stomach pain, nausea, or vomiting.

□ Do not take mineral oil while taking this medicine.

□ Call your doctor if your constipation is not relieved or if you develop rectal bleeding.

* * * * *

Doxepin HCl *(Oral Antidepressant-Anxiolytic)*
United States: Adapin, Sinequan
Canada: Sinequan

□ This medicine is used to help relieve the symptoms of depression and anxiety. It is important that you take the medicine regularly and that you do not miss any doses. The full effect of the medicine will not be noticed immediately, but may take from a few days to several weeks. Early signs of improvement are increased appetite, better sleep, increased energy and, later, improved mood. DO NOT STOP TAKING the medicine when you first feel better or you may feel worse in 3 or 4 days.

HOW TO USE THIS MEDICINE
□ This medicine may be taken with food unless otherwise directed.

SPECIAL INSTRUCTIONS
□ If you forget to take a dose, take it as soon as possible. However, if it is almost time for your next dose, do not take the missed dose. Instead, continue with your regular dosing schedule.

□ Any medicine has a few unwanted side effects. Because this medicine takes a few weeks to work, the side effects are the only thing that tell the doctor that the drug is being absorbed. Most of these side effects will go away as your body adjusts to the medicine.

□ In some people, this drug may cause dizziness or drowsiness. Do not drive a car or operate dangerous machinery or do jobs that require you to be alert until you know how you are going to react to this drug.

□ If this medicine causes dizziness, you should be careful going up and down stairs and you should not change positions too quickly. Get out of bed slowly in the morning and dangle your feet over the edge of the bed for a few minutes before standing up. Sit or lie down at the first sign of dizziness. Tell your doctor you have been dizzy and he may adjust your dose.

□ Do not drink alcoholic beverages while taking this drug without the approval of your doctor.

- ☐ It is important that you obtain the advice of your doctor or pharmacist before taking any other medicines, including pain relievers; sleeping pills; tranquilizers; other medicines for depression; cough, cold, or allergy medicines; or weight-reducing medicine.

- ☐ If your mouth becomes dry, suck a hard sour candy (sugarless) or ice chips, or chew gum. It is especially important to brush your teeth regularly if you develop a dry mouth.

- ☐ If you become constipated, try increasing the amount of bulk in your diet (for example, bran and salads), exercising more often, or drinking water.

- ☐ Call your doctor if you develop a sore throat, fever, mouth sores, eye pain or blurred vision, difficulty in urinating ("passing your water"), fast heartbeats, or a skin rash.

- ☐ Do not stop taking this medicine suddenly without your doctor's approval. When your doctor tells you to stop this medicine, you must follow these precautions for 1 week since some of the medicine will still be in your body.

- ☐ Carry an identification card indicating that you are taking this medicine. Always tell your dentist, pharmacist, and other doctors who are treating you that you are taking this medicine.

*　*　*　*　*

Doxycycline (Oral Antibiotic)
United States: Doxy-11, Doxychel, Vibramycin
Canada: Vibramycin

- ☐ This medicine is an antibiotic used to treat certain types of infections.

- ☐ IMPORTANT: If you have ever had an allergic reaction to tetracycline or any other antibiotic, tell your doctor or pharmacist before you take any of this medicine.

HOW TO USE THIS MEDICINE
- ☐ This medicine may be taken with food if it upsets your stomach. Call your doctor if you continue to have stomach upset.

- ☐ Take this drug with a full glass of water.

- ☐ For LIQUID MEDICINE
  - Shake the bottle well before using so that you can measure an accurate dose. (**United States:** Doxychel, Vibramycin Suspensions; **Canada:** Vibramycin Suspension)

SPECIAL INSTRUCTIONS
- ☐ It is important that you take **all** of this medicine plus any refills that your doctor told you to take. Do not stop taking this medicine earlier than your

doctor has recommended in spite of the fact that you may feel better. Otherwise, the infection may return.

☐ If you forget to take a dose, take it as soon as you remember and then continue with your regular schedule.

☐ Women who are pregnant, breast-feeding, or planning to become pregnant should tell their doctor before taking this medicine.

☐ Some antacids and some laxatives can make this medicine less effective if they are taken at the same time. If you must take them, they should be taken at least 2 to 3 hours after this medicine. If you have any questions, ask your pharmacist.

☐ If you must take iron products or vitamins containing iron, take them 2 hours before (or 3 hours after) this medicine.

☐ This medicine may make some people more sensitive to sunlight or sunlamps. When you begin taking this medicine, try to avoid getting too much sun until you see how you are going to react. If your skin does become more sensitive, try to stay out of direct sunlight. While in the sun, wear protective clothing and sunglasses. You may wish to ask your pharmacist about suitable sunscreen products. You may remain sensitive to sunlight and sunlamps for several weeks after you have stopped taking the drug. Check with your doctor if you become sunburned.

☐ Most people experience few or no side effects from their drugs. However, any medicine can sometimes cause unwanted effects. Call your doctor if you develop a dark-colored tongue, sore mouth, yellow-green stools or, in women, a vaginal discharge that was not present before you started taking this medicine.

☐ Store the medicine in a cool, dark place and keep it tightly closed.

☐ If, for some reason, you cannot take all of the medicine, discard the unused portion by flushing it down the toilet. Do not save this medicine for future use.

*   *   *   *   *

Doxylamine Succinate (*Oral Antihistamine*)
United States: Decapryn

☐ This medicine is used to help relieve the symptoms of certain types of allergic conditions, coughs and colds, and certain skin conditions.

HOW TO USE THIS MEDICINE
☐ This medicine may be taken with food or a glass of milk if it upsets your stomach.

SPECIAL INSTRUCTIONS
☐ If you forget to take a dose, take it as soon as possible. However, if it is almost time for your next dose, do not take the missed dose. Instead, continue with your regular dosing schedule.

□ In some people, this drug may initially cause dizziness or drowsiness. Do not drive a car or operate dangerous machinery or do jobs that require you to be alert until you know how you are going to react to the drug. If you become dizzy, you should be careful going up and down stairs. Sit or lie down at the first sign of dizziness. Tell your doctor if it continues.

□ Do not drink alcoholic beverages while taking this drug without the approval of your doctor.

□ If your mouth becomes dry, suck a hard sour candy (sugarless) or ice chips, or chew gum. It is especially important to brush your teeth regularly if you develop a dry mouth.

□ It is important that you obtain the advice of your doctor or pharmacist before taking pain relievers, nonprescription drugs, sleeping pills or tranquilizers, or other medicines for allergies.

□ Do not take this medicine more often or longer than recommended by your doctor.

□ Most people experience few or no side effects from their drugs. However, any medicine can sometimes cause unwanted effects. Call your doctor if you develop a skin rash, fast heartbeats, blurred vision, stomach pain, or difficulty in urinating ("passing your water").

*   *   *   *   *

Dydrogesterone (Oral Progestogen)
United States: Duphaston, Gynorest

□ This medicine is a hormone. It has many uses and the reason it was prescribed depends on your condition. If you do not understand why you are taking it, check with your doctor.

HOW TO USE THIS MEDICINE
□ The tablets may be taken after meals or with a snack if they upset your stomach.

SPECIAL INSTRUCTIONS
□ It is recommended that you do not smoke while you are taking this medicine because smoking may increase the incidence of heart attacks.

□ Diabetic patients should regularly check the sugar in their urine while they are taking this medicine.

□ Contact your doctor if any of the following side effects occur:
- Severe or persistent headaches
- Vomiting, dizziness, or fainting
- Blurred vision or slurred speech
- Pain in the calves of the legs or numbness in an arm or leg
- Chest pain, shortness of breath, or coughing of blood

- Lumps in the breast
- Severe depression
- A yellow color to the skin or eyes or dark-colored urine
- Severe abdominal pain
- Breakthrough vaginal bleeding

☐ Carry an identification card indicating that you are taking this medicine. Always tell your pharmacist, dentist, and other doctors who are treating you that you are taking this medicine.

* * * * *

Dyphylline (Oral Bronchodilator)
United States: Airet, Dilor, Lufyllin, Neothylline
Canada: Aerophylline, Dilin, Protophylline

☐ This medicine is used to help open up the bronchioles (air passages in the lungs) to make breathing easier.

☐ IMPORTANT: If you have ever had an allergic reaction to caffeine or any medicine for lung conditions, tell your doctor or pharmacist before you take any of this medicine.

HOW TO USE THIS MEDICINE
☐ It is best to take this medicine on an empty stomach with a glass of water. However, if it upsets your stomach, it may be taken with a glass of milk or a snack. Call your doctor if the stomach upset continues.

☐ It is very important that you take this medicine exactly as your doctor has prescribed and that you do not miss any doses. Try to take this medicine at the same time every day. Do not take extra tablets without your doctor's approval.

☐ This medicine must be swallowed whole. Do not crush, chew, or break it into pieces. (**United States:** Airet L.A.)

SPECIAL INSTRUCTIONS
☐ Do not change the dose of any other asthma or bronchitis medicines except on the advice of your doctor.

☐ If you forget to take a dose, take it as soon as possible. However, if it is almost time for your next dose, do not take the missed dose. Instead, continue with your regular dosing schedule.

☐ In some people, this drug may cause dizziness or drowsiness. Do not drive a car or operate dangerous machinery or do jobs that require you to be alert until you know how you are going to react to this drug.

☐ If you become dizzy, you should be careful going up and down stairs. Sit or lie down at the first sign of dizziness.

☐ It is important that you obtain the advice of your doctor or pharmacist before taking ANY other medicines including pain relievers, sleeping pills, tranquilizers or medicines for depression, cough/cold or allergy medicines, or weight-reducing medicines.

☐ Do not smoke while you are on this medicine because smoking can make the drug less effective.

☐ Avoid drinking large amounts of coffee, tea, cocoa, or cola drinks because you could be more sensitive to the caffeine in these beverages.

☐ Most people experience few or no side effects from their drugs. However, any medicine can sometimes cause unwanted effects. Call your doctor if you develop a skin rash, vomiting, stomach pain or red or black stools, fast heartbeats, confusion, unusual tiredness, restlessness, or thirst, increased urination ("passing your water"), or sputum that turns yellow or green in color.

*   *   *   *   *

Dyphylline (*Inhalation Bronchodilator*)
Canada: Protophylline

☐ This medicine is used to help open up the bronchioles (air passages in the lungs) to make breathing easier.

☐ IMPORTANT: If you have ever had an allergic reaction to caffeine or any medicine for lung conditions, tell your doctor or pharmacist before you take any of this medicine.

HOW TO USE THIS MEDICINE
☐ INSTRUCTIONS FOR USE
1. If troubled with sputum, try to clear your chest as completely as possible before using this medicine. This will help the drug to reach the lungs and will allow more thorough clearing of mucus during subsequent coughing.
2. Hold the inhaler upright during use so that the mouthpiece is at the bottom.
3. Shake the canister.
4. Breathe out fully and place the lips tightly around the mouthpiece and tilt the head slightly back.

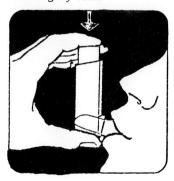

5. Start to breathe in slowly and press down firmly and fully on the valve at the middle of or early during inspiration ("breathing in") to release a "puff." Take the inhaler out of the mouth and close your mouth.

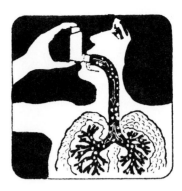

6. Hold your breath for a few seconds. Breathe out through your nose slowly.
7. If your doctor has prescribed a second dose, wait at least 30 seconds before shaking the container again and repeating this procedure.
8. Rinse your mouth with warm water after you have inhaled the medicine. This will help prevent your mouth and throat from becoming dry.
9. The mouthpiece of the inhaler should be kept clean and dry.
10. Failure to follow these instructions carefully can result in inadequate treatment.

☐ It is very important that you take this medicine exactly as your doctor has prescribed.

SPECIAL INSTRUCTIONS

☐ Do not change the dose of any other asthma or bronchitis medicines except on the advice of your doctor.

☐ If you forget to take a dose, take it as soon as possible. However, if it is almost time for your next dose, do not take the missed dose. Instead, continue with your regular dosing schedule.

☐ In some people, this drug may cause dizziness or drowsiness. Do not drive a car or operate dangerous machinery or do jobs that require you to be alert until you know how you are going to react to this drug.

☐ If you become dizzy, you should be careful going up and down stairs. Sit or lie down at the first sign of dizziness.

☐ It is important that you obtain the advice of your doctor or pharmacist before taking ANY other medicines including pain relievers, sleeping pills, tranquilizers or medicines for depression, cough/cold or allergy medicines, or weight-reducing medicines.

308

☐ Avoid drinking large amounts of coffee, tea, cocoa, or cola drinks because you could be more sensitive to the caffeine in these beverages.

☐ Most people experience few or no side effects from their drugs. However, any medicine can sometimes cause unwanted effects. Call your doctor if you develop a skin rash, vomiting, stomach pain or red or black stools, fast heartbeats, confusion, unusual tiredness, restlessness, or thirst, increased urination ("passing your water"), or sputum that turns yellow or green in color.

☐ Store the container in a cool place. Do not place the container in hot water or near radiators, stoves, or other sources of heat. Do not puncture, burn, or incinerate the container (even after it is empty).

*   *   *   *   *

Dyphylline (Rectal Bronchodilator)
Canada: Protophylline

☐ This medicine is used to help open up the bronchioles (air passages in the lungs) to make breathing easier.

☐ IMPORTANT: If you have ever had an allergic reaction to caffeine or any medicine for lung conditions, tell your doctor or pharmacist before you use any of this medicine.

HOW TO USE THIS MEDICINE
☐ Administration of SUPPOSITORIES
   - Remove the wrapper from the suppository.
   - Lie on your side and raise your knee to your chest.
   - Insert the suppository with the tapered (pointed) end first into the rectum.
   - Remain lying down for a few minutes so that the suppository will dissolve in the rectum.
   - Try to avoid having a bowel movement for at least 1 hour so that the drug will have time to work.

☐ It is very important that you use this medicine exactly as your doctor has prescribed and that you do not miss any doses. Do not use extra suppositories without your doctor's approval.

SPECIAL INSTRUCTIONS
☐ Do not change the dose of any other asthma or bronchitis medicines except on the advice of your doctor.

☐ If you forget a dose, insert it as soon as possible. However, if it is almost time for your next dose, do not use the missed dose. Instead, continue with your regular dosing schedule.

☐ In some people, this drug may cause dizziness or drowsiness. Do not drive a car or operate dangerous machinery or do jobs that require you to be alert until you know how you are going to react to this drug.

☐ If you become dizzy, you should be careful going up and down stairs. Sit or lie down at the first sign of dizziness.

☐ It is important that you obtain the advice of your doctor or pharmacist before taking ANY other medicines including pain relievers, sleeping pills, tranquilizers or medicines for depression, cough/cold or allergy medicines, or weight-reducing medicines.

☐ Do not smoke while you are on this medicine because smoking can make the drug less effective.

☐ Avoid drinking large amounts of coffee, tea, cocoa, or cola drinks because you could be more sensitive to the caffeine in these beverages.

☐ Most people experience few or no side effects from their drugs. However, any medicine can sometimes cause unwanted effects. Call your doctor if you develop a skin rash; vomiting; stomach pain or red or black stools; fast heartbeats; confusion; unusual tiredness, restlessness, or thirst; increased urination ("passing your water"); sputum that turns yellow or green in color; or rectal burning or pain that was not present before you started using the medicine.

* * * * *

Econazol Nitrate (*Vaginal Antifungal*)
Canada: Ecostatin

☐ This medicine is used to treat fungal infections of the vagina.

HOW TO USE THIS MEDICINE
☐ For VAGINAL OVULES
  • Remove the wrapper and dip the tablet into water quickly, just enough to moisten it.
  • Put the tablet into the applicator.
  • Insert the applicator into the vaginal canal and then depress the plunger.
  • Remove the applicator.
  • Wash the applicator with warm water and soap after each use.

SPECIAL INSTRUCTIONS
☐ It is important to use *all* of this medicine, plus any refills that your doctor told you to use. Do not stop using it earlier than your doctor has recommended in spite of the fact that your symptoms seem to have improved. Otherwise, the infection may return.

☐ If you forget a dose, insert it as soon as possible. However, if it is almost time for your next dose, do not insert the missed dose but continue with your regular schedule.

310

- [ ] During therapy, your doctor may recommend that you abstain from sexual intercourse or that your partner use a condom.

- [ ] Continue using this medicine even if you are having a menstrual period.

- [ ] Call your doctor if the condition for which this drug is being used persists or becomes worse or if you develop a constant irritation such as itching or burning that was not present before you started using this medicine.

- [ ] For external use only. Do not swallow.

*   *   *   *   *

Ecothiophate Iodide (*Ophthalmic Glaucoma Therapy*)
United States: Echodide, Phospholine Iodide
Canada: Phospholine Iodide

- [ ] This medicine is used to treat glaucoma and other eye conditions.

HOW TO USE THIS MEDICINE
- [ ] For EYE DROPS

INSTILLATION OF EYE DROPS

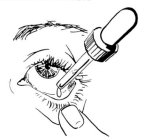

- If you have refrigerated the eye drops, they should be warmed before using. Hold the bottle between your hands for a few minutes. Do not put in hot water.
- The person administering the eye drops should wash his hands with soap and water.
- The eye drops must be kept clean. Do not touch the dropper against the face or anything else.
- Lie down or tilt your head backward and look at the ceiling.
- Gently pull down the lower lid of your eye to form a pouch.
- Hold the dropper in your other hand and approach the eye from the side. Place the dropper as close to the eye as possible without touching it.
- Place the prescribed number of drops into the pouch of the eye.
- Close your eyes. Do not rub them.
- Apply gentle pressure for a minute with your fingers to the bridge of the nose (inside corner of the eye) to prevent the eye drops from being drained from the eye.
- Blot excess solution around the eye with a tissue.

- ☐ If necessary, have someone else administer the eye drops for you.
- ☐ Do not use the eye drops if they change in color or have changed in any way since you purchased them.
- ☐ Keep the eye drop bottle tightly closed when not in use.
- ☐ Wash your hands after you have instilled the drops.
- ☐ Do not use the drug more frequently or in larger quantities than prescribed by your doctor.

SPECIAL INSTRUCTIONS

- ☐ IMPORTANT: If you have ever had an allergic reaction to an iodide medicine, tell your doctor or pharmacist before you use any of this drug.
- ☐ Vision may be blurred for a few minutes after using the eye medicine. Do not drive a car or operate dangerous machinery or do jobs that require you to be alert until vision has cleared.
  During the first 5 to 10 days of using this medicine, you may develop a headache or dimmed vision. This should disappear after you become used to the medicine. Unless otherwise directed, you may take ASA/aspirin to help relieve the headache.
- ☐ If you forget to use the medicine, use it as soon as possible. However, if it is almost time for your next dose, do not use the missed dose but continue with your regular schedule.
- ☐ Do not use this medicine at the same time as any other eye medicine without the approval of your doctor. Some medicines cannot be mixed.
- ☐ Contact your doctor if the condition for which you are using this medicine does not improve or if the eye becomes irritated by it for more than a few minutes. Many eye medicines sting for a short time immediately after use. Also call your doctor if you develop persistent diarrhea (loose bowel movements), muscle weakness, excessive sweating or flushing or difficulty in breathing.
- ☐ It is best to store these eye drops in the refrigerator because they will then be fresh for 3 months. If the eye drops are stored at room temperature, they should be thrown away after 1 month because they will not be fresh after 30 days.
- ☐ If you are routinely exposed to organophosphorus insecticides or pesticides such as parathion and malathion (for example, farmers, lawn service workers, aerial sprayers, or home users), you may be more sensitive to this medicine. It is advisable to wear a face mask when you are exposed to the insecticides and pesticides and to wash and change your clothes after exposure.
- ☐ Always tell any future doctors who are treating you that you have used this medicine.
- ☐ For external use only. Do not swallow.

* * * * *

Ephedrine-Aminacrine (*Nasal Decongestant-Antiseptic*)
Canada: Flavedrin Mild

☐ This medicine is used to help relieve nasal stuffiness.

HOW TO USE THIS MEDICINE
☐ For NOSE DROPS

INSTILLATION OF NOSE DROPS

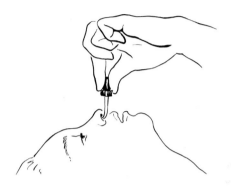

- Blow your nose gently before administering the drops.
- Sit in a chair and tilt your head backward or lie down on the bed with your head extending over the edge of the bed, or lie down and place a pillow under the shoulders so that the head is tipped backward.
- Insert the dropper into the nostril about $\frac{1}{3}$ inch and drop the prescribed number of drops into the nose.
- Try not to touch the inside of the nose with the dropper as it will probably make you sneeze and will contaminate the dropper.
- Remain in the same position for at least 5 minutes.

☐ For children:
- Let the head hang over the edge of a table, bed, or the mother's lap, and follow the procedure described above.

SPECIAL INSTRUCTIONS
☐ Do not use this medicine more often or longer than recommended by your doctor. If used for too long, this medicine may actually cause a type of congestion.

☐ Rinse the dropper in hot water after each use.

☐ If you forget to use the medicine, use it as soon as possible. However, if it is almost time for your next dose, do not use the missed dose but continue with your regular schedule.

☐ Do not use this medicine at the same time as any other nasal medicine without the approval of your doctor. Some medicines cannot be mixed.

313

☐ Contact your doctor if the condition for which you are using this medicine does not improve. Also call your doctor if you develop fast heartbeats, headache, dizziness, trembling, blurred vision, or drowsiness.

☐ For external use only. Do not swallow.

*   *   *   *   *

Epinephrine Bitartrate (*Ophthalmic—Glaucoma Therapy*)
United States: E½, E1, E2, Epitrate, Lyophrin, Murocoll, Mytrate
Canada: Epitrate

Epinephrine HCl
United States: Adrenaline Chloride, Epifrin, Glaucon, Mistura-E
Canada: Epifrin, Glaucon

Epinephrine Borate Complex
United States: Epinal, Eppy, Eppy/N
Canada: Epinal, Eppy/N

☐ This medicine is used in the treatment of glaucoma and other eye conditions.

HOW TO USE THIS MEDICINE

☐ For EYE DROPS

INSTILLATION OF EYE DROPS

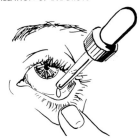

- The person administering the eye drops should wash his hands with soap and water.
- The eye drops must be kept clean. Do not touch the dropper against the face or anything else.
- Lie down or tilt your head backward and look at the ceiling.
- Gently pull down the lower lid of your eye to form a pouch.
- Hold the dropper in your other hand and approach the eye from the side. Place the dropper as close to the eye as possible without touching it.
- Place the prescribed number of drops into the pouch of the eye.
- Close your eyes. Do not rub them.

314

- Apply gentle pressure for a minute with your fingers to the bridge of the nose (inside corner of the eye) to prevent the eye drops from being drained from the eye.
- Blot excess solution around the eye with a tissue.

☐ If necessary, have someone else administer the eye drops for you.

☐ Do not use the eye drops if they have changed in color or have changed in any way since you purchased them.

☐ Keep the eye drop bottle tightly closed when not in use.

☐ Do not use the drug more frequently or in larger quantities than prescribed by your doctor.

SPECIAL INSTRUCTIONS

☐ Vision may be blurred for a few minutes after using the eye medicine. Do not drive a car or operate dangerous machinery or do jobs that require you to be alert until your vision has cleared.

☐ If you forget to use the medicine, use it as soon as possible. However, if it is almost time for your next dose, do not use the missed dose but continue with your regular schedule.

☐ Do not use this medicine at the same time as any other eye medicine without the approval of your doctor. Some medicines cannot be mixed.

☐ Contact your doctor if the condition for which you are using this medicine does not improve or if the eye becomes irritated by it for more than a few minutes. Many eye medicines sting for a short time immediately after use. Also call your doctor if you develop eye pain, fast heartbeats, paleness, trembling, or excessive sweating.

☐ Redness of the eye is normal and part of the response to the drug. A slight stinging sensation and pain may follow the first instillation of the medicine, but this should diminish with continued therapy. Taking ASA/aspirin or other mild pain killers will relieve the pain.

☐ For external use only.

* * * * *

Ergotamine Tartrate (*Inhalation Migraine Therapy*)
United States: Medihaler-Ergotamine
Canada: Medihaler-Ergotamine

☐ This medicine is used to treat migraine headaches and certain types of throbbing headaches.

HOW TO USE THIS MEDICINE

- Pull the cap from the mouthpiece.
- Shake well before using.

- Hold the inhaler upside down during use.
- Breathe out fully and place the mouthpiece well into the mouth and aim it at the back of the throat.

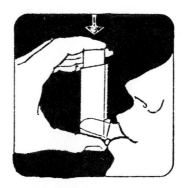

- Start to breathe in and press down on the vial.

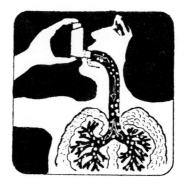

- Continue to breathe in until your lungs are completely filled.
- Release pressure on the vial and remove the inhaler from your mouth.
- Hold your breath as long as possible. Breathe out through your nose.
- Rinse your mouth with warm water after you have inhaled the medicine.
- This will help prevent your mouth and throat from becoming dry.
- Clean the plastic mouthpiece daily to keep it in good working order. Remove the metal vial and wash the mouthpiece with soap and hot water. Rinse well. Dry and replace the vial.

☐ A single inhalation should be taken at the first sign of a headache. The dose may be repeated in 5 minutes if the headache is not relieved. No more than 6 inhalations should be taken per day, and the interval between inhalations should be at least 5 minutes.

SPECIAL INSTRUCTIONS

☐ It may help to lie down in a darkened room after taking the drug.

☐ Do not take more of this medicine than your doctor has prescribed.

☐ Most people experience few or no side effects from their drugs. However, any medicine can sometimes cause unwanted effects. Call your doctor if you develop leg cramps, numbness or tingling in the fingers or toes, chest pain, stomach pain, or swelling or unusual weakness of the hands or legs.

*   *   *   *   *

Ergotamine Tartrate (*Oral Migraine Therapy*)
United States: Ergomar, Ergostat, Gynergen
Canada: Ergomar, Gynergen

Ergotamine Tartrate-Caffeine
United States: Cafergot, Cafermine, Cafertrate, Ergocaf, Migrastat
Canada: Cafergot

☐ This medicine is used to treat migraine headaches and certain types of throbbing headaches.

HOW TO USE THIS MEDICINE
☐ Take 2 tablets or capsules at the first sign of an attack and 1 tablet or capsule every $\frac{1}{2}$ hour until the attack is relieved. Do not take more than 6 tablets or capsules per day or 10 tablets or capsules per week. (**United States:** Cafergot, Cafermine, Cafertrate, Ergocaf, Gynergen, Migrastat; **Canada:** Cafergot, Gynergen)

☐ Place one tablet under the tongue at the onset of the attack. Allow the tablet to dissolve completely. Take another tablet every $\frac{1}{2}$ hour if needed. Do not take more than 3 tablets per day or 5 tablets per week. (**United States:** Ergomar, Ergostat; **Canada:** Ergomar)

SPECIAL INSTRUCTIONS
☐ It may help to lie down in a darkened room after taking the drug.

☐ Do not take more of this medicine than your doctor has prescribed.

☐ Most people experience few or no side effects from their drugs. However, any medicine can sometimes cause unwanted effects. Call your doctor if you develop leg cramps, numbness or tingling in the fingers or toes, chest pain, stomach pain, or swelling or unusual weakness of the hands or legs.

*   *   *   *   *

Erythrityl Tetranitrate (*Sublingual and Chewable Coronary Vasodilator*)
United States: Cardilate
Canada: Cardilate

☐ This medicine is used to help relieve a type of chest pain called angina.

☐ Carry this medicine with you at all times.

HOW TO USE THIS MEDICINE
- ☐ For SUBLINGUAL TABLETS
  - • This medicine should be used at the FIRST sign of an attack of angina. Do not wait until the pain becomes severe. Sit down or lie down as soon as you feel an attack of angina coming on.
  - • Then place a tablet UNDER YOUR TONGUE or in the pouch of your cheek until it is completely dissolved. Do NOT swallow or chew these tablets.
  - • Try not to swallow until the drug is dissolved and do not rinse the mouth for a few minutes. Do not eat, drink, or smoke while the tablet is dissolving.
  - • If your angina is not relieved within 5 to 10 minutes, you may dissolve a second tablet under your tongue, unless otherwise directed.
  - • If the angina continues for another 5 to 10 minutes, you may use a third tablet. If this does not relieve your chest pains, call your doctor immediately or go to the nearest hospital emergency department.

- ☐ CHEWABLE TABLETS
  - • This medicine should be used at the FIRST sign of an attack of angina. Do not wait until the pain becomes severe. Sit down or lie down as soon as you feel an attack of angina coming on.
  - • Then CHEW the tablet well and hold it in the mouth for 1 to 2 minutes without swallowing. Do not rinse the mouth for a few minutes.
  - • If your angina is not relieved within 5 to 10 minutes, you may chew a second tablet unless otherwise directed. If the angina continues for another 5 to 10 minutes, chew a third tablet. If this does not relieve your chest pains, call your doctor immediately or go to the nearest hospital emergency department.

HOW TO STORE THIS MEDICINE
- ☐ Store in a cool, dry place but not in the bathroom medicine cabinet or the refrigerator because these areas are very humid.

SPECIAL INSTRUCTIONS
- ☐ After using this medicine, you may get a headache or flushing which will usually disappear within a few minutes. This is a common side effect. If the headaches do not go away, tell your doctor.

- ☐ Try to relax and remain calm when you are taking the medicine. If you become dizzy or feel faint, breathe deeply and bend forward with your head between your knees. Always get up slowly after you have been sitting or lying down.

- ☐ Do not drink alcoholic beverages too soon after taking this medicine as it may make the dizziness and fainting worse.

- ☐ Some nonprescription drugs can aggravate your heart condition. Do not take any of the following without the approval of your doctor or pharmacist:

318

cough/cold or sinus products, asthma or allergy products, or diet or weight-reducing medicines.

☐ You may help prevent angina by taking a tablet 5 to 10 minutes before activities you know are likely to trigger attacks, such as strenuous exercise, emotional stress, a heavy meal, high altitudes, or exposure to cold. Let your doctor know what things usually cause your angina so that he can advise you about preventing attacks.

☐ Cigarette smoking can aggravate angina and is a special risk for people who have heart conditions.

☐ Most people experience few or no side effects from their drugs. However, any medicine can sometimes cause unwanted effects. Call your doctor if you develop a skin rash, fainting spells, nausea or vomiting, or a rapid pulse, or if your chest pain is not relieved.

☐ Carry an identification card indicating that you are taking this medicine. Always tell your pharmacist, dentist, and other doctors who are treating you that you are taking this medicine.

*   *   *   *   *

Erythrityl Tetranitrate (*Oral Coronary Vasodilator*)
United States: Cardilate
Canada: Cardilate

☐ This medicine is used to help prevent angina attacks and must be taken regularly as your doctor has prescribed. Do not miss any doses. It will not relieve an angina attack that has already started because it works too slowly.

HOW TO USE THIS MEDICINE
☐ It is best to take this medicine on an empty stomach 1 hour before (or 2 hours after) eating food.

☐ For ORAL TABLETS
  • If you forget to take a dose, take it as soon as possible. However, if your next dose is within 2 hours, do not take the missed dose but continue with your regular schedule.

HOW TO STORE THIS MEDICINE
☐ Store in a cool, dry place but not in the bathroom medicine cabinet or refrigerator because these areas are humid.

SPECIAL INSTRUCTIONS
☐ If you become dizzy or feel faint, breathe deeply and bend forward with your head between your knees. Always get up slowly after you have been sitting or lying down. Get out of bed slowly in the morning and dangle your feet over the edge of the bed for a few minutes before standing up. Do not drive a car

or operate dangerous machinery or do jobs that require you to be alert if you are dizzy or drowsy.

☐ Do not drink alcoholic beverages while you are taking this medicine as it may make the dizziness and fainting worse.

☐ Some nonprescription drugs can aggravate your heart condition. Do not take any of the following without the approval of your doctor or pharmacist: cough/cold or sinus products, asthma or allergy products, or diet or weight-reducing medicines.

☐ When you first start taking this medicine, you may get a headache or flushing. This is a common side effect and will usually disappear after you have taken the drug a few times. If the headaches do not go away or are severe, call your doctor.

☐ Cigarette smoking can aggravate angina and is a special risk for people who have angina.

☐ Most people experience few or no side effects from their drugs. However, any medicine can sometimes cause unwanted effects. Call your doctor if you develop a skin rash, fainting spells, nausea or vomiting, a rapid pulse, or if your chest pain is not relieved.

☐ Do not stop taking the medicine suddenly or it could cause an angina attack.

☐ Carry an identification card indicating that you are taking this medicine. Always tell your pharmacist, dentist, and other doctors who are treating you that you are taking this medicine.

*　*　*　*　*

Erythromycin (*Ophthalmic Antibiotic*)
United States: Ilotycin
Canada: Ilotycin

☐ This medicine is an antibiotic used to treat certain types of eye infections.

☐ IMPORTANT: If you have ever had an allergic reaction to erythromycin or any antibiotic medicine, tell your doctor or pharmacist before you use any of this drug.

HOW TO USE THIS MEDICINE
☐ For EYE OINTMENT

INSTILLATION OF EYE OINTMENT

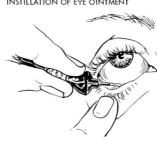

- The person administering the eye ointment should wash his hands with soap and water.
- The eye ointment must be kept clean. Do not touch the tube against the face or anything else.
- Lie down or tilt your head backward and look at the ceiling.
- Gently pull down the lower lid of your eye to form a pouch.
- Hold the tube in your other hand and place the tube as close as possible to the eye without touching it.
- Squeeze the prescribed amount of ointment (usually $\frac{1}{2}$ inch in adults) from the tube along the pouch.
- Close your eyes. Do not rub them.
- Wipe off any excess ointment around the eye with a tissue.
- Clean the tip of the ointment tube with a tissue.

☐ If necessary, have someone else administer the eye ointment for you.

☐ Keep the eye ointment tube tightly closed when not in use.

SPECIAL INSTRUCTIONS

☐ Vision may be blurred for a few minutes after using the eye medicine. Do not drive a car or operate dangerous machinery or do jobs that require you to be alert until your vision has cleared.

☐ Eye medicines should be used as prescribed by your doctor. Eye infections often clear rapidly after a few days of use of the medicine, but not always completely. It is important to use **all** of this medicine, plus any refills that your doctor told you to use. Do not stop using it earlier than your doctor has recommended in spite of the fact that your symptoms seem to have improved. Otherwise, the infection may return.

☐ If you forget to use the medicine, use it as soon as possible. However, if it is almost time for your next dose, do not use the missed dose but continue with your regular schedule.

☐ Do not use this medicine at the same time as any other eye medicine without the approval of your doctor. Some medicines cannot be mixed.

☐ Contact your doctor if the condition for which you are using this medicine does not improve or if the eye becomes irritated by it for more than a few minutes. Many eye medicines sting for a short time immediately after use.

☐ For external use only. Do not swallow.

*   *   *   *   *

Erythromycin (Oral Antibiotic)

United States: E-Mycin, Erythromycin Base, Ilotycin, Robimycin, RP-Mycin

Canada: E-Mycin, Erythromid, Ilotycin

Erythromycin Ethyl Succinate

United States: E.E.S., Pediamycin
Canada: E.E.S.

Erythromycin Stearate

United States: Bristamycin, Erythrocin Stearate, Ethril, Pfizer-E, SK-Erythromycin, Wyamycin
Canada: Erythrocin

Erythromycin Estolate

United States: Ilosone
Canada: Ilosone

☐ This medicine is an antibiotic used to treat certain types of infections.

☐ IMPORTANT: If you have ever had an allergic reaction to erythromycin or any other antibiotic, tell your doctor or pharmacist before you take any of this medicine.

HOW TO USE THIS MEDICINE

☐ For TABLETS AND CAPSULES

☐ It is best to take this medicine on an empty stomach at least 1 hour before (or 2 hours after) eating food. Take it with a full glass of water. If you develop stomach upset after taking the drug, take it with some crackers. Call your doctor if you continue to have stomach upset. (*United States:* Bristamycin, Erythrocin Stearate, Erythromycin Base, Ethril, Pfizer-E, SK-Erythromycin; *Canada:* Erythromid, Erythrocin Filmtabs)

☐ It is best to take this medicine immediately after meals (*United States:* E.E.S., Pediamycin; *Canada:* E.E.S.)

☐ These tablets have a special coating and must be swallowed whole. Do not crush, chew, or break them into pieces. Take them with a full glass of water on an empty stomach or with food. (*United States:* E-Mycin, Ilotycin, Robimycin, RP-Mycin; *Canada:* E-Mycin, Ilotycin)

☐ This medicine may be taken with a glass of water on an empty stomach or with food. (*United States:* Ilosone, Wyamycin; *Canada:* Erythrocin 250 mg., Ilosone)

☐ Take this medicine immediately before meals. (*Canada:* Erythrocin 500 mg B-PAC)

☐ Chew or crush these tablets well before swallowing. Do not swallow the tablets whole. (*United States:* E.E.S., Ilosone Chewable, Pediamycin; *Canada:* E.E.S., Ilosone Chewable)

☐ For LIQUID MEDICINES

    • Shake the bottle well before using so that you can measure an accurate dose. (*United States:* E.E.S. Liquid, Ilosone, Pediamycin, Wyamycin

Liquid; *Canada:* E.E.S., Ilosone Liquid, Drops & Suspension)
- If a dropper is used to measure the dose and you do not fully understand how to use it, check with your pharmacist.
- Store the bottle of medicine in a refrigerator unless otherwise directed.
- If there is a discard date on the bottle, throw away any unused medicine after that date. Do not take or save old medicine.

☐ Take this medicine at the proper time even if you skip a meal. If you forget to take a dose, take it as soon as you remember and then continue with your regular schedule.

SPECIAL INSTRUCTIONS

☐ It is important to take *all* of this medicine plus any refills that your doctor told you to take. Do not stop taking this medicine earlier than your doctor has recommended in spite of the fact that you may feel better. Otherwise, the infection may return.

☐ Most people experience few or no side effects from their drugs. However, any medicine can sometimes cause unwanted effects. Contact your doctor if you develop a dark-colored tongue, yellow-green stools or, in women, a vaginal discharge that was not present before you started taking the medicine.

☐ This medicine sometimes causes diarrhea (loose bowel movements). Call your doctor if the diarrhea becomes severe or does not go away after a few days.

☐ If you are taking ERYTHROMYCIN ESTOLATE and develop severe stomach cramps, pale-colored stools, nausea, vomiting, fever, or a yellow color to the skin or eyes, call your doctor. (*United States* and *Canada:* Ilosone)

☐ Women who are pregnant, breast-feeding, or planning to become pregnant should tell their doctor before taking this medicine.

☐ Call your doctor immediately if you think you may be allergic to the medicine or if you develop a skin rash, hives, itching, swelling of the face, or difficulty in breathing. If you cannot reach your doctor, phone a hospital emergency department.

☐ If for some reason you cannot take all of the medicine, discard the unused portion by flushing it down the toilet. Do not take or save old medicine.

*   *   *   *   *

Erythromycin (*Topical Antibiotic*)
United States: Ilotycin
Canada: Ilotycin

☐ This medicine is an antibiotic used to treat infections of the skin and to help control acne.

☐ IMPORTANT: If you have ever had an allergic reaction to an erythromycin medicine, tell your doctor or pharmacist before you use any of this drug.

HOW TO USE THIS MEDICINE

- Each time you apply the medicine, wash your hands and gently cleanse the skin area well with water unless otherwise directed by your doctor.
- Do not allow the skin to dry completely. Pat with a clean towel until almost dry.
- Apply a small amount of the drug to the affected area and spread lightly. Only the medicine that is actually touching the skin will work. A thick layer is not more effective than a thin layer. Do not bandage unless directed by your doctor.

☐ Do not use the drug more frequently or in larger quantities than prescribed by your doctor.

SPECIAL INSTRUCTIONS

☐ It is important to use *all* of this medicine, plus any refills that your doctor told you to use. Do not stop using it earlier than your doctor has recommended in spite of the fact that your symptoms seem to have improved. Otherwise, the infection may return.

☐ If you forget to apply the medicine, apply it as soon as possible. However, if it is almost time for your next dose, do not apply the missed dose but continue with your regular schedule.

☐ Do not apply cosmetics or lotions on top of the drug unless your doctor approves.

☐ Keep this preparation away from the eyes. If you should accidentally get some in your eyes, wash it away with water immediately.

☐ Call your doctor if the condition for which this drug is being used persists or becomes worse or if you develop a constant irritation such as itching or burning that was not present before you started using this medicine.

☐ For external use only. Do not swallow.

*   *   *   *   *

Esterified Estrogens (*Oral Estrogen*)

United States: Amnestrogen, Estabs, Estratab, Evex, Femogen, Menest

Canada: Climestrone, Estromed, Menotrol, Neo-Estrone

Esterified Estrogens–Methyltestosterone

United States: Estratest

☐ This medicine is a hormone. It has many uses and the reason it was prescribed depends on your condition. If you do not understand why you are taking it, check with your doctor.

HOW TO USE THIS MEDICINE

☐ The tablets may be taken after meals or with a snack if they upset your stomach.

SPECIAL INSTRUCTIONS

☐ Women who are pregnant, breast-feeding, or planning to become pregnant should tell their doctor before taking this medicine.

☐ It is recommended that you do not smoke while you are taking this medicine because smoking may increase the incidence of heart attacks.

☐ Diabetic patients should regularly check the sugar in their urine while they are taking this medicine.

☐ Contact your doctor if any of the following side effects occur:
  • Severe or persistent headaches
  • Vomiting, dizziness, or fainting
  • Blurred vision or slurred speech
  • Pain in the calves of the legs or numbness in an arm or leg
  • Chest pain, shortness of breath, or coughing of blood
  • Lumps in the breast
  • Severe depression
  • A yellow color to the skin or eyes or dark-colored urine
  • Severe abdominal pain
  • Vaginal bleeding

☐ Carry an identification card indicating that you are taking this medicine. Always tell your pharmacist, dentist, and other doctors who are treating you that you are taking this medicine.

* * * * *

Estradiol (Oral Estrogen)
United States: Estrace
Canada: Estrace

☐ This medicine is a hormone and is used to help relieve the symptoms of menopause or is used when the ovaries have been removed.

HOW TO USE THIS MEDICINE

☐ Take this medicine at the same time each day, for example, after the evening meal or at bedtime.

SPECIAL INSTRUCTIONS

☐ Women who are pregnant, breast-feeding, or planning to become pregnant should tell their doctor before taking this medicine.

☐ It is recommended that you do not smoke while you are taking this medicine because smoking may increase the incidence of heart attacks.

325

□ Contact your doctor if any of the following side effects occur:
  - Severe or persistent headaches
  - Vomiting, dizziness, or fainting
  - Blurred vision or slurred speech
  - Pain in the calves of the legs or numbness in an arm or leg
  - Chest pain, shortness of breath, or coughing up of blood
  - Lumps in the breast
  - Severe depression
  - A yellow color to the skin or eyes or dark-colored urine
  - Severe abdominal pain
  - Vaginal bleeding

□ Carry an identification card indicating that you are taking this medicine. Always tell your pharmacist, dentist, and other doctors who are treating you that you are taking this medicine.

* * * * *

Combination Estrogen-Progestogen Therapy (20 Day)

United States: Enovid-E, Enovid 5 mg., Norinyl 2 mg., Ortho Novum 10 mg., Ovulen

Canada: Enovid

□ This medicine is used as a birth control measure and to treat hormonal disorders. Some products are also used to treat certain types of menstrual problems.

HOW TO USE THIS MEDICINE

□ Take this medicine at the same time each day, for example, after the evening meal or at bedtime. It is important to take this medicine regularly.

□ If you are taking the drug for **birth control,** take the tablets as follows:
  1. During the first month of taking this medicine, it is important to use some additional form of birth control to help prevent pregnancy.
  2. The first day of menstruation is day **one.** Begin taking this medicine on day **five** of your menstrual cycle.

Day 5 of first cycle: Take 1st Tablet

SUN	MON	TUES	WED	THURS	FRI	SAT
MENSTRUATION				1	2	3
4	5	6	7	8	9	10
11	12	13	14	15	16	17
18	19	20				

3. Take one tablet every day for 20 days. Menstruation will usually start 1 to 3 days after the last tablet.
4. Do not take any tablets until day *five* of your menstrual cycle. Start a new 20-day cycle again on day *five.*
5. If you miss one daily dose, take it as soon as you remember and continue your regular schedule.
6. If you miss two daily doses, take 2 tablets daily for the next 2 days and then resume your normal schedule. It is advisable to use some additional form of birth control for the next 7 days to help avoid pregnancy.
7. If you miss 3 daily doses, stop taking the medicine and start a new schedule of tablets 7 days after the last dose was taken. An additional form of birth control should be used during the next 14 days of medication.

SPECIAL INSTRUCTIONS

☐ Contact your doctor at least once every 6 to 12 months so that you can be examined.

☐ In the summer, it is best to take the tablet at bedtime so that the highest levels of the drug are in your body during the night. This will help protect your skin from the sunlight which sometimes causes discolorations in women on this medicine.

☐ It is recommended that you do not smoke while you are taking this medicine because smoking may increase the incidence of heart attacks.

☐ Women who are breast-feeding, should tell their doctor before taking this medicine.

☐ Contact your doctor if any of the following side effects occur:
- Severe or persistent headaches.
- Vomiting, dizziness, or fainting.
- Blurred vision or slurred speech.
- Pain in the calves of the legs or numbness in an arm or leg.
- Chest pain, shortness of breath, or coughing of blood.
- Lumps in the breast.
- Severe depression.
- A yellow color to the skin or eyes or dark-colored urine.
- Severe abdominal pain.
- Breakthrough vaginal bleeding which persists after the third month of therapy. During the first 3 months of therapy, breakthrough bleeding may be expected, but you should keep taking the tablets and it will usually clear up in a day or two.
- If you miss 2 consecutive menstrual periods or if you think you are pregnant.

☐ Always tell your pharmacist, dentist, and other doctors who are treating you that you are taking this medicine.

* * * * *

327

Combination Estrogen-Progestogen Therapy (21 Day)

United States: Brevicon, Demulen, Enovid-E21, Loestrin 21 1/20, Loestrin 21 1.5/30, Lo/Ovral, Modicon, Minestrin 1/20, Norinyl 1 + 80, Norinyl 1/50 21-Day, Norlestrin-21 1/50, Norlestrin-21 2.5/50, Ortho-Novum 2 mg., Ortho-Novum 1/80 21, Ortho-Novum 1/50 21, Ortho-Novum 1/35, Ovral, Ovulen-21

Canada: Anoryol, Brevicon, Demulen, Enovid E, Loestrin 1.5/30, Logest 1.5/30, Logest 1/50, Min-Ovral, Norinyl 1 + 50, Norinyl 1 + 80, Norinyl-2, Norlestrin 1/50, Norlestria 2.5/50, Novinol-21, Ortho-Novum 1/80, Ortho-Novum 1/50, Ortho-Novum 2 mg., Ortho-Novum 5 mg., Ortho-Novum 0.5 mg., Ovral, Ovulen 1 mg., Ovulen 0.5 mg.

□ This medicine is used as a birth control measure and to treat hormonal disorders. Some products are also used to treat certain types of menstrual problems.

HOW TO USE THIS MEDICINE

□ Take this medicine at the same time each day, for example, after the evening meal or at bedtime. It is important to take this medication regularly.

□ If you are taking this drug for **birth control,** take the tablets as follows:
1. During the first month of taking this medicine it is important to use some additional form of birth control to help prevent pregnancy.
2. The first day of menstruation is day **one.** Begin taking this medication on day **five** of your menstrual cycle. Take the first tablet from the space marked with the corresponding day of the week. The day of the week that you take your first tablet is your regular starting day for future cycles.
3. Take one tablet every day for 3 weeks (21 days). Take it at the same time every day—preferably after dinner or at bedtime.
4. After finishing the package of 21 tablets wait 7 days. Do **not** take any tablets during these days. Your period will probably start about 3 days after you took the last tablet.
5. On the eighth day, start a new package of 21 tablets and again take one tablet daily. It is important to start taking your tablets on your regular starting day whether or not menstruation occurs as expected.
6. Repeat this 21 days on and 7 days off cycle.
7. If you miss one daily dose, take it as soon as you remember and continue your regular schedule.
8. If you miss two daily doses, take 2 tablets daily for the next 2 days and then resume your normal schedule. It is advisable to use some additional form of birth control for the next 7 days to help avoid pregnancy.
9. If you miss 3 daily doses, stop taking the medicine and throw away the remainder of the package. Start a new package of tablets 7 days after

If Menstruation Starts On	Start Tablets On
Sunday	Thursday
Monday	Friday
Tuesday	Saturday
Wednesday	Sunday
Thursday	Monday
Friday	Tuesday
Saturday	Wednesday

Day 5 of first cycle: Take 1st Tablet

SUN	MON	TUES	WED	THURS	FRI	SAT
MENSTRUATION				1	2	3
4	5	6	7	8	9	10
11	12	13	14	15	16	17
18	19	20	21	DO NOT TAKE		
ANY TABLETS FOR SEVEN DAYS				1	2	3

Start New Supply of Tablets

the last dose was taken. An additional form of birth control should be used during this time or until the start of the next menstrual period. Call your doctor if there is a chance that you may be pregnant.

SPECIAL INSTRUCTIONS

☐ Contact your doctor at least once every 6 to 12 months so that you can be examined.

☐ In the summer, it is best to take the tablet at bedtime so that the highest levels of the drug are in your body during the night. This will help protect your skin from the sunlight which sometimes causes discolorations in women on this medicine.

☐ It is recommended that you do not smoke while you are taking this medicine because smoking may increase the incidence of heart attacks.

☐ Women who are breast-feeding should tell their doctor before taking this medicine.

329

☐ Contact your doctor if any of the following side effects occur:
- Severe or persistent headaches.
- Vomiting, dizziness, or fainting.
- Blurred vision or slurred speech.
- Pain in the calves of the legs or numbness in an arm or leg.
- Chest pain, shortness of breath, or coughing of blood.
- Lumps in the breast.
- Severe depression.
- A yellow color to the skin or eyes or dark-colored urine.
- Severe abdominal pain.
- Breakthrough vaginal bleeding which persists after the third month of therapy. During the first 3 months of therapy, breakthrough bleeding may be expected, but you should keep taking the tablets and it will usually clear up in a day or two.
- If you miss 2 consecutive menstrual periods or if you think you are pregnant.

☐ Always tell your pharmacist, dentist, and other doctors who are treating you that you are taking this medicine.

* * * * *

Combination Estrogen-Progestogen Therapy (28 Day)

United States: Brevicon-28 Day, Demulen-28, Lo/Ovral-28, Loestrin 1.5/30, Loestrin Fe 1/20, Modicon 28, Norinyl 1 + 80 28-Day, Norinyl 1 + 50 28-Day, Norlestrin-28 1/50, Norlestrin Fe 1/50, Norlestrin Fe 2.5/50, Ortho-Novum 1/80 28, Ortho-Novum 1/50 28, Ortho-Novum 1/35, Ovcon-35, Ovcon-50, Ovral-28, Ovulen-28

Canada: Anoryol, Brevicon-28, Demulen, Loestrin 1.5/30, Logest 1.5/30, Logest 1/50, Min-Ovral-28, Modicon, Norinyl 1 + 50, Norinyl 1 + 80, Norinyl-2, Norlestrin-28 1/50, Norlestrin-28 2.5/50, Novinol-28, Ortho-Novum 1/50, Ovral 28, Ovulen 1 mg., Ovulen 0.5 mg.

☐ This medicine is used as a birth control measure and to treat hormonal disorders. Some products are also used to treat certain types of menstrual problems.

HOW TO USE THIS MEDICINE

☐ Take this medicine at the same time each day, for example, after the evening meal or at bedtime. It is important to take this medicine regularly.

☐ If you are taking this drug for **birth control,** take the tablets as follows:
1. During the first month of taking this medicine it is important to use some additional form of birth control to help prevent pregnancy.

330

If Menstruation Starts On	Start Tablets On
Sunday	Thursday
Monday	Friday
Tuesday	Saturday
Wednesday	Sunday
Thursday	Monday
Friday	Tuesday
Saturday	Wednesday

Day 5 of first cycle: Take 1st Tablet

SUN	MON	TUES	WED	THURS	FRI	SAT
MENSTRUATION				1	2	3
4	5	6	7	8	9	10
11	12	13	14	15	16	17
18	19	20	21	22	23	24
25	26	27	28	1	2	3

Start New Supply of Tablets

2. The first day of menstruation is day **one.** Begin taking this medication on day *five* of your menstrual cycle.
3. Take one tablet every day for 28 days. Take it at the same time every day—preferably after dinner or at bedtime. Take the tablets in numerical sequence. Do **not** miss a day between tablets. The first 21 tablets you take will contain active ingredients and the last 7 tablets contain no active ingredients. They are simply included to make it more convenient for you. You will probably have your period while you are taking these last 7 tablets.
4. After finishing the package, start a new package of 28 tablets the next day. Do **not** miss a day between finishing one package and starting another. It is important to take this medicine regularly whether or not menstruation occurs as expected.
5. If you miss one daily dose, take it as soon as you remember and continue your regular schedule.
6. If you miss two daily doses, take 2 tablets daily for the next 2 days and then resume your normal schedule. It is advisable to use some addi-

tional form of birth control for the next 7 days to help avoid pregnancy.

7. If you miss 3 daily doses, stop taking the medicine and throw away the remainder of the package. Start a new package of tablets 7 days after the last dose was taken. An additional form of birth control should be used during this time or until the start of the next menstrual period. Call your doctor if there is a chance that you may be pregnant.

SPECIAL INSTRUCTIONS

☐ Contact your doctor at least once every 6 to 12 months so that you can be examined.

☐ In the summer, it is best to take the tablet at bedtime so that the highest levels of the drug are in your body during the night. This will help protect your skin from the sunlight which sometimes causes discolorations in women on this medicine.

☐ It is recommended that you do not smoke while you are taking this medicine because smoking may increase the incidence of heart attacks.

☐ Women who are breast-feeding should tell their doctor before taking this medicine.

☐ Contact your doctor if any of the following side effects occur:
  • Severe or persistent headaches.
  • Vomiting, dizziness, or fainting.
  • Blurred vision or slurred speech.
  • Pain in the calves of the legs or numbness in an arm or leg.
  • Chest pain, shortness of breath, or coughing of blood.
  • Lumps in the breast.
  • Severe depression.
  • A yellow color to the skin or eyes or dark-colored urine.
  • Severe abdominal pain.
  • Breakthrough vaginal bleeding which persists after the third month of therapy. During the first 3 months of therapy, breakthrough bleeding may be expected, but you should keep taking the tablets and it will usually clear up in a day or two.
  • If you miss 2 consecutive menstrual periods or if you think you are pregnant.

☐ Always tell your pharmacist, dentist, and other doctors who are treating you that you are taking this medicine.

*   *   *   *   *

Conjugated Estrogens (*Oral Estrogen*)

United States: Kestrin, Menotab, Ovest, Premarin, Sodestrin, Sodestrin H

Canada: C.E.S., Oestrilin, Premarin

Conjugated Estrogens-Methyltestosterone *(Oral Estrogen-Androgen)*

United States: Premarin with M.T.

Canada: Oestrilin with Methyltestosterone, Premarin with Methyltestosterone

☐ This medicine is a hormone. It has many uses and the reason it was prescribed depends on your condition. If you do not understand why you are taking it, check with your doctor.

HOW TO USE THIS MEDICINE

☐ The tablets may be taken after meals or with a snack if they upset your stomach.

SPECIAL INSTRUCTIONS

☐ Women who are pregnant, breast-feeding, or planning to become pregnant should tell their doctor before taking this medicine.

☐ It is recommended that you do not smoke while you are taking this medicine because smoking may increase the incidence of heart attacks.

☐ Diabetic patients should regularly check the sugar in their urine while they are taking this medicine.

☐ Contact your doctor if any of the following side effects occur:
- Severe or persistent headaches
- Vomiting, dizziness, or fainting
- Blurred vision or slurred speech
- Pain in the calves of the legs or numbness in an arm or leg
- Chest pain, shortness of breath, or coughing of blood
- Lumps in the breast
- Severe depression
- A yellow color to the skin or eyes or dark-colored urine
- Severe abdominal pain
- Vaginal bleeding

☐ Call your doctor if you develop hoarseness, deepening of the voice, increase in facial hair, or acne. (**United States:** Premarin with M.T.; **Canada:** Oestrilin with Methyltestosterone, Premarin with M.T.)

☐ Carry an identification card indicating that you are taking this medicine. Always tell your pharmacist, dentist, and other doctors who are treating you that you are taking this medicine.

* * * * *

Conjugated Estrogens *(Vaginal Estrogen)*

United States: Premarin

Canada: Premarin

Estrone
Canada: Oestrilin

☐   This medicine is used to treat vaginal conditions.

HOW TO USE THIS MEDICINE

☐   For VAGINAL CREAM
1. Remove the cap from the tube of medicine.
2. Screw the applicator to the tube.
3. Gently squeeze the tube of cream to force the prescribed amount into the applicator.
4. Unscrew the applicator from the tube of medicine. Apply a small amount of cream to the outside of the applicator.
5. Hold the applicator by the cylinder and gently insert into the vaginal canal as far as it will comfortably go.
6. While still holding the cylinder, press the plunger gently to deposit the medicine.
7. While keeping the plunger depressed, remove the applicator from the vaginal canal.
8. After *each* use, take the applicator apart and wash it thoroughly with warm water and soap and rinse thoroughly.
9. Reassemble the applicator.

☐   For VAGINAL CONES
1. Remove the wrapper from the suppository. Dip the suppository into water quickly just to moisten it.
2. Insert the wide end of the suppository into the vaginal canal.

SPECIAL INSTRUCTIONS

☐   If you forget to apply the medicine, apply it as soon as possible. However, if it is almost time for your next dose, do not apply the missed dose but continue with your regular schedule.

☐   Call your doctor if the condition for which this drug is being used persists or becomes worse or if it causes a constant irritation such as itching or burning that was not present before you started using this medicine. Also call your doctor if you develop breast tenderness or vaginal bleeding.

☐   For external use only. Do not swallow.

*   *   *   *   *

Conjugated Estrogens (*Oral Estrogen*)
United States: Premarin
Canada: Premarin

334

Estrone

Canada: Oestrilin

□ This medicine is a hormone and is used to help relieve the symptoms of menopause or is used when the ovaries have been removed.

HOW TO USE THIS MEDICINE

□ Take this medicine at the same time each day, for example, after the evening meal or at bedtime.

SPECIAL INSTRUCTIONS

□ Women who are pregnant, breast-feeding, or planning to become pregnant should tell their doctor before taking this medicine.

□ It is recommended that you do not smoke while you are taking this medicine because smoking may increase the incidence of heart attacks.

□ Contact your doctor if any of the following side effects occur:
- Severe or persistent headaches
- Vomiting, dizziness, or fainting
- Blurred vision or slurred speech
- Pain in the calves of the legs or numbness in an arm or leg
- Chest pain, shortness of breath, or coughing of blood
- Lumps in the breast
- Severe depression
- A yellow color to the skin or eyes or dark-colored urine
- Severe abdominal pain
- Vaginal bleeding

□ Call your doctor if you develop breast tenderness or develop menstrual bleeding when you stop using this medicine. (**Canada:** Oestrilin)

□ Carry an identification card indicating that you are taking this medicine. Always tell your pharmacist, dentist, and other doctors who are treating you that you are taking this medicine.

* * * * *

Ethacrynic Acid (Oral Diuretic-Saluretic)

United States: Edecrin
Canada: Edecrin

□ This medicine is used to help rid the body of excess water and to decrease swelling. It is also used to treat high blood pressure. It is commonly called a "water pill."

□ IMPORTANT: If you have ever had an allergic reaction to sulfa drugs or thiazide diuretics, tell your doctor or pharmacist before taking any of this medicine.

HOW TO USE THIS MEDICINE

☐ Take the medicine with food, meals, or milk.

☐ Try to take it at the same time(s) every day so that you have a constant level of the medicine in your body. Do not miss any doses. Otherwise, you cannot expect the drug to work as well.

☐ When you first start taking this medicine, you will probably urinate ("pass your water") more often and in larger amounts than usual. Therefore, if you are to take one dose every day, take it in the morning after breakfast. If you are to take more than one dose every day, take the last dose 6 hours before bedtime so that you will not have to get up during the night to go to the bathroom. This effect will usually lessen after you have taken the drug for awhile.

SPECIAL INSTRUCTIONS

☐ If you forget to take a dose, take it as soon as possible. However, if it is almost time for your next dose, do not take the missed dose. Instead, continue with your regular dosing schedule.

☐ Women who are pregnant, breast-feeding, or planning to become pregnant should tell their doctor before taking this medicine.

☐ This medicine normally causes your body to lose potassium. The body has warning signs to let you know if too much potassium is being lost. Call your doctor if you become unusually thirsty or if you develop leg cramps, unusual weakness, fatigue, vomiting, confusion, or irregular pulse.

☐ If your doctor recommends that you eat foods that are high in potassium, one or more of the foods listed in Appendix A should be eaten daily. All of these foods are rich in potassium. Your goal should be to take in 1000 to 2000 mg. of potassium (approximately 25.6 to 51 mEq) each day. The calorie content and sodium content are included for your convenience in meal planning. CHANGE YOUR DIET ONLY IF YOUR DOCTOR TELLS YOU TO.

☐ If this medicine causes dizziness, you should be careful going up and down stairs and you should not change positions too rapidly. Get out of bed slowly in the morning and dangle your feet over the edge of the bed for a few minutes before standing up. Sit down or lie down at the first sign of dizziness. Tell your doctor you have been dizzy. Be careful drinking alcoholic beverages while taking this medicine because they could make the dizziness worse. Do not drive a car or operate dangerous machinery or do jobs that require you to be alert if you are dizzy.

☐ In order to help prevent dizziness and fainting, your doctor may also recommend that you avoid strenuous exercises, standing for long periods of time (especially in hot weather), or hot showers or hot baths.

☐ This medicine may make some people more sensitive to sunlight and sunlamps. When you begin taking this medicine, try to avoid getting too much sun until you see how you are going to react. If you skin does become more sensitive to sunlight, tell your doctor and try to stay out of direct sun-

light. While in the sun, wear protective clothing and sunglasses. You may wish to ask your pharmacist about suitable sunscreen products. Check with your doctor if you become sunburned.

☐ Call your doctor immediately if you think you may be allergic to the medicine or if you develop a skin rash, hives, itching, swelling of the face, or difficulty in breathing. If you cannot reach your doctor, phone a hospital emergency department.

☐ Most people experience few or no side effects from their drugs. However, any medicine can sometimes cause unwanted effects. Call your doctor if you develop sharp stomach pain, diarrhea, chest pain, sharp joint pain, sore throat and fever, "ringing or buzzing" or a feeling of fullness in the ears, black stools, easy bruising or bleeding, a yellow color to the skin or eyes, or a sudden weight gain of 5 pounds or more.

* * * * *

Ethambutol HCl (*Oral Tuberculostatic Agent*)
United States: Myambutol
Canada: Myambutol

☐ This medicine is used to prevent or help the body overcome tuberculosis. Because tuberculosis (TB) heals very slowly, it may be necessary for you to take this medicine for a long time.

☐ It is very important that you keep taking this medicine for the full length of time that your doctor has prescribed. Do not stop taking the medicine earlier than your doctor has recommended in spite of the fact that you may feel better. DO NOT MISS ANY DOSES and DO NOT RUN OUT OF THIS MEDICINE.

☐ The most important thing you can do to protect others from catching your TB is to take your medicine regularly and to cover your coughs and sneezes with a double-ply tissue. This will reduce the spray of germs into the air. Covering your mouth with the bare hand does no good.

HOW TO USE THIS MEDICINE
☐ This medicine may be taken with food if it upsets your stomach.

SPECIAL INSTRUCTIONS
☐ If you forget to take a dose, take it as soon as you can remember and then continue with your regular schedule. However, if it is almost time for your next dose, omit the dose you forgot.

☐ Women who are pregnant, breast-feeding, or planning to become pregnant should tell their doctor before taking this medicine.

☐ Check with your doctor immediately if you develop blurred vision, eye pain, any loss of vision, or changes in your ability to see red or green objects. He may want you to have your eyes checked.

- Most people experience few or no side effects from their drugs. However, any medicine can sometimes cause unwanted effects. Call your doctor if you develop a skin rash, chills, pain or a burning feeling in the joints, or numbness or tingling in the hands or feet.

* * * * *

Ethchlorvynol (*Oral Hypnotic*)
United States: Placidyl
Canada: Placidyl

- This medicine is used to cause sleep.

HOW TO USE THIS MEDICINE
- It is best to take this medicine with food or a glass of milk to help prevent dizziness and stomach upset.

SPECIAL INSTRUCTIONS
- Sleeping medicines are only useful for a short time. If used for too long, they lose their effectiveness. Do not take any more of this medicine than your doctor has prescribed and do not stop taking this medicine suddenly without the approval of your doctor.

- Women who are pregnant, breast-feeding, or planning to become pregnant should tell their doctor before taking this medicine.

- In some people, this drug may cause dizziness or drowsiness. Do not drive a car or operate dangerous machinery or do jobs that require you to be alert until you know how you are going to react to this drug.

- If you become dizzy, you should be careful going up and down stairs. Sit or lie down at the first sign of dizziness.

- Do not drink alcoholic beverages while taking this drug without the approval of your doctor.

- It is important that you obtain the advice of your doctor or pharmacist before taking ANY other medicines including pain relievers, sleeping pills, tranquilizers or medicines for depression, or cough/cold or allergy medicines.

- Go to bed after you have taken this medicine. Do not smoke in bed after you have taken it.

- Call your doctor immediately if you think you may be allergic to the medicine or if you develop a skin rash, hives, itching, swelling of the face, or difficulty in breathing. If you cannot reach your doctor, phone a hospital emergency department.

- Most people experience few or no side effects from their drugs. However, any medicine can sometimes cause unwanted effects. Call your doctor if you develop slow heartbeats, bothersome sleepiness or laziness during the day,

338

dark-colored urine or a yellow color to the skin or eyes, easy bruising or bleeding, changes in eyesight, numbness or tingling in the hands or feet, or unusual nervousness.

* * * * *

Ethinamate (Oral Sedative)
United States: Valmid

☐ This medicine is used to cause sleep.

HOW TO USE THIS MEDICINE
☐ It is best to take this medicine with a glass of water 20 minutes before going to bed. Go to bed after you have taken this medicine. Do not smoke in bed after you have taken it.

SPECIAL INSTRUCTIONS
☐ Sleeping medicines are only useful for a short time. If used for too long, they losse their effectiveness. Do not take any more of this medicine than your doctor has prescribed and do not stop taking this medicine suddenly without the approval of your doctor.

☐ In some people, this drug may cause dizziness or drowsiness. Do not drive a car or operate dangerous machinery or do jobs that require you to be alert until you know how you are going to react to this drug.

☐ If you become dizzy, you should be careful going up and down stairs. Sit or lie down at the first sign of dizziness.

☐ Do not drink alcoholic beverages while taking this drug without the approval of your doctor.

☐ It is important that you obtain the advice of your doctor or pharmacist before taking ANY other medicines including pain relievers, sleeping pills, tranquilizers or medicines for depression, or cough/cold or allergy medicines.

☐ Call your doctor immediately if you think you may be allergic to the medicine or if you develop a skin rash, hives, itching, swelling of the face, or difficutly in breathing. If you cannot reach your doctor, phone a hospital emergency department.

☐ Most people experience few or no side effects from their drugs. However, any medicine can sometimes cause unwanted effects. Call your doctor if you develop slow heartbeats, easy bruising or bleeding, or unusual nervousness.

* * * * *

Ethinyl Estradiol (Oral Estrogen)
United States: Estinyl, Feminone
Canada: Estinyl

Ethinyl Estradiol-Methyltestosterone (*Oral Estrogen-Androgen*)
United States: Gynetone, Test-Estrin
Canada: Mepilin

☐ This medicine is a hormone and is used to help relieve the symptoms of menopause or is used if the ovaries have been removed.

HOW TO USE THIS MEDICINE
☐ The tablets may be taken after meals or with a snack if they upset your stomach.

SPECIAL INSTRUCTIONS
☐ Women who are pregnant, breast-feeding, or planning to become pregnant should tell their doctor before taking this medicine.

☐ It is recommended that you do not smoke while you are taking this medicine because smoking may increase the incidence of heart attacks.

☐ Diabetic patients should regularly check the sugar in their urine while they are taking this medicine.

☐ Contact your doctor if any of the following side effects occur:
  • Severe or persistent headaches
  • Vomiting, dizziness, or fainting
  • Blurred vision or slurred speech
  • Pain in the calves of the legs or numbness in an arm or leg
  • Chest pain, shortness of breath, or coughing of blood
  • Lumps in the breast
  • Severe depression
  • A yellow color to the skin or eyes or dark-colored urine
  • Severe abdominal pain
  • Vaginal bleeding

☐ Call your doctor if you develop hoarseness, deepening of the voice, increase in facial hair, or acne. (***United States:*** Gynetone; ***Canada:*** Mepilin)

☐ Carry an identification card indicating that you are taking this medicine. Always tell your pharmacist, dentist, and other doctors who are treating you that you are taking this medicine.

*   *   *   *   *

Ethionamide (*Oral Antituberculous Agent*)
United States: Trecator-SC

☐ This medicine is used to prevent or help the body overcome tuberculosis. Because tuberculosis (TB) heals very slowly, it may be necessary for you to take this medicine for a long time.

□ It is very important that you keep taking this medicine for the full length of time that your doctor has prescribed. Do not stop taking the medicine earlier than your doctor has recommended in spite of the fact that you may feel better. DO NOT MISS ANY DOSES and DO NOT RUN OUT OF THIS MEDICINE.

□ The most important thing you can do to protect others from catching your TB is to take your medicine regularly and to cover your coughs and sneezes with a double-ply tissue. This will reduce the spray of germs into the air. Covering your mouth with the bare hand does no good.

HOW TO USE THIS MEDICINE

□ This medicine may be taken with food if it upsets your stomach.

SPECIAL INSTRUCTIONS

□ If you forget to take a dose, take it as soon as you can remember and then continue with your regular schedule. However, if it is almost time for your next dose, do not take the dose you forgot.

□ It is recommended that you avoid the use of alcoholic beverages while you are taking this medicine.

□ Check with your doctor if you develop blurred vision or any changes in your eyesight. He may want you to have your eyes checked.

□ If this medicine causes dizziness, you should be careful going up and down stairs and you should not change positions too rapidly. Get out of bed slowly in the morning and dangle your feet over the edge of the bed for a few minutes before standing up. Sit down or lie down at the first sign of dizziness. Tell your doctor you have been dizzy. Do not drive a car or operate dangerous machinery if you are dizzy. Avoid hot showers and baths because they could make you dizzy.

□ Most people experience few or no side effects from their drugs. However, any medicine can sometimes cause unwanted effects. Call your doctor if you develop numbness or tingling in the hands or feet, a skin rash, sore throat or fever, vomiting, unusual tiredness or weakness, dark-colored urine, or a yellow color in the skin or eyes.

*   *   *   *   *

Ethoheptazine Citrate
United States: Zactane

□ This medicine is used to help relieve pain.

HOW TO USE THIS MEDICINE

□ Take this medicine with food or a glass of water.

SPECIAL INSTRUCTIONS

☐ It is important that you obtain the advice of your doctor or pharmacist before taking **any** other medicines including pain relievers, sleeping pills, tranquilizers, or medicines for depression, coughs, colds, or allergies.

☐ Do not drink alcoholic beverages while taking this drug without the approval of your doctor.

☐ If you feel nauseated when you first start taking the medicine, it may help if you lie down for a few minutes.

☐ In some people, this drug may cause dizziness or drowsiness. Do not drive a car or operate dangerous machinery or do jobs that require you to be alert until you know how you are going to react to this drug.

☐ If you become dizzy, you should be careful going up and down stairs. Sit or lie down at the first sign of dizziness.

☐ Most people experience few or no side effects from their drugs. However, any medicine can sometimes cause unwanted effects. Call your doctor if you develop a skin rash, headaches, blurred vision, fainting spells, or unusual nervousness.

*   *   *   *   *

Ethopropazine HCl (*Oral Antiparkinsonism Agent*)
United States: Parsidol
Canada: Parsitan

☐ This medicine is used to improve muscle control and relieve muscle spasm in Parkinson's disease and certain other medical conditions.

HOW TO USE THIS MEDICINE

☐ Take this medicine with food or immediately after meals to help prevent stomach upset, unless otherwise directed.

☐ If you forget to take a dose, take it as soon as possible. However, if your next dose is within 2 hours, do not take the missed dose but continue with your regular schedule.

SPECIAL INSTRUCTIONS

☐ If your mouth becomes dry, suck a hard sour candy (sugarless) or ice chips, or chew gum. It is especially important to brush your teeth regularly if you develop a dry mouth.

☐ In some people, this drug may cause dizziness, drowsiness, or blurred vision during the first 2 weeks of using this drug. This will usually go away as your body adjusts to this medicine. Do not drive a car or operate dangerous machinery or do jobs that require you to be alert until you know how you are going to react to this drug.

342

- [ ] If you become dizzy, you should be careful going up and down stairs. Sit or lie down at the first sign of dizziness.

- [ ] If your eyes become more sensitive to sunlight, it may help to wear sunglasses.

- [ ] Do not take antacids or diarrhea medicines within 1 hour of taking this medicine as it could make this medicine less effective.

- [ ] A desire to urinate ("pass your water") with an inability to do so is not an uncommon effect with this drug. Urinating each time before the drug is taken may help relieve this problem. Call your doctor if it continues.

- [ ] Do not drink alcoholic beverages while taking this drug without the approval of your doctor.

- [ ] It is important that you obtain the advice of your doctor or pharmacist before taking pain relievers, nonprescription drugs, sleeping pills, tranquilizers, or medicine for depression while you are taking this drug.

- [ ] You may become more sensitive to heat because your body may perspire less while you are taking this medicine. Be careful not to become overheated during exercise or in hot weather.

- [ ] Most people experience few or no side effects from their drugs. However, any medicine can sometimes cause unwanted effects. Call your doctor if you develop a skin rash, eye pain, dizziness or fainting, fast heartbeats, constipation, sore throat, fever or mouth sores, dark-colored urine, a yellow color to the skin or eyes, or unusual tiredness, or if you become confused.

* * * * *

Ethosuximide (Oral Anticonvulsant)
United States: Zarontin
Canada: Zarontin

- [ ] This medicine is used to help control convulsions and seizures. It is commonly used in the treatment of epilepsy.

- [ ] IMPORTANT: If you have ever had an allergic reaction to an anticonvulsant or seizure medicine, tell your doctor or pharmacist before you take any of this medicine.

HOW TO USE THIS MEDICINE
- [ ] Take this medicine with food if it upsets your stomach. Call your doctor if you continue to have stomach upset.

- [ ] It is very important that you take this medicine regularly and that you do not miss any doses. Try to take the medicine at the same time(s) every day. This is the only way that you can receive the full benefit of the medicine. If you forget to take this medicine, the amount of medicine in your blood will go down and you may have seizures.

SPECIAL INSTRUCTIONS

☐ If you forget to take a dose, take it as soon as possible. However, if it is almost time for your next dose, do not take the missed dose. Instead, continue with your regular dosing schedule. Do not double doses.

☐ Do not stop taking this medicine suddenly or change the amount you are taking without the approval of your doctor.

☐ Avoid swimming alone or taking part in high-risk sports in which a sudden seizure could cause injury.

☐ In some people, this drug may cause dizziness or drowsiness. Do not drive a car or operate dangerous machinery or do jobs that require you to be alert until you know how you are going to react to this drug. If you become dizzy, you should be careful going up and down stairs. Sit or lie down at the first sign of dizziness.

☐ If this medicine is for a child, do not let him (her) ride a bike or climb trees until you can determine how he (she) is going to react to the medicine. Children could hurt themselves if they participated in these activities if they were dizzy.

☐ Do not drink alcoholic beverages while taking this drug without the approval of your doctor.

☐ It is important that you obtain the advice of your doctor or pharmacist before taking pain relievers, nonprescription drugs, sleeping pills, tranquilizers, or medicines for depression while you are taking this drug.

☐ Women who are pregnant, breast-feeding, or planning to become pregnant should tell their doctor before taking this medicine.

☐ Most people experience few or no side effects from their drugs. However, any medicine can sometimes cause unwanted effects. Call your doctor if you develop a sore throat, fever or mouth sores, skin rash, swollen glands, easy bruising or bleeding, or if you become depressed.

☐ Do not go without this medicine between prescription refills. Call your pharmacist 2 or 3 days before you will run out of the medicine.

☐ Carry an identification card indicating that you are taking this medicine. Always tell your pharmacist, dentist, and other doctors who are treating you that you are taking this medicine,

* * * * *

Ethotoin (*Oral Anticonvulsant*)
United States: Peganone

☐ This medicine is used to help control convulsions and seizures. It is commonly used in the treatment of epilepsy.

344

☐ IMPORTANT: If you have ever had an allergic reaction to an anticonvulsant or seizure medicine, tell your doctor or pharmacist before you take any of this medicine.

HOW TO USE THIS MEDICINE

☐ Take this medicine with food if it upsets your stomach. Call your doctor if you continue to have stomach upset.

☐ It is very important that you take this medicine regularly and that you do not miss any doses. Try to take the medicine at the same time(s) every day. This is the only way that you can receive the full benefit of the medicine. If you forget to take this medicine, the amount of medicine in your blood will go down and you may have seizures.

SPECIAL INSTRUCTIONS

☐ If you forget to take a dose, take it as soon as possible. However, if it is almost time for your next dose, do not take the missed dose. Instead, continue with your regular dosing schedule. Do not double doses.

☐ Do not stop taking this medicine suddenly or change the amount you are taking without the approval of your doctor.

☐ Avoid swimming alone or taking part in high-risk sports in which a sudden seizure could cause injury.

☐ In some people, this drug may cause dizziness or drowsiness. Do not drive a car or operate dangerous machinery or do jobs that require you to be alert until you know how you are going to react to this drug. If you become dizzy, you should be careful going up and down stairs. Sit or lie down at the first sign of dizziness.

☐ If this medicine is for a child, do not let him (her) ride a bike or climb trees until you can determine how he (she) is going to react to the medicine. Children could hurt themselves if they participated in these activities if they were dizzy.

☐ Do not drink alcohol beverages while taking this drug without the approval of your doctor.

☐ It is important that you obtain the advice of your doctor or pharmacist before taking pain relievers, nonprescription drugs, sleeping pills, tranquilizers, or medicines for depression while you are taking this drug.

☐ This medicine may cause your urine to turn pink or red-brown in color. this is not unusual.

☐ Women who are pregnant, breast-feeding, or planning to become pregnant should tell their doctor before taking this medicine.

☐ Most people experience few or no side effects from their drugs. However, any medicine can sometimes cause unwanted effects. Call your doctor if you develop a sore throat, fever or mouth sores, skin rash, persistent headache, slurred speech, fast eye movements, joint pain, swollen glands, difficulty in walking, easy bruising or bleeding, or a yellow color to the skin or eyes.

□ Do not go without this medicine between prescription refills. Call your pharmacist 2 or 3 days before you will run out of the medicine.

□ Carry an identification card indicating that you are taking this medicine. Always tell your pharmacist, dentist, and other doctors who are treating you that you are taking this medicine,

*　*　*　*　*

Ethoxazene HCl (*Oral Urinary Analgesic*)
United States: Serenium

□ This medicine is used to help relieve pain associated with infections of the urinary tract.

HOW TO USE THIS MEDICINE
□ It is best to take this medicine with meals.

SPECIAL INSTRUCTIONS
□ If you forget to take a dose, take it as soon as you remember and then continue with your regular schedule.

□ This medicine may cause your urine to turn orange-red in color. This is not an unusual effect. Protect your undergarments while you are taking this medicine because your urine could cause staining.

□ Most people experience few or no side effects from their drugs. However, any medicine can sometimes cause unwanted effects. Call your doctor if you develop a skin rash or a yellow color to your skin or eyes.

□ If for some reason you cannot take all of the medicine, throw away the unused portion by flushing it down the toilet. Do not take or save old medicine.

*　*　*　*　*

Ethylestrenol (*Oral Anabolic Steroid*)
United States: Maxibolin
Canada: Maxibolin

□ This medicine is similar to a hormone which is normally produced by the body. This medicine has many uses and the reason it was prescribed depends upon your condition. If you do not understand why you are taking it, check with your doctor.

HOW TO USE THIS MEDICINE
□ Take this drug after meals or with a snack if it upsets your stomach.

□ It is very important that you take this drug as your doctor has prescribed.

346

- ☐ Women who are pregnant, breast-feeding, or planning to become pregnant should tell their doctor before taking this medicine.

- ☐ Diabetic patients should regularly check the sugar in the urine and report any abnormal results to their doctor.

- ☐ Carry an identification card indicating that you are taking this medicine. Always tell your pharmacist, dentist, and other doctors who are treating you that you are taking this medicine.

- ☐ Most people experience few or no side effects from their drugs. However, any medicine can sometimes cause unwanted effects. Call your doctor if you develop swelling of the hands, legs, or ankles; sore throat and fever; acne; unusual restlessness; dark-colored urine; or a yellow color to the skin or eyes. Women should call their doctor if they develop menstrual problems, hoarseness or a deepening of the voice, baldness, or increased facial hair.

* * * * *

Etidronate Disodium (*Oral Paget's Disease Therapy*)
United States: Didronel
Canada: Didronel

- ☐ This medicine is used to strengthen the bones in certain conditions.

HOW TO USE THIS MEDICINE
- ☐ Take this medicine on an empty stomach 2 hours before a meal. Take it with fruit juice or water and do not eat anything for 2 hours after you have taken it.

SPECIAL INSTRUCTIONS
- ☐ It is important that your diet contain an adequate amount of calcium and vitamin D. Follow any diet instructions that your doctor has recommended.

- ☐ Most people experience few or no side effects from their drugs. However, any medicine can sometimes cause unwanted effects. Call your doctor if you develop severe nausea, stomach cramps, or diarrhea (loose bowel movements).

- ☐ Do not stop taking this medicine without your doctor's approval and do not go without medicine between prescription refills. Call your pharmacist 2 or 3 days before you will run out of the medicine.

* * * * *

Fenfluramine HCl (*Oral Anorexiant*)
United States: Pondimin
Canada: Ponderal, Pondimin

- ☐ This medicine is used to help reduce the appetite in weight reduction programs. It can help you develop new eating habits and is only useful for a short time. Do not take any more of this medicine than your doctor has prescribed and do not stop taking this medicine suddenly without the approval of your doctor.

HOW TO USE THIS MEDICINE
☐ Take this medicine on an empty stomach 1 hour before a meal.

SPECIAL INSTRUCTIONS
☐ If you forget to take a dose, take it as soon as possible. However, if it is almost time for your next dose, do not take the missed dose. Instead, continue with your regular dosing schedule.

☐ It is very important that you follow the diet prescribed by your doctor.

☐ If your mouth becomes dry, suck a hard sour candy (sugarless) or ice chips, or chew gum. It is especially important to brush your teeth regularly if you develop a dry mouth.

☐ In some people, this drug may cause dizziness or drowsiness. Do not drive a car or operate dangerous machinery or do jobs that require you to be alert until you know how you are going to react to this drug. Therefore, you should be careful going up and down stairs. Sit or lie down at the first sign of dizziness.

☐ Do not drink alcoholic beverages while taking this drug without the approval of your doctor.

☐ It is important that you obtain the advice of your doctor or pharmacist before taking ANY other medicines including pain relievers, sleeping pills, tranquilizers or medicines for depression, cough/cold or allergy medicines, or other weight-reducing medicines.

☐ Most people experience few or no side effects from their drugs. However, any medicine can sometimes cause unwanted effects. Call your doctor if you develop a skin rash, diarrhea, sore throat, fever or mouth sores, unusual nervousness, difficulty in urinating ("passing your water"), palpitations, or nightmares, or if you become depressed or confused.

☐ Carry an identification card indicating that you are taking this medicine. Always tell your pharmacist, dentist, and other doctors who are treating you that you are taking this medicine,

*   *   *   *   *

Fenoprofen Calcium (*Oral Anti-inflammatory-Analgesic*)
United States: Nalfon
Canada: Nalfon

☐ This medicine is used to help relieve pain, redness, stiffness, and swelling in certain kinds of arthritis.

348

- IMPORTANT: If you have ever had an allergic reaction to aspirin or any other medicine for arthritis, tell your doctor or pharmacist before you take any of this medicine.

- It is very important that you take this medicine regularly and that you DO NOT MISS ANY DOSES. If you miss a dose, the level of the medicine in your body will fall and the drug will not be as effective. Only if the level of the drug is high enough can it decrease the inflammation and swelling in your joints and help prevent further damage.

- The full benefit of this medicine may not be noticed immediately, but may take from a few days to 3 weeks.

HOW TO USE THIS MEDICINE

- It is best to take this medicine on an empty stomach at least 1 hour before (or 2 hours after) food unless otherwise directed. If you develop stomach upset, take the medicine with food or immediately after meals. Call your doctor if you continue to have stomach upset.

SPECIAL INSTRUCTIONS

- In some people, this drug may cause dizziness or drowsiness. Do not drive a car or operate dangerous machinery or do jobs that require you to be alert until you know how you are going to react to this drug.

- If you become dizzy, you should be careful going up and down stairs. Sit or lie down at the first sign of dizziness.

- If you forget to take a dose, take it as soon as possible. However, if it is almost time for your next dose, do not take the missed dose. Instead, continue with your regular dosing schedule.

- While you are taking this medicine, do not drink alcoholic beverages or take aspirin without the permission of your doctor. It is usually safe to take acetaminophen for the occasional headache. Check with your pharmacist.

- Call your doctor immediately if you think you may be allergic to the medicine or if you develop a skin rash, hives, itching, swelling of the face, or difficulty in breathing. If you cannot reach your doctor, phone a hospital emergency department.

- Most people experience few or no side effects from their drugs. However, any medicine can sometimes cause unwanted effects. Call your doctor if you develop a skin rash, sore throat or fever, "ringing" or "buzzing" in the ears, fast heartbeats, swelling of the legs or ankles or sudden weight gain, blurred vision or changes in your eyesight, red or black stools, or severe stomach pain.

- Carry an identification card indicating that you are taking this medicine. Always tell your dentist, pharmacist, and other doctors who are treating you that you are taking this medicine.

*　*　*　*　*

Fenoterol HBr (*Inhalation Bronchodilator*)
Canada: Berotec Inhaler

☐ This medicine is used to help open the bronchioles (air passages in the lungs) to make breathing easier.

☐ IMPORTANT: If you have ever had an allergic reaction to any cough/cold, allergy, heart, or weight-reducing medicines, tell your doctor or pharmacist before you take any of this medicine.

HOW TO USE THIS MEDICINE
☐ INSTRUCTIONS FOR USE

1. If you are troubled with sputum, try to clear your chest as completely as possible before using this medicine. This will help the drug to reach the lungs and will allow more thorough clearing of mucus during subsequent coughing.
2. Hold the inhaler upright during use so that the mouthpiece is at the bottom.
3. Shake the canister.
4. Breathe out fully and place the lips tightly around the mouthpiece and tilt the head slightly back.

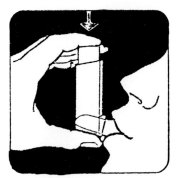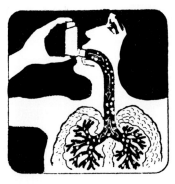

5. Start to breathe in slowly and press down firmly and fully on the valve at the middle of or early during inspiration ("breathing in") to release a "puff." Take the inhaler out of your mouth and close your mouth.
6. Hold your breath for a few seconds. Breathe out through your nose slowly.
7. If your doctor has prescribed a second dose, wait at least 30 seconds before shaking the container again and repeating this procedure.
8. Rinse your mouth with warm water after you have inhaled the medicine. This will help prevent your mouth and throat from becoming dry.
9. The mouthpiece of the inhaler should be kept clean and dry.
10. Failure to follow these instructions carefully can result in inadequate treatment.

SPECIAL INSTRUCTIONS

□ Do not change the dose of your regular asthma or bronchitis medicines except on the advice of your doctor.

□ Store the container in a cool place. Do not place the container in hot water or near radiators, stoves, or other sources of heat. Do not puncture, burn, or incinerate the container (even when it is empty).

□ Call your doctor if the medicine does not relieve your breathing problems, or if your sputum turns yellow or green in color.

□ Most people experience few or no side effects from their drugs. However, any medicine can sometimes cause unwanted effects. Call your doctor if you develop chest pain, headaches, sweating, palpitations, or dizziness.

* * * * *

Fenoterol HBr (Oral Bronchodilator)
Canada: Berotec

□ This medicine is used to help open the bronchioles (air passages in the lungs) to make breathing easier.

□ IMPORTANT: If you have ever had an allergic reaction to any cough/cold, allergy, heart, or weight-reducing medicines, tell your doctor or pharmacist before taking any of this medicine.

HOW TO USE THIS MEDICINE
□ This medicine may be taken with food or a glass of water.

SPECIAL INSTRUCTIONS
□ Do not change the dose of your regular asthma or bronchitis medicines except on the advice of your doctor.

□ Call your doctor if the medicine does not relieve your breathing problems, or if your sputum turns yellow or green in color.

□ Most people experience few or no side effects from their drugs. However, any medicine can sometimes cause unwanted effects. Call your doctor if you develop chest pain, headaches, sweating, palpitations, or dizziness.

* * * * *

Ferrous Fumarate (Oral Anemia Therapy)
United States: Feostat, Fumasorb, Fumerin, Ircon, Laud-Iron, Palm-iron, Toleron

Canada: Feroton, Fersamal, Hematon, Novofumar, Palafer

351

Ferrous Fumarate-Vitamin C

United States: C-Ron, C-Ron Forte, C-Ron Freckles, Cytoferin, Ferancee, Ferosorb-C, Ferrobid Duracap, Fumaral, Irolong, Iron W/C, Palmiron-C, Vitron-C

☐ This medicine is an iron supplement used to "build up" the blood and to treat some forms of anemia.

HOW TO USE THIS MEDICINE

☐ Do not take this medicine within 1 hour of bedtime. It is best to take this medicine with a glass of water on an empty stomach 1 hour before (or 2 hours after) eating food. However, if stomach upset occurs, it may be taken with a small amount of food. Call your doctor if the stomach upset continues.

☐ The following medicine has a special coating and must be swallowed whole. Do not crush, chew, or break it into pieces. (*United States:* Fumaral Spancap, Irolong Granucaps)

☐ The following tablets may be chewed before swallowed. (*United States:* C-Ron Freckles, Feostat, Ferancee, Ferosorb-C, Toleron, Vitron-C)

☐ Liquid medicines may cause staining of the teeth. In order to prevent this, mix the medicine with water or fruit juice and drink the medicine through a straw. Follow the dose with a drink of plain water or fruit juice. If stains do occur on the teeth, they may be removed by brushing the teeth with a small amount of sodium bicarbonate (baking soda) or hydrogen peroxide.

SPECIAL INSTRUCTIONS

☐ Do not take antacids within 1 hour of taking this medicine as they make this medicine less effective.

☐ This medicine may cause the stools to turn black or dark green in color. This is not unusual.

☐ Occasionally, this medicine may cause constipation or diarrhea. Call your doctor if this becomes troublesome.

☐ If your doctor recommends that you eat foods high in iron, good sources include brewer's yeast, eggs, dried beans, dried fruits, oysters, organ meats (liver, hearts, and kidneys), fish, poultry, cereals, green vegetables, and dark molasses.

☐ Store this medicine in a tightly capped container as it is sensitive to air and moisture.

☐ Keep this medicine out of the reach of children. Children may think it is candy and could become seriously ill if they swallowed several of the tablets or capsules.

*   *   *   *   *

Ferrous Gluconate (*Oral Anemia Therapy*)
United States: Fergon
Canada: Fergon, Fertinic, Novoferrogluc

Ferrous Gluconate-Polysorbate 20
United States: Simron
Canada: Sym-Fer

□ This medicine is an iron supplement used to "build up" the blood and to treat some forms of anemia.

HOW TO USE THIS MEDICINE

□ Do not take this medicine within 1 hour of bedtime. It is best to take this medicine with a glass of water on an empty stomach 1 hour before (or 2 hours after) eating food. However, if stomach upset occurs, it may be taken with a small amount of food. Call your doctor if the stomach upset continues.

□ Liquid medicines may cause staining of the teeth. In order to prevent this, mix the medicine with water or fruit juice and drink the medicine through a straw. Follow the dose with a drink of plain water or fruit juice. If stains do occur on the teeth, they may be removed by brushing the teeth with a small amount of sodium bicarbonate (baking soda) or hydrogen peroxide.

SPECIAL INSTRUCTIONS

□ Do not take antacids within 1 hour of taking this medicine as they make this medicine less effective.

□ This medicine may cause the stools to turn black or dark green in color. This is not unusual.

□ Occasionally, this medicine may cause constipation or diarrhea. Call your doctor if this becomes troublesome.

□ If your doctor recommends that you eat food high in iron, good sources include brewer's yeast, eggs, dried beans, dried fruits, oysters, organ meats (liver, hearts, and kidneys), fish, poultry, cereals, green vegetables, and dark molasses.

□ Store this medicine in a tightly capped container as it is sensitive to air and moisture.

□ Keep this medicine out of the reach of children. Children may think it is candy and could become seriously ill if they swallowed several of the tablets or capsules.

*   *   *   *   *

Ferrous Succinate (*Oral Anemia Therapy*)
Canada: Cerevon

☐ This medicine is an iron supplement used to "build up" the blood and to treat some forms of anemia.

HOW TO USE THIS MEDICINE

☐ Do not take this medicine within 1 hour of bedtime. It is best to take this medicine with a glass of water on an empty stomach 1 hour before (or 2 hours after) eating food. However, if stomach upset occurs, it may be taken with a small amount of food. Call your doctor if the stomach upset continues.

☐ If your doctor has prescribed the liquid medicine, drink a glass of water or fruit juice after taking the dose.

SPECIAL INSTRUCTIONS

☐ Do not take antacids within 1 hour of taking this medicine as they make this medicine less effective.

☐ This medicine may cause the stools to turn black or dark green in color. This is not unusual.

☐ Occasionally, this medicine may cause constipation or diarrhea. Call your doctor if this becomes troublesome.

☐ If your doctor recommends that you eat foods high in iron, good sources include brewer's yeast, eggs, dried beans, dried fruits, oysters, organ meats (liver, hearts, and kidneys), fish, poultry, cereals, green vegetables, and dark molasses.

☐ Store this medicine in a tightly capped container as it is sensitive to air and moisture.

☐ Keep this medicine out of the reach of children. Children may think it is candy and could become seriously ill if they swallowed several of the tablets or capsules.

*　*　*　*　*

Ferrous Sulfate (*Oral Anemia Therapy*)
United States: Feosol, Fer-In-Sol, Fero-Gradumet, Mol-Iron
Canada: Fer-In-Sol, Fero-Grad, Fesofor, Novoferrosulfa, Slow-Fe

☐ This medicine is an iron supplement used to "build up" the blood and to treat some forms of anemia.

HOW TO USE THIS MEDICINE

☐ Do not take this medicine within 1 hour of bedtime. It is best to take this medicine with a glass of water on an empty stomach 1 hour before (or 2 hours after) eating food. However, if stomach upset occurs, it may be taken with some food. Call your doctor if the stomach upset continues.

- [ ] The following medicine has a special coating and must be swallowed whole. Do not crush, chew, or break it into pieces. (**United States:** Feosol Spansules, Feo-Gradumets, Mol-Iron Chronosules; **Canada:** Fero-Grad, Fesofor Spansules, Novoferrosulfa, Slow-Fe)

- [ ] Children who are unable to swallow the capsule may be given the following medicine by opening the capsule and mixing the contents with a spoonful of soft food (applesauce or custard). (**Canada:** Fesofor)

- [ ] For DROPS (**United States:** Feosol Elixir, Fer-In-Sol; **Canada:** Fer-In-Sol)
  - The pharmacist will explain the correct method of measuring the medicine with the dropper.
  - Give the drops in water or fruit juice (**not milk**) and preferably between meals.
  - Follow the dose with a drink of plain water or fruit juice.

- [ ] Liquid medicine may cause staining of the teeth. In order to prevent this, mix the medicine with water or fruit juice and drink the medicine through a straw. Follow the dose with a drink of plain water or fruit juice. If stains do occur on the teeth, they may be removed by brushing the teeth with a small amount of sodium bicarbonate (baking soda) or hydrogen peroxide.

SPECIAL INSTRUCTIONS

- [ ] Do not take antacids within 1 hour of taking this medicine as they make this medicine less effective.

- [ ] This medicine may cause the stools to turn black or dark green in color. This is not unusual.

- [ ] Occasionally, this medicine may cause constipation or diarrhea. Call your doctor if this becomes troublesome.

- [ ] If your doctor recommends that you eat food high in iron, good sources include brewer's yeast, eggs, dried beans, dried fruits, oysters, organ meats (liver, hearts, and kidneys), fish, poultry, cereals, green vegetables, and dark molasses.

- [ ] Store this medicine in a tightly capped container as it is sensitive to air and moisture.

- [ ] Keep this medicine out of the reach of children. Children may think it is candy and could become seriously ill if they swallowed several of the tablets or capsules.

* * * * *

Flavoxate (*Oral Antispasmodic*)
United States: Urispas

- [ ] This medicine is used to help relieve muscle spasm of the urinary tract and difficult urination.

HOW TO USE THIS MEDICINE

☐ It is best to take this medicine on an empty stomach with a glass of water. However, if it upsets your stomach, it may be taken with a glass of milk or a snack. Call your doctor if the stomach upset continues.

SPECIAL INSTRUCTIONS

☐ If you forget to take a dose, take it as soon as possible. However, if it is almost time for your next dose, do not take the missed dose. Instead, continue with your regular dosing schedule.

☐ In some people, this drug may cause dizziness, drowsiness, or blurred vision. Do not drive a car or operate dangerous machinery or do jobs that require you to be alert until you know how you are going to react to this drug.

☐ If you become dizzy, you should be careful going up and down stairs.

☐ Sit or lie down at the first sign of dizziness.

☐ It is best to avoid alcoholic beverages while taking this drug unless you have the approval of your doctor.

☐ It is important that you obtain the advice of your doctor or pharmacist before taking ANY other medicines including pain relievers, sleeping pills, tranquilizers or medicines for depression, cough/cold or allergy medicines, or weight-reducing medicines.

☐ If your mouth becomes dry, suck a hard sour candy (sugarless) or ice chips, or chew gum. It is especially important to brush your teeth regularly if you develop a dry mouth.

☐ Most people experience few or no side effects from their drugs. However, any medicine can sometimes cause unwanted effects. Call your doctor if you develop eye pain or changes in vision, a skin rash, fast heartbeats or chest pain, sore throat, fever, or confusion.

*   *   *   *   *

Flucytosine (Oral Antifungal)
United States: Ancobon
Canada: Ancotil

☐ This medicine is used to treat certain types of fungal infections.

HOW TO USE THIS MEDICINE

☐ If you are taking more than 1 capsule for a dose, it may help to space them out over a period of 15 minutes in order to help prevent stomach upset.
☐ If you forget to take a dose, take it as soon as possible. However, if it is almost time for your next dose, do not take the missed dose. Instead, continue with your regular dosing schedule.

356

□ It is important to take **all** of this medicine plus any refills that your doctor told you to take. Do not stop taking it earlier than your doctor has recommended in spite of the fact that you may feel better. Otherwise, the infection may return.

□ Most people experience few or no side effects from their drugs. However, any medicine can sometimes cause unwanted effects. Call your doctor if you develop a skin rash, sore throat, fever or mouth sores, easy bruising or bleeding, unusual tiredness, or severe vomiting or diarrhea.

* * * * *

Fludrocortisone Acetate (*Oral Corticosteroid*)
United States: Florinef
Canada: Florinef

□ This medicine is similar to cortisone, which is a hormone normally produced by the body. This medicine is used in the treatment of certain conditions to help correct the hormone levels if the body is not producing enough of its own.

HOW TO USE THIS MEDICINE
□ Take this medicine with food or a glass of milk in order to help prevent stomach upset. Call your doctor if you develop stomach upset or stomach pain or heartburn (especially if it awakens you during the night). Do not try to treat this yourself.

□ If your doctor has prescribed only ONE dose of this medicine every day, it is best to take it before 9 A.M. or with breakfast.

□ If you forget to take a dose, take it as soon as possible. However, if it is almost time for your next dose, do not take the missed dose. Instead, continue with your regular dosing schedule.

SPECIAL INSTRUCTIONS
□ Women who are pregnant, breast-feeding, or planning to become pregnant should tell their doctor before taking this medicine.

□ It is best not to drink alcoholic beverages while you are taking this medicine because the combination can cause stomach problems.

□ Do not take any more of this medicine than your doctor has prescribed and do not stop taking this medicine suddenly without the approval of your doctor. It may be necessary for your doctor to slowly reduce your dose since your body becomes used to this medicine and it might be harmful if you suddenly did not receive this medicine.

□ Do not take aspirin or medicines containing aspirin without the approval of your doctor.

☐ While you are taking this medicine you may gain some weight. This could be due to an increase in your appetite or increased water in your system. Your doctor may prescribe a special diet to decrease the number of calories you eat and/or to lower the amount of sodium or increase the amount of potassium in your diet. Follow any diet that your doctor may order.

☐ You may find that you bruise more easily. Try to protect yourself from all injuries to prevent bruising.

☐ Diabetic patients should regularly check the sugar in their urine and report any unusual levels to their doctor.

☐ Carry an identification card indicating that you are taking this medicine. Always tell your pharmacist, dentist, and other doctors who are treating you that you are taking this medicine. If you have an acute infection, injury or operation, or dental surgery within 1 year of taking this medicine, it is important to tell your doctor.

☐ Most people experience few or no side effects from their drugs. However, any medicine can sometimes cause unwanted effects. Call your doctor if you develop swelling of the legs or ankles, sudden weight gain of 5 pounds or more, stomach pain, red or black stools, severe headaches, unusual weakness, a wound which does not heal, eye pain or blurred vision, or menstrual problems.

* * * * *

Flumethasone Pivalate (*Topical Anti-inflammatory*)
United States: Locorten
Canada: Locacorten

Flumethasone Pivalate-Clioquinol (*Topical Anti-inflammatory-Antifungal-Antibacterial*)
Canada: Locacorten-Vioform

☐ This medicine is used to help relieve the symptoms of redness, swelling, and itching of certain types of skin conditions.

☐ IMPORTANT: If you have ever had an allergic reaction to iodine medicine, tell your doctor or pharmacist before you use any of this drug. (**Canada:** Locacorten-Vioform)

HOW TO USE THIS MEDICINE
☐ For CREAM and OINTMENT
  • Each time you apply the medicine, wash your hands and gently cleanse the skin area well with water unless otherwise directed by your doctor.

Do not allow the skin to dry completely. Pat with a clean towel until slightly damp.

Apply a small amount of the drug to the affected area and spread lightly. Only the medicine that is actually touching the skin will work. A thick layer is not more effective than a thin layer. Do not bandage unless directed by your doctor.

☐ Keep this medicine away from the hair, nails, and clothing because it may cause staining. (**Canada:** Locacorten-Vioform)

☐ Do not use the drug more frequently or in larger quantities than prescribed by your doctor. Overuse of this medicine may cause you to absorb too much of the drug and increase the risk of side effects.

SPECIAL INSTRUCTIONS

☐ If you forget to apply the medicine, apply it as soon as possible. However, if it is almost time for your next dose, do not apply the missed dose but continue with your regular schedule.

☐ Do not use this medicine for any other skin problems without checking with your doctor.

☐ Do not apply cosmetics or lotions on top of the drug unless your doctor approves.

☐ Call your doctor if the condition for which this drug is being used persists or becomes worse or if you have a constant irritation such as itching or burning that was not present before you started using this medicine. Also call your doctor if you develop abnormal lines or thinning of the skin, especially under the arms or between the legs.

☐ Store in a cool place but do not freeze.

☐ For external use only. Do not swallow.

☐ Tell future doctors that you have used this medicine.

* * * * *

Flumethasone Pivalate-Clioquinol (*Ear Corticosteroid-Antiseptic*)

Canada: Locacorten-Vioform

☐ This medicine is used to help relieve the pain, redness, and itching of certain types of ear conditions.

☐ IMPORTANT: If you have ever had an allergic reaction to an iodine medicine, tell your doctor or pharmacist before you use any of this drug.

HOW TO USE THIS MEDICINE

☐ For EAR DROPS

INSTILLATION OF EAR DROPS

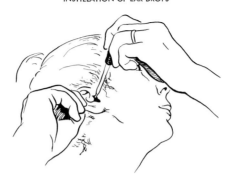

- Warm the ear drops to body temperature by holding the bottle in your hands for a few minutes. Do NOT heat the drops in hot water.
- The person administering the ear drops should wash his hands with soap and water.
- The ear drops must be kept clean. Do not touch the dropper against the ear or anything else.
- Tilt your head or lie on your side so that the ear to be treated is facing up.
- In ADULTS, hold the ear lobe up and back.
- In CHILDREN, hold the ear lobe down and back.
- Place the prescribed number of drops into the ear. Do not insert the dropper into the ear as it may cause injury.
- Remain in the same position for a short time (2 minutes) after you have administered the drops.
- Dry the ear lobe if there are any drops on it.

☐ If necessary, have someone else administer the ear drops for you.

☐ Do not use the ear drops if they have changed in color or have changed in any way since you purchased them.

☐ Keep the bottle tightly closed when not in use.

☐ Keep this medicine away from the hair, skin, nails or clothing because it may cause staining. (**Canada:** Locacorten-Vioform)

☐ Do not use the drug more frequently or in larger quantities than prescribed by your doctor.

SPECIAL INSTRUCTIONS

☐ This medicine should be used as long as your doctor has prescribed. Do not stop using it earlier than your doctor has recommended in spite of the fact that you may feel better.

☐ If you forget to use the medicine, use it as soon as possible. However, if it is almost time for your next dose, do not use the missed dose but continue with your regular schedule.

☐ Do not use this medicine at the same time as any other ear medicine without the approval of your doctor. Some medicines cannot be mixed.

☐ Call your doctor if the condition for which you are using this medicine persists or becomes worse or if the medicine causes itching or burning for more than a few minutes after instillation.

☐ For external use only. Do not swallow.

*   *   *   *   *

Flunisolide (*Nasal Allergic Rhinitis Therapy*)
Canada: Rhinalar

☐ This medicine is used in the treatment of hay fever to help relieve the symptoms of nasal stuffiness and "runny nose."

HOW TO USE THIS MEDICINE
☐ INSTRUCTIONS FOR USE
- Blow your nose gently.
- Sit upright with the head slightly back.
- Shake the canister.
- Insert the nozzle firmly into the nostril. The nozzle should be aimed upward and outward to obtain the best results. Close the other nostril by pressing your finger on the side of it.
- With the mouth closed, begin breathing in and press down on the valve of the container.
- Hold your breath for a few seconds.
- Repeat for the other nostril if necessary.

☐ It is very important that you use this nasal spray regularly as your doctor has prescribed. It will not relieve your symptoms immediately. It is NOT like ordinary nasal decongestants that you take only when you feel it is necessary.

SPECIAL INSTRUCTIONS
☐ If you forget to take a dose, take it as soon as possible. However, if it is almost time for your next dose, do not take the missed dose. Instead, continue with your regular dosing schedule.

☐ Do not take any more of this medicine than your doctor has prescribed and do not stop taking this medicine suddenly without the approval of your doctor. It may be necessary for your doctor to slowly reduce your dose since your body becomes used to this medicine and it might be harmful if you suddenly did not receive this medicine.

☐ Carry an identification card indicating that you are taking this medicine. Always tell your pharmacist, dentist, and other doctors who are treating you that you are taking this medicine.

- [ ] Store the container in a cool place. Do not place the container in hot water or near radiators, stoves, or other sources of heat. Do not puncture, burn, or incinerate the container (even after it is empty).

- [ ] Most people experience few or no side effects from their drugs. However, any medicine can sometimes cause unwanted effects. Call your doctor if you develop soreness in the mouth or throat, a bad taste in the mouth that will not go away, burning or soreness of the nose, or nosebleeds.

*   *   *   *   *

Fluocinolone Acetonide (*Topical Corticosteroid*)
United States: Fluonid, Synalar, Synemol
Canada: Dermalar, Synalar, Synamol, Viaderm-F.A.

Fluocinolone Acetonide-Clioquinol
Canada: Synaform

- [ ] This medicine is used to help relieve redness, itching, swelling and inflammation of certain types of skin conditions.

- [ ] IMPORTANT: If you have ever had an allergic reaction to iodine medicine, tell your doctor or pharmacist before you use any of this drug. (**Canada:** Synaform)

HOW TO USE THIS MEDICINE

- [ ] For CREAM and OINTMENT (**United States:** Fluonid, Synalar, Synemol Creams and Ointments; **Canada:** Synaform, Synalar Creams and Ointments)
  - Each time you apply the medicine, wash your hands and gently cleanse the skin area well with water unless otherwise directed by your doctor.
  - Do not allow the skin to dry completely. Pat with a clean towel until slightly damp.
  - Apply a small amount of the drug to the affected area and spread lightly. Only the medicine that is actually touching the skin will work. A thick layer is not more effective than a thin layer. Do not bandage unless directed by your doctor.

- [ ] For SOLUTIONS (**United States:** Fluonid, Synalar Solutions; **Canada:** Synalar, Synamol Solutions)
  - Each time you apply the medicine, wash your hands with water unless otherwise directed by your doctor. Do not allow the skin to dry completely. Pat with a clean towel until slightly damp.
  - Apply a small amount of the drug, drop by drop, to the affected area and spread lightly. Do not bandage unless otherwise directed by your doctor.
  - In hairy areas, the hair should be parted before applying in order to get the medicine right on the skin.

362

☐ For OCCLUSIVE DRESSINGS (*Canada:* Synalar, Synamol Occlusive Dressing)

- Cleanse the affected area well with soap and water before applying cream, unless otherwise directed by your doctor.
- Apply a very small amount to the area and gently rub it in until it disappears.
- Reapply the cream and leave a thin film over the affected area.
- Cover with a dressing as directed by your doctor.

☐ Avoid getting this medicine on hair or fabrics as it may stain them. (*Canada:* Synaform)

☐ Do not use the drug more frequently or in larger quantities than prescribed by your doctor.

SPECIAL INSTRUCTIONS

☐ If you forget to apply the medicine, apply it as soon as possible. However, if it is almost time for your next dose, do not apply the missed dose but continue with your regular schedule.

Do not use this medicine for any other skin problems without checking with your doctor.

☐ Do not apply cosmetics or lotions on top of the drug unless your doctor approves.

☐ Call your doctor if the condition for which this drug is being used persists or becomes worse or if you have a constant irritation such as itching or burning that was not present before you started using this medicine. Also call your doctor if you develop abnormal lines or thinning of the skin, especially under the arms or between the legs.

☐ Store in a cool place but do not freeze.

☐ For external use only. Do not swallow.

☐ Tell future doctors that you have used this medicine.

* * * * *

Fluocinonide (*Topical Corticosteroid*)
United States: Lidex, Topsyn Gel
Canada: Lidemol, Lidex, Topsyn Gel

☐ This medicine is used to help relieve redness, swelling, and itching of certain types of skin conditions.

HOW TO USE THIS MEDICINE

☐ For GEL

- Each time you apply the medicine, wash your hands and gently cleanse the skin area well with water unless otherwise directed by your doctor.

Do not allow the skin to dry completely. Pat with a clean towel until slightly damp.
  • Apply a small amount of the drug to the affected area and spread lightly. Only the medicine that is actually touching the skin will work. A thick layer is not more effective than a thin layer. Do not bandage unless directed by your doctor.

☐ Do not use the drug more frequently or in larger quantities than prescribed by your doctor. Overuse of this medicine may cause you to absorb too much of the drug and increase the risk of side effects.

☐ Keep the medicine away from the eyes, nose, and mouth.

SPECIAL INSTRUCTIONS

☐ If you forget to apply the medicine, apply it as soon as possible. However, if it is almost time for your next dose, do not apply the missed dose but continue with your regular schedule.

☐ Do not use this medicine for any other skin problems without checking with your doctor.

☐ Do not apply cosmetics or lotions on top of the drug unless your doctor approves.

☐ Call your doctor if the condition for which this drug is being used persists or becomes worse or if you have a constant irritation such as itching or burning that was not present before you started using this medicine. Also call your doctor if you develop abnormal lines or thinning of the skin, especially under the arms or between the legs.

☐ Store in a cool place but do not freeze.

☐ For external use only. Do not swallow.

☐ Tell future doctors that you have used this medicine.

*   *   *   *   *

Fluorometholone (*Ophthalmic Corticosteroid*)
United States: FML Liquifilm
Canada: FML Liquifilm

☐ This medicine is used to help relieve the pain, redness, and itching of certain types of eye conditions.

HOW TO USE THIS MEDICINE
☐ For EYE DROPS
  • The person administering the eye drops should wash his hands with soap and water.
  • The eye drops must be kept clean. Do not touch the dropper against the face or anything else.

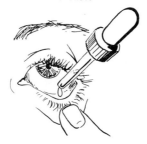

- Lie down or tilt your head backward and look at the ceiling.
- Shake the bottle well before using.
- Gently pull down the lower lid of your eye to form a pouch.
- Hold the dropper in your other hand and approach the eye from the side. Place the dropper as close to the eye as possible without touching it.
- Place the prescribed number of drops into the pouch of the eye.
- Close your eyes. Do not rub them.
- Apply gentle pressure for a minute with your fingers to the bridge of the nose (inside corner of the eye) to prevent the eye drops from being drained from the eye.
- Blot excess solution around the eye with a tissue.

☐ If necessary, have someone else administer the eye drops for you.

☐ Do not use the eye drops if they have changed in color or have changed in any way since you purchased them.

☐ Keep the eye drop bottle tightly closed when not in use.

☐ Do not use the drug more frequently or in larger quantities than prescribed by your doctor.

SPECIAL INSTRUCTIONS

☐ This medicine should be used as long as prescribed by your doctor. Do not stop using it earlier than your doctor has recommended in spite of the fact that your symptoms seem to have improved.

☐ If you forget to use the medicine, use it as soon as possible. However, if it is almost time for your next dose, do not use the missed dose but continue with your regular schedule.

☐ Do not use this medicine at the same time as any other eye medicine without the approval of your doctor. Some medicines cannot be mixed.

☐ Contact your doctor if the condition for which you are using this medicine does not improve or if the eye becomes irritated by it for more than a few minutes. Many eye medicines sting for a short time immediately after use.

☐ For external use only. Do not swallow.

*　　*　　*　　*　　*

Fluorometholone (*Topical Corticosteroid*)
United States: Oxylone

☐ This medicine is used to help relieve redness, swelling, and itching of certain types of skin conditions.

HOW TO USE THIS MEDICINE
☐ For CREAM
- Each time you apply the medicine, wash your hands and gently cleanse the skin area well with water unless otherwise directed by your doctor. Do not allow the skin to dry completely. Pat with a clean towel until slightly damp.
- Apply a small amount of the drug to the affected area and spread lightly. Only the medicine that is actually touching the skin will work. A thick layer is not more effective than a thin layer. Do not bandage unless directed by your doctor.

☐ Do not use the drug more frequently or in larger quantities than prescribed by your doctor. Overuse of this medicine may cause you to absorb too much of the drug and increase the risk of side effects.

☐ Keep the medicine away from the eyes, nose, and mouth.

SPECIAL INSTRUCTIONS
☐ If you forget to apply the medicine, apply it as soon as possible. However, if it is almost time for your next dose, do not apply the missed dose but continue with your regular schedule.

☐ Do not use this medicine for any other skin problems without checking with your doctor.

☐ Do not apply cosmetics or lotions on top of the drug unless your doctor approves.

☐ Call your doctor if the condition for which this drug is being used persists or becomes worse or if you have a constant irritation such as itching or burning that was not present before you started using this medicine. Also call your doctor if you develop abnormal lines or thinning of the skin, especially under the arms or between the legs.

☐ Store in a cool place but do not freeze.

☐ For external use only. Do not swallow.

☐ Tell future doctors that you have used this medicine.

* * * * *

Fluorouracil (*Topical Antineoplastic*)
United States: Efudex, Fluoroplex
Canada: Efudex, Fluoroplex

☐ This medicine is used in certain types of skin conditions to help slow the rate of growth of some of the skin cells.

HOW TO USE THIS MEDICINE

☐ For CREAM and SOLUTION

- Each time you apply the medicine, wash your hands and gently cleanse the skin area well with water unless otherwise directed by your doctor. Do not allow the skin to dry completely. Pat with a clean towel until almost dry.
- Apply a small amount of the drug to the affected area and spread lightly. Only the medicine that is actually touching the skin will work. A thick layer is not more effective than a thin layer. Do not bandage unless directed by your doctor.

☐ It is best to apply this medicine with a cotton-tipped applicator (Q-Tip) or to put on a plastic glove. If you do decide to apply it with your fingers, WASH YOUR HANDS IMMEDIATELY AFTERWARDS.

☐ Be very careful when using this medicine and keep it away from the eyes, nose, or mouth. If you should get some medicine in these areas, wash it off immediately.

☐ Do not use the drug more frequently or in larger quantities than prescribed by your doctor.

SPECIAL INSTRUCTIONS

☐ It is important to keep your doctor appointments so that your progress can be monitored.

☐ If you forget to apply the medicine, apply it as soon as possible. However, if it is almost time for your next dose, do not apply the missed dose but continue with your regular schedule.

☐ While using this medicine and for 1 to 2 months after you have stopped using it, you may be more sensitive to sunlight. Do not use sunlamps and wear protective clothing. Check with your doctor if you get a sunburn.

☐ You will probably notice that after you have used this medicine for 1 to 2 weeks, the treated area will become red and may peel. This is expected and you should continue using the medicine unless directed otherwise.

☐ Sometimes a pink smooth scar will form over the treated area. The scar usually fades after 1 to 2 months. Call your doctor if you have any questions.

☐ Call your doctor if you develop redness and swelling of untreated skin, a sore throat, or fever.

☐ For external use only. Do not swallow.

* * * * *

Fluoxymesterone (*Oral Anabolic Steroid*)
United States: Halotestin, Ora-Testryl
Canada: Halotestin, Oratestin

☐ This medicine is similar to a hormone which is normally produced by the body. This medicine has many uses and the reason it was prescribed depends upon your condition. If you do not understand why you are taking it, check with your doctor.

HOW TO USE THIS MEDICINE
☐ Take the drug after meals or with a snack if it upsets your stomach.

☐ It is very important that you take this drug as your doctor has prescribed.

SPECIAL INSTRUCTIONS
☐ Women who are pregnant, breast-feeding, or planning to become pregnant should tell their doctor before taking this medicine.

☐ Diabetic patients should regularly check the sugar in the urine and report any abnormal results to their doctor.

☐ Carry an identification card indicating that you are taking this medicine. Always tell your pharmacist, dentist, and other doctors who are treating you that you are taking this medicine.

☐ Most people experience few or no side effects from their drugs. However, any medicine can sometimes cause unwanted effects. Call your doctor if you develop swelling of the hands, legs, or ankles; sore throat and fever; acne; unusual restlessness; dark-colored urine; or a yellow color to the skin or eyes. Women should call their doctor if they develop menstrual problems, hoarseness or a deepening of the voice, baldness, or increased facial hair.

* * * * *

Fluphenazine HCl (*Oral Antipsychotic-Antianxiety*)
United States: Permitil, Prolixin
Canada: Moditen

☐ This medicine is used to help treat certain types of mental and emotional problems. Check with your doctor if you do not fully understand why you are taking it.

☐ IMPORTANT: If you have ever had an allergic reaction to a phenothiazine medicine, tell your doctor or pharmacist before you take any of this medicine.

HOW TO USE THIS MEDICINE
☐ This medicine may be taken with food or a full glass of water.

368

- ☐ If a dropper or a dispensing spoon is used to measure the dose and you do not fully understand how to use it, check with your pharmacist. (**United States:** Permitil Drops and Permitil Elixir)

- ☐ These tablets must be swallowed whole. Do not crush, chew, or break them into pieces. (**United States:** Permitil Chronotabs)

- ☐ Store the liquid medicine in a cool dark place and do not get the liquid on your skin or clothing. (**United States:** Permitil, Prolixin; **Canada:** Moditen)

- ☐ Do not take this medicine at the same time as antacids or diarrhea medicine. Try to space them at least 1 hour apart.

- ☐ The effect of the medicine may not be noticed immediately but may take from 2 to 4 weeks. Be patient. Take the medicine regularly and try not to miss any doses.

- ☐ Do not stop taking this medicine suddenly without the approval of your doctor.

SPECIAL INSTRUCTIONS

- ☐ If you forget to take a dose, take it as soon as possible. However, if it is almost time for your next dose, do not take the missed dose. Instead, continue with your regular dosing schedule.

- ☐ Any medicine has a few unwanted side effects. Because this medicine takes a few weeks to work, the side effects show the doctor that the drug is being absorbed. Many of these side effects will go away as your body adjusts to the medicine.

- ☐ Women who are pregnant, breast-feeding, or planning to become pregnant should tell their doctor before taking this medicine.

- ☐ In some people, this drug may cause dizziness or drowsiness. Do not drive a car or operate dangerous machinery or do jobs that require you to be alert until you know how you are going to react to this drug.

- ☐ If this medicine causes dizziness, you should be careful going up and down stairs and you should not change positions too rapidly. Get out of bed slowly in the morning and dangle your feet over the edge of the bed for a few minutes before standing up. Sit down or lie down at the first sign of dizziness. Tell your doctor you have been dizzy. Avoid hot showers and baths because they could make you dizzy.

- ☐ Do not drink alcoholic beverages while taking this drug without the approval of your doctor.

- ☐ This medicine may make some people more sensitive to sunlight and sunlamps. When you begin taking this medicine, try to avoid getting too much sun until you see how you are going to react. If your skin does become more sensitive to sunlight, tell your doctor and try to stay out of direct sunlight. While in the sun, wear protective clothing and sunglasses. You may wish to ask your pharmacist about suitable sunscreen products. Check with your doctor if you become sunburned.

- [ ] If your mouth becomes dry, suck a hard sour candy (sugarless) or ice chips, or chew gum. It is especially important to brush your teeth regularly if you develop a dry mouth.

- [ ] It is important that you obtain the advice of your doctor or pharmacist before taking **any** other medicines including pain relievers, sleeping pills, other tranquilizers or medicines for depression, cough/cold or allergy medicines, weight-reducing medicines, or laxatives.

- [ ] This medicine may cause your urine to turn pink, red, or red-brown in color. This is not unusual.

- [ ] In hot weather or during exercise, be careful not to become overheated. You may be more sensitive to heat since this medicine may affect your body's ability to regulate temperature.

- [ ] If you become constipated, try increasing the amount of bulk in your diet (for example, bran and salads), exercising more often, or drinking more water. Call your doctor if the constipation continues.

- [ ] Call your doctor if you develop a sore throat, fever, mouth sores, skin rash, changes in eyesight, rapid heartrate, a yellow color in the eyes or skin, unusual weakness or unusual movements of the face, tongue, or hands, or difficulty in urinating ("passing your water"). Also call your doctor if you become restless or unable to sit still or sleep.

- [ ] Carry an identification card indicating that you are taking this medicine. Always tell your pharmacist, dentist, and other doctors who are treating you that you are taking this medicine.

* * * * *

Fluprednisolone (*Oral Corticosteroid*)
United States: Alphadrol

- [ ] This medicine is similar to cortisone, which is a hormone normally produced by the body. This medicine is used to help decrease inflammation and this then relieves pain, redness, and swelling. It is used in the treatment of certain kinds of arthritis, severe allergies, or skin conditions.

HOW TO USE THIS MEDICINE
- [ ] Take this medicine with food or a glass of milk in order to help prevent stomach upset. Call your doctor if you develop stomach upset or stomach pain or heartburn (especially if it awakens you during the night). Do not try to treat this yourself.

- [ ] If your doctor has prescribed only ONE dose of this medicine every day, it is best to take it before 9 A.M. or with breakfast.

- [ ] If you forget to take a dose, take it as soon as possible. However, if it is

370

almost time for your next dose, do not take the missed dose. Instead, continue with your regular dosing schedule.

SPECIAL INSTRUCTIONS

☐ Women who are pregnant, breast-feeding, or planning to become pregnant should tell their doctor before taking this medicine.

☐ It is best not to drink alcoholic beverages while you are taking this medicine because the combination can cause stomach problems.

☐ Do not take any more of this medicine than your doctor has prescribed and do not stop taking this medicine suddenly without the approval of your doctor. It may be necessary for your doctor to slowly reduce your dose since your body becomes used to this medicine and it might be harmful if you suddenly did not receive this medicine.

☐ Do not take aspirin or medicines containing aspirin without the approval of your doctor.

☐ While you are taking this medicine you may gain some weight. This could be due to an increase in your appetite or increased water in your system. Your doctor may prescribe a special diet to decrease the number of calories you eat and/or to lower the amount of sodium or increase the amount of potassium in your diet. Follow any diet that your doctor may order.

☐ You may find that you bruise more easily. Try to protect yourself from all injuries to prevent bruising.

☐ Diabetic patients should regularly check the sugar in their urine and report any unusual levels to their doctor.

☐ Carry an identification card indicating that you are taking this medicine. Always tell your pharmacist, dentist, and other doctors who are treating you that you are taking this medicine. If you have an acute infection, injury or operation, or dental surgery within 1 year of taking this medicine, it is important to tell your doctor.

☐ Most people experience few or no side effects from their drugs. However, any medicine can sometimes cause unwanted effects. Call your doctor if you develop stomach pain, sore throat, fever, swelling of the legs or ankles, a wound which does not heal, eye pain or blurred vision, frequent urination ("passing your water"), nightmares or depression, muscle cramps, red or black stools, puffing of the face, or menstrual problems.

*   *   *   *   *

Flurandrenolide (*Topical Anti-inflammatory*)
United States: Cordran
Canada: Drenison

371

Flurandrenolide-Clioquinol (*Topical Anti-inflammatory–Antifungal–Antibacterial*)
Canada: Dreniform

- ☐ This medicine is used to help relieve redness, swelling and itching, and inflammation of certain types of skin conditions.

- ☐ IMPORTANT: If you have ever had an allergic reaction to iodine medicine, tell your doctor or pharmacist before you use any of this drug. (**Canada:** Dreniform)

HOW TO USE THIS MEDICINE
- ☐ For CREAM, OINTMENT, and LOTION
  - Each time you apply the medicine, wash your hands and gently cleanse the skin area well with water unless otherwise directed by your doctor. Do not allow the skin to dry completely. Pat with a clean towel until slightly damp.
  - Apply a small amount of the drug to the affected area and spread lightly. Only the medicine that is actually touching the skin will work. A thick layer is not more effective than a thin layer. Do not bandage unless directed by your doctor.

- ☐ Shake the liquid preparation well before using. (**United States:** Cordran Lotion)

- ☐ The liquid preparation may cause a slight temporary stinging sensation after it is applied.

- ☐ Do not use the drug more frequently or in larger quantities than prescribed by your doctor. Overuse of this medicine may cause you to absorb too much of the drug and increase the risk of side effects.

- ☐ Keep the medicine away from the eyes, nose, and mouth.

- ☐ Keep this medicine away from the hair, nails, and clothing because it may cause staining. (**Canada:** Dreniform)

SPECIAL INSTRUCTIONS
- ☐ If you forget to apply the medicine, apply it as soon as possible. However, if it is almost time for your next dose, do not apply the missed dose but continue with your regular schedule.

- ☐ Do not use this medicine for any other skin problems without checking with your doctor.

- ☐ Do not apply cosmetics or lotions on top of the drug unless your doctor approves.

- ☐ Call your doctor if the condition for which this drug is being used persists or becomes worse or if you have a constant irritation such as itching or burning that was not present before you started using this medicine. Also call your doctor if you develop abnormal lines or thinning of the skin, especially under the arms or between the legs.

- ☐ Store in a cool place but do not freeze.
- ☐ For external use only. Do not swallow.
- ☐ Tell future doctors that you have used this medicine.

*   *   *   *   *

Flurazepam (*Oral Hypnotic*)
United States: Dalmane
Canada: Dalmane

- ☐ This medicine is used to cause sleep.
- ☐ IMPORTANT: If you have ever had an allergic reaction to a sleeping pill or tranquilizer, tell your doctor or pharmacist before you take any of this medicine.

HOW TO USE THIS MEDICINE
- ☐ This medicine may be taken with food or a full glass of water.
- ☐ It may take 2 or 3 nights before you will notice the full benefit of this medicine.

SPECIAL INSTRUCTIONS
- ☐ Sleeping medicines are only useful for a short time. If used for too long, they lose their effectiveness. Do not take any more of this medicine than your doctor has prescribed and do not stop taking this medicine suddenly without the approval of your doctor.
- ☐ Women who are pregnant, breast-feeding, or planning to become pregnant should tell their doctor before taking this medicine.
- ☐ In some people, this drug may cause dizziness or drowsiness. Do not drive a car or operate dangerous machinery or do jobs that require you to be alert until you know how you are going to react to this drug.
- ☐ If you become dizzy, you should be careful going up and down stairs. Sit or lie down at the first sign of dizziness.
- ☐ Do not drink alcoholic beverages while taking this drug without the approval of your doctor.
- ☐ It is important that you obtain the advice of your doctor or pharmacist before taking ANY other medicines including pain relievers, sleeping pills, tranquilizers or medicines for depression, cough/cold medicines, or allergy medicines.
- ☐ Call your doctor immediately if you think you may be allergic to the medicine or if you develop a skin rash, hives, itching, swelling of the face, or difficulty

in breathing. If you cannot reach your doctor, phone a hospital emergency department.

☐ Most people experience few or no side effects from their drugs. However, any medicine can sometimes cause unwanted effects. Call your doctor if you develop a sore throat, fever or mouth sores, fast heartbeats, bothersome sleepiness during the day, dark-colored urine or a yellow color to the skin or eyes, nightmares, or depression.

* * * * *

Folic Acid (*Oral Anemia Therapy*)
United States: Folic Acid
Canada: Folvite, Novofolacid

☐ This medicine is used to treat anemia.

☐ Do not take this medicine without the consent of your doctor.

* * * * *

Framycetin Sulfate (*Ophthalmic Antibiotic*)
Canada: Soframycin

☐ This medicine is an antibiotic used to treat certain types of eye infections.

☐ IMPORTANT: If you have ever had an allergic reaction to any antibiotic medicines, tell your doctor or pharmacist before you use any of this drug.

HOW TO USE THIS MEDICINE
☐ For EYE DROPS

INSTILLATION OF EYE DROPS

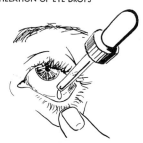

• The person administering the eye drops should wash his hands with soap and water.
• The eye drops must be kept clean. Do not touch the dropper against the face or anything else.
• Lie down or tilt your head backward and look at the ceiling.
• Gently pull down the lower lid of your eye to form a pouch.
• Hold the dropper in your other hand and approach the eye from the

374

side. Place the dropper as close to the eye as possible without touching it.
- Place the prescribed number of drops into the pouch of the eye.
- Close your eyes. Do not rub them.
- Apply gentle pressure for a minute with your fingers to the bridge of the nose (inside corner of the eye) to prevent the eye drops from being drained from the eye.
- Blot excess solution around the eye with a tissue.
- If necessary, have someone else administer the eye drops for you.
- Do not use the eye drops if they have changed in color or have changed in any way since you purchased them.
- Keep the eye drop bottle tightly closed when not in use.

☐ For EYE OINTMENT

INSTILLATION OF EYE OINTMENT

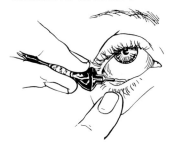

- The person administering the eye ointment should wash his hands with soap and water.
- The eye ointment must be kept clean. Do not touch the tube against the face or anything else.
- Lie down or tilt your head backward and look at the ceiling.
- Gently pull down the lower lid of your eye to form a pouch.
- Hold the tube in your other hand and place the tube as close as possible to the eye without touching it.
- Squeeze the prescribed amount of ointment (usually $\frac{1}{2}$ inch in adults) from the tube along the pouch.
- Close your eyes. Do not rub them.
- Wipe off any excess ointment around the eye with a tissue.
- Clean the tip of the ointment tube with a tissue.
- If necessary, have someone else administer the eye ointment for you.
- Keep the eye ointment tube tightly closed when not in use.
- Do not use the drug more frequently or in larger quantities than prescribed by your doctor.

SPECIAL INSTRUCTIONS

☐ Vision may be blurred for a few minutes after using the eye medicine. Do not drive a car or operate dangerous machinery or do jobs that require you to be alert until your vision has cleared.

☐ It is important to use **all** of this medicine, plus any refills that your doctor told you to use. Do not stop using it earlier than your doctor has recommended in spite of the fact that your symptoms seem to have improved. Otherwise, the infection may return.

☐ If you forget to use the medicine, use it as soon as possible. However, if it is almost time for your next dose, do not use the missed dose but continue with your regular schedule.

☐ Contact your doctor if the condition for which you are using this medicine does not improve or if the eye becomes irritated by it for more than a few minutes. Many eye medicines sting for a short time immediately after use.

☐ Do not use this medicine at the same time as any other eye medicine without the approval of your doctor. Some medicines cannot be mixed.

☐ For external use only. Do not swallow.

* * * * *

Framycetin Sulfate (*Topical Antibiotic*)
Canada: Soframycin

☐ This medicine is an antibiotic used to treat and help prevent skin infections.

HOW TO USE THIS MEDICINE
☐ For OINTMENT
- Each time you apply the medicine, wash your hands and gently cleanse the skin area well with water unless otherwise directed by your doctor. Do not allow the skin to dry completely. Pat with a clean towel until almost dry.
- Apply a small amount of the drug to the affected area and spread lightly. Only the medicine that is actually touching the skin will work. A thick layer is not more effective than a thin layer. Do not bandage unless directed by your doctor.

☐ Do not use the drug more frequently or in larger quantities than prescribed by your doctor.

SPECIAL INSTRUCTIONS
☐ It is important to use **all** of this medicine, plus any refills that your doctor told you to use. Do not stop using it earlier than your doctor has recommended in spite of the fact that your symptoms seem to have improved. Otherwise, the infection may return.

☐ If you forget to apply the medicine, apply it as soon as possible. However, if it is almost time for your next dose, do not apply the missed dose but continue with your regular schedule.

☐ Do not apply cosmetics or lotions on top of the drug unless your doctor approves.

376

- [ ] Keep this preparation away from the eyes. If you should accidentally get some in your eyes, wash it away with water immediately.
- [ ] Call your doctor if the condition for which this drug is being used persists or becomes worse or if you develop a constant irritation such as itching or burning that was not present before you started using this medicine.
- [ ] For external use only. Do not swallow.

* * * * *

Furazolidone (Oral Antidiarrheal)
United States: Furoxone

- [ ] This medicine is used to treat diarrhea and certain types of infections.
- [ ] IMPORTANT: If you have ever had an allergic reaction to nitrofurantoin or nitrofurazone, tell your doctor or pharmacist before you take any of this medicine.

HOW TO USE THIS MEDICINE
- [ ] Take the medicine with a glass of water.
- [ ] For LIQUID MEDICINE
  - Shake the bottle well before using so that you can measure an accurate dose.

SPECIAL INSTRUCTIONS
- [ ] If you are on this medicine for longer than 5 days, avoid eating any of the following foods in order to avoid unpleasant side effects: broad beans, avocados, bananas, canned figs, raisins, licorice, chocolate, aged cheeses, pickled herring, chicken livers, yeast extracts and fermented products, soy sauce, meat tenderizers, beer, wine (especially Chianti), and excessive amounts of coffee, tea, or cola.
- [ ] Do not drink alcoholic beverages while you are taking this medicine and for at least 5 days after you have stopped taking it. Otherwise, you may experience unpleasant side effects.
- [ ] This medicine may cause your urine to turn brown in color. This is not an unusual effect.
- [ ] This medicine can interact with other prescription medicines. If you visit another doctor or your dentist, it is extremely important that you tell them that you are taking or have been taking this medicine before they prescribe any other drugs for you.
- [ ] It is recommended that you avoid self-medicating with other drugs, especially certain nasal sprays and cold and hay fever remedies, without first checking with your doctor or pharmacist.

- Most people experience few or no side effects from their drugs. However, any medicine can sometimes cause unwanted effects. Call your doctor if you develop nausea, vomiting, pounding headache, chest pain, or faintness, or if the diarrhea persists.

* * * * *

Furosemide (*Oral Diuretic*)
United States: Lasix
Canada: Furoside, Lasix, Neo-Renal, Novosemide, Uritol

- This medicine is used to help rid the body of excess water and to decrease swelling. It is also used to treat high blood pressure. It is commonly called a "water pill."

- IMPORTANT: If you have ever had an allergic reaction to sulfa drugs or thiazide diuretics, tell your doctor or pharmacist before taking any of this medicine.

HOW TO USE THIS MEDICINE
- Take the medicine with food, meals, or milk.

- Try to take it at the same time(s) every day so that you have a constant level of the medicine in your body. Do not miss any doses. Otherwise, you cannot expect the drug to work as well.

- When you first start taking this medicine, you will probably urinate ("pass your water") more often and in larger amounts than usual. Therefore, if you are to take one dose every day, take it in the morning after breakfast. If you are to take more than one dose every day, take the last dose 6 hours before bedtime so that you will not have to get up during the night to go to the bathroom. This effect will usually lessen after you have taken the drug for awhile.

- If a dropper or special measuring spoon is used to measure a dose and you do not fully understand how to use it, check with your pharmacist. (**United States** and **Canada:** Lasix Solution)

SPECIAL INSTRUCTIONS
- Do not take large doses of aspirin or other salicylates without the approval of your doctor while you are taking this drug.

- If you forget to take a dose, take it as soon as possible. However, if it is almost time for your next dose, do not take the missed dose. Instead, continue with your regular dosing schedule.

- Women who are pregnant, breast-feeding, or planning to become pregnant should tell their doctor before taking this medicine.

- This medicine normally causes your body to lose potassium. The body has warning signs to let you know if too much potassium is being lost. Call your

378

doctor if you become unusually thirsty or if you develop leg cramps, unusual weakness, fatigue, vomiting, confusion, or irregular pulse.

☐ If your doctor recommends that you eat foods that are high in potassium, one or more of the foods listed in Appendix A should be eaten daily. All of these foods are rich in potassium. Your goal should be to take in 1000 to 2000 mg. of potassium (approximately 25.6 to 51 mEq) each day. The calorie content and sodium content are included for your convenience in meal planning. CHANGE YOUR DIET ONLY IF YOUR DOCTOR TELLS YOU TO.

☐ If this medicine causes dizziness, you should be careful going up and down stairs and you should not change positions too rapidly. Get out of bed slowly in the morning and dangle your feet over the edge of the bed for a few minutes before standing up. Sit down or lie down at the first sign of dizziness. Tell your doctor you have been dizzy. Be careful drinking alcoholic beverages while taking this medicine because they could make the dizziness worse. Do not drive a car or operate dangerous machinery or do jobs that require you to be alert if you are dizzy.

☐ In order to help prevent dizziness and fainting, your doctor may also recommend that you avoid strenuous exercises, standing for long periods of time (especially in hot weather), or hot showers or hot baths.

☐ This medicine may make some people more sensitive to sunlight and sunlamps. When you begin taking this medicine, try to avoid getting too much sun until you see how you are going to react. If your skin does become more sensitive to sunlight, tell your doctor and try to stay out of direct sunlight. While in the sun, wear protective clothing and sunglasses. You may wish to ask your pharmacist about suitable sunscreen products. Check with your doctor if you become sunburned.

☐ Call your doctor immediately if you think you may be allergic to the medicine or if you develop a skin rash, hives, itching, swelling of the face, or difficulty in breathing. If you cannot reach your doctor, phone a hospital emergency department.

☐ Most people experience few or no side effects from their drugs. However, any medicine can sometimes cause unwanted effects. Call your doctor if you develop a sore throat, fever, "ringing or buzzing" or a feeling of fullness in the ears, sharp stomach pain, chest pain, sharp joint pain, easy bruising or bleeding, a yellow color to the skin or eyes, or a sudden weight gain of 5 pounds or more.

* * * * *

Gamma Benzene Hexachloride (*See Lindane*)

* * * * *

379

Gentamicin Sulfate (*Eye/Ear Antibiotic*)

United States: Garamycin Ophthalmic Solution and Ointment

Canada: Garamycin Ophthalmic Solution and Ointment, Garamycin Otic

- ☐ This medicine is an antibiotic used to treat certain types of eye and ear infections.

- ☐ IMPORTANT: If you have ever had an allergic reaction to gentamicin or any antibiotic medicine, tell your doctor or pharmacist before you use any of this drug.

HOW TO USE THIS MEDICINE

- ☐ For EYE OINTMENT

INSTALLATION OF EYE OINTMENT

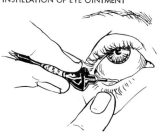

- The person administering the eye ointment should wash his hands with soap and water.
- The eye ointment must be kept clean. Do not touch the tube against the face or anything else.
- Lie down or tilt your head backward and look at the ceiling.
- Gently pull down the lower lid of your eye to form a pouch.
- Hold the tube in your other hand and place the tube as close as possible to the eye without touching it.
- Squeeze the prescribed amount of ointment (usually $\frac{1}{2}$ inch in adults) from the tube along the pouch.
- Close your eyes. Do not rub them.
- Wipe off any excess ointment around the eye with a tissue.
- Clean the tip of the ointment tube with a tissue.
- If necessary, have someone else administer the eye ointment for you.
- Keep the eye ointment tube tightly closed when not in use.

- ☐ For EYE DROPS

INSTALLATION OF EYE DROPS

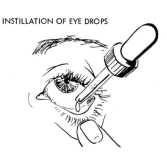

- The person administering the eye drops should wash his hands with soap and water.
- The eye drops must be kept clean. Do not touch the dropper against the face or anything else.
- Lie down or tilt your head backward and look at the ceiling.
- Gently pull down the lower lid of your eye to form a pouch.
- Hold the dropper in your other hand and approach the eye from the side. Place the dropper as close to the eye as possible without touching it.
- Place the prescribed number of drops into the pouch of the eye.
- Close your eyes. Do not rub them.
- Apply gentle pressure for a minute with your fingers to the bridge of the nose (inside corner of the eye) to prevent the eye drops from being drained from the eye.
- Blot excess solution around the eye with a tissue.
- If necessary, have someone else administer the eye drops for you.
- Do not use the eye drops if they have changed in color or have changed in any way since you purchased them.
- Keep the eye drop bottle tightly closed when not in use.

☐ For EAR DROPS

INSTILLATION OF EAR DROPS

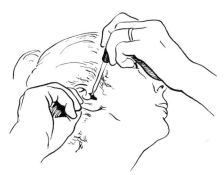

- Warm the ear drops to body temperature by holding the bottle in your hands for a few minutes. Do NOT heat the drops in hot water.
- The person administering the ear drops should wash his hands with soap and water.
- The ear drops must be kept clean. Do not touch the dropper against the ear or anything else.
- Tilt your head or lie on your side so that the ear to be treated is facing up.
- In ADULTS, hold the ear lobe up and back.
  In CHILDREN, hold the ear lobe down and back.
- Place the prescribed number of drops into the ear. Do not insert the dropper into the ear as it may cause injury.
- Remain in the same position for a short time (2 minutes) after you have administered the drops.
- Dry the ear lobe if there are any drops on it.

381

- If necessary, have someone else administer the ear drops for you.
- Do not use the ear drops if they have changed in color or have changed in any way since you purchased them.
- Keep the bottle tightly closed when not in use.

SPECIAL INSTRUCTIONS

☐ Vision may be blurred for a few minutes after using the eye medicine. Do not drive a car or operate dangerous machinery or do jobs that require you to be alert until your vision has cleared.

☐ It is important to use **all** of this medicine, plus any refills that your doctor told you to use. Do not stop using it earlier than your doctor has recommended in spite of the fact that your symptoms seem to have improved. Otherwise, the infection may return.

☐ If you forget to use the medicine, use it as soon as possible. However, if it is almost time for your next dose, do not use the missed dose but continue with your regular schedule.

☐ Do not use this medicine at the same time as any other eye or ear medicine without the approval of your doctor. Some medicines cannot be mixed.

☐ Call your doctor if the condition for which you are using this medicine persists or becomes worse or if the medicine causes itching or burning for more than a few minutes after instillation.

☐ For external use only. Do not swallow.

*　*　*　*　*

Gentamicin Sulfate (*Topical Antibiotic*)
United States: Garamycin
Canada: Garamycin

☐ This medicine is an antibiotic used to treat infections of the skin.

☐ IMPORTANT: If you have ever had an allergic reaction to gentamicin or any antibiotic medicine, tell your doctor or pharmacist before you use any of this drug.

HOW TO USE THIS MEDICINE

- Each time you apply the medicine, wash your hands and gently cleanse the skin area well with water unless otherwise directed by your doctor. Do not allow the skin to dry completely. Pat with a clean towel until almost dry.
- Apply a small amount of the drug to the affected area and spread lightly. Only the medicine that is actually touching the skin will work. A thick layer is not more effective than a thin layer. Do not bandage unless directed by your doctor.

☐ Do not use the drug more frequently or in larger quantities than prescribed by your doctor.

382

SPECIAL INSTRUCTIONS

☐ It is important to use **all** of this medicine, plus any refills that your doctor told you to use. Do not stop using it earlier than your doctor has recommended in spite of the fact that your symptoms seem to have improved. Otherwise, the infection may return.

☐ If you forget to apply the medicine, apply it as soon as possible. However, if it is almost time for your next dose, do not apply the missed dose but continue with your regular schedule.

☐ Do not apply cosmetics or lotions on top of the drug unless your doctor approves.

☐ Keep this preparation away from the eyes. If you should accidentally get some in your eyes, wash it away with water immediately.

☐ Call your doctor if the condition for which this drug is being used persists or becomes worse or if you develop a constant irritation such as itching or burning that was not present before you started using this medicine. Also call your doctor if you develop redness or swelling.

☐ Store in a cool place.

☐ For external use only. Do not swallow.

* * * * *

Gitalin (*See Digitoxin*)

* * * * *

Glucose Oxidase Reagent (*Glucosuria Diagnostic Aid*)
United States: Diastix
Canada: Diastix

☐ This preparation is used to test for the presence of glucose (sugar) in the urine.

☐ Testing procedure:
  1. Dip the end of the strip in the urine or briefly pass the strip through the urine stream.
  2. Tap the edge of the strip to remove excess urine.
  3. At exactly 30 seconds, compare the test side of the strip to the closest matching color block to find the concentration of glucose in the urine.

☐ For further information, refer to the package insert which accompanies this medicine.*

* * * * *

*Diastix (Package Insert), Ames Company Division, Miles Laboratories, Ltd., Rexdale, Ontario.

Glucose Oxidase Reagent (*Glucosuria Diagnostic Aid*)
United States: Clinistix
Canada: Clinistix

☐ This preparation is used to detect the presence of glucose (sugar) in the urine.

☐ The **Index Urine Test** is a test with Clinistix Reagent Strips on urine passed 2 hours after the main meal of the day, usually the evening meal. It is used as an indicator to help you and your doctor in the control of your condition.

☐ Directions for use:

Test urine 2 hours after your main meal:

- Moisten the red end of Clinistix by passing it once through the urine stream or by dipping it in a urine sample. Remove the strip immediately.
- Exactly 10 seconds after wetting, compare the test area with the matching color block on the bottle label.
- Record the test result on the report form:
  N (for negative) if no purple color develops
  L (for light) if color matches **light** block
  M (for medium) if color matches **medium** block
  D (for dark) if color matches **dark** block

☐   For further information, refer to the package insert which accompanies this medicine.*

* * * * *

Glutamic Acid (*Oral Gastric Acidifier*)
United States: Acidulin
Canada: Acidulin

☐ This medicine is used in certain conditions to supply the stomach with acid that it needs to digest food.

HOW TO USE THIS MEDICINE
☐ Take the medicine with meals or immediately after meals.

SPECIAL INSTRUCTIONS
☐ It is important that you follow the diet your doctor has prescribed.

☐ Most people experience few or no side effects from their drugs. However, any medicine can sometimes cause unwanted effects. Call your doctor if you

*Clinistix (Package Insert), Ames Company Division, Miles Laboratories, Ltd., Rexdale, Ontario.

384

develop stomach pain, red or black stools, headaches, deep breathing, nausea, vomiting, or diarrhea.

* * * * *

Glutethimide (*Oral Sedative Hypnotic*)
United States: Rolathimide
Canada: Doriden

☐ This medicine is used to cause sleep.

HOW TO USE THIS MEDICINE
☐ Take the medicine with food or a glass of water.

☐ If you are taking this medicine to help you sleep, take it at bedtime and no later than 4 hours before your usual time of arising. Otherwise, it will cause drowsiness during the day.

SPECIAL INSTRUCTIONS
☐ Sleeping medicines are only useful for a short time. If used for too long, they lose their effectiveness. Do not take any more of this medicine than your doctor has prescribed and do not stop taking this medicine suddenly without the approval of your doctor.

☐ Women who are pregnant, breast-feeding, or planning to become pregnant should tell their doctor before taking this medicine.

☐ In some people, this drug may cause dizziness or drowsiness. Do not drive a car or operate dangerous machinery or do jobs that require you to be alert until you know how you are going to react to this drug.

☐ If you become dizzy, you should be careful going up and down stairs. Sit or lie down at the first sign of dizziness.

☐ Do not drink alcoholic beverages while taking this drug without the approval of your doctor.

☐ It is important that you obtain the advice of your doctor or pharmacist before taking ANY other medicines including pain relievers, sleeping pills, tranquilizers or medicines for depression, cough/cold medicines, or allergy medicines.

☐ Call your doctor immediately if you think you may be allergic to the medicine or if you develop a skin rash, hives, itching, swelling of the face, or difficulty in breathing. If you cannot reach your doctor, phone a hospital emergency department.

☐ Most people experience few or no side effects from their drugs. However, any medicine can sometimes cause unwanted effects. Call your doctor if you

385

develop a sore throat, fever or mouth sores, slow heartbeats, bothersome sleepiness or laziness during the day, easy bruising or bleeding, unusual nervousness, stomach pain, or nightmares.

*   *   *   *   *

Glyburide (Oral Hypoglycemic)
Canada: Diabeta, Euglucon

☐ This medicine is used in the treatment of diabetes. When you have diabetes, the body either is not producing enough insulin or is not able to use what is produced. Insulin is needed for the body's proper use of food, especially sugar. In a diabetic patient, the sugar in the blood can build up to dangerous levels and is passed out in the urine. Your doctor has prescribed this medicine to help keep your blood sugar at nearly normal levels.

HOW TO USE THIS MEDICINE
☐ This medicine must ALWAYS be taken with food or immediately after a meal.

☐ It is very important that you take this medicine exactly as your doctor has prescribed. Do not miss any doses. Try to take this medicine at the same time every day. Do not take extra tablets without your doctor's approval.

☐ Do not take this medicine at bedtime unless your doctor tells you to.

☐ If you forget to take a dose, take it as soon as possible. However, if it is almost time for your next dose, do not take the missed dose. Instead, continue with your regular dosing schedule.

SPECIAL INSTRUCTIONS
☐ Women who are pregnant, breast-feeding, or planning to become pregnant should tell their doctor before taking this medicine.

☐ This medicine may make some people more sensitive to sunlight and sunlamps. When you begin taking this medicine try to avoid getting too much sun until you see how you are going to react. If your skin does become more sensitive to sunlight, tell your doctor and try to stay out of direct sunlight. While in the sun, wear protective clothing and sunglasses. You may wish to ask your pharmacist about suitable sunscreen products. Check with your doctor if you become sunburned.

☐ Most people experience few or no side effects from their drugs. However, any medicine can sometimes cause unwanted effects. Call your doctor if you develop a skin rash, sore throat, fever, mouth sores, dark-colored urine, a yellow color to the skin or eyes, easy bruising or bleeding, unusual tiredness, diarrhea, or light-colored stools.

GENERAL INSTRUCTIONS FOR DIABETIC PATIENTS
☐ Keep a regular schedule of daily activities. Eat, exercise, and take your insulin at approximately the same time every day.

386

☐ The diet that your doctor has prescribed has been carefully planned especially for you. It is to your advantage to follow it very closely.

☐ Test your urine regularly for sugar and if your doctor recommends, test it for acetone.

☐ Learn the signs of hypoglycemia (low blood sugar). When this happens, your urine sugar will be negative. Hypoglycemia may occur if you delay or skip a meal, exercise too much, become sick or emotionally upset, take too much insulin, drink alcohol, or take certain drugs. If you develop sweating, drowsiness, headache, unusual hunger, dizziness, nausea, nervousness, blurred vision, weakness, shaking, or trembling, eat or drink any of the following:

- 2 sugar cubes or 2 teaspoons of sugar in water
- 4 ounces orange juice
- 4 ounces regular ginger ale, cola beverages, or any other sweetened carbonated beverage. Do NOT use low-calorie or diet beverages
- 2 teaspoons honey or corn syrup
- 4 Lifesaver candies

Artificial sweeteners are of no use. Call your doctor if any of the above items do not relieve your symptoms in about 15 minutes.

☐ Always carry sugar cubes or hard candy in case you have a hypoglycemic (low blood sugar) reaction.

☐ Before you purchase any nonprescription medicine (for example, cough and cold medicines), ask your pharmacist if the medicine is safe for diabetic patients to use. Some nonprescription medicines have very high sugar contents which could interfere with the control of your diabetes. Aspirin and medicines containing salicylates or vitamin C could affect your urine test results. Check with your pharmacist.

☐ Ask your doctor if it is safe for you to drink alcoholic beverages because the combination may cause low blood sugar as well as a pounding headache, flushing, upset stomach, dizziness, or sweating.

☐ Take special care of your feet.

- Wash your feet daily and dry them well.
- Check your feet daily for minor injuries. Bring these to the attention of your doctor immediately.
- Wear clean shoes and stockings and choose shoes that fit well.
- If you develop corns or calluses, soak your feet in lukewarm water for about 10 minutes. Then rub them off gently with a pumice stone. Never use a knife to cut corns or calluses on your feet. Do NOT use commercial corn removers or commercial arch supports.
- Soften dry skin by rubbing with oil or lotion.
- Trim your toenails straight across with a file or nail cutter. Do not cut your own toenails if your eyesight is poor.
- Do not wear garters or socks with tight elastic tops. Do NOT sit with your knees crossed.
- Do not warm your feet with a hot water bottle or a heating pad. Use

loose bed socks instead. If your feet are cold under normal conditions, tell your doctor. Your circulation may be poor and your doctor can offer advice.

- Call your doctor if you injure your toes or feet. Cuts and scratches in the diabetic person can become infected easily and take longer to heal. Do not apply iodine or strong antiseptics to the feet at any time.

☐ Call your doctor immediately if you develop any of the following symptoms of hyperglycemia (high blood sugar): high urine sugar, acetone in urine, drowsiness, hunger, unusual thirst, fast breathing, nausea, confusion, a flushed dry skin, increase in urination (''passing your water''), or a fruity odor to the breath. These symptoms may occur if you take too little insulin, miss a dose, overeat, or if you have a fever or infection.

☐ Call your doctor if you become sick and have a fever, an infection, nausea, or vomiting.

☐ Carry an identification card or wear a bracelet indicating that you have diabetes and that you are taking this medicine. Always tell your pharmacist, dentist, and other doctors who are treating you that you are taking this medicine,

*   *   *   *   *

Glycopyrrolate (Oral Anticholinergic)
United States: Robinul, Robinul Forte
Canada: Robinul, Robinul Forte

☐ This medicine is used to help relax muscles of the stomach and bowels and to decrease the amount of acid formed in the stomach.

☐ IMPORTANT: If you have ever had an allergic reaction to atropine or any other drug used to relax the stomach or bowels, tell your doctor or pharmacist before you take any of this medicine.

HOW TO USE THIS MEDICINE
☐ Take this medicine approximately 30 minutes before a meal unless otherwise directed.

☐ If you miss a dose of this medicine, do not take the missed dose and do not double the next dose.

SPECIAL INSTRUCTIONS
☐ If your mouth becomes dry, suck a hard sour candy (sugarless) or ice chips, or chew gum. It is especially important to brush your teeth regularly if you develop a dry mouth.

☐ In some people, this drug may cause dizziness or drowsiness. Do not drive a car or operate dangerous machinery or do jobs that require you to be alert until you know how you are going to react to this drug.

- ☐ If you become dizzy, you should be careful going up and down stairs. Sit or lie down at the first sign of dizziness. Tell your doctor you have been dizzy.

- ☐ A desire to urinate ("passing your water") with an inability to do so is not an uncommon effect with this drug. Urinating each time before taking the drug may help relieve this problem. Call your doctor if it continues.

- ☐ You may become more sensitive to heat because your body may perspire less while you are taking this drug. Be careful not to become overheated during exercise or in hot weather.

- ☐ Do not take antacids within 1 hour of taking this medicine as they could make this medicine less effective.

- ☐ If you become constipated, try increasing the amount of bulk in your diet (for example, bran and salads), exercising more often, or drinking more water. Call your doctor if the constipation continues.

- ☐ If your eyes become more sensitive to sunlight, it may help to wear sunglasses.

- ☐ Most people experience few or no side effects from their drugs. However, any medicine can sometimes cause unwanted effects. Call your doctor if you develop a skin rash, diarrhea, unusual restlessness, flushing, or eye pain.

* * * * *

Gold Salts (*See Sodium Aurothiomalate*)

* * * * *

Griseofulvin (*Oral Antifungal-Antibiotic*)
United States: Fulvicin U/F, Grisactin, Grifulvin V, Grisowen
Canada: Fulvicin-U/F, Grisovin-FP

- ☐ This medicine is used to treat certain types of fungal infections.

HOW TO USE THIS MEDICINE
- ☐ Shake the liquid preparation well before using. (**United States:** Grivulfin V Suspension)

- ☐ This medicine should be taken with food in order to help prevent headache.

SPECIAL INSTRUCTIONS
- ☐ IMPORTANT: If you have ever had an allergic reaction to a penicillin medicine, tell your doctor or pharmacist before you use any of this drug.

- ☐ Women who are pregnant, breast-feeding, or planning to become pregnant should tell their doctor before taking this medicine.

- ☐ It is important to take **all** of this medicine plus any refills that your doctor told you to take. Do not stop taking it earlier than your doctor has recommended in spite of the fact that you may feel better. Otherwise, the infection may return.

☐ If you forget to take a dose, take it as soon as possible. However, if it is almost time for your next dose, do not take the missed dose. Instead, continue with your regular dosing schedule.

☐ If appropriate, your doctor will recommend a special diet to help increase the effect of the drug.

☐ Do not drink alcoholic beverages while taking this drug without the approval of your doctor.

☐ This medicine may make some people more sensitive to sunlight and sunlamps. When you begin taking this medicine, try to avoid getting too much sun until you see how you are going to react. If your skin does become more sensitive to sunlight, tell your doctor and try to stay out of direct sunlight. While in the sun, wear protective clothing and sunglasses. You may wish to ask your pharmacist about suitable sunscreen products. Check with your doctor if you become sunburned.

☐ In some people, this drug may cause dizziness or drowsiness. Do not drive a car or operate dangerous machinery or do jobs that require you to be alert until you know how you are going to react to this drug.

☐ Call your doctor immediately if you think you may be allergic to the medicine or if you develop a skin rash, hives, itching, swelling of the face, or difficulty in breathing. If you cannot reach your doctor, phone a hospital emergency department.

☐ Most people experience few or no side effects from their drugs. However, any medicine can sometimes cause unwanted effects. Call your doctor if you develop a skin rash, sore throat, fever or mouth sores, numbness or tingling in hands or feet, or a white coating on the tongue.

* * * * *

Guaifenesin (*Oral Expectorant*)

United States: Anti-Tuss, Glycotuss, Robitussin

Canada: Balminil Expectorant, Robitussin, Tussanca

☐ This medicine is used to help relieve dry irritating coughs.

☐ IMPORTANT: If you have ever had an allergic reaction to a guaifenesin or cough medicine, tell your doctor or pharmacist before you take any of this medicine.

HOW TO USE THIS MEDICINE

☐ Do not chew the tablets and do not let them dissolve in your mouth. Swallow them whole.

☐ Do not dilute the syrup. The soothing effect of the syrup will be enhanced if you do not drink liquids immediately after taking the medicine.

SPECIAL INSTRUCTIONS

- ☐ In some people, this drug may cause drowsiness. Do not drive a car or operate dangerous machinery or do jobs that require you to be alert until you know how you are going to react to this drug.

- ☐ Call your doctor if the cough lasts longer than 1 week or if you develop a fever, skin rash, or persistent headache.

- ☐ Do not use this medicine for more than 1 week without the advice of your doctor.

* * * * *

Guanethidine Sulfate (*Oral Antihypertensive*)
United States: Ismelin Sulfate
Canada: Ismelin

Guanethidine Sulfate-Hydrochlorothiazide
Canada: Ismelin-Esidrix

- ☐ This medicine is used to lower the blood pressure.

- ☐ Hypertension (high blood pressure) is a long-term condition and it will probably be necessary for you to take the drug for a long time in spite of the fact that you feel better. It is very important that you take this medicine as your doctor has directed and that you do not miss any doses. Otherwise, you cannot expect the drug to keep your blood pressure down.

HOW TO USE THIS MEDICINE

- ☐ Try to take the medicine at the same time(s) every day.

- ☐ Take this medicine with food or milk. If possible, avoid taking it at bedtime in order to avoid having to urinate ("pass your water") during the night. (**Canada:** Ismelin-Esidrix)

SPECIAL INSTRUCTIONS

- ☐ If you forget to take a dose, take it as soon as possible. However, if it is almost time for your next dose, do not take the missed dose. Instead, continue with your regular dosing schedule.

- ☐ Women who are pregnant, breast-feeding, or planning to become pregnant should tell their doctor before taking this medicine.

- ☐ This medicine may cause dizziness or fainting if you get up quickly from a lying or sitting position. Get up slowly, especially in the morning. It is advisable to dangle your feet over the edge of the bed in the morning for a few minutes before getting up. Sit or lie down at the first sign of dizziness. Tell you doctor you have been dizzy.

- ☐ Do not drive a car, operate dangerous machinery, or do jobs that require you to be alert if you are dizzy or have blurred vision.

- [ ] In order to help prevent dizziness and fainting, it is also recommended that you avoid strenuous exercises and standing for long periods of time, especially if the weather is hot. Be careful of the amount of alcohol you drink and avoid hot showers and baths while taking this medicine.

- [ ] If your mouth becomes dry, suck a hard sour candy (sugarless) or ice chips, or chew gum. It is especially important to brush your teeth regularly if you develop a dry mouth.

- [ ] Follow any special diet your doctor may have ordered. He may want you to limit the amount of salt in your food.

- [ ] Some nonprescription drugs can aggravate your condition. Do not take any of the following without the approval of your doctor or pharmacist: cough, cold or sinus products; asthma or allergy products; or diet or weight-reducing medicines.

- [ ] Most people experience few or no side effects from their drugs. However, any medicine can sometimes cause unwanted effects. Call your doctor if you develop severe diarrhea (loose bowel movements), swelling of the legs or ankles, sudden weight gain of 5 pounds or more, chest pains, or difficulty in breathing.

- [ ] Call your doctor if you develop muscle weakness or sharp joint pain. (**Canada:** Ismelin-Esidrix)

- [ ] Carry an identification card indicating that you are taking this medicine. Always tell your pharmacist, dentist, and other doctors who are treating you that you are taking this medicine.

- [ ] Do not stop taking this medicine without your doctor's approval and do not go without medicine between prescription refills. Call your pharmacist 2 or 3 days before you will run out of the medicine.

* * * * *

Halcinonide (*Topical Corticosteroid*)
United States: Halog
Canada: Halog

- [ ] This medicine is used to help relieve redness, swelling and itching, and inflammation of certain types of skin conditions.

HOW TO USE THIS MEDICINE
- [ ] For CREAM, OINTMENT, and SOLUTION
    - Each time you apply the medicine, wash your hands and gently cleanse the skin area well with water unless otherwise directed by your doctor. Do not allow the skin to dry completely. Pat with a clean towel until slightly damp.

392

- Apply a small amount of the drug to the affected area and spread lightly. Only the medicine that is actually touching the skin will work. A thick layer is not more effective than a thin layer. Do not bandage unless directed by your doctor.

☐ The liquid preparation may cause a slight temporary stinging sensation after it is applied.

☐ Do not use the drug more frequently or in larger quantities than prescribed by your doctor. Overuse of this medicine may cause you to absorb too much of the drug and increase the risk of side effects.

☐ Keep the medicine away from the eyes, nose, and mouth.

SPECIAL INSTRUCTIONS

☐ If you forget to apply the medicine, apply it as soon as possible. However, if it is almost time for your next dose, do not apply the missed dose but continue with your regular schedule.

☐ Do not use this medicine for any other skin problems without checking with your doctor.

☐ Do not apply cosmetics or lotions on top of the drug unless your doctor approves.

☐ Call your doctor if the condition for which this drug is being used persists or becomes worse or if you have a constant irritation such as itching or burning that was not present before you started using this medicine. Also call your doctor if you develop abnormal lines or thinning of the skin, especially under the arms or between the legs.

☐ Store in a cool place but do not freeze.

☐ For external use only. Do not swallow.

☐ Tell future doctors that you have used this medicine.

*　*　*　*　*

Haloperidol (*Oral Antipsychotic-Antiemetic*)
United States: Haldol
Canada: Haldol

☐ This medicine has many uses and the reason it was prescribed depends upon your condition. Check with your doctor if you do not fully understand why you are taking it.

HOW TO USE THIS MEDICINE

☐ This medicine may be taken with food or a full glass of water.

393

☐ For LIQUID MEDICINE
- The liquid medicine may be taken in juices, milk, food, or water.
- If a dropper or a dispensing spoon is used to measure the dose and you do not fully understand how to use it, check with your pharmacist.
- Do not get the liquid on your skin or clothing.
- Store in a dark place.

SPECIAL INSTRUCTIONS

☐ The full benefit of the medicine may not be noticed immediately but may take a few weeks. Be patient. Take the medicine regularly and try not to miss any doses.

☐ If you forget to take a dose, take it as soon as possible. However, if your next dose is within 6 hours, do not take the missed dose but continue with your regular schedule.

☐ Do not stop taking this medicine suddenly without the approval of your doctor.

☐ If your mouth becomes dry, suck a hard sour candy (sugarless) or ice chips, or chew gum. It is especially important to brush your teeth regularly if you develop a dry mouth.

☐ Do not drink alcoholic beverages while taking this drug without the approval of your doctor.

☐ It is important that you obtain the advice of your doctor or pharmacist before taking ANY other medicines including pain relievers, sleeping pills, tranquilizers or medicines for depression, cough/cold medicines, allergy medicines, or weight-reducing medicines.

☐ In some people, this drug may cause drowsiness, especially after any increase in your dose. Do not drive a car or operate dangerous machinery or do jobs that require you to be alert until you know how you are going to react to this drug.

☐ If this medicine causes dizziness, you should be careful going up and down stairs and you should not change positions too rapidly. Get out of bed slowly in the morning and dangle your feet over the edge of the bed for a few minutes before standing up. Sit down or lie down at the first sign of dizziness. Tell your doctor you have been dizzy.

☐ Most people experience few or no side effects from their drugs. However, any medicine can sometimes cause unwanted effects. Call your doctor if you develop a sore throat; fever; mouth sores; skin rash; unusual tiredness; unusual movements of the face, tongue, or hands; stiffness of the arms or legs; or difficulty in urinating ("passing your water").

☐ Carry an identification card indicating that you are taking this medicine. Always tell your pharmacist, dentist, and other doctors who are treating you that you are taking this medicine.

*   *   *   *   *

394

Haloprogin (*Topical Antifungal-Antimonilial*)
United States: Halotex
Canada: Halotex

☐ This medicine is used to treat fungal infections of the skin.

HOW TO USE THIS MEDICINE

- Each time you apply the medicine, wash your hands and gently cleanse the skin area well with water unless otherwise directed by your doctor. Do not allow the skin to dry completely. Pat with a clean towel until almost dry.
- Apply a small amount of the drug to the affected area and spread lightly. Only the medicine that is actually touching the skin will work. A thick layer is not more effective than a thin layer. Do not bandage unless directed by your doctor.

☐ Do not use the drug more frequently or in larger quantities than prescribed by your doctor.

SPECIAL INSTRUCTIONS

☐ It is important to use **all** of this medicine, plus any refills that your doctor told you to use. Do not stop using it earlier than your doctor has recommended in spite of the fact that your symptoms seem to have improved. Otherwise, the infection may return.

☐ If you forget to apply the medicine, apply it as soon as possible. However, if it is almost time for your next dose, do not apply the missed dose but continue with your regular schedule.

☐ Do not apply cosmetics or lotions on top of the drug unless your doctor approves.

☐ Keep this preparation away from the eyes. If you should accidentally get some in your eyes, wash it away with water immediately.

☐ Call your doctor if the condition for which this drug is being used persists or becomes worse or if you develop a constant irritation such as itching or burning that was not present before you started taking this medicine.

☐ For external use only. Do not swallow.

* * * * *

Hema-Combistix (*Diagnostic Aid*)
United States: Hema-Combistix
Canada: Hema-Combistix

☐ This preparation is used to test for various chemicals in the urine.
☐ Testing procedure:
1. Moisten the test end of the strip in urine.
2. Touch the tip of the strip against the edge of the urine container to remove excess urine.

3. Compare the test areas with the color charts after waiting the correct amount of time:

   a. protein and pH—read immediately
   b. glucose   —wait 10 seconds
   c. blood   —wait 30 seconds

☐ For further information, refer to the package insert which accompanies this medicine.*

*   *   *   *   *

Heptabarbital (*Oral Sedative-Hypnotic*)
Canada: Medomin

☐ This medicine is used to cause sleep.

☐ IMPORTANT: If you have ever had an allergic reaction to a barbiturate medicine, tell your doctor or pharmacist before you take any of this medicine.

HOW TO USE THIS MEDICINE
☐ This medicine may be taken with food or a full glass of water.

SPECIAL INSTRUCTIONS
☐ Sleeping medicines are only useful for a short time. If used for too long, they lose their effectiveness. Do not take any more of this medicine than your doctor has prescribed and do not stop taking this medicine suddenly without the approval of your doctor.

☐ Women who are pregnant, breast-feeding, or planning to become pregnant should tell their doctor before taking this medicine.

☐ In some people, this drug may cause dizziness or drowsiness. Do not drive a car or operate dangerous machinery or do jobs that require you to be alert until you know how you are going to react to this drug.

☐ If you become dizzy, you should be careful going up and down stairs. Sit or lie down at the first sign of dizziness.

☐ Do not drink alcoholic beverages while taking this drug without the approval of your doctor.

☐ It is important that you obtain the advice of your doctor or pharmacist before taking ANY other medicines including pain relievers, sleeping pills, tranquilizers or medicines for depression, cough/cold or allergy medicines.

☐ Go to bed after you have taken the medicine. Do not smoke in bed after you have taken it.

*Hema-Combistix (Package Insert), Ames Company Division, Miles Laboratories, Ltd., Rexdale, Ontario.

- [ ] Do not store this medicine at the bedside and keep it out of the reach of children.

- [ ] Call your doctor immediately if you think you may be allergic to the medicine or if you develop a skin rash, hives, itching, swelling of the face, or difficulty in breathing. If you cannot reach your doctor, phone a hospital emergency department.

- [ ] Most people experience few or no side effects from their drugs. However, any medicine can sometimes cause unwanted effects. Call your doctor if you develop a sore throat, bothersome sleepiness or laziness during the day, nightmares, staggering walk, unusual nervousness, a yellow color to the skin or eyes, easy bruising or, slow heartbeats.

*　*　*　*　*

Hetacillin (Oral Antibiotic)
United States: Versapen, Versapen-K

- [ ] This medicine is an antibiotic used to treat certain types of infections.

- [ ] IMPORTANT: If you have ever had an allergic reaction to penicillin or any other antibiotic, tell your doctor or pharmacist before you take any of this medicine.

HOW TO USE THIS MEDICINE
- [ ] It is best to take this medicine on an empty stomach 1 hour before (or 2 hours after) meals or food unless otherwise directed by your doctor. Take it at the proper time even if you skip a meal.

- [ ] Take this medicine with a full glass of water.

- [ ] For LIQUID MEDICINE
    - If you were prescribed a SUSPENSION, shake the bottle well before using so that you can measure an accurate dose. Store the bottle of medicine in the refrigerator. (**United States** and **Canada:** Versapen Suspension)
    - If there is a discard date on the bottle, throw away any unused medicine after that date.
    - If a dropper is used to measure a dose and you do not fully understand how to use it, check with your pharmacist. (**United States:** Versapen Drops)

SPECIAL INSTRUCTIONS
- [ ] It is important to take **all** of this medicine plus any refills that your doctor told you to take. Do not stop taking this medicine earlier than your doctor has recommended in spite of the fact that you may feel better. Otherwise, the infection may return.

□ If you forget to take a dose, take it as soon as you remember and then continue with your regular schedule.

□ Women who are breast-feeding should tell their doctor before taking this medicine.

□ Most people experience few or no side effects from their drugs. However, any medicine can sometimes cause unwanted effects. Call your doctor if you develop a dark-colored tongue, yellow-green stools or, in women, a vaginal discharge that was not present before you started taking this medication.

□ This medicine sometimes causes diarrhea (loose bowel movements). Call your doctor if the diarrhea becomes severe or lasts for more than 2 days.

□ Call your doctor immediately if you think you may be allergic to the medicine or if you develop a skin rash, hives, itching, swelling of the face, or difficulty in breathing. If you cannot reach your doctor, phone a hospital emergency department.

□ If for some reason you cannot take all of the medicine, throw away the unused portion by flushing it down the toilet. Do not take or save old medicine.

* * * * *

Hexachlorophene Compound (*Topical Antibacterial-Detergent*)
United States: Hexamead-PH, Phisohex, Soy-Dome Cleanser, WescoHex
Canada: Phisohex

□ This medicine is used to cleanse the skin.

HOW TO USE THIS MEDICINE
□ Instructions for use:
  • Apply the medicine to wet skin or a wet sponge and add more water to form a lather while washing.
  • After using this medicine, rinse the treated area thoroughly with water.

SPECIAL INSTRUCTIONS
□ Do not use this medicine on open cuts, burns, and wounds or leave it in contact with these areas for a long time.

□ Stop using the cleanser if you develop a skin rash, redness, swelling, or an infection.

□ Keep away from the eyes.

□ For external use only. Do not swallow.

* * * * *

398

Hexobarbital (*Oral Hypnotic*)
United States: Sombulex

- [ ] This medicine is used to cause sleep.

- [ ] IMPORTANT: If you have ever had an allergic reaction to a barbiturate medicine, tell your doctor or pharmacist before you take any of this medicine.

HOW TO USE THIS MEDICINE
- [ ] This medicine may be taken with food or a full glass of water.

SPECIAL INSTRUCTIONS
- [ ] Sleeping medicines are only useful for a short time. If used for too long, they lose their effectiveness. Do not take any more of this medicine than your doctor has prescribed and do not stop taking this medicine suddenly without the approval of your doctor.

- [ ] Women who are pregnant, breast-feeding, or planning to become pregnant should tell their doctor before taking this medicine.

- [ ] In some people, this drug may cause dizziness or drowsiness. Do not drive a car or operate dangerous machinery or do jobs that require you to be alert until you know how you are going to react to this drug.

- [ ] If you become dizzy, you should be careful going up and down stairs. Sit or lie down at the first sign of dizziness.

- [ ] Do not drink alcoholic beverages while taking this drug without the approval of your doctor.

- [ ] It is important that you obtain the advice of your doctor or pharmacist before taking ANY other medicines including pain relievers, sleeping pills, tranquilizers or medicines for depression, cough/cold medicines, or allergy medicines.

- [ ] Since you are taking this medicine to help you sleep, take it about 20 minutes before you want to go to sleep. Go to bed after you have taken it. Do not smoke in bed after you have taken it.

- [ ] Do not store this medicine at the bedside and keep it out of the reach of children.

- [ ] Call your doctor immediately if you think you may be allergic to the medicine or if you develop a skin rash, hives, itching, swelling of the face, or difficulty in breathing. If you cannot reach your doctor, phone a hospital emergency department.

- [ ] Most people experience few or no side effects from their drugs. However, any medicine can sometimes cause unwanted effects. Call your doctor if you develop a sore throat, bothersome sleepiness or laziness during the day, nightmares, staggering walk, unusual nervousness, a yellow color to the skin or eyes, easy bruising, or slow heartbeats.

*   *   *   *   *

Hexocyclium (*Oral Antispasmodic*)
United States: Tral

☐ This medicine is used to help relax muscles of the stomach and bowels as well as to decrease the amount of acid formed in the stomach.

☐ IMPORTANT: If you have ever had an allergic reaction to atropine or any other drug used to relax the stomach or bowels, tell your doctor or pharmacist before you take any of this medicine.

HOW TO USE THIS MEDICINE

☐ Take this medicine approximately 30 minutes before a meal unless otherwise directed.

☐ If you miss a dose of this medicine, do not take the missed dose and do not double the next dose.

☐ This medicine must be swallowed whole. Do not crush, chew, or break it into pieces. (*United States:* Tral Gradumets)

SPECIAL INSTRUCTIONS

☐ If your mouth becomes dry, suck a hard sour candy (sugarless) or ice chips, or chew gum. It is especially important to brush your teeth regularly if you develop a dry mouth.

☐ In some people, this drug may cause dizziness or drowsiness. Do not drive a car or operate dangerous machinery or do jobs that require you to be alert until you know how you are going to react to this drug.

☐ If you become dizzy, you should be careful going up and down stairs. Sit or lie down at the first sign of dizziness. Tell your doctor you have been dizzy.

☐ A desire to urinate ("pass your water") with an inability to do so is not an uncommon effect with this drug. Urinating each time before taking the drug may help relieve this problem. Call your doctor if it continues.

☐ You may become more sensitive to heat because your body may perspire less while you are taking this drug. Be careful not to become overheated during exercise or in hot weather.

☐ Do not take antacids within 1 hour of taking this medicine because they could make this medicine less effective.

☐ If you become constipated, try increasing the amount of bulk in your diet (for example, bran and salads), exercising more often, or drinking more water. Call your doctor if the constipation continues.

☐ If your eyes become more sensitive to sunlight, it may help to wear sunglasses.

☐ Most people experience few or no side effects from their drugs. However, any medicine can sometimes cause unwanted effects. Call your doctor if you develop a skin rash, diarrhea, unusual restlessness, flushing, or eye pain.

* * * * *

400

Homatropine HBr (*Ophthalmic Mydriatic-Cycloplegic*)

United States: Homatrocel, Isopto Homatropine

Canada: Isopto Homatropine

☐ This medicine is used to treat conditions of the eye. The drug will cause the pupil of the eye to dilate (become larger in size). This is a normal effect of the drug.

☐ IMPORTANT: If you have ever had an allergic reaction to bromide medicine, tell your doctor or pharmacist before you use any of this drug.

HOW TO USE THIS MEDICINE

☐ For EYE DROPS

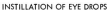

INSTILLATION OF EYE DROPS

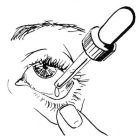

- The person administering the eye drops should wash his hands with soap and water.
- The eye drops must be kept clean. Do not touch the dropper against the face or anything else.
- Lie down or tilt your head backward and look at the ceiling.
- Gently pull down the lower lid of your eye to form a pouch.
- Hold the dropper in your other hand and approach the eye from the side. Place the dropper as close to the eye as possible without touching it.
- Place the prescribed number of drops into the pouch of the eye.
- Close your eyes. Do not rub them.
- Apply gentle pressure for a minute with your fingers to the bridge of the nose (inside corner of the eye) to prevent the eye drops from being drained from the eye.
- Blot excess solution around the eye with a tissue.

☐ If necessary, have someone else administer the eye drops for you.

☐ Do not use the eye drops if they have changed in color or have changed in any way since being purchased.

SPECIAL INSTRUCTIONS

☐ Vision may be blurred for a few minutes after using the eye medicine. Do not drive a car or operate dangerous machinery or do jobs that require you to be alert until your vision has cleared.

401

- ☐ If you forget to use the medicine, use it as soon as possible. However, if it is almost time for your next dose, do not use the missed dose but continue with your regular schedule.

- ☐ Do not use this medicine at the same time as any other eye medicine without the approval of your doctor. Some medicines cannot be mixed.

- ☐ If your eyes become more sensitive to light, it may help to wear sunglasses.

- ☐ Contact your doctor if the condtion for which you are using this medicine does not improve or if the eye becomes irritated by it for more than a few minutes. Many eye medicines sting for a short time immediately after use. Also call your doctor if you develop eye pain, a skin rash, flushing, dryness of the skin, a fast pulse, or fever.

- ☐ Always tell any future doctors who are treating you that you have used this medicine.

- ☐ Keep the container tightly closed and store in a cool place.

- ☐ For external use only. Do not swallow.

*　*　*　*　*

Hydralazine HCl (*Oral Antihypertensive*)
United States: Apresoline, Dralzine, Rolazine
Canada: Apresoline

- ☐ This medicine is used to lower the blood pressure.

- ☐ Hypertension (high blood pressure) is a long-term condition, and it will probably be necessary for you to take the drug for a long time in spite of the fact that you feel better. It is very important that you take this medicine as your doctor has directed and that you do not miss any doses. Otherwise, you cannot expect the drug to keep your blood pressure down.

HOW TO USE THIS MEDICINE
- ☐ This medicine may be taken with food.

- ☐ Try to take the medicine at the same time(s) every day.

SPECIAL INSTRUCTIONS
- ☐ If you forget to take a dose, take it as soon as possible. However, if it is almost time for your next dose, do not take the missed dose. Instead, continue with your regular dosing schedule.

- ☐ Do not drive a car, operate dangerous machinery, or do jobs that require you to be alert if you are dizzy. Sit or lie down at the first sign of dizziness. Tell your doctor you have been dizzy.

- ☐ In order to help prevent dizziness, it is also recommended that you avoid strenuous exercises and standing for long periods of time, especially if the

402

weather is hot. Be careful of the amount of alcohol you drink and avoid hot showers and baths while taking this medicine.

☐ Follow any special diet your doctor may have ordered. He may want you to limit the amount of salt in your food.

☐ Headaches may occur during the first few days of therapy, but they usually disappear within the first week. If they continue, call your doctor.

☐ Some nonprescription drugs can aggravate your condition. Do not take any of the following without the approval of your doctor or pharmacist: cough, cold, or sinus products; asthma or allergy products; or diet or weight-reducing medicines.

☐ Most people experience few or no side effects from their drugs. However, any medicine can sometimes cause unwanted effects. Call your doctor if you develop sore throat, fever, unusual tiredness, muscle or joint pain, skin rash, chest pains, swelling of the legs or ankles, sudden weight gain of 5 pounds or more, or numbness or tingling in the hands or feet.

☐ Carry an identification card indicating that you are taking this medicine. Always tell your pharmacist, dentist, and other doctors who are treating you that you are taking this medicine.

☐ Do not stop taking this medicine without your doctor's approval and do not go without medicine between prescription refills. Call your pharmacist 2 or 3 days before you will run out of the medicine.

* * * * *

Hydrochlorothiazide (*Oral Diuretic-Antihypertensive*)

United States: Diaqua, Esidrix, Hydrodiuril, Hydro-Z, Lexxor, Oretic

Canada: Diuchlor H, Esidrix, Hydro-Aquil, HydroDiuril, Natrimax, Neo-Codema, Novohydrazide, Urozide

☐ This medicine is used to help rid the body of excess water and to decrease swelling. It is also used to treat high blood pressure. It is commonly called a "water pill."

☐ IMPORTANT: If you have ever had an allergic reaction to sulfa drugs or thiazide diuretics, tell your doctor or pharmacist before taking any of this medicine.

HOW TO USE THIS MEDICINE

☐ Take the medicine with food, meals, or milk.

☐ Try to take it at the same time(s) every day so that you have a constant level of the medicine in your body. Do not miss any doses. Otherwise, you cannot expect the drug to work as well.

403

☐ When you first start taking this medicine, you will probably urinate ("pass your water") more often and in larger amounts than usual. Therefore, if you are to take one dose every day, take it in the morning after breakfast. If you are to take more than one dose every day, take the last dose 6 hours before bedtime so that you will not have to get up during the night to go to the bathroom. This effect will usually lessen after you have taken the drug for awhile.

SPECIAL INSTRUCTIONS

☐ If you forget to take a dose, take it as soon as possible. However, if it is almost time for your next dose, do not take the missed dose. Instead, continue with your regular dosing schedule.

☐ Women who are pregnant, breast-feeding, or planning to become pregnant should tell their doctor before taking this medicine.

☐ This medicine normally causes your body to lose potassium. The body has warning signs to let you know if too much potassium is being lost. Call your doctor if you become unusually thirsty or if you develop leg cramps, unusual weakness, fatigue, vomiting, confusion, or irregular pulse.

☐ If your doctor recommends that you eat foods that are high in potassium, one or more of the foods listed in Appendix A should be eaten daily. All of these foods are rich in potassium. Your goal should be to take in 1000 to 2000 mg. of potassium (approximately 25.6 to 51 mEq) each day. The calorie content and sodium content are included for your convenience in meal planning. CHANGE YOUR DIET ONLY IF YOUR DOCTOR TELLS YOU TO.

☐ If this medicine causes dizziness, you should be careful going up an down stairs and you should not change positions too rapidly. Get out of bed slowly in the morning and dangle your feet over the edge of the bed for a few minutes before standing up. Sit down or lie down at the first sign of dizziness. Tell your doctor you have been dizzy. Be careful drinking alcoholic beverages while taking this medicine because they could make the dizziness worse. Do not drive a car or operate dangerous machinery or do jobs that require you to be alert if you are dizzy.

☐ In order to help prevent dizziness and fainting, your doctor may also recommend that you avoid strenuous exercises, standing for long periods of time (especially in hot weather), or hot showers or hot baths.

☐ This medicine may make some people more sensitive to sunlight and sunlamps. When you begin taking this medicine, try to avoid getting too much sun until you see how you are going to react. If your skin does become more sensitive to sunlight, tell your doctor and try to stay out of direct sunlight. While in the sun, wear protective clothing and sunglasses. You may wish to ask your pharmacist about suitable sunscreen products. Check with your doctor if you become sunburned.

☐ Call your doctor immediately if you think you may be allergic to the medicine

404

or if you develop a skin rash, hives, itching, swelling of the face, or difficulty in breathing. If you cannot reach your doctor, phone a hospital emergency department.

☐ Most people experience few or no side effects from their drugs. However, any medicine can sometimes cause unwanted effects. Call your doctor if you develop a sore throat, fever, sharp stomach pain, chest pain, sharp joint pain, easy bruising or bleeding, a yellow color to the skin or eyes, or a sudden weight gain of 5 pounds or more.

* * * * *

Hydrocodone Bitartrate (*Oral Antitussive*)
United States: Codone, Dicodid
Canada: Corutol DH, Hycodan, Robidone

☐ This medicine is used to help relieve dry irritating coughs.

☐ IMPORTANT: If you have ever had an allergic reaction to hydrocodone or codeine medicine, tell your doctor or pharmacist before you take any of this medicine.

HOW TO USE THIS MEDICINE

☐ Do not dilute the syrup. The soothing effect will be enhanced if you do not drink liquid immediately after taking the medicine. (**Canada:** Corutol DH, Robidone)

☐ Swallow the tablets whole and take them with some food or milk to help prevent stomach upset.

SPECIAL INSTRUCTIONS

☐ In some people, this drug may cause dizziness or drowsiness. Do not drive a car or operate dangerous machinery or do jobs that require you to be alert until you know how you are going to react to this drug.

☐ If this medicine causes dizziness, you should be careful going up and down stairs and you should not change positions too rapidly. Get out of bed slowly in the morning and dangle your feet over the edge of the bed for a few minutes before standing up. Sit down or lie down at the first sign of dizziness. Tell your doctor you have been dizzy. Avoid hot showers and baths because they could make you dizzy.

☐ Do not drink alcoholic beverages while taking this drug without the approval of your doctor.

☐ It is important that you obtain the advice of your doctor or pharmacist before taking pain relievers, nonprescription drugs, sleeping pills, tranquilizers, or medicines for depression while you are taking this drug.

☐ If your mouth becomes dry, suck a hard sour candy (sugarless) or ice chips, or chew gum. It is especially important to brush your teeth regularly if you develop a dry mouth.

☐ If you do feel nauseated when you first start taking this medicine, it may help to lie down for a few minutes.

☐ Call your doctor if the cough lasts longer than 1 week or if you develop a fever, skin rash, or persistent headache.

☐ Most people experience few or no side effects from their drugs. However, any medicine can sometimes cause unwanted effects. Call your doctor if you develop a skin rash, shortness of breath, slow or fast heartbeats, fainting, or difficulty in urinating ("passing your water").

☐ Do not use this medicine for more than 1 week without the advice of your doctor.

*   *   *   *   *

Hydrocodone and Phenyltoloxamine-Resin Complexes
(Oral Antitussive)

United States: Tussionex

Canada: Tussionex

☐ This medicine is used to help relieve dry irritating coughs.

☐ IMPORTANT: If you have ever had an allergic reaction to hydrocodone or codeine medicine, tell your doctor or pharmacist before you take any of this medicine.

HOW TO USE THIS MEDICINE

☐ Shake the bottle well before using so that you can measure an accurate dose.

☐ Do not dilute the medicine and do not drink other liquids after taking this medicine.

SPECIAL INSTRUCTIONS

☐ In some people, this drug may cause dizziness or drowsiness. Do not drive a car or operate dangerous machinery or do jobs that require you to be alert until you know how you are going to react to this drug.

☐ If this medicine causes dizziness, you should be careful going up and down stairs and you should not change positions too rapidly. Get out of bed slowly in the morning and dangle your feet over the edge of the bed for a few minutes before standing up. Sit down or lie down at the first sign of dizziness. Tell your doctor you have been dizzy. Avoid hot showers and baths because they could make you dizzy.

☐ Do not drink alcoholic beverages while taking this drug without the approval of your doctor.

☐ It is important that you obtain the advice of your doctor or pharmacist before taking pain relievers, nonprescription drugs, sleeping pills, tranquilizers, or medicines for depression while you are taking this drug.

- [ ] If your mouth becomes dry, suck a hard sour candy (sugarless) or ice chips, or chew gum. It is especially important to brush your teeth regularly if you develop a dry mouth.

- [ ] If you do feel nauseated when you first start taking this medicine, it may help to lie down for a few minutes.

- [ ] Call your doctor if the cough lasts longer than 1 week or if you develop a fever, skin rash, or persistent headache.

- [ ] Most people experience few or no side effects from their drugs. However, any medicine can sometimes cause unwanted effects. Call your doctor if you develop a skin rash, shortness of breath, slow or fast heartbeats, fainting, or difficulty in urinating ("passing your water").

- [ ] Do not use this medicine for more than 1 week without the advice of your doctor.

*   *   *   *   *

Hydrocortisone (*Eye/Ear Corticosteroid*)

United States: Hydro-Cortone Acetate Ophthalmic, Optef
Canada: Cortamed, Cortril

- [ ] This medicine is used to help relieve the pain, redness, and swelling of certain types of eye and ear conditions.

HOW TO USE THIS MEDICINE

- [ ] Shake this medicine well before using. (**United States:** Hydro-Cortone Acetate Ophthalmic; **Canada:** Cortamed)

- [ ] For EYE DROPS

INSTILLATION OF EYE DROPS

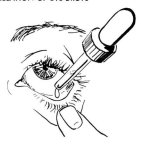

- The person administering the eye drops should wash his hands with soap and water.
- The eye drops must be kept clean. Do not touch the dropper against the face or anything else.
- Lie down or tilt your head backward and look at the ceiling.
- Gently pull down the lower lid of your eye to form a pouch.

407

- Hold the dropper in your other hand and approach the eye from the side. Place the dropper as close to the eye as possible without touching it.
- Place the prescribed number of drops into the pouch of the eye.
- Close your eyes. Do not rub them.
- Apply gentle pressure for a minute with your fingers to the bridge of the nose (inside corner of the eye) to prevent the eye drops from being drained from the eye.
- Blot excess solution around the eye with a tissue.
- If necessary, have someone else administer the eye drops for you.
- Do not use the eye drops if they change in color or change in any way after being purchased.
- Keep the eye drop bottle tightly closed when not in use.

☐ For EAR DROPS

INSTILLATION OF EAR DROPS

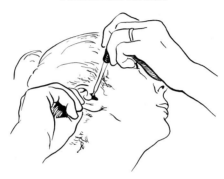

- Warm the ear drops to body temperature by holding the bottle in your hands for a few minutes. Do NOT heat the drops in hot water.
- The person administering the ear drops should wash his hands with soap and water.
- The ear drops must be kept clean. Do not touch the dropper against the ear or anything else.
- Tilt you head or lie on your side so that the ear to be treated is facing up.
- In ADULTS, hold the ear lobe up and back.
  In CHILDREN, hold the ear lobe down and back.
- Place the prescribed number of drops into the ear. Do not insert the dropper into the ear as it may cause injury.
- Remain in the same position for a short time (2 minutes) after you have administered the drops.
- Dry the ear lobe if there are any drops on it.

☐ For EAR DROPS AFTER APPLICATION OF EAR WICK (*Canada:* Cortamed)

- Warm the medicine to body temperature by holding it in your hands for a few minutes.

408

- Tilt your head to the side or lie on your side so that the ear to be treated is uppermost.
- Drop the prescribed amount of medicine into the ear canal.
- Do not use the solution if it is discolored or if it appears to have changed in any way since you purchased it.
  - Keep the wick moist and replace with a clean wick as directed by your doctor.
- If necessary, have someone else administer the ear drops for you.
- Do not use the ear drops if they change in color or change in any way after being purchased.
- Keep the bottle tightly closed when not in use.

☐ For EYE OINTMENT

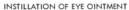

INSTILLATION OF EYE OINTMENT

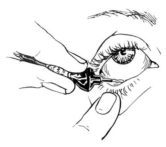

- The person administering the eye ointment should wash his hands with soap and water.
- The eye ointment must be kept clean. Do not touch the tube against the face or anything else.
- Lie down or tilt your head backward and look at the ceiling.
- Gently pull down the lower lid of your eye to form a pouch.
- Hold the tube in your other hand and place the tube as close as possible to the eye without touching it.
- Squeeze the prescribed amount of ointment (usually $\frac{1}{2}$ inch in adults) from the tube along the pouch.
- Close your eyes. Do not rub them.
- Wipe off any excess ointment around the eye with a tissue.
  - Clean the tip of the ointment tube with a tissue.
- If necessary, have someone else administer the eye ointment for you.
- Keep the eye ointment tube tightly closed when not in use.

☐ Do not use this drug more frequently or in larger quantities than prescribed by your doctor.

SPECIAL INSTRUCTIONS

☐ This medicine should be used as long as prescribed by your doctor. Do not stop using it earlier than your doctor has recommended in spite of the fact that your symptoms seem to have improved.

☐ If you forget to use the medicine, use it as soon as possible. However, if it is almost time for your next dose, do not use the missed dose, but continue with your regular schedule.

☐ Vision may be blurred for a few minutes after using the eye medicine. Do not drive a car or operate dangerous machinery or do jobs that require you to be alert until your vision has cleared.

☐ Do not use this medicine at the same time as any other eye or ear medicine without the approval of your doctor. Some medicines cannot be mixed.

☐ Call your doctor if the condition for which you are using this medicine persists or becomes worse or if the medicine causes itching or burning for more than a few minutes after instillation.

☐ For external use only. Do not swallow.

* * * * *

Hydrocortisone (*Oral Corticosteroid*)
United States: Cortef, Hydrocortone
Canada: Cortef, Cortone, Hydrocortone

☐ This medicine is similar to cortisone, which is a hormone normally produced by the body. This medicine is used to help decrease inflammation which then relieves pain, redness, and swelling. It is used in the treatment of certain kinds of arthritis as well as severe allergies or skin conditions.

HOW TO USE THIS MEDICINE
☐ Take this medicine with food or a glass of milk in order to help prevent stomach upset. Call your doctor if you develop stomach upset or stomach pain or heartburn (especially if it awakens you during the night). Do not try to treat this yourself.

☐ If your doctor has prescribed only ONE dose of this medicine every day, it is best to take it before 9 A.M. or with breakfast.

☐ If you forget to take a dose, take it as soon as possible. However, if it is almost time for your next dose, do not take the missed dose. Instead, continue with your regular schedule.

☐ Shake the bottle well before using so that you can measure an accurate dose. (**Canada** and **United States:** Cortef Fluid)

SPECIAL INSTRUCTIONS
☐ Women who are pregnant, breast-feeding, or planning to become pregnant should tell their doctor before taking this medicine.

☐ It is best not to drink alcoholic beverages while you are taking this medicine because the combination can cause stomach problems.

410

- [ ] Do not take any more of this medicine than your doctor has prescribed and do not stop taking this medicine suddenly without the approval of your doctor. It may be necessary for your doctor to slowly reduce your dose since your body becomes used to this medicine and it might be harmful if you suddenly did not receive this medicine.

- [ ] Do not take aspirin or medicines containing aspirin without the approval of your doctor.

- [ ] While you are taking this medicine, you may gain some weight. This could be due to an increase in your appetite or increased water in your system. Your doctor may prescribe a special diet to decrease the number of calories you eat and/or to lower the amount of sodium or increase the amount of potassium in your diet. Follow any diet that your doctor may order.

- [ ] You may find that you bruise more easily. Try to protect yourself from all injuries to prevent bruising.

- [ ] Diabetic patients should regularly check the sugar in their urine and report any unusual levels to their doctor.

- [ ] Carry an identification card indicating that you are taking this medicine. Always tell your pharmacist, dentist, and other doctors who are treating you that you are taking this medicine. If you have an acute infection, injury, or operation or dental surgery within 1 year of taking this medicine, it is important to tell your doctor.

- [ ] Most people experience few or no side effects from their drugs. However, any medicine can sometimes cause unwanted effects. Call your doctor if you develop stomach pain, sore throat, fever, swelling of the legs or ankles, a wound which does not heal, eye pain or blurred vision, frequent urination ("passing your water"), nightmares or depression, muscle cramps, red or black stools, puffing of the face, or menstrual problems.

* * * * *

Hydrocortisone Retention Enema (*Rectal Glucocorticoid*)
United States: Cortenema, Rectoid
Canada: Cortenema

- [ ] This medicine is used to help relieve inflammation of the rectum and bowels.

HOW TO USE THIS MEDICINE
- [ ] This medicine should be used in the evening before going to bed. It is best to use it right after a bowel movement.

- [ ] Administration of ENEMA
  - Shake enema bottle well before using.
  - Lie on your left side and raise your knee to your chest.
  - Remove the protective cover from the tip of the bottle.

411

- Carefully insert the tip of the bottle into the rectum.
- Slowly compress the container and use all of the solution.
- After instillation of the enema, remain in the same position (lie on left side) for at least 30 minutes.
- Try to avoid having a bowel movement or expelling the solution for at least 1 hour (preferably all night).

SPECIAL INSTRUCTIONS

☐ Women who are pregnant, breast-feeding, or planning to become pregnant should tell their doctor before taking this medicine.

☐ It is best not to drink alcoholic beverages while you are using this medicine because the combination can cause stomach problems.

☐ Do not use any more of this medicine than your doctor has prescribed and do not stop using this medicine suddenly without the approval of your doctor. It may be necessary for your doctor to slowly reduce your dose since your body becomes used to this medicine and it might be harmful if you suddenly did not receive this medicine.

☐ Do not take aspirin or medicines containing aspirin without the approval of your doctor.

☐ While you are using this medicine you may gain some weight. This could be due to an increase in your appetite or increased water in your system. Your doctor may prescribe a special diet to decrease the number of calories you eat and/or to lower the amount of sodium or increase the amount of potassium in your diet. Follow any diet that your doctor may order.

☐ You may find that you bruise more easily. Try to protect yourself from all injuries to prevent bruising.

☐ Diabetic patients should regularly check the sugar in their urine and report any unusual levels to their doctor.

☐ Carry an identification card indicating that you are taking this medicine. Always tell your pharmacist, dentist, and other doctors who are treating you that you are taking this medicine. If you have an acute infection, injury, operation, or dental surgery within 1 year of taking this medicine, it is important to tell your doctor.

☐ Most people experience few or no side effects from their drugs. However, any medicine can sometimes cause unwanted effects. Call your doctor if you develop stomach pain, sore throat, fever, swelling of the legs or ankles, a wound which does not heal, eye pain or blurred vision, frequent urination ("passing your water"), nightmares or depression, muscle cramps, red or black stools, puffing of the face, or menstrual problems.

☐ Also call your doctor if the suppository causes pain, burning, itching, blistering, or rectal bleeding that was not present before you started using the medicine.

*   *   *   *   *

Hydrocortisone Suppositories (*Rectal Glucocorticoid*)
Canada: Cortiment, Rectacort

☐ This medicine is used to help relieve inflammation of the rectum and bowels.

HOW TO USE THIS MEDICINE

☐ This medicine should be used in the evening before going to bed. It is best to use it right after a bowel movement.

☐ Administration of SUPPOSITORIES
   • Remove the wrapper from the suppository.
   • Lie on your side and raise your knee to your chest.
   • Insert the suppository with the tapered (pointed) end first into the rectum.
   • Remain lying down for a few minutes so that the suppository will dissolve in the rectum.
   • Try to avoid having a bowel movement for at least 1 hour so that the drug will have time to work.

SPECIAL INSTRUCTIONS

☐ Women who are pregnant, breast-feeding, or planning to become pregnant should tell their doctor before taking this medicine.

☐ It is best not to drink alcoholic beverages while you are taking this medicine because the combination can cause stomach problems.

☐ Do not use any more of this medicine than your doctor has prescribed and do not stop using this medicine suddenly without the approval of your doctor. It may be necessary for your doctor to slowly reduce your dose since your body becomes used to this medicine and it might be harmful if you suddenly did not receive this medicine.

☐ Do not take aspirin or medicines containing aspirin without the approval of your doctor.

☐ While you are using this medicine you may gain some weight. This could be due to an increase in your appetite or increased water in your system. Your doctor may prescribe a special diet to decrease the number of calories you eat and/or to lower the amount of sodium or increase the amount of potassium in your diet. Follow any diet that your doctor may order.

☐ You may find that you bruise more easily. Try to protect yourself from all injuries to prevent bruising.

☐ Diabetic patients should regularly check the sugar in their urine and report any unusual levels to their doctor.

☐ Carry an identification card indicating that you are using this medicine. Always tell your pharmacist, dentist, and other doctors who are treating you that you are taking this medicine. If you have an acute infection, injury, operation, or dental surgery within 1 year of taking this medicine, it is important to tell your doctor.

□ Most people experience few or no side effects from their drugs. However, any medicine can sometimes cause unwanted effects. Call your doctor if you develop stomach pain, sore throat, fever, swelling of the legs or ankles, a wound which does not heal, eye pain or blurred vision, frequent urination ("passing your water"), nightmares or depression, muscle cramps, red or black stools, puffing of the face, or menstrual problems.

□ Also call your doctor if the suppository causes pain, burning, itching, blistering, or rectal bleeding that was not present before you started using the medicine.

*   *   *   *   *

Hydrocortisone (*Topical Corticosteroid*)

United States: Cetacort, Cort-Dome, Cortef, Cortril, Dermacort, Eldecort, Epicort, Heb-Cort, Hexaderm Cream Modified, Hydrocortone Acetate, Hytone, Microcort, Nutracort, Relecort, Texacort, Ulcort

Canada: Cort-Dome, Cortef, Corticreme, Cortril, Emo-Cort, Hydro-Cortilean, Manticor, Microcort, Novohydrocort, Nutracort, Unicort, Westcort

□ This medicine is used to help relieve redness, swelling, itching, and inflammation of certain types of skin conditions.

HOW TO USE THIS MEDICINE

□ For CREAM, OINTMENT, and LOTION

- Each time you apply the medicine, wash your hands and gently cleanse the skin area well with water unless otherwise directed by your doctor. Do not allow the skin to dry completely. Pat with a clean towel until slightly damp.
- Apply a small amount of the drug to the affected area and spread lightly. Only the medicine that is actually touching the skin will work. A thick layer is not more effective than a thin layer. Do not bandage unless directed by your doctor.

□ For LIQUID MEDICINE

- Shake the liquid preparation well before using. (**United States:** Cetacort, Cort-Dome, Dermacort, Epicort, Heb-Cort, Microcort, Nutracort, Texacort; **Canada:** Cort-Dome, Manticor)
- The liquid preparation may cause a slight temporary stinging sensation after it is applied.

□ Do not use the drug more frequently or in larger quantities than prescribed by your doctor. Overuse of this medicine may cause you to absorb too much of the drug and increase the risk of side effects.

□ Keep the medicine away from the eyes, nose, and mouth.

414

SPECIAL INSTRUCTIONS

☐ If you forget to apply the medicine, apply it as soon as possible. However, if it is almost time for your next dose, do not apply the missed dose but continue with your regular schedule.

☐ Do not use this medicine for any other skin problems without checking with your doctor.

☐ Do not apply cosmetics or lotions on top of the drug unless your doctor approves.

☐ Call your doctor if the condition for which this drug is being used persists or becomes worse or if you have a constant irritation such as itching or burning that was not present before you started using this medicine. Also call your doctor if you develop abnormal lines or thinning of the skin, especially under the arms or between the legs.

☐ Store in a cool place but do not freeze.

☐ For external use only. Do not swallow.

☐ Tell future doctors that you have used this medicine.

*   *   *   *   *

Hydroflumethiazide (*Oral Diuretic-Antihypertensive*)
United States: Diucardin, Saluron

☐ This medicine is used to help rid the body of excess water and to decrease swelling. It is also used to treat high blood pressure. It is commonly called a "water pill."

☐ IMPORTANT: If you have ever had an allergic reaction to sulfa drugs or thiazide diuretics, tell your doctor or pharmacist before taking any of this medicine.

HOW TO USE THIS MEDICINE

☐ Take the medicine with food, meals, or milk.

☐ Try to take it at the same time(s) every day so that you have a constant level of the medicine in your body. Do not miss any doses. Otherwise, you cannot expect the drug to work as well.

☐ When you first start taking this medicine, you will probably urinate ("pass your water") more often and in larger amounts than usual. Therefore, if you are to take one dose every day, take it in the morning after breakfast. If you are to take more than one dose every day, take the last dose 6 hours before bedtime so that you will not have to get up during the night to go to the bathroom. This effect will usually lessen after you have taken the drug for awhile.

415

SPECIAL INSTRUCTIONS

- ☐ If you forget to take a dose, take it as soon as possible. However, if it is almost time for your next dose, do not take the missed dose. Instead, continue with your regular dosing schedule.

- ☐ Women who are pregnant, breast-feeding, or planning to become pregnant should tell their doctor before taking this medicine.

- ☐ This medicine normally causes your body to lose potassium. The body has warning signs to let you know if too much potassium is being lost. Call your doctor if you become unusually thirsty or if you develop leg cramps, unusual weakness, fatigue, vomiting, confusion, or irregular pulse.

- ☐ If your doctor recommends that you eat foods that are high in potassium, one or more of the foods listed in Appendix A should be eaten daily. All of these foods are rich in potassium. Your goal should be to take in 1000 to 2000 mg. of potassium (approximately 25.6 to 51 mEq) each day. The calorie content and sodium content are included for your convenience in meal planning. CHANGE YOUR DIET ONLY IF YOUR DOCTOR TELLS YOU TO.

- ☐ If this medicine causes dizziness, you should be careful going up and down stairs and you should not change positions too rapidly. Get out of bed slowly in the morning and dangle your feet over the edge of the bed for a few minutes before standing up. Sit down or lie down at the first sign of dizziness. Tell your doctor you have been dizzy. Be careful drinking alcoholic beverages while taking this medicine because they could make the dizziness worse. Do not drive a car or operate dangerous machinery or do jobs that require you to be alert if you are dizzy.

- ☐ In order to help prevent dizziness and fainting, your doctor may also recommend that you avoid strenuous exercises, standing for long periods of time (especially in hot weather), or hot showers or hot baths.

- ☐ This medicine may make some people more sensitive to sunlight and sunlamps. When you begin taking this medicine, try to avoid getting too much sun until you see how you are going to react. If your skin does become more sensitive to sunlight, tell your doctor and try to stay out of direct sunlight. While in the sun, wear protective clothing and sunglasses. You may wish to ask your pharmacist about suitable sunscreen products. Check with your doctor if you become sunburned.

- ☐ Call your doctor immediately if you think you may be allergic to the medicine or if you develop a skin rash, hives, itching, swelling of the face, or difficulty in breathing. If you cannot reach your doctor, phone a hospital emergency department.

- ☐ Most people experience few or no side effects from their drugs. However, any medicine can sometimes cause unwanted effects. Call your doctor if you

416

develop a sore throat, fever, sharp stomach pain, chest pain, sharp joint pain, easy bruising or bleeding, a yellow color to the skin or eyes, or a sudden weight gain of 5 pounds or more.

* * * * *

Hydromorphone (*Oral Analgesic*)
United States: Dilaudid
Canada: Dilaudid

☐ This medicine is used to help relieve pain.

HOW TO USE THIS MEDICINE
☐ This medicine may be taken with food or a glass of water.

☐ Do not take any more of this medicine than your doctor has prescribed. The drug could become habit-forming or you could take an overdose if you take it more often or longer than prescribed.

☐ Do not wait to take this medicine until the pain becomes severe. This medicine works best if you take it at the beginning of the pain. Call your doctor if you feel you need it more often than he prescribed.

SPECIAL INSTRUCTIONS
☐ Do not drink alcoholic beverages while taking this drug without the approval of your doctor.

☐ It is important that you obtain the advice of your doctor or pharmacist before taking ANY other medicines including other pain relievers, sleeping pills, tranquilizers or medicines for depression, cough/cold or allergy medicines, or weight-reducing medicines.

☐ In some people, this drug may cause dizziness or drowsiness. Do not drive a car or operate dangerous machinery or do jobs that require you to be alert until you know how you are going to react to this drug.

☐ If you become dizzy, you should be careful going up and down stairs. Sit or lie down at the first sign of dizziness. Get up slowly if you have been lying or sitting down.

☐ If you do feel nauseated when you first start taking this medicine, it may help if you lie down for a few minutes.

☐ If you become constipated, try increasing the amount of bulk in your diet (for example, bran and salads), exercising more often, or drinking more water. Call your doctor if the constipation continues.

☐ Most people experience few or no side effects from their drugs. However, any medicine can sometimes cause unwanted effects. Call your doctor if you

develop shortness of breath, a slow heartbeat, unusual nervousness, stomach pain, or difficulty in urinating ("passing your water").

☐ Always tell your dentist, pharmacist, and other doctors who are treating you that you are taking this medicine.

* * * * *

Hydromorphone (*Rectal Analgesic*)
United States: Dilaudid
Canada: Dilaudid

☐ This medicine is used to help relieve pain.

HOW TO USE THIS MEDICINE

☐ Administration of SUPPOSITORIES
- Remove the wrapper from the suppository.
- Lie on your side and raise your knee to your chest.
- Insert the suppository with the tapered (pointed) end first into the rectum.
- Remain lying down for a few minutes so that the suppository will dissolve in the rectum.
- Try to avoid having a bowel movement for at least one hour so that the drug will have time to work.

☐ Do not use any more of this medicine than your doctor has prescribed and do not stop using this medicine suddenly without the approval of your doctor.

☐ Do not wait to take this medicine until the pain becomes severe. This medicine works best if you use it at the beginning of the pain. Call your doctor if you feel you need it more often than he prescribed.

SPECIAL INSTRUCTIONS

☐ Do not drink alcoholic beverages while taking this drug without the approval of your doctor.

☐ It is important that you obtain the advice of your doctor or pharmacist before taking ANY other medicines including other pain relievers, sleeping pills, tranquilizers or medicines for depression, cough/cold or allergy medicines, or weight-reducing medicines.

☐ In some people, this drug may cause dizziness or drowsiness. Do not drive a car or operate dangerous machinery or do jobs that require you to be alert until you know how you are going to react to this drug.

☐ If you become dizzy, you should be careful going up and down stairs. Sit or lie down at the first sign of dizziness. Get up slowly if you have been lying or sitting down.

☐ If you do feel nauseated when you first start taking the medicine, it may help if you lie down for a few minutes.

☐ If you become constipated, try increasing the amount of bulk in your diet (for example, bran and salads), exercising more often, or drinking more water. Call your doctor if the constipation continues.

☐ Most people experience few of no side effects from their drugs. However, any medicine can sometimes cause unwanted effects. Call your doctor if you develop shortness of breath, slow heartbeats, unusual nervousness, stomach pain, or difficulty in urinating ("passing your water").

☐ Always tell your dentist, pharmacist, and other doctors who are treating you that you are taking this medicine.

*　*　*　*　*

Hydroquinone (*Topical Demelanizing Agent*)
United States: Eldopaque, Eldoquin
Canada: Eldopaque, Eldoquin

Hydroquinone-Titanium Dioxide
Canada: Meltex

☐ This medicine is used to lighten dark patches on the skin.

HOW TO USE THIS MEDICINE
☐ For CREAM, OINTMENT, and LOTION
  • Cleanse the area well with soap and water unless otherwise directed by your doctor.
  • Apply the medicine and rub into the skin well.
  • Cover the treated area with the preparation.
  • At bedtime, remove makeup and the medicine by washing thoroughly with soap and water.
  • Apply the medicine again and rub in well.

☐ Do not use the drug more frequently, in larger quantities, or for a longer period of time than prescribed by your doctor.

SPECIAL INSTRUCTIONS
☐ Use this medicine every 12 hours until the desired color of skin has been achieved; then use only occasionally to maintain the color. (**United States:** and **Canada:** Eldoquin)

☐ Test this medicine first by rubbing in a small amount of cream into an area about the size of a quarter on the inside of the upper arm. If redness or itching develops within 24 hours, you should not use this product.

☐ Discontinue using this medicine if a rash or irritation develops.

□ Do not use this medicine near the eyes, on open cuts or wounds, or on a sunburn.

□ For external use only.

*   *   *   *   *

Hydroxycloroquine Sulfate (*Oral Antimalarial-Anti-Inflam-matory*)
United States: Plaquenil Sulfate
Canada: Plaquenil Sulfate

□ This medicine has many uses and the reason it was prescribed depends upon your condition. If you do not understand why you are taking it, check with your doctor.

HOW TO USE THIS MEDICINE
□ Take this medicine immediately before or after meals or with food in order to help prevent stomach upset.

□ It is very important that you take this medicine exactly as your doctor has prescribed and that you do not miss any doses. Try to take this medicine at the same time every day. Do not take extra tablets without your doctor's approval. Take the medicine for the full treatment.

SPECIAL INSTRUCTIONS
□ If you forget to take a dose, take it as soon as possible. However, if it is almost time for your next dose, do not take the missed dose. Instead, continue with your regular dosing schedule.

□ Women who are pregnant, breast-feeding, or planning to become pregnant should tell their doctor before taking this medicine.

□ This medicine may cause the urine to turn rusty-yellow or brown in color. This is not unusual.

□ If you find that your eyes become more sensitive to light, it may help to wear sunglasses.

□ Most people experience few or no side effects from their drugs. However, any medicine can sometimes cause unwanted effects. Call your doctor if you develop muscle weakness, blurred vision, night blindness or any changes in eyesight or hearing, a skin rash, sore throat, fever or mouth sores, blue-black color to skin or nails, numbness or tingling in the hands or feet, or unusual bruising or bleeding.

□ Keep this medicine well out of the reach of children.

*   *   *   *   *

420

Hydroxyurea (*Oral Antineoplastic*)
United States: Hydrea
Canada: Hydrea

- [ ] This medicine is used in certain medical conditions to help slow down the growth and reproduction of some of the body's cells.

HOW TO USE THIS MEDICINE

- [ ] It is best to take this medicine 1 hour before breakfast or 2 hours after dinner in order to help prevent nausea or vomiting.
- [ ] If you are unable to swallow capsules, the capsules may be opened and the powder may be mixed with a glass of water.
- [ ] It is very important that you take this medicine exactly as your doctor has prescribed and that you do not miss any doses. Try to take this medicine at the same time every day.
- [ ] Even if you become nauseated or lose your appetite, do not stop taking the medicine but check with your doctor.
- [ ] If you miss a dose of this medicine, do not take the missed dose and do not double your next dose. Check with your doctor.

SPECIAL INSTRUCTIONS

- [ ] Always keep your doctor appointments so that your doctor can watch your progress.
- [ ] If your doctor has prescribed some other medicines for you, it is important that you take them in the right order and that you do not miss them.
- [ ] Unless otherwise directed, drink plenty of fluids (2 to 3 quarts daily) while you are taking this medicine. This will help your kidneys handle the medicine and help prevent kidney problems.
- [ ] Men and women should take appropriate birth control measures to avoid conception while taking this medicine.
- [ ] Always tell your pharmacist, dentist, and other doctors who are treating you that you are taking this medicine. This is especially important if you plan to have surgery or any vaccinations.
- [ ] This is a very strong medicine. In addition to its benefits, there may be some unwanted effects even for a short time after you stop taking the medicine. Call your doctor if you develop unusual bruising or bleeding, sore throat, fever or mouth sores, a skin rash, diarrhea (loose bowel movements), severe vomiting, stomach or joint pain, loss of appetite, or if you become confused or have difficulty or pain in urinating ("passing your water").

*   *   *   *   *

Hydroxyzine HCl (*Oral Antianxiety Agent*)

United States: Atarax, Vistaril
Canada: Atarax

☐ This medicine has several uses, and the reason it was prescribed depends upon your condition. Check with your doctor if you do not fully understand why you are taking it.

HOW TO USE THIS MEDICINE

☐ This medicine may be taken with food or a full glass of water.

☐ For LIQUID MEDICINE

   • Shake the bottle well before using so that you can measure an accurate dose. (**United States:** Vistaril Suspension)

SPECIAL INSTRUCTIONS

☐ If you forget to take a dose, take it as soon as possible. However, if it is almost time for your next dose, do not take the missed dose. Instead, continue with your regular dosing schedule.

☐ Do not drink alcoholic beverages while taking this drug without the approval of your doctor.

☐ It is important that you obtain the advice of your doctor or pharmacist before taking ANY other medicines including pain relievers, sleeping pills, tranquilizers or medicines for depression, cough/cold or allergy medicines, or weight-reducing medicines.

☐ If your mouth becomes dry, suck a hard sour candy (sugarless) or ice chips, or chew gum. It is especially important to brush your teeth regularly if you develop a dry mouth.

☐ In some people, this drug may cause drowsiness. Do not drive a car or operate dangerous machinery or do jobs that require you to be alert until you know how you are going to react to this drug.

☐ Do not take any more of this medicine than your doctor has prescribed.

☐ Most people experience few or no side effects from their drugs. However, any medicine can sometimes cause unwanted effects. Call your doctor if you develop a skin rash, sore throat, fever, mouth sores, or tremors.

*   *   *   *   *

Hyoscine HBr (*Ophthalmic Mydriatic-Cycloplegic*)

United States: Isopto Hyoscine, Scopolamine HBr Ophthalmic, Scopolamine 0.2% S.O.P.

☐ This medicine is used to treat conditions of the eye. The drug will cause the pupil of the eye to dilate (become larger in size). This is a normal effect of the drug.

422

HOW TO USE THIS MEDICINE

☐ For EYE DROPS

INSTILLATION OF EYE DROPS

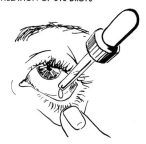

- The person administering the eye drops should wash his hands with soap and water.
- The eye drops must be kept clean. Do not touch the dropper against the face or anything else.
- Lie down or tilt your head backward and look at the ceiling.
- Gently pull down the lower lid of your eye to form a pouch.
- Hold the dropper in your other hand and approach the eye from the side. Place the dropper as close to the eye as possible without touching it.
- Place the prescribed number of drops into the pouch of the eye.
- Close your eyes. Do not rub them.
- Apply gentle pressure for a minute with your fingers to the bridge of the nose (inside corner of the eye) to prevent the eye drops from being drained from the eye.
- Blot excess solution around the eye with a tissue.
- If necessary, have someone else administer the eye drops for you.
- Do not use the eye drops if they have changed in color or have changed in any way since being purchased.
- Keep the eye drop bottle tightly closed when not in use.

☐ For EYE OINTMENT

INSTILLATION OF EYE OINTMENT

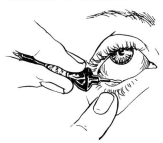

- The person administering the eye ointment should wash his hands with soap and water.
- The eye ointment must be kept clean. Do not touch the tube against the face or anything else.
- Lie down or tilt your head backward and look at the ceiling.
- Gently pull down the lower lid of your eye to form a pouch.
- Hold the tube in your other hand and place the tube as close as possible to the eye without touching it.
- Squeeze the prescribed amount of ointment (usually $\frac{1}{2}$ inch in adults) from the tube along the pouch.
- Close your eyes. Do not rub them.
- Wipe off any excess ointment around the eye with a tissue.
- Clean the tip of the ointment tube with a tissue.
- If necessary, have someone else administer the eye ointment for you.
- Keep the eye ointment tube tightly closed when not in use.

SPECIAL INSTRUCTIONS

☐ Vision may be blurred for a few minutes after using the eye medicine. Do not drive a car or operate dangerous machinery or do jobs that require you to be alert until your vision has cleared.

☐ If you forget to use the medicine, use it as soon as possible. However, if it is almost time for your next dose, do not use the missed dose but continue with your regular schedule.

☐ Do not use this medicine at the same time as any other eye medicine without the approval of your doctor. Some medicines cannot be mixed.

☐ If your eyes become more sensitive to light, it may help to wear sunglasses.

☐ Contact your doctor if the condition for which you are using this medicine does not improve or if the eye becomes irritated by it for more than a few minutes. Many eye medicines sting for a short time immediately after use. Also call your doctor if you develop eye pain, a skin rash, flushing, dryness of the skin, a fast pulse, or fever.

☐ Do not use the drug more frequently or in larger quantities than prescribed by your doctor.

☐ Always tell any future doctors who are treating you that you are using this medicine.

☐ For external use only. Do not swallow.

$$* \quad * \quad * \quad * \quad *$$

Ibuprofen (*Oral Analgesic-Anti-inflammatory*)
United States: Motrin
Canada: Amersol, Motrin

☐ This medicine is used to help relieve pain, redness, stiffness, and swelling in certain kinds of arthritis and other medical conditions.

- ☐ IMPORTANT: If you have ever had an allergic reaction to aspirin or any other medicine for arthritis, tell your doctor or pharmacist before you take any of this medicine.

- ☐ It is very important that you take this medicine regularly and that you DO NOT MISS ANY DOSES. If you miss a dose, the level of the medicine in your body will fall and the drug will not be as effective. Only if the level of the drug is high enough can it decrease the inflammation and swelling in your joints and help prevent further damage.

- ☐ The full benefit of this medicine may not be noticed immediately but may take from 1 to 2 weeks.

HOW TO USE THIS MEDICINE

- ☐ It is best to take this medicine on an empty stomach at least 1 hour before (or 2 hours after) eating food unless otherwise directed. If you develop stomach upset, take the medicine with food or immediately after meals. Call your doctor if you continue to have stomach upset.

SPECIAL INSTRUCTIONS

- ☐ If this medicine causes dizziness, you should be careful going up and down stairs and you should not change positions too rapidly. Get out of bed slowly in the morning and dangle your feet over the edge of the bed for a few minutes before standing up. Sit down or lie down at the first sign of dizziness. Tell your doctor you have been dizzy. Do not drive a car or operate dangerous machinery if you are dizzy. Avoid hot showers and baths because they could make you dizzy.

- ☐ If you forget to take a dose, take it as soon as possible. However, if it is almost time for your next dose, do not take the missed dose. Instead, continue with your regular dosing schedule.

- ☐ While you are taking this medicine, do not drink alcoholic beverages or take aspirin without the permission of your doctor. It is usually safe to take acetaminophen for the occasional headache. Check with your pharmacist.

- ☐ Call your doctor immediately if you think you may be allergic to the medicine or if you develop a skin rash, hives, itching, swelling of the face, or difficulty in breathing. If you cannot reach your doctor, phone a hospital emergency department.

- ☐ Most people experience few or no side effects from their drugs. However, any medicine can sometimes cause unwanted effects. Call your doctor if you develop a skin rash, sore throat or fever, "ringing" or "buzzing" in the ears, swelling of the legs or ankles or sudden weight gain, blurred vision or changes in your eyesight, red or black stools, or severe stomach pain.

- ☐ Carry an identification card indicating that you are taking this medicine. Always tell your pharmacist, dentist, and other doctors who are treating you that you are taking this medicine.

* * * * *

425

Idoxuridine (*Ophthalmic Antiviral*)

United States: Dendrid, Herplex Liquifilm, Stoxil Ophthalmic
Canada: Herplex Liquifilm, Stoxil

☐ This medicine is used to treat viral infections of the eye.

HOW TO USE THIS MEDICINE

☐ For EYE DROPS

INSTILLATION OF EYE DROPS

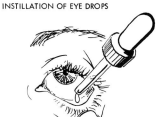

- The person administering the eye drops should wash his hands with soap and water.
- The eye drops must be kept clean. Do not touch the dropper against the face or anything else.
- Lie down or tilt your head backward and look at the ceiling.
- Gently pull down the lower lid of your eye to form a pouch.
- Hold the dropper in your other hand and approach the eye from the side. Place the dropper as close to the eye as possible without touching it.
- Place the prescribed number of drops into the pouch of the eye.
- Close your eyes. Do not rub them.
- Apply gentle pressure for a minute with your fingers to the bridge of the nose (inside corner of the eye) to prevent the eye drops from being drained from the eye.
- Blot excess solution around the eye with a tissue.
- If necessary, have someone else administer the eye drops for you.
- Do not use the eye drops if they have changed in color or have changed in any way since being purchased.
- Keep the eye drop bottle tightly closed when not in use.

☐ For EYE OINTMENT

INSTILLATION OF EYE OINTMENT

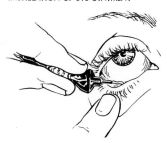

426

- The person administering the eye ointment should wash his hands with soap and water.
- The eye ointment must be kept clean. Do not touch the tube against the face or anything else.
- Lie down or tilt your head backward and look at the ceiling.
- Gently pull down the lower lid of your eye to form a pouch.
- Hold the tube in your other hand and place the tube as close as possible to the eye without touching it.
- Squeeze the prescribed amount of ointment (usually $\frac{1}{2}$ inch in adults) from the tube along the pouch.
- Close your eyes. Do not rub them.
- Wipe off any excess ointment around the eye with a tissue.
- Clean the tip of the ointment tube with a tissue.
- If necessary, have someone else administer the eye ointment for you.
- Keep the eye ointment tube tightly closed when not in use.
- Do not use the drug more frequently or in larger quantities than prescribed by your doctor.

SPECIAL INSTRUCTIONS

☐ Vision may be blurred for a few minutes after using the eye medicine. Do not drive a car or operate dangerous machinery or do jobs that require you to be alert until your vision has cleared.

☐ If you forget to use the medicine, use it as soon as possible. However, if it is almost time for your next dose, do not use the missed dose but continue with your regular schedule.

☐ The eyes may become sensitive to the light while using this medicine. Wearing sunglasses in brightly lit areas will help to relieve this problem.

☐ It is important to keep the eye surface covered with this medicine. Use the medicine regularly *exactly* as your doctor advises.

☐ Continue to use this medicine until your doctor tells you otherwise, despite the fact that the infection may appear to have disappeared.

☐ Do not use this medicine at the same time as any other eye medicine without the approval of your doctor. Some medicines cannot be mixed.

☐ Contact your doctor if the condition for which you are using this medicine does not improve or if the eye becomes irritated by it for more than a few minutes. Many eye medicines sting for a short time immediately after use.

☐ Store this eye medicine in a cool place and protect from light.

☐ For external use only.

* * * * *

Idoxuridine (*Topical Antiviral*)
Canada: Herplex-D Liquifilm

☐ This medicine is used to treat viral infections of the skin.

427

HOW TO USE THIS MEDICINE

☐ For SOLUTION

  • Apply the prescribed number of drops of solution to cover the sore. The medicine should also cover the immediately surrounding area to help prevent spreading.
  • **Never** contaminate the dropper and solution by touching the sore with the dropper.
  • It is important to keep the affected area covered with this medicine. Use the medicine regularly **exactly** as your doctor advises.

SPECIAL INSTRUCTIONS

☐ Continue to use this medicine until your doctor tells you otherwise, despite the fact that the infection may appear to have disappeared.

☐ Store this medicine in a cool place and protect from light.

☐ For external use only.

*　*　*　*　*

Imipramine HCl (*Oral Antidepressant*)

United States: Antipress, Janimine, Ropramine, SK-Pramine, Tofranil

Canada: Impril, Novopramine, Praminil, Tofranil

Imipramine Pamoate
United States: Tofranil-PM

☐ This medicine is used to help relieve the symptoms of depression. It is important that you take the medicine regularly and that you do not miss any doses. The full effect of the medicine will not be noticed immediately but may take from a few days to several weeks. Early signs of improvement are increased appetite, better sleep, increased energy and later improved mood. DO NOT STOP TAKING the medicine when you first feel better or you may feel worse in 3 or 4 days.

☐ This medicine has also been used in children to treat bed-wetting.

HOW TO USE THIS MEDICINE

☐ This medicine may be taken with food unless otherwise directed.

SPECIAL INSTRUCTIONS

☐ If you forget to take a dose, take it as soon as possible. However, if it is almost time for your next dose, do not take the missed dose. Instead, continue with your regular dosing schedule.

☐ Any medicine has a few unwanted side effects. Because this medicine takes a few weeks to work, the side effects are the only thing that tell the doctor that the drug is being absorbed. Most of these side effects will go away as your body adjusts to the medicine.

- [ ] Women who are pregnant, breast-feeding, or planning to become pregnant should tell their doctor before taking this medicine.

- [ ] In some people, this drug may cause dizziness or drowsiness. Do not drive a car or operate dangerous machinery or do jobs that require you to be alert until you know how you are going to react to this drug.

- [ ] If this medicine causes dizziness, you should be careful going up and down stairs and you should not change positions too quickly. Get out of bed slowly in the morning and dangle your feet over the edge of the bed for a few minutes before standing up. Sit or lie down at the first sign of dizziness. Tell your doctor you have been dizzy and he may adjust your dose.

- [ ] Do not drink alcoholic beverages while taking this drug without the approval of your doctor.

- [ ] It is important that you obtain the advice of your doctor or pharmacist before taking any other medicines, including pain relievers, sleeping pills, tranquilizers, other medicines for depression, cough/cold or allergy medicines, or weight-reducing medicine.

- [ ] If your mouth becomes dry, suck a hard candy (sugarless) or ice chips, or chew gum. It is especially important to brush your teeth regularly if you develop a dry mouth.

- [ ] If you become constipated, try increasing the amount of bulk in your diet (for example, bran, salads), exercising more often, or drinking water.

- [ ] Call your doctor if you develop a sore throat, fever, mouth sores, eye pain or blurred vision, difficulty in urinating ("passing your water"), fast heartbeats, or a skin rash.

- [ ] Do not stop taking this medicine suddenly without your doctor's approval. When your doctor tells you to stop this medicine, you must follow these precautions for 1 week since some of the medicine will still be in your body.

- [ ] Carry an identification card indicating that you are taking this medicine. Always tell your pharmacist, dentist, and other doctors who are treating you that you are taking this medicine.

*　*　*　*　*

Indomethacin (Oral Anti-inflammatory–Analgesic)
United States: Indocin
Canada: Indocid

- [ ] This medicine is used to help relieve pain, redness, stiffness, and swelling in certain kinds of arthritis and other medical conditions.

☐ IMPORTANT: If you have ever had an allergic reaction to aspirin or any other medicine for arthritis, tell your doctor or pharmacist before you take any of this medicine.

☐ It is very important that you take this medicine regularly and that you DO NOT MISS ANY DOSES. If you miss a dose, the level of the medicine in your body will fall and the drug will not be as effective. Only if the level of the drug is high enough can it decrease the inflammation in your joints and help prevent further damage.

☐ The full benefit of this medicine may not be noticed immediately but may take from a few days to 4 weeks.

HOW TO USE THIS MEDICINE

☐ Always take this medicine with food or a glass of milk or immediately after meals to help prevent stomach upset.

SPECIAL INSTRUCTIONS

☐ Women who are pregnant, breast-feeding, or planning to become pregnant should tell their doctor before taking this medicine.

☐ In some people, this drug may cause dizziness or drowsiness. Do not drive a car or operate dangerous machinery or do jobs that require you to be alert until you know how you are going to react to this drug.

☐ If you become dizzy, you should be careful going up and down stairs. Sit or lie down at the first sign of dizziness.

☐ If you forget to take a dose of this medicine, do not take the missed dose and do not double the next dose. Instead, continue with your regular dosing schedule.

☐ This medicine initially may cause headaches which usually will disappear with continued use of the medicine. Call your doctor if they continue.

☐ While taking this medicine, do not drink alcoholic beverages or take aspirin without the permission of your doctor. It is usually safe to take acetaminophen for the occasional headache. Check with your pharmacist.

☐ Call your doctor immediately if you think you may be allergic to the medicine or if you develop a skin rash, hives, itching, swelling of the face, or difficulty in breathing. If you cannot reach your doctor, phone a hospital emergency department.

☐ Most people experience few or no side effects from their drugs. However, any medicine can sometimes cause unwanted effects. Call your doctor if you develop a skin rash, sore throat, fever or mouth sores, "ringing" or "buzzing" in the ears, diarrhea (loose bowel movements), stomach pain, easy bruising, red or black stools, blurred vision, swelling of the legs or ankles, or a yellow color to the skin and eyes, or if you become depressed.

- [ ] Carry an identification card indicating that you are taking this medicine. Always tell your pharmacist, dentist, and other doctors who are treating you that you are taking this medicine.

* * * * *

Indomethacin (*Rectal Anti-inflammatory–Analgesic*)
Canada: Indocid

- [ ] This medicine is used to help relieve pain, redness, stiffness, and swelling in certain kinds of arthritis and other medical conditions.

- [ ] IMPORTANT: If you have ever had an allergic reaction to aspirin or any other medicine for arthritis, tell your doctor or pharmacist before you take any of this medicine.

- [ ] It is very important that you take this medicine regularly and that you DO NOT MISS ANY DOSES. If you miss a dose, the level of the medicine in your body will fall and the drug will not be as effective. Only if the level of the drug is high enough can it decrease the inflammation and swelling in your joints and help prevent further damage.

- [ ] The full benefit of this medicine may not be noticed immediately but may take from a few days to 4 weeks.

HOW TO USE THIS MEDICINE
- [ ] Administration of SUPPOSITORIES
  - Remove the wrapper from the suppository.
  - Lie on your side and raise your knee to your chest.
  - Insert the suppository with the tapered (pointed) end first into the rectum.
  - Remain lying down for a few minutes so that the suppository will dissolve in the rectum.
  - Try to avoid having a bowel movement for at least 1 hour so that the drug will have time to work.

SPECIAL INSTRUCTIONS
- [ ] Women who are pregnant, breast-feeding, or planning to become pregnant should tell their doctor before taking this medicine.

- [ ] In some people, this drug may cause dizziness or drowsiness. Do not drive a car or operate dangerous machinery or do jobs that require you to be alert until you know how you are going to react to this drug.

- [ ] If you become dizzy, you should be careful going up and down stairs. Sit or lie down at the first sign of dizziness.

- [ ] If you forget to use a dose of this medicine, do not use the missed dose and do not double the next dose. Instead, continue with your regular dosing schedule.

☐ This medicine initially may cause headaches which usually will disappear with continued use of the medicine. Call your doctor if they continue.

☐ While you are using this medicine, do not drink alcoholic beverages or take aspirin without the permission of your doctor. It is usually safe to take acetaminophen for the occasional headache. Check with your pharmacist.

☐ Call your doctor immediately if you think you may be allergic to the medicine or if you develop a skin rash, hives, itching, swelling of the face, or difficulty in breathing. If you cannot reach your doctor, phone a hospital emergency department.

☐ Most people experience few or no side effects from their drugs. However, any medicine can sometimes cause unwanted effects. Call your doctor if you develop a skin rash, sore throat, fever or mouth sores, "ringing" or "buzzing" in the ears, diarrhea (loose bowel movements), stomach pain, easy bruising, red or black stools, blurred vision, swelling of the legs or ankles, or a yellow color to the skin and eyes, or if you become depressed. Also call your doctor if you develop bleeding from the rectum which was not present before you started using this medicine.

☐ Carry an identification card indicating that you are taking this medicine. Always tell your dentist, pharmacist, and other doctors who are treating you that you are taking this medicine.

* * * * *

Insulin (*Diabetes Mellitus Therapy*)

☐ Insulin is a hormone which is naturally produced by the body. It is needed for the body's proper use of food, especially sugar. With diabetes, the body either does not produce enough insulin or may not be able to use what is produced. As a result, the sugar in the blood can build up to dangerous levels and is passed out in the urine. Your doctor has prescribed this medicine to help keep your blood sugar at nearly normal levels.

HOW TO USE THIS MEDICINE

☐ There are several different types of insulin preparations available. Use only the type prescribed for you by your doctor. Always read the label carefully. NEVER change from one type or brand to another without instructions from your doctor.

☐ Doses of insulin are prescribed in UNITS. Always use the syringe which matches the strength of insulin you are using. If you do not, you will measure the wrong amount of insulin. For example, use a 100-Unit syringe with 100-Unit (commonly called U-100) insulin.

STERILIZATION OF NEEDLES AND SYRINGES

☐ Glass insulin syringes and metal needles may be used repeatedly if they are sterilized each time.

432

☐ Sterilize the needle and syringe by one of the following methods:

1. *Sterilizing in boiling water*
   a. Remove the plunger from the barrel of the syringe. Place the plunger, barrel, and needle on clean guaze in a shallow heat-proof dish and cover with distilled water. Another method is to place the plunger, barrel, and needle in a kitchen sieve and immerse in water. Carefully pass the needle through a hole in the sieve. All parts should be immersed in water, but none of the parts should touch the bottom of the pan.
   b. Boil for 5 minutes.
   c. Allow the parts to cool. Carefully with tweezers or tongs, remove the plunger by its top and the needle by the thick end. Attach the needle to the syringe.
   d. Push the plunger in and out to remove all water from the syringe.
   e. Do not allow the needle to touch a table or your hands as the needle will become contaminated.

2. *Sterilizing in alcohol*
   a. Draw alcohol into the syringe. Immerse the syringe in alcohol and leave for about 10 minutes.
   b. Eject all alcohol and let the syringe dry in the air for a few minutes. It must be completely dry before it is used.
   c. Rubbing alcohol should be used. This is important because alcohol can irritate your skin and may alter the insulin in your vial. Alcohol is very flammable. You must *never* heat it.

3. *Storage in alcohol*
   a. Store the syringe and needle in a commercially available case filled with isopropyl alcohol 91%.
   b. It is also necessary to sterilize the syringe and needle in boiling water at least once a week.

4. *Disposable syringes and needles*
   a. Disposable syringes and needles are presterilized and the sterilization step is eliminated. They may be used only once and should not be reused.
   b. After using each needle, replace the plastic cap. Snap off the needle and throw it away in a special container so that other people do not injure themselves when handling garbage.

ADMINISTRATION OF INSULIN

☐ To withdraw the correct dose of insulin from the vial, follow these steps:
1. Flip off the plastic protective cap. Do not remove the rubber stopper or the metal ring. Be careful not to cut yourself with the metal.
2. Wipe the surface of the rubber stopper with an antiseptic sponge or swab with rubbing alcohol.

3. Pull out the plunger to the same number of units of insulin you will be taking. This will put air in the syringe.

4. With Protamine Zinc Insulin, NPH Insulin, Semilente Insulin, Lente Insulin, and Ultralente Insulin, mix the contents of the vial by rotating the vial in the palms of the hands. This is necessary in order to be able to withdraw an accurate dose. Do **not** shake the vial.

5. Insert the needle into the center of the rubber stopper. Inject the air in the syringe into the vial. Hold the vial upside down. Withdraw the required amount of insulin by pulling back the plunger. Keep the point of the needle below the surface of the insulin in the vial. If air bubbles appear in the syringe, push the plunger back in. Withdraw the dose again. Do **not** inject a dose containing air bubbles because air bubbles will prevent measurement of an accurate dose.

6. Remove the needle from the rubber stopper.

7. Check to be sure that the dose you have withdrawn is correct. Then lay down the syringe. Make sure the needle does not touch anything.

☐ Cleanse the site of injection with soap and water. Rub with a piece of absorbent cotton soaked with alcohol.

☐ Gently grab a fold of skin between the thumb and index finger. Insert the needle into the loose tissue under the skin of the arm, leg, or abdomen. Release the fold of skin.

☐ Pull back the plunger of the syringe slightly. If blood enters the syringe, the needle has entered a blood vessel. If this happens, withdraw the needle and select a new site.

☐ Slowly inject the dose.

☐ Remove the needle and gently press the area with a piece of cotton. Do not rub. Rotate the injection site every day as advised by your doctor, pharmacist, or nurse (Fig. 6).

☐ Do not use this insulin if it turns cloudy. (**United States:** Iletin-Regular; **Canada:** Insulin-Toronto, Sulphated)

SPECIAL INSTRUCTIONS

☐ Do not use insulin after the expiration date which appears on the label. If you have not yet opened the vial, you may be able to exchange it at your pharmacy.

☐ All unopened bottles of insulin should be stored in the refrigerator. Do not freeze. Do not expose to direct sunlight or extreme heat. The bottle you are using at present may be stored at room temperature for 1 month, after which time any unused insulin should be thrown out. If you do not use a complete bottle of insulin in 1 month, you should refrigerate it and warm the bottle before use by holding it in your hands for a few minutes. It is best not to inject cold insulin.

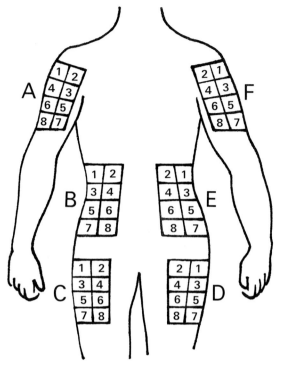

Figure 6. *Rotation of insulin injection sites.*

☐ If your doctor wants you to mix 2 different types of insulin, it is best that you ALWAYS mix them in the same order.

☐ Once you have injected your insulin, it is essential that you do **not** skip meals.

☐ If you exercise in active sports, it is best to inject the insulin into the abdomen or arm rather than the leg muscles because the leg muscles may absorb the medicine too quickly. Vigorous exercise may increase your requirements for carbohydrates or decrease your insulin requirements. Review this with your doctor.

GUIDELINES FOR AIR TRAVEL

☐ If you are traveling, carry some of your insulin and syringes in your hand luggage so that if your luggage is lost, you will not be without your insulin. It is a good idea to carry an extra vial, syringe, and needle in event of breakage. Take along an extra supply of insulin and syringes when traveling in foreign countries. In some countries abroad, there may be slight differences in potency of some of the insulins manufactured in those countries. Remember: Insulin 100 Units is not used in Europe. If you need new supplies, you will have to use 40- or 80-Unit insulin AND the corresponding 40- or 80-Unit syringes.

435

□ If you must take insulin during your flight, always make sure that the next meal (for example, breakfast) is ready before you take your dose.

□ If you must take a dose of insulin while you are in an airplane, inject less air into the vial than you usually use. Try injecting about half as much air as the number of units of insulin you intend to withdraw from the bottle. The reason for this is that in an airplane flying at an altitude over 10,000 feet, there is considerably more pressure in the insulin vial than in the cabin of the plane. Therefore, it is not necessary to inject as much air into the insulin bottle.

CROSSING TIME ZONES

□ If you are crossing time zones in your air travel, your meal times and insulin injection times may have to be altered. It is usually only necessary to make these adjustments on the day going and the day coming back.

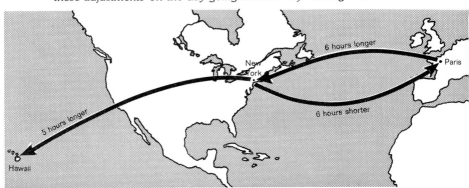

When you are traveling, the day becomes shorter going east and longer going west. Going east, New York to Paris, the day is six hours shorter; Hawaii to New York, five hours shorter. Going west, Paris to New York, the day is six hours longer; New York to Hawaii, five hours longer. Flying north to south doesn't make much difference, because generally one crosses only one time zone. (From Krall, L. P., (Ed.): Joslin Diabetes Manual, 11th Ed. Philadelphia, Lea & Febiger, 1978.)

□ Do not change your insulin dose when traveling without first checking with your doctor who treats your diabetes. He may suggest a slightly different procedure depending on your special needs.

□ As you cross time zones in an airplane, keep your watch set according to the departure time. (This is not necessary when traveling by ship because the time changes occur more slowly.)

□ IF YOU ARE FLYING *EAST*
    • If your day is shortened by 3 or more hours, you will probably require less insulin on the day of departure. Your doctor will calculate how much less insulin you should take depending upon your condition and the time difference between the two points of travel.
    • When you arrive at your destination, take your insulin and meals at the

436

usual times. Set your watch to the time of the country you are in. ALWAYS USE NEW LOCAL TIMES.

☐ IF YOU ARE FLYING *WEST*
- Take your usual dose of insulin the morning before the flight.
- If your day is lengthened by 3 or more hours, you will probably require a few extra units of regular insulin or a few extra units of long-acting insulin. Your doctor will calculate how much more insulin you should take depending upon your condition and the time difference between the two points of travel. Your doctor can tell you the correct time to take this "catch-up" dose of insulin.
- This extra insulin will have to be balanced with extra food. Your doctor, nurse, or dietitian can tell you what time to eat extra food as well as the type and amount of food to eat.

☐ When you arrive at your destination, take your insulin and meals at the usual times. Set your watch to the time of the country you are in. ALWAYS USE NEW LOCAL TIMES.

GENERAL INSTRUCTIONS FOR DIABETIC PATIENTS

☐ Keep a regular schedule of daily activities. Eat, exercise, and take your insulin at approximately the same time every day.

☐ The diet that your doctor has prescribed has been carefully planned especially for you. It is to your advantage to follow it very closely.

☐ Test your urine regularly for sugar and if your doctor recommends, test it for acetone.

☐ Learn the signs of hypoglycemia (low blood sugar). When this happens, your urine sugar will be negative. Hypoglycemia may occur if you delay or skip a meal, exercise too much, become sick or emotionally upset, take too much insulin, drink alcohol, or take certain drugs. If you develop sweating, drowsiness, headache, unusual hunger, dizziness, nausea, nervousness, blurred vision, weakness, shaking, or trembling, eat or drink any of the following:
- 2 sugar cubes or 2 teaspoons of sugar in water
- 4 ounces orange juice
- 4 ounces regular ginger ale, cola beverages, or any other sweetened carbonated beverage. Do NOT use low-calorie or diet beverages.
- 2 to 3 teaspoons honey or corn syrup
- 4 Lifesaver candies

Artificial sweeteners are of no use. Call your doctor if one of the above does not relieve your symptoms in about 15 minutes.

☐ Always carry sugar cubes or hard candy in case you have a hypoglycemic (low blood sugar) reaction.

☐ Before you purchase any nonprescription medicine (for example, cough and cold medicines), ask your pharmacist if the medicine is safe for diabetic patients to use. Some nonprescription medicines have very high sugar contents which could interfere with the control of your diabetes. Aspirin and

437

medicines containing salicylates or vitamin C could affect your urine test results. Check with your pharmacist.

☐ Ask your doctor if it is safe for you to drink alcoholic beverages because without care the combination could cause low blood sugar (see Appendix E).

☐ Take special care of your feet.
- Wash your feet daily and dry them well.
- Check your feet daily for minor injuries. Bring these to the attention of your doctor immediately.
- Wear clean shoes and stockings and choose shoes that fit well.
- If you develop corns or calluses, soak your feet in lukewarm water for about 10 minutes. Then rub then off gently with a pumice stone. Never use a knife to cut corns or calluses on your feet. Do NOT use commercial corn removers or commercial arch supports.
- Soften dry skin by rubbing with oil or lotion.
- Trim your toenails straight across with a file or a nail cutter. Do not cut your own toenails if your eyesight is poor.
- Do not wear garters or socks with tight elastic tops. Do NOT sit with your knees crossed.
- Do not warm your feet with a hot water bottle or a heating pad. Use loose bed socks instead. If your feet are cold under normal conditions, tell your doctor. Your circulation may be poor and your doctor can offer advice.
- Call your doctor if you injure your toes or feet. Cuts and scratches in the diabetic patient can become infected easily and take longer to heal. Do not apply iodine or strong antiseptics to the feet at any time.

☐ Call your doctor immediately if you develop any of the following symptoms of hyperglycemia (high blood sugar): high urine sugar, acetone in urine, drowsiness, hunger, unusual thirst, fast breathing, nausea, confusion, a flushed dry skin, increase in urination ("passing your water"), or a fruity odor to the breath. These symptoms may occur if you take too little insulin, miss a dose, overeat, or have a fever or infection.

☐ Call your doctor if you become sick and have a fever, an infection, nausea, or vomiting.

☐ Carry an identification card or wear a bracelet indicating that you are a diabetic and that you are taking this medicine. Always tell your pharmacist, dentist, and other doctors who are treating you that you are taking this medicine.

* * * * *

Iodinated Glycerol (*Oral Expectorant*)
United States: Organidin
Canada: Organidin

☐ This medicine is used to help relieve dry irritating coughs and to thin the sputum.

438

☐ IMPORTANT: If you have ever had an allergic reaction to iodide medicine, tell your doctor or pharmacist before you take any of this medicine.

HOW TO USE THIS MEDICINE
☐ Take the medicine with a little liquid.

SPECIAL INSTRUCTIONS
☐ Women who are pregnant, breast-feeding, or planning to become pregnant should tell their doctor before taking this medicine.

☐ Call your doctor if the cough lasts longer than 1 week or if you develop a fever, skin rash, or persistent headache.

☐ Most people experience few or no side effects from their drugs. However, any medicine can sometimes cause unwanted effects. Call your doctor if you develop a sore throat, "runny nose," metallic taste, stomach pain, mouth sores, or swollen glands.

☐ Do not use this medicine for more than 1 week without the advice of your doctor.

* * * * *

Iodochlorhydroxyquin (*See Clioquinol*)

Isoamyl Nitrite (*See Amyl Nitrate*)

Isocarboxazid (*Oral Antidepressant*)
United States: Marplan
Canada: Marplan

☐ This medicine is used to help relieve the symptoms of depression. It is important that you take the medicine regularly and that you do not miss any doses. The full effect of the medicine will not be noticed immediately but may take from a few days to several weeks. Early signs of improvement are increased appetite, better sleep, increased energy and, later, improved mood. DO NOT STOP TAKING the medicine when you first feel better or you may feel worse in 3 or 4 days.

HOW TO USE THIS MEDICINE
☐ It is best to take this medicine with a glass of water.

☐ While taking this medicine and for at least 2 weeks after your treatment ends, you must be very careful about your diet. You must not eat any of the following foods or beverages because you could experience a very unpleasant reaction (severe headache, nausea, vomiting, and chest pains):

- Aged and natural cheese (for example, cheddar, blue, Camembert, Stilton, Gruyère, Brie, Swiss, and Emmenthaler). In general, avoid food in which aging is used to increase the flavor. Cream cheese, processed cheese, and cottage cheese are safe to eat.
- Sour cream or yogurt.
- Wines, especially Chianti and other heavy red wines.
- Alcoholic beverages, including sherry and beer.
- Canned figs or raisins.
- Yeast extracts (such as Marmite or Bovril) or meat extracts.
- Chicken livers.
- Broad beans (also called fava beans).
- Fermented sausage (such as fermented bolognas and salamis, pepperoni, and summer sausage).
- Pickled or kippered herring.
- Meats prepared with tenderizers.
- Avocados, bananas.
- Soya sauce.
- Chocolate.
- Excessive amounts of caffeine (for example, coffee, tea, cola beverages).

SPECIAL INSTRUCTIONS

☐ If you forget to take a dose, take it as soon as possible. However, if your next dose is within 2 hours, do not take the missed dose but continue with your regular schedule.

☐ Any medicine has a few unwanted side effects. Because this medicine takes a few weeks to work, the side effects are the only thing that tell the doctor that the drug is being absorbed. Most of these side effects will go away as your body adjusts to the medicine.

☐ In some people, this drug may cause dizziness or drowsiness. Do not drive a car or operate dangerous machinery or do jobs that require you to be alert until you know how you are going to react to this drug.

☐ If this medicine causes dizziness, you should be careful going up and down stairs and you should not change positions too quickly. Get out of bed slowly in the morning and dangle your feet over the edge of the bed for a few minutes before standing up. Sit or lie down at the first sign of dizziness. Tell your doctor you have been dizzy.

☐ It is important that you obtain the advice of your doctor or pharmacist before taking any other medicines, including pain relievers, sleeping pills, tranquilizers, other medicines for depression, cough/cold or allergy medicines, or weight-reducing medicine.

☐ If your mouth becomes dry, suck a hard sour candy (sugarless) or ice chips, or chew gum. It is especially important to brush your teeth regularly if you develop a dry mouth.

☐ This medicine may make some people more sensitive to sunlight and sunlamps. When you begin taking this medicine, try to avoid getting too much sun until you see how you are going to react. If your skin does become more sensitive to sunlight, tell your doctor and try to stay out of direct sunlight. While in the sun, wear protective clothing and sunglasses. You may wish to ask your pharmacist about suitable sunscreen products. Check with your doctor if you become sunburned.

☐ If you become constipated, try increasing the amount of bulk in your diet (for example, bran, salads), exercising more often, or drinking water.

☐ Call your doctor immediately if you develop frequent or severe headaches, chest pains, rapid heart rate, nausea, or vomiting. If you cannot reach your doctor, call a hospital emergency department.

☐ Most people experience few or no side effects from their drugs. However, any medicine can sometimes cause unwanted effects. Call your doctor if you develop a skin rash, fever, fainting, difficulty in urinating ("passing your water"), swelling of the legs and ankles, eye pain, or changes in ability to see red and green colors.

☐ Do not stop taking this medicine suddenly without your doctor's approval. Have your prescriptions refilled before you are completely out of this medicine so that you will not miss any doses. When your doctor tells you to stop this medicine, you must follow these precautions for 2 weeks since some of the medicine will still be in your body.

☐ Carry an identification card indicating that you are taking this medicine. Always tell your dentist, pharmacist, and other doctors who are treating you that you are taking this medicine.

* * * * *

Isoetharine (Inhalation Bronchodilator)
United States: Bronkometer

☐ This medicine is used to help open the bronchioles (air passages in the lungs) to make breathing easier.

☐ IMPORTANT: If you have ever had an allergic reaction to any cough/cold, allergy, heart, or weight-reducing medicines, tell your doctor or pharmacist before you take any of this medicine.

HOW TO USE THIS MEDICINE
☐ INSTRUCTIONS FOR USE
    1. If troubled with sputum, try to clear your chest as completely as possible before using this medicine. This will help the drug to reach

441

the lungs and will allow more thorough clearing of mucus during subsequent coughing.
2. Hold the inhaler upright during use so that the mouthpiece is at the bottom.
3. Shake the canister.
4. Breathe out fully and place the lips tightly around the mouthpiece and tilt the head slightly back.

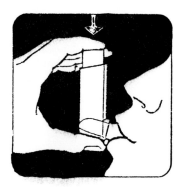

5. Start to breathe in slowly and press down firmly and fully on the valve at the middle of or early during inspiration ("breathing in") to release a "puff." Take the inhaler out of the mouth and close the lips.

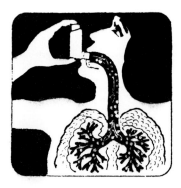

6. Hold your breath for a few seconds. Breathe out through your nose slowly.
7. If your doctor has prescribed a second dose, wait at least 30 seconds before shaking the container again and repeating this procedure.
8. Rinse your mouth with warm water after you have inhaled the medicine. This will help prevent your mouth and throat from becoming dry.
9. The mouthpiece of the inhaler should be kept clean and dry.
10. Failure to follow these instructions carefully can result in inadequate treatment.

SPECIAL INSTRUCTIONS

☐ Do not change the dose of your regular asthma or bronchitis medicines except on the advice of your doctor.

☐ Store the container in a cool place. Do not place the container in hot water or near radiators, stoves, or other sources of heat. Do not puncture, burn, or incinerate the container (even when it is empty).

☐ Call your doctor if the medicine does not relieve your breathing problems, or if your sputum turns yellow or green in color.

☐ Most people experience few or no side effects from their drugs. However, any medicine can sometimes cause unwanted effects. Call your doctor if you develop chest pain, headaches, palpitations, or dizziness.

* * * * *

Isoflurophate (*Ophthalmic Miotic*)
United States: Floropryl Ophthalmic

HOW TO USE THIS MEDICINE

☐ For EYE OINTMENT

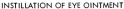

INSTILLATION OF EYE OINTMENT

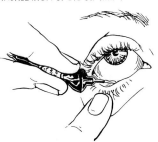

- The person administering the eye ointment should wash his hands with soap and water.
- The eye ointment must be kept clean. Do not touch the tube against the face or anything else.
- Lie down or tilt your head backward and look at the ceiling.
- Gently pull down the lower lid of your eye to form a pouch.
- Hold the tube in your other hand and place the tube as close as possible to the eye without touching it.
- Squeeze the prescribed amount of ointment (usually $\frac{1}{2}$ inch in adults) from the tube along the pouch.
- Close your eyes. Do not rub them.
- Wipe off any excess ointment around the eye with a tissue.
- Clean the tip of the ointment tube with a tissue.

443

☐ If necessary, have someone else administer the eye ointment for you.

☐ Keep the eye ointment tube tightly closed when not in use. Do not use the drug more frequently or in larger quantities than prescribed by your doctor.

SPECIAL INSTRUCTIONS

☐ If you are routinely exposed to organophosphorus insecticides or pesticides such as parathion and malathion (e.g., farmers, lawn service workers, aerial sprayers, or home users) you may be more sensitive to this medicine. It is advisable to wear a face mask when you are exposed to the insecticides and pesticides and to wash and change your clothes after exposure.

☐ Vision may be blurred for a few minutes after using the eye medicine. Do not drive a car or operate dangerous machinery or do jobs that require you to be alert until your vision has cleared.

☐ During the first few days of using the eye drops, you may experience aching in the eyes and head. This is not unusual and should disappear. Call your doctor if the pain persists.

☐ If you forget to use the medicine, use it as soon as possible. However, if it is almost time for your next dose, do not use the missed dose but continue with your regular schedule.

☐ Do not use this medicine at the same time as any other eye medicine without the approval of your doctor. Some medicines cannot be mixed.

☐ Contact your doctor if the condition for which you are using this medicine does not improve or if the eye becomes irritated by it for more than a few minutes. Many eye medicines sting for a short time immediately after use. Also call your doctor if you develop excessive sweating, flushing, stomach cramps, diarrhea (loose bowel movements), difficulty in breathing, difficulty in urinating ("passing your water"), or muscle weakness.

☐ Always tell any future doctors who are treating you that you have used this medicine.

☐ For external use only. Do not swallow.

*   *   *   *   *

Isoniazid (Oral Antituberculous Agent)

United States: Hyzyd, Laniazid, Niconyl, Nydrazid, Rolazid, Teebaconin

Canada: Isotamine, Rimifon

☐ This medicine is used to prevent or help the body overcome tuberculosis. Because tuberculosis (TB) heals very slowly, it may be necessary for you to take this medicine for a long time.

444

□ It is very important that you keep taking this medicine for the full length of time that your doctor has prescribed. Do not stop taking the medicine earlier than your doctor has recommended in spite of the fact that you may feel better. DO NOT MISS ANY DOSES and DO NOT RUN OUT OF THIS MEDICINE.

□ The most important thing you can do to protect others from catcing your TB is to take your medicine regularly and to cover your coughs and sneezes with a double-ply tissue. This will reduce the spray of germs into the air. Covering your mouth with the bare hand does no good.

HOW TO USE THIS MEDICINE
□ This medicine may be taken with food if it upsets your stomach.

SPECIAL INSTRUCTIONS
□ If you forget to take a dose, take it as soon as you remember and then continue with your regular schedule. However, if it is almost time for your next dose, do not take the dose you forgot.

□ Women who are pregnant, breast-feeding, or planning to become pregnant should tell their doctor before taking this medicine.

□ It is best to avoid taking this medicine at the same time as antacids containing aluminum. If you must take the antacid, take it at least 1 hour after this medicine. Check with your pharmacist if you have any questions.

□ It is recommended that you avoid the use of alcoholic beverages while you are taking this medicine.

□ Check with your doctor if you develop blurred vision or any changes in your eyesight. He may want you to have your eyes checked.

□ Most people experience few or no side effects from their drugs. However, any medicine can sometimes cause unwanted effects. Call your doctor if you develop numbness or tingling in the hands or feet, a skin rash, sore throat or fever, vomiting, loss of appetite, unusual tiredness or weakness, dark-colored urine or a yellow color in the skin or eyes.

*   *   *   *   *

Isopropamide (*Oral Anticholinergic*)
United States: Darbid
Canada: Darbid

□ This medicine is used to help relax muscles of the stomach and bowels as well as to decrease the amount of acid formed in the stomach.

□ IMPORTANT: If you have ever had an allergic reaction to atropine or iodides or any other drug used to relax the stomach or bowels, tell your doctor or pharmacist before you take any of this medicine.

HOW TO USE THIS MEDICINE

- ☐ Take this medicine approximately 30 minutes before a meal unless otherwise directed.

- ☐ If you miss a dose of this medicine, do not take the missed dose and do not double the next dose.

SPECIAL INSTRUCTIONS

- ☐ Women who are pregnant, breast-feeding, or planning to become pregnant should tell their doctor before taking this medicine.

- ☐ If your mouth becomes dry, suck a hard sour candy (sugarless) or ice chips, or chew gum. It is especially important to brush your teeth regularly if you develop a dry mouth.

- ☐ In some people, this drug may cause dizziness or drowsiness. Do not drive a car or operate dangerous machinery or do jobs that require you to be alert until you know how you are going to react to this drug.

- ☐ If you become dizzy, you should be careful going up and down stairs. Sit or lie down at the first sign of dizziness. Tell your doctor you have been dizzy.

- ☐ A desire to urinate ("pass your water") with an inability to do so is not an uncommon effect with this drug. Urinating each time before taking the drug may help relieve this problem. Call your doctor if it continues.

- ☐ You may become more sensitive to heat because your body may perspire less while you are taking this drug. Be careful not to become overheated during exercise or in hot weather.

- ☐ Do not take antacids within 1 hour of taking this medicine as they could make this medicine less effective.

- ☐ If you become constipated, try increasing the amount of bulk in your diet (for example, bran and salads), exercising more often, or drinking more water. Call your doctor if the constipation continues.

- ☐ If your eyes become more sensitive to sunlight, it may help to wear sunglasses.

- ☐ Most people experience few or no side effects from their drugs. However, any medicine can sometimes cause unwanted effects. Call your doctor if you develop a skin rash, diarrhea, unusual restlessness, flushing, or eye pain.

*　*　*　*　*

Isopropamide-Prochlorperazine (*Oral Anticholinergic-Antianxiety*)

United States: Combid

Canada: Combid

- ☐ This medicine is used to help relax muscles of the stomach and bowels as well as to decrease the amount of acid formed in the stomach.

446

- ☐ IMPORTANT: If you have ever had an allergic reaction to atropine, iodides, or phenothiazine medicines or any other drug used to relax the stomach or bowels, tell your doctor or pharmacist before you take any of this medicine.

HOW TO USE THIS MEDICINE

- ☐ Take this medicine approximately 30 minutes before a meal unless otherwise directed.

- ☐ This medicine must be swallowed whole. Do not crush, chew, or break it into pieces. (**United States** and **Canada:** Combid Spansules)

- ☐ If you miss a dose of this medicine, do not take the missed dose and do not double the next dose.

SPECIAL INSTRUCTIONS

- ☐ Women who are pregnant, breast-feeding, or planning to become pregnant should tell their doctor before taking this medicine.

- ☐ If your mouth becomes dry, suck a hard sour candy (sugarless) or ice chips, or chew gum. It is especially important to brush you teeth regularly if you develop a dry mouth.

- ☐ In some people, this drug may cause dizziness or drowsiness. Do not drive a car or operate dangerous machinery or do jobs that require you to be alert until you know how you are going to react to this drug.

- ☐ If this medicine causes dizziness, you should be careful going up and down stairs and you should not change positions too rapidly. Get out of bed slowly in the morning and dangle your feet over the edge of the bed for a few minutes before standing up. Sit down or lie down at the first sign of dizziness. Tell your doctor you have been dizzy. Avoid hot showers and baths because they could make you dizzy.

- ☐ Do not drink alcoholic beverages while taking this drug without the approval of your doctor.

- ☐ It is important that you obtain the advice of your doctor or pharmacist before taking pain relievers, nonprescription drugs, sleeping pills, tranquilizers, or medicine for depression while you are taking this drug.

- ☐ Do not take any more of this medicine than your doctor has prescribed and do not stop taking this medicine suddenly without the approval of your doctor.

- ☐ A desire to urinate ("pass your water") with an inability to do so is not an uncommon effect with this drug. Urinating each time before taking the drug may help relieve this problem. Call your doctor if it continues.

- ☐ You may become more sensitive to heat because your body may perspire less while you are taking this drug. Be careful not to become overheated during exercise or in hot weather.

- ☐ Do not take antacids within 1 hour of taking this medicine because they could make this medicine less effective.

☐ If you become constipated, try increasing the amount of bulk in your diet (for example, bran and salads), exercising more often, or drinking more water. Call your doctor if the constipation continues.

☐ This medicine may make some people more sensitive to sunlight and sun-lamps. When you begin taking this medicine, try to avoid getting too much sun until you see how you are going to react. If your skin does become more sensitive to sunlight, tell your doctor and try to stay out of direct sunlight. While in the sun, wear protective clothing and sunglasses. You may wish to ask your pharmacist about suitable sunscreen products. Check with your doctor if you become sunburned.

☐ Most people experience few or no side effects from their drugs. However, any medicine can sometimes cause unwanted effects. Call your doctor if you develop a skin rash; diarrhea; unusual restlessness; flushing or eye pain; a yellow color to the skin or eyes; unusual movements or trembling of the face, tongue, or hands; or a shuffling walk.

*   *   *   *   *

Isoproterenol (*Inhalation Bronchodilator*)
United States: Isuprel, Iprenol, Medihaler-Iso, Norisodrine Aerotrol
Canada: Isuprel, Medihaler-Iso

Isoproterenol-Phenylephrine
United States: Duo-Medihaler, Duohaler
Canada: Isuprel-Neo Mistometer, Duo-Medihaler

Isoproterenol-Cyclopentamine
Canada: Aerolone Compound

☐ This medicine is used to help open up the bronchioles (air passages in the lungs) and make breathing easier.

☐ IMPORTANT: If you have *ever* had an allergic reaction to any cough/cold, allergy, heart, or weight-reducing medicines, tell your doctor or pharmacist before you take any of this medicine.

HOW TO USE THIS MEDICINE
☐ Instructions for use of Mistometer: (*United States:* Isuprel; *Canada:* Isuprel, Isuprel-Neo Mistometer)
    1. Pull the cap from the mouthpiece.
    2. Pull the white mouthpiece off the bottle, turn it sideways, and fit the hole in the flattened end onto the metal spout (valve stem) of the bottle.
    3. During use, the mistometer must always be turned upside down as it does **not** operate properly in the upright position.

4. Hold the assembled unit between the thumb and index finger.
5. Breathe out completely. Invert the bottle and close your lips around the open end of the mouthpiece. Breathe in deeply while firmly pressing down on the bottle. Breathe out through the nose.
6. Wait one full minute if a second dose is necessary.
7. Replace the mouthpiece and cap on the bottle to protect it at all times.
8. Run warm or cold water through the mouthpiece after each use to clean it. You may sanitize it by washing it in alcohol.

☐ Instructions for use of Medihaler: (**United States** and **Canada:** Duo-Medihaler, Medihaler-Iso)

1. Before use, remove the dustcap and shake the Medihaler.
2. Hold the Medihaler with the metal vial (contains the medicine) upside down. (**United States** and **Canada:** Medihaler-Iso)
   Hold the Medihaler upright. (**United States** and **Canada:** Duo-Medihaler)
3. Breathe out fully and place the mouthpiece well into the mouth, aimed at the back of the throat.
4. Start to breathe in slowly and press the vial firmly down into the adapter at the middle of inspiration ("breathing in"). This releases **one** dose.
5. Continue to breathe in until your lungs are completely filled.
6. Release pressure on the vial and remove the unit from your mouth.
7. Hold your breath as long as possible, then breathe out slowly.
8. The mouthpiece should be kept clean. Remove the metal vial and rinse the oral adapter with running water. Dry and replace the vial.

☐ Instructions for use of Nebulizer: (**Canada:** Aerolone Compound)

1. Place a small amount of solution in the nebulizer.
2. Aim the mouthpiece, through the mouth, at the back of the throat. Keep about two inches away from the mouth.

☐ Instructions for use of Aerotrol: (**United States:** Norisodrine Aerotrol)

1. Remove the white plastic mouthpiece from the bottle.
2. Pull the plastic connector sleeve out from mouthpiece to expose the connecting slot.
3. Insert the bottle's spray head into the slot of the connector sleeve.
4. Insert the mouthpiece deep in your mouth. The bottle must be held right side up as indicated by the arrow on the label.
5. Breathe out completely. Close the lips firmly around the mouthpiece. Take a deep breath through the mouthpiece and press down on the spray head at the same time.
6. Hold your breath for a few seconds, then remove the mouthpiece and breathe out slowly.
7. The mouthpiece should be washed regularly.

☐ Start with one inhalation. If two inhalations are required to relieve the attack, wait one minute after the first inhalation before taking a second inhalation.

(**United States:** Medihaler-Iso; **Canada:** Isuprel-Neo Mistometer, Medihaler-Iso)

☐ Do not use more than two inhalations in one hour. If after three doses of the medicine you do not get relief of your attack, do not use any more inhalations for that attack. Contact your doctor immediately. (**United States:** Norisodrine Aerotrol)

SPECIAL INSTRUCTIONS

☐ Do not change the dose of your regular asthma or bronchitis medicines except on the advice of your doctor.

☐ The medicine may cause your saliva to turn pink or red in color. This is not an unusual effect.

☐ Rinse your mouth after you have inhaled the medicine. This will help prevent your mouth and throat from becoming dry.

☐ Do not use the solution if it turns pink or brown in color.

☐ Store in a cool place. Do not place the container in hot water or near radiators, stoves, or other sources of heat. Do not puncture, burn, or incinerate the container (even when it is empty).

☐ Call your doctor if the medicine does not relieve your breathing problems.

☐ Most people experience few or no side effects from their drugs. However, any medicine can sometimes cause unwanted effects. Call your doctor if you develop swollen glands, skin rash, dizziness, sweating, or chest pain.

* * * * *

Isoproterenol (*Sublingual Bronchodilator*)
United States: Isuprel
Canada: Isuprel

☐ This medicine is used to help open up the bronchioles (air passages in the lungs) to make breathing easier.

☐ IMPORTANT: If you have ever had an allergic reaction to any cough/cold, allergy, heart, or weight-reducing medicines, tell your doctor or pharmacist before you take any of this medicine.

HOW TO USE THIS MEDICINE

☐ Place the tablet under your tongue or in the pouch of your cheek. Do not swallow until the tablet has completely dissolved.

☐ Rinse your mouth or brush your teeth after the tablet has dissolved in order to wash the medicine off the teeth.

SPECIAL INSTRUCTIONS

☐ Do not change the dose of your regular asthma or bronchitis medicines except on the advice of your doctor.

- ☐ It is not unusual to have a little flushing of the face or a faster heartbeat just after you take the medicine.
- ☐ The medicine may cause your saliva to turn pink or red in color.
- ☐ Call your doctor if the medicine does not relieve your breathing problems.
- ☐ Most people experience few or no side effects from their drugs. However, any medicine can sometimes cause unwanted effects. Call your doctor if you develop swollen glands, skin rash, dizziness, sweating, or chest pain.

* * * * *

Isosorbide Dinitrate (*Sublingual and Chewable Coronary Vasodilator*)

United States: Iso-Bid, Isordil, Isotrate, Onset, Sorbitate

Canada: Coronex, Isordil

- ☐ This medicine is used to help relieve a type of chest pain called angina.
- ☐ Carry this medicine with you at all times.

HOW TO USE THIS MEDICINE

- ☐ SUBLINGUAL TABLETS
  - This medicine should be used at the FIRST sign of an attack of angina. Do not wait until the pain becomes severe. Sit down or lie down as soon as you feel an attack of angina coming on.
  - Then place a tablet UNDER YOUR TONGUE or in the pouch of your cheek until it is completely dissolved. Do NOT swallow or chew these tablets.
  - Try not to swallow until the drug is dissolved and do not rinse the mouth for a few minutes. Do not eat, drink, or smoke while the tablet is dissolving.
  - If your angina is not relieved within 5 to 10 minutes, you may dissolve a second tablet under your tongue, unless otherwise directed.
  - If the angina continues for another 5 to 10 minutes, you may use a third tablet. If this does not relieve your chest pains, call your doctor immediately or go to the nearest hospital emergency department.

- ☐ CHEWABLE TABLETS
  - This medicine should be used at the FIRST sign of an attack of angina. Do not wait until the pain becomes severe. Sit down or lie down as soon as you feel an attack of angina coming on.
  - Then CHEW the tablet well and hold it in the mouth for 1 to 2 minutes without swallowing. Do not rinse the mouth for a few minutes.
  - If your angina is not relieved within 5 to 10 minutes, you may chew a second tablet unless otherwise directed. If the angina continues for another 5 to 10 minutes, chew a third tablet. If this does not relieve your chest pains, call your doctor immediately or go to the nearest hospital emergency department.

451

HOW TO USE THIS MEDICINE

☐ Store in a cool, dry place but not in the bathroom medicine cabinet or the refrigerator because these areas are very humid.

SPECIAL INSTRUCTIONS

☐ After using this medicine, you may get a headache or flushing which will usually disappear within a few minutes. This is a common side effect. If the headaches do not go away, tell your doctor.

☐ Try to relax and remain calm when you are taking the medicine. If you become dizzy or feel faint, breathe deeply and bend forward with your head between your knees. Always get up slowly after you have been sitting or lying down.

☐ Do not drink alcoholic beverages too soon after taking this medicine as they may make the dizziness and fainting worse.

☐ Some nonprescription drugs can aggravate your heart condition. Do not take any of the following without the approval of your doctor or pharmacist: cough, cold, or sinus products; asthma or allergy products; or diet or weight-reducing medicines.

☐ You may help prevent angina by taking a tablet 5 to 10 minutes before activities you know are likely to trigger attacks, such as strenuous exercise, emotional stress, a heavy meal, high altitudes, or exposure to cold. Let your doctor know what things usually cause your angina so that he can advise you about preventing attacks.

☐ Cigarette smoking can aggravate angina and is a special risk for people who have heart conditions.

☐ Most people experience few or no side effects from their drugs. However, any medicine can sometimes cause unwanted effects. Call your doctor if you develop a skin rash, fainting spells, nausea or vomiting, or a rapid pulse, or if your chest pain is not relieved.

☐ Carry an identification card indicating that you are taking this medicine. Always tell your pharmacist, dentist, and other doctors who are treating you that you are taking this medicine.

*   *   *   *   *

Isosorbide Dinitrate (Oral and Sustained Release Coronary Vasodilator)

United States: Iso-Bid, Isordil Tembids, Isordil Titradose, Isotrate Timecelles, Laserdil, Sorbide-10, Sorbitrate, Sorbitrate SA

Canada: Coronex, Isordil

☐ This medicine is used to help prevent angina attacks and must be taken regularly as your doctor has prescribed. Do not miss any doses. It will not relieve an angina attack that has already started because it works too slowly.

452

HOW TO USE THIS MEDICINE

- [ ] It is best to take this medicine on an empty stomach 1 hour before (or 2 hours after) eating food.

- [ ] SUSTAINED RELEASE MEDICINE
  - Swallow this medicine whole. Do not crush, chew, or break it into pieces. (**United States:** Iso-Bid, Isordil Tembids, Isotrate Timecelles, Sorbide T.D., Sorbitrate SA)
  - If you do forget to take a dose, take it as soon as possible. However, if your next dose is within 6 hours, do not take the missed dose but continue with your regular schedule.

- [ ] ORAL TABLETS
  - If you forget to take a dose, take it as soon as possible. However, if your next dose is within 2 hours, do not take the missed dose but continue with your regular schedule.

HOW TO STORE THIS MEDICINE

- [ ] Store in a cool, dry place but not in the bathroom medicine cabinet or refrigerator because these areas are humid.

SPECIAL INSTRUCTIONS

- [ ] If you become dizzy or feel faint, breathe deeply and bend forward with your head between your knees. Always get up slowly after you have been sitting or lying down. Get out of bed slowly in the morning and dangle your feet over the edge of the bed for a few minutes before standing up. Do not drive a car or operate dangerous machinery or do jobs that require you to be alert if you are dizzy or drowsy.

- [ ] Do not drink alcoholic beverages while you are taking this medicine because they may make the dizziness and fainting worse.

- [ ] Some nonprescription drugs can aggravate your heart condition. Do not take any of the following without the approval of your doctor or pharmacist: cough, cold, or sinus products; asthma or allergy products; or diet or weight-reducing medicines.

- [ ] When you first start taking this medicine, you may get a headache or flushing. This is a common side effect and will usually disappear after you have taken the drug a few times. If the headaches do not go away or are severe, call your doctor.

- [ ] Cigarette smoking can aggravate angina and is a special risk for people who have angina.

- [ ] Most people experience few or no side effects from their drugs. However, any medicine can sometimes cause unwanted effects. Call your doctor if you develop a skin rash, fainting spells, nausea or vomiting, or a rapid pulse, or if your chest pain is not relieved.

- [ ] Do not stop taking the medicine suddenly or it could cause an angina attack.

□ Carry an identification card indicating that you are taking this medicine. Always tell your pharmacist, dentist, and other doctors who are treating you that you are taking this medicine.

* * * * *

Isoxsuprine HCl (*Oral Uterine Relaxant and Peripheral Vasodilator*)

United States: Vasodilan, Vasoprine

Canada: Vasodilan

□ This medicine is used to improve the circulation of blood in the body.

HOW TO USE THIS MEDICINE

□ This medicine may be taken with food or on an empty stomach.

□ If you forget to take a dose, take it as soon as possible. However, if it is almost time for your next dose, do not take the missed dose. Instead, continue with your regular dosing schedule.

SPECIAL INSTRUCTIONS

□ Women who are pregnant, breast-feeding, or planning to become pregnant should tell their doctor before taking this medicine.

□ If this medicine causes dizziness, you should be careful going up and down stairs and you should not change positions too rapidly. Get out of bed slowly in the morning and dangle your feet over the edge of the bed for a few minutes before standing up. Sit down or lie down at the first sign of dizziness. Tell your doctor you have been dizzy. Do not drive a car or operate dangerous machinery if you are dizzy. Avoid hot showers and baths because they could make you dizzy.

□ Some nonprescription drugs can aggravate your condition. Do not take any of the following without the approval of your doctor or pharmacist: cough, cold, or sinus products; asthma or allergy products; or diet or weight-reducing medicines.

□ Do not drink alcoholic beverages while taking this drug without the approval of your doctor.

□ The activity of this drug is improved if you keep warm. Avoid getting cold or exposing yourself to a cold environment.

□ Most people experience few or no side effects from their drugs. However, any medicine can sometimes cause unwanted effects. Call your doctor if you develop a skin rash, fainting spells, nausea or vomiting, or a fast heart rate.

* * * * *

454

Kanamycin Sulfate (*Oral Antibiotic*)
United States: Kantrex
Canada: Kantrex

☐ This medicine is an antibiotic used to treat certain types of infections.

☐ IMPORTANT: If you have ever had an allergic reaction to any antibiotics, tell your doctor or pharmacist before you take any of this medicine.

HOW TO USE THIS MEDICINE
☐ This medicine may be taken either with meals or on an empty stomach.

SPECIAL INSTRUCTIONS
☐ It is important to take *all* of this medicine plus any refills that your doctor told you to take. Do not stop taking it earlier than your doctor has recommended in spite of the fact that you may feel better. Otherwise, the infection may return.

☐ If you forget to take a dose, take it as soon as you remember and then continue with your regular schedule.

☐ Most people experience few or no side effects from their drugs. However, any medicine can sometimes cause unwanted effects. Call your doctor if you develop "ringing" or "buzzing" in the ears or difficulty hearing, become dizzy, or if you become very thirsty or urinate ("pass your water") less frequently or in smaller amounts than normal.

☐ Call your doctor immediately if you think you may be allergic to the medicine or if you develop a skin rash, hives, itching, swelling of the face, or difficulty in breathing. If you cannot reach your doctor, phone a hospital emergency department.

☐ If for some reason you cannot take all of the medicine, throw away the unused portion by flushing it down the toilet. Do not take or save old medicine.

*　*　*　*　*

Kaolin-Pectin Preparations (*Oral Antidiarrheal*)
United States: Kaomead, Kaopectate, Pargel
Canada: Donnagel-MB, Kao-Con, Kaopectate

☐ This medicine is used in the treatment of diarrhea.

HOW TO USE THIS MEDICINE
☐ Shake the liquid medicine well before using so that you can measure an accurate dose.

- ☐ Do not take any more of this medicine than your doctor has prescribed.
- ☐ Call your doctor if you develop a fever or if the diarrhea persists.
- ☐ If you are taking any other medicines, check with your pharmacist to see if the other medicines have to be taken at a different time.

* * * * *

Kaolin-Pectin-Belladonna Alkaloids (*Oral Antidiarrheal*)
United States: Donnagel, Kaodonna, Kaomead w/Belladonna
Canada: Donnagel

Kaolin-Pectin-Belladonna Alkaloids-Paregoric
United States: Amogel PG, Donnagel-PG, Kaodonna-PG, Ru-K-N
Canada: Donnagel-PG

- ☐ This medicine is used in the treatment of diarrhea.

HOW TO USE THIS MEDICINE
- ☐ Shake the liquid medicine well before using so that you can measure an accurate dose.

SPECIAL INSTRUCTIONS
- ☐ Do not take any more of this medicine than your doctor has prescribed.
- ☐ If you are taking any other medicines, check with your pharmacist to see if the other medicines have to be taken at a different time.
- ☐ If your mouth becomes dry, suck a hard sour candy (sugarless) or ice chips, or chew gum. It is especially important to brush your teeth regularly if you develop a dry mouth.
- ☐ If this medicine causes blurred vision, do not drive a car or operate dangerous machinery or do jobs that require you to be alert.
- ☐ This medicine may make you perspire less and become more sensitive to heat. Be careful not to get overheated during exercise or in hot weather.
- ☐ Most people experience few or no side effects from their drugs. However, any medicine can sometimes cause unwanted effects. Call your doctor if you develop difficulty in urinating ("passing your water"), eye pain, fast heartbeats, or dizziness.
- ☐ Call your doctor if you develop a fever or if the diarrhea persists.

* * * * *

Kaolin-Pectin-Paregoric *(Oral Antidiarrheal)*
United States: Parepectolin, Pecto-Kalin
Canada: Parepectolin

☐ This medicine is used in the treatment of diarrhea.

HOW TO USE THIS MEDICINE
☐ Shake the liquid medicine well before using to that you can measure an accurate dose.

☐ Store the liquid medicine in a refrigerator but do not freeze.

SPECIAL INSTRUCTIONS
☐ Do not take any more of this medicine than your doctor has prescribed. The drug could become habit-forming or you could take an overdose if you take it more often or longer than prescribed.

☐ If you are taking any other medicines, check with your pharmacist to see if the other medicines have to be taken at a different time.

☐ Do not drink alcoholic beverages while taking this drug without the approval of your doctor.

☐ In some people, this drug may cause dizziness or drowsiness. Do not drive a car or operate dangerous machinery or do jobs that require you to be alert until you know how you are going to react to this drug.

☐ If you become dizzy, you should be careful going up and down stairs. Sit or lie down at the first sign of dizziness.

☐ Call your doctor if you develop a fever or if the diarrhea persists.

* * * * *

Keto-Diastix *(Diagnostic Aid)*
United States: Keto-Diastix
Canada: Keto-Diastix

☐ This preparation is used to detect the presence of glucose (sugar) and ketones in the urine.

☐ Testing procedure:
1. Dip the test end of the strip in urine or pass through the urine stream.
2. Tap the edge of the strip against the bottle to remove excess urine.
3. Compare the test side of the test area to the appropriate color charts. Read at 15 seconds for ketones and at 30 seconds for glucose.

457

- [ ] For further information, refer to the package insert which accompanies this medication.*

*   *   *   *   *

Ketoprofen (*Oral Anti-inflammatory–Analgesic*)
Canada: Orudis

- [ ] This medicine is used to help relieve pain, redness, stiffness, and swelling in certain kinds of arthritis.
- [ ] IMPORTANT: If you have ever had an allergic reaction to aspirin or any other medicine for arthritis, tell your doctor or pharmacist before you take any of this medicine.
- [ ] It is very important that you take this medicine regularly and that you DO NOT MISS ANY DOSES. If you miss a dose, the level of the medicine in your body will fall and the drug will not be as effective. Only if the level of the drug is high enough can it decrease the inflammation and swelling in your joints and help prevent further damage.
- [ ] The full benefit of this medicine may not be noticed immediately but may take from a few days to 3 weeks.

HOW TO USE THIS MEDICINE
- [ ] It is best to take this medicine on an empty stomach at least 1 hour before (or 2 hours after) food unless otherwise directed. If you develop stomach upset, take the medicine with food or immediately after meals. Call your doctor if you continue to have stomach upset.

SPECIAL INSTRUCTIONS
- [ ] In some people, this drug may cause dizziness or drowsiness. Do not drive a car or operate dangerous machinery or do jobs that require you to be alert until you know how you are going to react to this drug.
- [ ] If you become dizzy, you should be careful going up and down stairs. Sit or lie down at the first sign of dizziness.
- [ ] If you forget to take a dose, take it as soon as possible. However, if it is almost time for your next dose, do not take the missed dose. Instead, continue with your regular dosing schedule.
- [ ] While you are taking this medicine, do not drink alcoholic beverages or take aspirin without the permission of your doctor. It is usually safe to take acetaminophen for the occasional headache. Check with your pharmacist.
- [ ] If you become constipated, try increasing the amount of bulk in your diet (for example, bran and salads), exercising more often, or drinking more water. Call your doctor if the constipation continues.

*Keto-Diastix (Package Insert), Ames Company Division, Miles Laboratories, Ltd., Rexdale, Ontario.

☐ Call your doctor immediately if you think you may be allergic to the medicine or if you develop a skin rash, hives, itching, swelling of the face, or difficulty in breathing. If you cannot reach your doctor, phone a hospital emergency department.

☐ Most people experience few or no side effects from their drugs. However, any medicine can sometimes cause unwanted effects. Call your doctor if you develop a skin rash, sore throat or fever, "ringing" or "buzzing" in the ears, fast heartbeats, swelling of the legs or ankles, sudden weight gain, sore tongue or mouth sores, red or black stools, or severe stomach pain.

☐ Carry an identification card indicating that you are taking this medicine. Always tell your pharmacist, dentist, and other doctors who are treating you that you are taking this medicine.

*   *   *   *   *

Lactobacillus Acidophilus (Oral Flora Modifier)
United States: Bacid, Dofus, Lactinex
Canada: Bacid

☐ This medicine is used in the treatment of diarrhea.

HOW TO USE THIS MEDICINE
☐ Take this medicine with one-half glass of milk or tomato juice.

☐ For infants, the medicine may be mixed with cereal, food, milk, or tomato juice.

SPECIAL INSTRUCTIONS
☐ This medicine must be stored in the refrigerator.

☐ Call your doctor if you develop a fever or if the diarrhea persists.

*   *   *   *   *

Lactulose (Oral Laxative)
United States: Cephulac, Duphalac
Canada: Cephulac, Chronulac

☐ This medicine is used in the treatment of certain conditions to reduce the amount of ammonia in the blood or to cause a laxative effect.

HOW TO USE THIS MEDICINE
☐ Take this medicine with a little water.

☐ If you forget to take a dose, take it as soon as possible. However, if it is almost time for your next dose, do not take the missed dose. Instead, continue with your regular dosing schedule.

SPECIAL INSTRUCTIONS

☐ Do not take any laxatives while you are taking this medicine unless otherwise directed.

☐ Check with your doctor if you develop stomach cramps or diarrhea which do not go away as your body adjusts to the medicine.

* * * * *

Lanatoside C (*See Digitoxin*)

* * * * *

Levodopa (*Oral Antiparkinsonian Agent*)
United States: Bendopa, Dopar, Larodopa
Canada: Larodopa, Levopa

Levodopa-Carbidopa
United States: Sinemet
Canada: Sinemet

Levodopa-Benserazide
Canada: Prolopa

☐ This medicine is used in the treatment of Parkinson's disease.

HOW TO USE THIS MEDICINE

☐ Take the drug with food to help prevent stomach upset.

☐ This medicine must be swallowed whole. Do not crush, chew, or break it open. (**Canada:** Prolopa)

☐ If you forget to take a dose of this medicine, take it as soon as possible. However, if your next dose is within 2 hours, do not take the missed dose and do not double doses. Instead, continue with your regular schedule.

SPECIAL INSTRUCTIONS

☐ It is very important that you take this medicine exactly as your doctor has prescribed and that you do not miss any doses. Try to take this medicine at the same time every day. Do not take extra tablets without your doctor's approval.

☐ In some people, this drug may cause dizziness or drowsiness. Do not drive a car or operate dangerous machinery or do jobs that require you to be alert until you know how you are going to react to this drug.

☐ If this medicine causes dizziness, you should be careful going up and down stairs and you should not change positions too rapidly. Get out of bed slowly in the morning and dangle your feet over the edge of the bed for a few

460

minutes before standing up. Sit down or lie down at the first sign of dizziness. Avoid hot showers and baths because they could make you dizzy.

□ If your mouth becomes dry, suck a hard sour candy (sugarless) or ice chips, or chew gum. It is especially important to brush your teeth regularly if you develop a dry mouth.

□ This medicine may cause the urine to turn red in color and then turn black upon being exposed to air. The sweat may also be darker in color. This is not an unusual effect and you should not become alarmed.

□ Some nonprescription drugs can aggravate your condition. Do not take any of the following without the approval of your doctor or pharmacist: cough, cold, or sinus products; asthma or allergy products; or diet or weight-reducing medicines.

□ Do not take vitamins containing vitamin B_6 (pyridoxine) without the approval of your doctor. Vitamin B_6 can reduce the effect of this medicine. Do not eat unusually large amounts of the following foods which contain vitamin B_6: peas, beans, avocados, tuna, sweet potatoes, pork, dry skim milk, beef liver, oatmeal, or fortified cereals. (**United States:** Bendopa, Dopar, Larodopa; **Canada:** Larodopa, Levodopa)

□ As your condition improves, it is important to gradually resume physical activities. This will give your body a chance to adjust to the drug and help prevent you from injuring yourself by falling.

□ Most people experience few or no side effects from their drugs. However, any medicine can sometimes cause unwanted effects. Call your doctor if you develop a sore throat; fever; mouth sores; unusual movements of the hands, face, or tongue; fast heartbeats; unusual weakness; vomiting; muscle twitching or eye twitching; difficulty in urinating ("passing your water"); or depression; or if the medicine seems to stop working (after at least 1 year of treatment).

□ Carry an identification card indicating that you are taking this medicine. Always tell your dentist and other doctors who are treating you that you are taking this medicine.

□ Do not stop taking this medicine without your doctor's approval and do not go without medicine between prescription refills. Call your pharmacist for a refill 2 or 3 days before you run out of the medicine.

* * * * *

Levopropoxyphene (*Oral Antitussive*)
United States: Novrad

□ This medicine is used to help relieve dry irritating coughs.

HOW TO USE THIS MEDICINE
□ Shake the bottle well before using so that you can measure an accurate dose.

□ Take the capsules with a glass of water.

461

- ☐ In some people, this drug may cause drowsiness. Do not drive a car or operate dangerous machinery or do jobs that require you to be alert until you know how you are going to react to this drug.

- ☐ Do not drink alcoholic beverages while taking this drug without the approval of your doctor.

- ☐ Call your doctor if the cough lasts longer than 1 week or if you develop a fever, skin rash, or persistent headache.

- ☐ Do not use this medicine for more than 1 week without the permission of your doctor.

* * * * *

Levorphanol Tartrate (*Oral Analgesic*)
United States: Levo-Dromoran
Canada: Levo-Dromoran

- ☐ This medicine is used to help relieve pain.

HOW TO USE THIS MEDICINE

- ☐ This medicine may be taken with food or a glass of water.

- ☐ Do not take any more of this medicine than your doctor has prescribed. The drug could become habit-forming or you could take an overdose if you take it more often or longer than prescribed.

- ☐ Do not wait to take this medicine until the pain becomes severe. This medicine works best if you take it at the beginning of the pain. Call your doctor if you feel you need it more often than he prescribed.

SPECIAL INSTRUCTIONS

- ☐ Do not drink alcoholic beverages while taking this drug without the approval of your doctor.

- ☐ It is important that you obtain the advice of your doctor or pharmacist before taking ANY other medicines including other pain relievers, sleeping pills, tranquilizers or medicines for depression, cough/cold or allergy medicines, or weight-reducing medicines.

- ☐ In some people, this drug may cause dizziness or drowsiness. Do not drive a car or operate dangerous machinery or do jobs that require you to be alert until you know how you are going to react to this drug.

- ☐ If you become dizzy, you should be careful going up and down stairs. Sit or lie down at the first sign of dizziness. Get up slowly if you have been lying or sitting down.

- ☐ If you do feel nauseated when you first start taking the medicine, it may help if you lie down for a few minutes.

☐ If you become constipated, try increasing the amount of bulk in your diet (for example, bran and salads), exercising more often, or drinking more water. Call your doctor if the constipation continues.

☐ Most people experience few or no side effects from their drugs. However, any medicine sometimes can cause unwanted effects. Call your doctor if you develop shortness of breath, slow heartbeats, unusual nervousness, stomach pain, or difficulty in urinating ("passing your water").

☐ Always tell your dentist, pharmacist, and other doctors who are treating you that you are taking this medicine.

*　*　*　*　*

Lidocaine (Oral Anesthetic)
United States: Xylocaine Viscous
Canada: Xylocaine Viscous

☐ This medicine is used to help relieve pain.

☐ IMPORTANT: If you have ever had an allergic reaction to lidocaine, "freezing," or any "caine" type of medicine, tell your doctor or pharmacist before you use any of this drug.

HOW TO USE THIS MEDICINE
☐ Instructions for use: (**United States** and **Canada:** Xylocaine Viscous)
  • Shake the bottle well before using.
  • Avoid taking food for at least 60 minutes after taking this medicine; otherwise, you may have difficulty in swallowing the food.
  • You should not take more than 2 tablespoonfuls of medicine every 6 hours or 4 fluid ounces in one day unless otherwise directed.

SPECIAL INSTRUCTIONS
☐ Call your doctor if the condition for which this drug is being used persists or becomes worse or if you have a constant irritation such as itching or burning that was not present before you started using this medicine. Also call your doctor if you develop a slow heartbeat, fainting, tremors, or difficulty in breathing.

*　*　*　*　*

Lidocaine (Topical Anesthetic)
United States: Lida-Mantle, Xylocaine Ointment
Canada: Xylocaine Ointment, Xylocaine Topical Spray

☐ This medicine is used to help relieve pain and itching of skin conditions.

☐ IMPORTANT: If you have ever had an allergic reaction to lidocaine or any "caine" type of medicine, tell your doctor or pharmacist before you use any of this drug.

463

HOW TO USE THIS MEDICINE

☐ For TOPICAL SPRAY
- Spray the affected area from a distance of approximately 6 inches.
- Do not inhale vapors or spray near food.
- Do not place the medicine container in hot water or near radiators, stoves, or other sources of heat. Do not puncture or incinerate the container (even when empty). Do not store at temperatures greater than 120°F (49°C).

☐ For OINTMENT
- Cleanse the affected area well with water unless otherwise directed by your doctor.
- For *nipple soreness:* It is important for you to cleanse the nipple area thoroughly before each feeding.
- *Application to broken or burned skin:* Apply to area with a sterile gauze pad after cleaning as directed by your doctor.

SPECIAL INSTRUCTIONS

☐ Call your doctor if the condition for which this drug is being used persists or becomes worse or if you have a constant irritation such as itching or burning that was not present before you started using this medicine. Also call your doctor if you develop a slow heartbeat, fainting, or tremors.

☐ For external use only. Do not swallow.

* * * * *

Lincomycin Hydrochloride *(Oral Antibiotic)*
United States: Lincocin
Canada: Lincocin

☐ This medicine is an antibiotic used to treat certain types of infections.

☐ IMPORTANT: If you have ever had an allergic reaction to any antibiotics, tell your doctor or pharmacist before you take any of this medicine.

HOW TO USE THIS MEDICINE

☐ It is best to take this medicine on an empty stomach at least 1 hour before (or 2 hours after) eating food. Take it at the proper time even if you skip a meal.

☐ Take capsules with a full glass of water. Do not eat or drink anything but water for 1 to 2 hours before and after taking this medicine.

SPECIAL INSTRUCTIONS

☐ It is important to take *all* of this medicine plus any refills that your doctor told you to take. Do not stop taking it earlier than your doctor has recommended in spite of the fact that you may feel better. Otherwise, the infection may return.

☐ If you forget to take a dose, take it as soon as you remember and then continue with your regular schedule.

☐ Most people experience few or no side effects from their drugs. However, any medicine can sometimes cause unwanted effects. Call your doctor if you develop a skin rash, fever, severe stomach cramps, or severe diarrhea (loose bowel movements) that may be accompanied by blood or mucus.

☐ Do not self-treat any diarrhea (loose bowel movements) without first checking with your doctor or pharmacist. Some antidiarrheal products can cancel the effect of this antibiotic and may make your diarrhea worse or last longer.

☐ If for some reason you cannot take all of the medicine, throw away the unused portion by flushing it down the toilet. Do not take or save old medicine.

*   *   *   *   *

Lindane (*Topical Scabicide–Pediculicide*)
United States: Kwell
Canada: Kwellada

☐ This medicine is used to treat scabies and lice infections.

HOW TO USE THIS MEDICINE

☐ Instructions for use (for scabies). (***United States:*** Kwell Cream or Lotion; ***Canada:*** Kwellada Cream or Lotion):
  • Take a hot soapy bath or shower using a lot of soap to cleanse the skin well.
  • Dry the skin well and apply a thin layer of cream or lotion over the entire skin surface.
  • Leave on for 12 to 24 hours and then wash thoroughly.
  • Put on freshly laundered or dry-cleaned clothing in order to prevent reinfestation.

☐ Instructions for use (for lice):
  • Take a hot soapy bath or shower using lots of soap to cleanse skin well.
  • Dry the skin well.
  • Apply the medicine to the infested areas and surrounding areas.
  • Leave on for 12 to 24 hours.
  • Wash thoroughly again and put on freshly laundered or dry-cleaned clothing in order to prevent reinfestation.

☐ Instructions for use (as shampoo) (***United States:*** Kwell Shampoo; ***Canada:*** Kwellada Shampoo):
  • Wet hair thoroughly with warm water.
  • Pour 2 tablespoonfuls onto the affected area and work into a good lather.

- Rub vigorously for at least 4 minutes, being sure to cover all hair areas.
- Rinse hair thoroughly and rub with a dry towel.
- Comb with a fine-tooth comb.
- This shampoo may also be used to clean combs and brushes to prevent spread of the infection.
- Do not let other members of the family use your comb.
- Do **not** use the shampoo as a regular shampoo routine.

SPECIAL INSTRUCTIONS

☐ Disinfect combs and brushes immediately after using.

☐ Put on freshly laundered clean clothing after each application of the medicine. Use fresh towels and fresh bed sheets after each application. Launder or dry-clean contaminated clothing.

☐ Keep this medicine away from the eyes, mouth, or open wounds. If some does get in the eyes, flush it away with water immediately.

☐ Call your doctor if the condition for which this drug is being used persists or becomes worse or if you develop a constant irritation such as itching or burning that was not present before you started using this medicine. Also call your doctor if you develop muscle cramps, seizures, fast heartbeats, vomiting, or unusual nervousness.

☐ Do not use this drug more frequently or for a longer period than prescribed by your doctor.

☐ For external use only. Do not swallow.

* * * * *

Liothyronine Sodium (*Oral Hypothyroidism Therapy*)
United States: Cytomel
Canada: Cytomel

☐ This medicine is a hormone which is used to treat conditions in which the body is not producing enough thyroid hormone.

HOW TO USE THIS MEDICINE

☐ It is very important that you take this medicine exactly as your doctor has prescribed and that you do not miss any doses. Try to take this medicine at the same time every day.

☐ If you forget to take a dose, take it as soon as possible. However, if it is almost time for your next dose, do not take the missed dose. Instead, continue with your regular dosing schedule.

☐ Do not take any more of this medicine than your doctor has prescribed and do not stop taking this medicine suddenly without the approval of your doctor.

SPECIAL INSTRUCTIONS

☐ It is important that you obtain the advice of your doctor or pharmacist before taking ANY other medicines including pain relievers, sleeping pills, tranquilizers or medicines for depression, cough/cold or allergy medicines, or weight-reducing medicines.

☐ Most people experience few or no side effects from their drugs. However, any medicine can sometimes cause unwanted effects. Call your doctor if you develop chest pain, shortness of breath, leg cramps, skin rash, fast heartbeats, trembling, diarrhea, sensitivity to heat, unusual nervousness, sweating, or weight loss.

*   *   *   *   *

Liotrix (*Oral Hypothyroidism Therapy*)
United States: Euthroid, Thyrolar
Canada: Thyrolar

☐ This medicine is a hormone which is used to treat conditions in which the body is not producing enough thyroid hormone.

HOW TO USE THIS MEDICINE

☐ It is very important that you take this medicine exactly as your doctor has prescribed and that you do not miss any doses. Try to take this medicine at the same time every day.

☐ If you forget to take a dose, take it as soon as possible. However, if it is almost time for your next dose, do not take the missed dose. Instead, continue with your regular dosing schedule.

☐ Do not take any more of this medicine than your doctor has prescribed and do not stop taking this medicine suddenly without the approval of your doctor.

SPECIAL INSTRUCTIONS

☐ It is important that you obtain the advice of your doctor or pharmacist before taking ANY other medicines including pain relievers, sleeping pills, tranquilizers or medicines for depression, cough/cold or allergy medicines, or weight-reducing medicines.

☐ Most people experience few or no side effects from their drugs. However, any medicine can sometimes cause unwanted effects. Call your doctor if you develop chest pain, shortness of breath, leg cramps, skin rash, fast heartbeats, trembling, diarrhea, sensitivity to heat, unusual nervousness, sweating, or weight loss.

*   *   *   *   *

Lithium Carbonate (*Oral Antimanic Agent*)

United States: Eskalith, Lithane, Lithobid, Lithonate, Lithotabs, PFI-Lithium

Canada: Carbolith, Lithane

Lithium Citrate

United States: Lithonate-S

☐ This medicine is used to help relieve the symptoms of certain types of emotional conditions. It is important that you take the medicine regularly and that you do not miss any doses. The full effect of the medicine may not be noticed immediately, but may take from a few days to several weeks. DO NOT STOP TAKING THE MEDICINE when you first feel better or you will feel worse in a few days.

HOW TO USE THIS MEDICINE

☐ Take the medicine with food or milk to help prevent stomach upset.

☐ This medicine must be swallowed whole. Do not crush, chew, or break it into pieces. (*United States:* Lithobid)

☐ If you forget to take a dose, take it as soon as possible. However, if your next dose is within 2 hours, do not take the missed dose but continue with your regular schedule.

SPECIAL INSTRUCTIONS

☐ Unless otherwise directed, try to drink at least 8 to 10 glasses of water or other liquids every day while you are taking this medicine.

☐ Use a normal amount of table salt in your diet.

☐ If your mouth becomes dry, suck a hard sour candy (sugarless) or ice chips, or chew gum. It is especially important to brush your teeth regularly if you develop a dry mouth.

☐ In some people, this drug may cause dizziness or drowsiness. Do not drive a car or operate dangerous machinery or do jobs that require you to be alert until you know how you are going to react to this drug.

☐ If this medicine causes dizziness, you should be careful going up and down stairs and you should not change positions too rapidly. Get out of bed slowly in the morning and dangle your feet over the edge of the bed for a few minutes before standing up. Sit down or lie down at the first sign of dizziness. Tell your doctor you have been dizzy. In order to help prevent dizziness and fainting, your doctor may also recommend that you avoid strenuous exercises, standing for long periods of time (especially in hot weather), or hot showers or hot baths.

468

- [ ] Do not drink large quantities of beverages containing caffeine (coffee, tea, colas) while taking this medicine. These beverages can lower the effect of this medicine and make it less helpful.

- [ ] Some nonprescription drugs should not be taken at the same time as this medicine. Do not take any of the following without the approval of your doctor or pharmacist: asthma or allergy products, laxatives, sodium bicarbonate (baking soda), or caffeine products.

- [ ] The only time NOT to take your lithium is the morning before every lithium blood test. Otherwise, your blood test will give an inaccurate reading.

- [ ] Most people experience few or no side effects from their drugs. However, any medicine can sometimes cause unwanted effects. Call your doctor if you develop diarrhea, increased desire to urinate ("pass your water"), vomiting, slurred speech, trembling of the hands, unusual weakness, "ringing" or "buzzing" in the ears, swelling of the hands or feet, or lack of coordination.

- [ ] Check with your doctor if you develop an infection, fever, or excessive perspiration.

- [ ] Always keep your doctor appointments so that he can watch your progress.

- [ ] Carry an identification card indicating that you are taking this medicine. Always tell your pharmacist, dentist, and other doctors who are treating you that you are taking this medicine.

- [ ] Do not stop taking this medicine without your doctor's approval and do not go without medicine between prescription refills. Call your pharmacist 2 or 3 days before you will run out of the medicine.

*　*　*　*　*

Lomustine (Oral Antineoplastic)
United States: CeeNu
Canada: CeeNu

- [ ] This medicine is used in certain medical conditions to help slow down the growth and reproduction of some of the body's cells.

HOW TO USE THIS MEDICINE
- [ ] In order that you receive the correct dose, there may be 2 or more different colored capsules in the container. Take all of the capsules at once in 1 dose. (United States: CeeNu)

- [ ] It is best to take this medicine 1 hour before breakfast or 2 hours after supper in order to help prevent nausea or vomiting.

- [ ] Even if you become nauseated or lose your appetite, do not stop taking the medicine but check with your doctor. The nausea will usually disappear within 24 hours and your appetite will usually return in a few days.

□ Always keep your doctor appointments so that your doctor can watch your progress.

□ If your doctor has prescribed some other medicines for you, it is important that you take them in the right order and that you do not miss them.

□ Men and women should take appropriate birth control measures while taking this medicine in order to avoid conception.

□ This medicine may cause a temporary loss of hair. Brush your hair gently and no more often than necessary. After your treatment is finished, your hair should grow back in.

□ Always tell your pharmacist, dentist, and any other doctors who are treating you that you are taking this medicine. This is especially important if you plan to have surgery or any vaccinations.

□ This is a very strong medicine. In addition to its benefits, there may be some unwanted effects, even for a short time after you stop taking the medicine. Call your doctor if you develop unusual bruising or bleeding, sore throat, fever or mouth sores, a skin rash, or a yellow color to the skin or eyes.

□ Store this medicine in the refrigerator but do not freeze.

*   *   *   *   *

Loperamide (*Oral Antidiarrheal*)
United States: Imodium
Canada: Imodium

□ This medicine is used in the treatment of diarrhea.

HOW TO USE THIS MEDICINE
□ This medicine may be taken with food or a glass of water.

□ If you miss a dose of this medicine, do not take the missed dose and do not double your next dose.

SPECIAL INSTRUCTIONS
□ Do not take any more of this medicine than your doctor has prescribed.

□ In some people, this drug may cause dizziness or drowsiness. Do not drive a car or operate dangerous machinery or do jobs that require you to be alert until you know how you are going to react to this drug.

□ If you become dizzy, you should be careful going up and down stairs. Sit or lie down at the first sign of dizziness.

□ If your mouth becomes dry, suck a hard sour candy (sugarless) or ice chips, or chew gum. It is especially important to brush your teeth regularly if you develop a dry mouth.

☐ Call your doctor if you develop a fever or if the diarrhea continues.

☐ Most people experience few or no side effects from their drugs. However, any medicine can sometimes cause unwanted effects. Call your doctor if you develop a skin rash, bloating, constipation, nausea, vomiting, or stomach pain.

* * * * *

Lorazepam (*Oral Anxiolytic-Sedative*)
United States: Ativan
Canada: Ativan

☐ This medicine is used to help relieve anxiety and tension. It is also used to help relax muscles as well as to treat some other conditions. Check with your doctor if you do not fully understand why you are using it.

☐ IMPORTANT: If you have ever had an allergic reaction to a benzodiazepine medicine, tell your doctor or pharmacist before you take any of this medicine.

HOW TO USE THIS MEDICINE
☐ This medicine may be taken with food or a full glass of water.

SPECIAL INSTRUCTIONS
☐ If you forget to take a dose, take it as soon as possible. However, if it is almost time for your next dose, do not take the missed dose. Instead, continue with your regular dosing schedule.

☐ Women who are pregnant, breast-feeding, or planning to become pregnant should tell their doctor before taking this medicine.

☐ In some people, this drug may cause dizziness or drowsiness. Do not drive a car or operate dangerous machinery or do jobs that require you to be alert until you know how you are going to react to this drug.

☐ If you become dizzy, you should be careful going up and down stairs. Sit or lie down at the first sign of dizziness.

☐ Do not drink alcoholic beverages while taking this drug without the approval of your doctor.

☐ It is important that you obtain the advice of your doctor or pharmacist before taking ANY other medicines including pain relievers, sleeping pills, tranquilizers or medicines for depression, cough/cold or allergy medicines, or weight-reducing medicines.

☐ Do not take any more of this medicine than your doctor has prescribed because the drug could become habit-forming. Do not stop taking this medicine suddenly without the approval of your doctor.

☐ Most people experience few or no side effects from their drugs. However, any medicine can sometimes cause unwanted effects. Call your doctor if you

develop a sore throat, fever, mouth sores, a staggering walk, a yellow color to the skin or eyes, slow heartbeats, shortness of breath, unusual tiredness, nervousness, or stomach pain.

*   *   *   *   *

Loxapine (Oral Psychotic)
United States: Daxolin, Loxitane
Canada: Loxapac

☐ This medicine is used to treat certain types of emotional conditions.

HOW TO USE THIS MEDICINE
☐ This medicine may be taken with food or a full glass of water.
☐ For LIQUID MEDICINE
   • If a dropper or a dispensing spoon is used to measure the dose and you do not fully understand how to use it, check with your pharmacist. (**United States:** Loxitane C; **Canada:** Loxapac Oral Concentrate)
   • Mix the liquid with orange or grapefruit juice just before you take it.
   • If there is a discard date on the bottle, throw away any unused medicine after that date. Do not take or save old medicine.

SPECIAL INSTRUCTIONS
☐ If you forget to take a dose, take it as soon as possible. However, if your next dose is within 3 hours, do not take the missed dose but continue with your regular schedule.

☐ In some people, this drug may cause drowsiness which usually will go away after you have taken the medicine for a while. Do not drive a car or operate dangerous machinery or do jobs that require you to be alert until you know how you are going to react.

☐ If this medicine causes dizziness, you should be careful going up and down stairs and you should not change positions too rapidly. Get out of bed slowly in the morning and dangle your feet over the edge of the bed for a few minutes before standing up. Sit down or lie down at the first sign of dizziness. Tell your doctor you have been dizzy. Do not drive a car or operate dangerous machinery if you are dizzy. Avoid hot showers and baths because they could make you dizzy.

☐ If your mouth becomes dry, suck a hard sour candy (sugarless) or ice chips, or chew gum. It is especially important to brush your teeth regularly if you develop a dry mouth.

☐ Do not drink alcoholic beverages while taking this drug without the approval of your doctor.

☐ It is important that you obtain the advice of your doctor or pharmacist before taking *any* other medicines including pain relievers, sleeping pills, other tran-

472

quilizers or medicines for depression, cough/cold or allergy medicines, or weight-reducing medicines.

☐ Do not take any more of this medicine than your doctor has prescribed and do not stop taking this medicine suddenly without the approval of your doctor.

☐ Most people experience few or no side effects from their drugs. However, any medicine can sometimes cause unwanted effects. Call you doctor if you develop a skin rash; difficulty in urinating ("passing your water"); unusual movements of the hands, face, or tongue; or a fast heart rate.

*   *   *   *   *

Lypressin (*Nasal Antidiuretic Hormone Analogue*)
United States: Diapid

☐ This medicine is used in certain conditions to help decrease the amount of water excreted in the urine and to decrease the thirst.

HOW TO USE THIS MEDICINE
☐ For NOSE SPRAY

- Blow the nose gently.
- Sit upright with the head upright.
- Hold the spray bottle upright and insert the nozzle of the bottle into the nostril. Close the other nostril by pressing the finger on the side.
- Squeeze the bottle once firmly to deliver a short spray.
- Repeat for the other nostril if prescribed.

☐ It is best not to use this spray more than 2 or 3 times in each nostril at any one time because this usually will waste some of the drug.

SPECIAL INSTRUCTIONS
☐ Your doctor may limit the amount of liquids you should drink.

☐ Call your doctor immediately if you think you may be allergic to the medicine or if you develop a skin rash, hives, itching, swelling of the face, or difficulty in breathing. If you cannot reach your doctor, phone a hospital emergency department.

☐ Most people experience few or no side effects from their drugs. However, any medicine can sometimes cause unwanted effects. Call your doctor if you develop swelling of the legs or ankles, shortness of breath, nasal congestion or nasal soreness, heartburn, diarrhea, or stomach cramps.

☐ Do not use this medicine after the discard date.

*   *   *   *   *

473

Magaldrate (*Oral Antacid*)

United States: Riopan

Canada: Riopan

Magaldrate-Dimethylpolysiloxane (*Oral Antacid-Antiflatulent*)

Canada: Rioplus

☐ This medicine is an antacid which is used to reduce the acidity of the stomach contents. It is used for helping relieve the symptoms of heartburn as well as in the treating of peptic ulcer, "reflux," or hiatus hernia.

HOW TO USE THIS MEDICINE

☐ For LIQUID MEDICINE

- Shake the bottle well before using so that you can measure an accurate dose. The dose may be followed with a sip of water. (**United States:** Riopan Suspension; **Canada:** Riopan Suspension, Rioplus Suspension)
- Store in a cool place but do not freeze.

☐ For CHEWABLE TABLETS

- The tablets may be chewed or dissolved slowly in the mouth. Follow with a glass of water. Do not swallow the tablets. (**United States** and **Canada:** Riopan Chewable)

☐ For TABLETS

- Swallow these tablets with a glass of water. (**United States:** Riopan Swallow Tablets)

SPECIAL INSTRUCTIONS

☐ Do not take this medicine more often than recommended by your doctor.

☐ If you are taking this medicine because you have an ULCER, you will have to have this antacid very often. This is because your stomach must not be without food or this medicine for usually more than 2 hours at a time. You must follow any diet prescribed by your doctor and continue to take this medicine even if your pain fades. If you stop the antacid too early, your ulcer may not be fully healed and could quickly return. It is best to avoid smoking as well as coffee, tea, alcohol, spices, and aspirin because all of these agents can irritate the stomach. Check with your pharmacist before you take any nonprescription drugs.

☐ If you are taking this medicine because you have REFLUX or HIATUS HERNIA, it is usually best to avoid overeating, to limit the amount of fluids you drink during a meal, to reduce the amount of fats you eat, and to keep your shoulders elevated about 30° in bed.

☐ If you are on a low-sodium diet, do not switch to another antacid without the advice of your doctor.

474

☐ Most people experience few or no side effects from their drugs. However, any medicine can sometimes cause unwanted effects. Call your doctor if you develop stomach pain which lasts more than 3 days, loss of appetite, tremors, weakness, or bone pain.

*　*　*　*　*

Magnesium-Aluminum Preparations (*Oral Antacid*)

United States: Aludrox, Alurex, Alurex No. 2, A-M-T, Creamalin, Delcid, Estomul-M, Kolantyl, Kudrox, Maalox, Magnagel, Magnatril, Neosorb Plus, Neutralox, Pama, Trisogel, WinGel

Canada: Buffergel, Chemdrox, Chemlox, Creamalin, Gelusil, Maalox, Neutralca-S, Univol

Magnesium-Aluminum-Calcium Preparations

United States: Camalox
Canada: Camalox

☐ This medicine is an antacid which is used to reduce the acidity of the stomach contents. It is used for helping relieve the symptoms of heartburn as well as in the treating of peptic ulcer, "reflux," or hiatus hernia.

HOW TO USE THIS MEDICINE

☐ For LIQUID MEDICINE
- Shake the bottle well before using so that you can measure an accurate dose. The dose may be followed with a sip of water.
- Store in a cool place but do not freeze.

☐ For CHEWABLE TABLETS
- The tablets may be chewed or dissolved slowly in the mouth. Follow with a glass of water. Do not swallow the tablets.

☐ For TABLETS
- Swallow these tablets with a glass of water.

SPECIAL INSTRUCTIONS

☐ Do not take this medicine more often than recommended by your doctor.

☐ If you are taking this medicine because you have an ULCER, you will have to have this antacid very often. This is because your stomach must not be without food or this medicine for usually more than 2 hours at a time. You must follow any diet prescribed by your doctor and continue to take this medicine even if your pain fades. If you stop the antacid too early, your ulcer may not be fully healed and could quickly return. It is best to avoid smoking as well as coffee, tea, alcohol, spices, and aspirin because all of these agents can irritate the stomach. Check with your pharmacist before you take any nonprescription drugs.

□ If you are taking this medicine because you have REFLUX or HIATUS HER-NIA, it is usually best to avoid overeating, to limit the amount of fluids you drink during a meal, to reduce the amount of fats you eat, and to keep your shoulders elevated about 30° in bed.

□ Most people experience few or no side effects from their drugs. However, any medicine can sometimes cause unwanted effects. Call your doctor if you develop stomach pain which lasts more than 3 days, loss of appetite, tremors, weakness, or bone pain.

*　*　*　*　*

Magnesium-Aluminum-Dimethylpolysiloxane Preparations
(*Oral Antacid-Antiflatulent*)
> *Canada:* Chemgastric, Diovol, Maalox-Plus

Magnesium-Aluminum-Simethicone Preparations
> *United States:* Di-Gel, Gelusil, Gelusil-M, Gelusil-II, Maalox Plus, Mylanta, Mylanta-II, Silain-Gel
> *Canada:* Mylanta

Aluminum-Dimethylpolysiloxane Preparations
> *Canada:* Amphojel 65

□ This medicine is an antacid which is used to reduce the acidity of the stomach contents and to relieve excess gas in the stomach and intestines. It is used for helping relieve the symptoms of heartburn as well as in the treating of peptic ulcer, "reflux," or hiatus hernia.

HOW TO USE THIS MEDICINE

□ For LIQUID MEDICINE
  • Shake the bottle well before using so that you can measure an accurate dose. The dose may be followed with a sip of water.
  • Store in a cool place but do not freeze.

□ For CHEWABLE TABLETS
  • The tablets may be chewed or dissolved slowly in the mouth. Follow with a glass of water. Do not swallow the tablets.

□ For TABLETS
  • Swallow these tablets with a glass of water.

476

SPECIAL INSTRUCTIONS

- ☐ Do not take this medicine more often than recommended by your doctor.

- ☐ If you are taking this medicine because you have an ULCER, you will have to have this antacid very often. This is because your stomach must not be without food or this medicine for usually more than 2 hours at a time. You must follow any diet prescribed by your doctor and continue to take this medicine even if your pain fades. If you stop the antacid too early, your ulcer may not be fully healed and could quickly return. It is best to avoid smoking as well as coffee, tea, alcohol, spices, and aspirin because all of these agents can irritate the stomach. Check with your pharmacist before you take any nonprescription drugs.

- ☐ If you are taking this medicine because you have REFLUX or HIATUS HER- NIA, it is usually best to avoid overeating, to limit the amount of fluids you drink during a meal, to reduce the amount of fats you eat, and to keep your shoulders elevated about 30° in bed.

- ☐ Most people experience few or no side effects from their drugs. However, any medicine can sometimes cause unwanted effects. Call your doctor if you develop stomach pain which lasts more than 3 days, loss of appetite, trem- ors, weakness, or bone pain.

*   *   *   *   *

Magnesium Glucoheptonate Solution (*Oral Magnesium Supplement*)

Canada: Magnesium-Rougier

- ☐ This medicine is a magnesium supplement.
- ☐ Take this medicine before eating food.
- ☐ It is recommended that patients taking this medicine avoid drinking alcoholic beverages because the combination may cause undesired side effects.
- ☐ Do not use this medicine more often than recommended by your doctor.

*   *   *   *   *

Magnesium Salicylate (*Oral Analgesic–Anti-inflammatory*)

United States: Analate, Arthrin, Lorisal, Magan, Mobidin

- ☐ This medicine is used to help relieve pain, reduce fever, and relieve redness and swelling in certain kinds of arthritis.

- ☐ IMPORTANT: If you have a stomach ulcer or if you have ever had an allergic reaction to aspirin, tell your doctor or pharmacist before you take any of this medicine.

477

HOW TO USE THIS MEDICINE

☐ This medicine may be taken with food or a full glass of water.

☐ Do not take this medicine if it smells strongly like vinegar since this means the medicine is not fresh.

☐ Do not take this medicine regularly for more than 10 days without consulting your doctor and do not administer it to children under 12 years of age for more than 5 days without your doctor's approval.

SPECIAL INSTRUCTIONS

☐ Do not take any other medicines containing aspirin while you are taking this medicine because it could result in too high a dose.

☐ Women who are pregnant, breast-feeding, or planning to become pregnant should tell their doctor before taking this medicine.

☐ If you are taking this medicine for arthritis, it is very important that you take it regularly and that you DO NOT MISS ANY DOSES. If you miss a dose, the level of the medicine in your body will fall and the drug will not be as effective. Only if the level of the drug is high enough can it decrease the inflammation in your joints and help prevent further damage. If you forget to take a dose, take it as soon as possible. However, if it is almost time for your next dose, do not take the missed dose. Instead, continue with your regular dosing schedule.

☐ It is best not to drink alcoholic beverages while you are taking this medicine since the combination can cause stomach problems.

☐ Most people experience few or no side effects from their drugs. However, any medicine can sometimes cause unwanted effects. Call your doctor if you develop "ringing" or "buzzing" in the ears, skin rash, stomach pain, red or black stools, dizziness, fever, sweating, wheezing, or shortness of breath.

☐ Call your doctor if the medicine does not relieve your symptoms.

*   *   *   *   *

Maprotiline (*Oral Antidepressant*)
Canada: Ludiomil

☐ This medicine is used to help relieve the symptoms of depression. It is important that you take the medicine regularly and that you do not miss any doses. The full effect of the medicine may not be noticed immediately, but may take from a few days to four weeks. Early signs of improvement are increased appetite, better sleep, increased energy, and later improved mood. DO NOT STOP TAKING the medicine when you first feel better or you will feel worse in 3 or 4 days.

☐ This medicine has also been used in children to treat bed-wetting.

HOW TO USE THIS MEDICINE

☐ This medicine may be taken with food unless otherwise directed.

SPECIAL INSTRUCTIONS

☐ If you forget to take a dose, take it as soon as possible. However, if it is almost time for your next dose, do not take the missed dose. Instead, continue with your regular dosing schedule.

☐ Any medicine has a few unwanted side effects. Because this medicine takes a few weeks to work, the side effects are the only thing that tell the doctor that the drug is being absorbed. Most of these side effects will go away as your body adjusts to the medicine.

☐ Women who are pregnant, breast-feeding, or planning to become pregnant should tell their doctor before taking this medicine.

☐ In some people, this drug may cause dizziness or drowsiness. Do not drive a car or operate dangerous machinery or do jobs that require you to be alert until you know how you are going to react to this drug.

☐ If this medicine causes dizziness, you should be careful going up and down stairs and you should not change positions too quickly. Get out of bed slowly in the morning and dangle your feet over the edge of the bed for a few minutes before standing up. Sit or lie down at the first sign of dizziness. Tell your doctor you have been dizzy.

☐ Do not drink alcoholic beverages while taking this drug without the approval of your doctor.

☐ It is important that you obtain the advice of your doctor or pharmacist before taking any other medicines, including pain relievers, sleeping pills, tranquilizers, other medicines for depression, cough/cold or allergy medicines, or weight-reducing medicine.

☐ If your mouth becomes dry, suck a hard sour candy (sugarless) or ice chips, or chew gum. It is especially important to brush your teeth regularly if you develop a dry mouth.

☐ This medicine may make some people more sensitive to sunlight and sunlamps. When you begin taking this medicine, try to avoid getting too much sun until you see how you are going to react. If your skin does become more sensitive to sunlight, tell your doctor and try to stay out of direct sunlight. While in the sun, wear protective clothing and sunglasses. You may wish to ask your pharmacist about suitable sunscreen products. Check with your doctor if you become sunburned.

☐ If you become constipated, try increasing the amount of bulk in your diet (for example, bran and salads), exercising more often, or drinking water.

☐ Call your doctor if you develop a sore throat, fever, mouth sores, eye pain or blurred vision, difficulty in urinating ("passing your water"), fast heartbeats, dark-colored urine or a yellow color to the skin or eyes, a skin rash, or nightmares.

☐ Do not stop taking this medicine suddenly without your doctor's approval. When your doctor tells you to stop this medicine, you must follow these precautions for 2 weeks since some of the medicine may still be in your body.

☐ Carry an identification card indicating that you are taking this medicine. Always tell your pharmacist, dentist, and other doctors who are treating you that you are taking this medicine.

*   *   *   *   *

Mazindol (*Oral Anorexiant*)
United States: Sanorex
Canada: Sanorex

☐ This medicine is used to help reduce the appetite in weight-reduction programs. It can help you develop new eating habits and is only useful for a short time. Do not take any more of this medicine than your doctor has prescribed and do not stop taking this medicine suddenly without the approval of your doctor.

HOW TO USE THIS MEDICINE
☐ This medicine may be taken with food or a glass of water.

☐ Do not take the medicine late in the day or it may cause insomnia (difficulty in sleeping).

SPECIAL INSTRUCTIONS
☐ If you forget to take a dose, take it as soon as possible. However, if it is almost time for your next dose, do not take the missed dose. Instead, continue with your regular dosing schedule.

☐ It is very important that you follow the diet prescribed by your doctor.

☐ If your mouth becomes dry, suck a hard sour candy (sugarless) or ice chips, or chew gum. It is especially important to brush your teeth regularly if you develop a dry mouth.

☐ In some people, this drug may cause dizziness or drowsiness. Do not drive a car or operate dangerous machinery or do jobs that require you to be alert until you know how you are going to react to this drug. Therefore, you should be careful going up and down stairs. Sit or lie down at the first sign of dizziness.

☐ Most people experience few or no side effects from their drugs. However, any medicine can sometimes cause unwanted effects. Call your doctor if you develop a skin rash, sore throat, fever or mouth sores, unusual nervousness, palpitations or pounding heartbeats, or nightmares, or if you become depressed.

☐ It is important that you obtain the advice of your doctor or pharmacist before taking ANY other medicines including pain relievers, sleeping pills, tranquil-

480

izers or medicines for depression, cough/cold or allergy medicines, or other weight-reducing medicines.

□ Carry an identification card indicating that you are taking this medicine. Always tell your pharmacist, dentist, and other doctors who are treating you that you are taking this medicine.

* * * * *

Mebendazole (Oral Anthelmintic)
United States: Vermox
Canada: Vermox

□ This medicine is used to treat worm infections.

HOW TO USE THIS MEDICINE
□ Chew the tablets well before swallowing. Follow with a glass of water.

SPECIAL INSTRUCTIONS
□ Do not take any more of this medicine than your doctor has prescribed, but it is important that you do not miss any doses. Otherwise, the infection will not be eliminated.

□ It is not necessary to take a laxative or change your diet unless your doctor recommends that you do so.

□ Most people experience few or no side effects from their drugs. However, any medicine can sometimes cause unwanted effects. Call your doctor if you develop a skin rash, itching, or hives.

GENERAL INSTRUCTIONS
□ Good personal hygiene is very important to prevent reinfection.

□ It is recommended that you have a shower every morning in order to remove any eggs in the anal area that have appeared during the night.

□ Wash your hands frequently, especially before handling food or anything that will be put into the mouth. Wash your hands after urination and bowel movements.

□ Keep your nails short and clean and avoid biting them. Do not put your fingers in your mouth or nose.

□ On the day of therapy, change the bed linen, underwear, and nightclothes. Wash or dry-clean them immediately.

□ Do not scratch the affected area.

□ Disinfect the toilet seat and bathtub daily.

* * * * *

Mecamylamine HCl (*Oral Ganglionic Blocking Agent*)
United States: Inversine

☐ This medication is used to lower the blood pressure.

☐ Hypertension (high blood pressure) is a long-term condition, and it will probably be necessary for you to take the drug for a long time in spite of the fact
that you feel better. It is very important that you take this medicine as your
doctor has directed and that you do not miss any doses. Otherwise, you
cannot expect the drug to keep your blood pressure down.

HOW TO USE THIS MEDICINE

☐ It is best to take this medicine after eating food.

☐ Try to take the medicine at the same time(s) every day.

SPECIAL INSTRUCTIONS

☐ If you forget to take a dose, take it as soon as possible. However, if it is
almost time for your next dose, do not take the missed dose. Instead, continue with your regular dosing schedule.

☐ In some people, this drug causes blurred vision or dizziness. Do not drive a
car or operate dangerous machinery or do jobs that require you to be alert
until you know how you are going to react.

☐ If this medicine causes dizziness, you should be careful going up and down
stairs and you should not change positions too rapidly. Get out of bed slowly
in the morning and dangle your feet over the edge of the bed for a few
minutes before standing up. Sit or lie down at the first sign of dizziness. Tell
your doctor you have been dizzy. Your doctor may also want you to avoid
strenuous exercise, standing for long periods of time (especially in hot
weather), hot showers, and hot baths.

☐ If your mouth becomes dry, suck a hard sour candy (sugarless) or ice chips,
or chew gum. It is especially important to brush your teeth regularly if you
develop a dry mouth.

☐ Some nonprescription drugs can aggravate your condition. Do not take any
of the following without the approval of your doctor or pharmacist: cough,
cold, or sinus products; asthma or allergy products, or diet or weight-reducing medicines.

☐ Do not drink alcoholic beverages while taking this drug without the approval
of your doctor.

☐ If constipation should occur while you are taking this medicine, check with
your doctor rather than treating yourself with laxatives.

☐ Most people experience few or no side effects from their drugs. However,
any medicine can sometimes cause unwanted effects. Call your doctor if you
develop diarrhea (loose bowel movements), swelling of the legs or ankles,
sudden weight gain of 5 pounds or more, chest pains, or difficulty in breath-

482

ing, or if you urinate ("pass your water") less frequently or in smaller amounts than usual.

☐ Carry an identification card indicating that you are taking this medicine. Always tell your pharmacist, dentist, and other doctors who are treating you that you are taking this medicine.

☐ Do not stop taking this medicine without your doctor's approval and do not go without medicine between prescription refills. Call your pharmacist 2 or 3 days before you will run out of the medicine.

* * * * *

Meclizine HCl (*Oral Antiemetic*)
United States: Antivert, Bonine
Canada: Bonamine

☐ This medicine is used to help control nausea, vomiting, dizziness, and motion sickness.

HOW TO USE THIS MEDICINE
☐ These tablets can be taken without water. Place the tablet in the mouth and either let it dissolve, chew it, or swallow it whole. (**Canada:** Bonamine)

☐ Chew the tablets completely before swallowing. (**United States:** Antivert Chewable, Bonine)

SPECIAL INSTRUCTIONS
☐ Women who are breast-feeding should tell their doctor before taking this medicine.

☐ In some people, this drug may cause drowsiness. Do not drive a car or operate dangerous machinery or do jobs that require you to be alert until you know how you are going to react to this drug.

☐ If your mouth becomes dry, suck a hard sour candy (sugarless) or ice chips, or chew gum. It is especially important to brush your teeth regularly if you develop a dry mouth.

☐ Do not drink alcoholic beverages while taking this drug without the approval of your doctor.

☐ It is important that you obtain the advice of your doctor or pharmacist before taking pain relievers, nonprescription drugs, sleeping pills, tranquilizers, or medicines for depression while you are taking this drug.

☐ Most people experience few or no side effects from their drugs. However, any medicine can sometimes cause unwanted effects. Call your doctor if you develop a skin rash, sore throat, fever, or mouth sores.

* * * * *

Meclizine-Niacin (*Oral Vertigo Therapy*)
Canada: Antivert

☐ This medicine is used to treat nausea, vomiting, and dizziness.

HOW TO USE THIS MEDICINE
☐ It is best to take this medicine before meals.

☐ This medicine usually causes some flushing, tingling, and itching of the skin. This is a normal side effect, but if it becomes bothersome, take the medicine with some food or after meals. Tell your doctor.

SPECIAL INSTRUCTIONS
☐ Women who are breast-feeding should tell their doctor before taking this medicine.

☐ If your mouth becomes dry, suck a hard sour candy (sugarless) or ice chips, or chew gum. It is especially important to brush your teeth regularly if you develop a dry mouth.

☐ In some people, this drug may cause drowsiness or blurred vision. Do not drive a car or operate dangerous machinery or do jobs that require you to be alert until you know how you are going to react to this drug.

☐ Do not drink alcoholic beverages while taking this drug without the approval of your doctor.

☐ Call your doctor immediately if you think you may be allergic to the medicine or if you develop a skin rash, hives, itching, swelling of the face, or difficulty in breathing. If you cannot reach your doctor, phone a hospital emergency department.

☐ Most people experience few or no side effects from their drugs. However, any medicine can sometimes cause unwanted effects. Call your doctor if you develop a sore throat, fever, or mouth sores.

*   *   *   *   *

Medrogestone (*Oral Progestogen*)
Canada: Colprone

☐ This medicine is a hormone and is used to treat menstrual problems.

HOW TO USE THIS MEDICINE
☐ The tablets may be taken after meals or with a snack if they upset your stomach.

SPECIAL INSTRUCTIONS
☐ It is recommended that you do not smoke while you are taking this medicine because smoking may increase the incidence of heart attacks.

484

☐ Women who are pregnant, breast-feeding, or planning to become pregnant should tell their doctor before taking this medicine.

☐ Diabetic patients should regularly check the sugar in their urine while they are taking this medicine.

☐ Contact your doctor if any of the following side effects occur:
- Severe or persistent headaches
- Vomiting, dizziness, or fainting
- Blurred vision or slurred speech
- Pain in the calves of the legs or numbness in an arm or leg
- Chest pain, shortness of breath, or coughing of blood
- Lumps in the breast
- Severe depression
- A yellow color to the skin or eyes or dark-colored urine
- Severe abdominal pain
- Breakthrough vaginal bleeding

☐ Carry an identification card indicating that you are taking this medicine. Always tell your pharmacist, dentist, and other doctors who are treating you that you are taking this medicine.

*   *   *   *   *

Medroxyprogesterone Acetate (Oral Progestogen)
United States: Amen, Provera
Canada: Provera

☐ This medicine is a hormone and is used to treat menstrual problems.

HOW TO USE THIS MEDICINE
☐ The tablets may be taken after meals or with a snack if they upset your stomach.

SPECIAL INSTRUCTIONS
☐ It is recommended that you do not smoke while you are taking this medicine because smoking may increase the incidence of heart attacks.

☐ Women who are pregnant, breast-feeding, or planning to become pregnant should tell their doctor before taking this medicine.

☐ Diabetic patients should regularly check the sugar in their urine while they are taking this medicine.

☐ Contact your doctor if any of the following side effects occur:
- Severe or persistent headaches
- Vomiting, dizziness, or fainting
- Blurred vision or slurred speech
- Pain in the calves of the legs or numbness in an arm or leg

485

- Chest pain, shortness of breath, or coughing of blood
- Lumps in the breast
- Severe depression
- A yellow color to the skin or eyes or dark-colored urine
- Severe abdominal pain
- Breakthrough vaginal bleeding

☐ Carry an identification card indicating that you are taking this medicine. Always tell your pharmacist, dentist, and other doctors who are treating you that you are taking this medicine.

* * * * *

Medrysone Suspension (*Ophthalmic Corticosteroid*)
United States: HMS Liquifilm
Canada: HMS Liquifilm

☐ This medicine is used to help relieve the pain, redness, and itching of certain types of eye conditions.

HOW TO USE THIS MEDICINE
☐ For EYE DROPS

INSTILLATION OF EYE DROPS

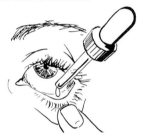

- The person administering the eye drops should wash his hands with soap and water.
- The eye drops must be kept clean. Do not touch the dropper against the face or anything else.
- Lie down or tilt your head backward and look at the ceiling.
- Shake the bottle well before using.
- Gently pull down the lower lid of your eye to form a pouch.
- Hold the dropper in your other hand and approach the eye from the side. Place the dropper as close to the eye as possible without touching it.
- Place the prescribed number of drops into the pouch of the eye.
- Close your eyes. Do not rub them.
- Apply gentle pressure for a minute with your fingers to the bridge of the nose (inside corner of the eye) to prevent the eye drops from being drained from the eye.
- Blot excess solution around the eye with a tissue.

☐ If necessary, have someone else administer the eye drops for you.

☐ Do not use the eye drops if they have changed in color or have changed in any way since being purchased.

☐ Keep the eye drop bottle tightly closed when not in use.

☐ Do not use the drug more frequently or in larger quantities than prescribed by your doctor.

SPECIAL INSTRUCTIONS

☐ This medicine should be used as long as prescribed by your doctor. Do not stop using it earlier than your doctor has recommended in spite of the fact that your symptoms seem to have improved.

☐ If you forget to use the medicine, use it as soon as possible. However, if it is almost time for your next dose, do not use the missed dose but continue with your regular schedule.

☐ Do not use this medicine at the same time as any other eye medicine without the approval of your doctor. Some medicines cannot be mixed.

☐ Contact your doctor if the condition for which you are using this medicine does not improve or if the eye becomes irritated by it for more than a few minutes. Many eye medicines sting for a short time immediately after use.

☐ For external use only. Do not swallow.

* * * * *

Mefenamic Acid (Oral Analgesic)
United States: Ponstel
Canada: Ponstan

☐ This medicine is used to help relieve pain.

☐ IMPORTANT: If you have ever had an allergic reaction to mefenamic acid, tell your doctor or pharmacist before you take any of this medicine.

HOW TO USE THIS MEDICINE

☐ Take this medicine with food or immediately after a meal.

☐ Do not take this medicine for longer than one week unless otherwise directed.

SPECIAL INSTRUCTIONS

☐ In some people, this drug may cause dizziness or drowsiness. Do not drive a car or operate dangerous machinery or do jobs that require you to be alert until you know how you are going to react to this drug.

☐ If you become dizzy, you should be careful going up and down stairs. Sit or lie down at the first sign of dizziness.

☐ Most people experience few or no side effects from their drugs. However, any medicine can sometimes cause unwanted effects. Call your doctor if you develop a skin rash, sore throat, fever or mouth sores, vomiting, diarrhea, shortness of breath, any changes in your eyesight, easy bruising, or bleeding.

* * * * *

Megestrol Acetate (Oral Antineoplastic)
United States: Megace
Canada: Megace

☐ This medicine is used in certain medical conditions to help slow down the growth and reproduction of some of the body's cells.

HOW TO USE THIS MEDICINE
☐ It is best to take this medicine on an empty stomach at least 1 hour before (or 2 hours after) eating food. Take it at the proper time even if you skip a meal.

☐ It is very important that you take this medicine exactly as your doctor has prescribed and that you do not miss any doses. Try to take this medicine at the same time every day. Do not take extra tablets without your doctor's approval.

SPECIAL INSTRUCTIONS
☐ Always keep your doctor appointments so that your doctor can watch your progress.

☐ Always tell your pharmacist, dentist, and other doctors who are treating you that you are taking this medicine.

☐ Men and women should take appropriate birth control measures to avoid conception while taking this medicine.

* * * * *

Melphalan (Oral Antineoplastic)
United States: Alkeran
Canada: Alkeran

☐ This medicine is used in certain medical conditions to help slow down the growth and reproduction of some of the body's cells.

HOW TO USE THIS MEDICINE
☐ Take this medicine with meals or food if you develop nausea or vomiting.

☐ It is very important that you take this medicine exactly as your doctor has prescribed and that you do not miss any doses. Try to take this medicine at the same time every day.

488

- ☐ Even if you become nauseated or lose your appetite, do not stop taking the medicine but check with your doctor.
- ☐ If you miss a dose of this medicine, do not take the missed dose and do not double your next dose. Check with your doctor.

SPECIAL INSTRUCTIONS

- ☐ Always keep your doctor appointments so that your doctor can watch your progress.
- ☐ If your doctor has prescribed some other medicines for you, it is important that you take them in the right order and that you do not miss them.
- ☐ Unless otherwise directed, drink plenty of fluids (2 to 3 quarts daily) while you are taking this medicine. This will help your kidneys handle the medicine and help prevent kidney problems.
- ☐ This medicine rarely may cause a temporary loss of hair. Brush your hair gently and no more often than necessary. After your treatment is finished, your hair should grow back in.
- ☐ Always tell your pharmacist, dentist, and any other doctors who are treating you that you are taking this medicine. This is especially important if you plan to have surgery or any vaccinations.
- ☐ Men and women should take appropriate birth control measures to avoid conception while taking this medicine.
- ☐ This is a very strong medicine. In addition to its benefits, there may be some unwanted effects, even for a short time after you stop taking the medicine. Call your doctor if you develop unusual bruising or bleeding, black "tarry" stools, skin rash, sore throat, fever or mouth sores, stomach or joint pain, swelling of the legs or ankles, shortness of breath, or difficulty in urinating ("passing your water").

* * * * *

Mepenzolate Bromide (*Oral Anticholinergic*)
United States: Cantil

- ☐ This medicine is used to help relax muscles of the stomach and bowels and to decrease the amount of acid formed in the stomach.
- ☐ IMPORTANT: If you have ever had an allergic reaction to atropine or bromides or any other drug used to relax the stomach or bowels, tell your doctor or pharmacist before you take any of this medicine.

HOW TO USE THIS MEDICINE

- ☐ Take this medicine with food unless otherwise directed.
- ☐ If you miss a dose of this medicine, do not take the missed dose and do not double the next dose.

489

SPECIAL INSTRUCTIONS

☐ If your mouth becomes dry, suck a hard sour candy (sugarless) or ice chips, or chew gum. It is especially important to brush your teeth regularly if you develop a dry mouth.

☐ In some people, this drug may cause dizziness or drowsiness. Do not drive a car or operate dangerous machinery or do jobs that require you to be alert until you know how you are going to react to this drug.

☐ If you become dizzy, you should be careful going up and down stairs. Sit or lie down at the first sign of dizziness. Tell your doctor you have been dizzy.

☐ A desire to urinate ("pass your water") with an inability to do so is not an uncommon effect with this drug. Urinating each time before taking the drug may help relieve this problem. Call your doctor if it continues.

☐ You may become more sensitive to heat because your body may perspire less while you are taking this drug. Be careful not to become overheated during exercise or in hot weather.

☐ Do not take antacids within 1 hour of taking this medicine as they could make this medicine less effective.

☐ If you become constipated, try increasing the amount of bulk in your diet (for example, bran and salads), exercising more often, or drinking more water. Call your doctor if the constipation continues.

☐ If your eyes become more sensitive to sunlight, it may help to wear sunglasses.

☐ Most people experience few or no side effects from their drugs. However, any medicine can sometimes cause unwanted effects. Call your doctor if you develop a skin rash, diarrhea, unusual restlessness, flushing, or eye pain.

* * * * *

Meperidine HCl (*Pethidine HCl*) (*Oral Analgesic*)
United States: Demerol
Canada: Demerol

☐ This medicine is used to help relieve pain.

HOW TO USE THIS MEDICINE

☐ This medicine may be taken with food or a glass of water.

☐ For LIQUID MEDICINE
   • Mix the dose of medicine with a half glass of water just before you take it unless otherwise directed. This will help prevent the medicine from numbing your mouth and throat.

☐ Do not take any more of this medicine than your doctor has prescribed. The drug could become habit-forming or you could take an overdose if you take it more often or longer than prescribed.

490

☐ Do not wait to take this medicine until the pain becomes severe. This medicine works best if you take it at the beginning of the pain. Call your doctor if you feel you need it more often than he prescribed.

SPECIAL INSTRUCTIONS

☐ Do not drink alcoholic beverages while taking this drug without the approval of your doctor.

☐ It is important that you obtain the advice of your doctor or pharmacist before taking ANY other medicines including other pain relievers, sleeping pills, tranquilizers or medicines for depression, cough/cold or allergy medicines, or weight-reducing medicines.

☐ In some people, this drug may cause dizziness or drowsiness. Do not drive a car or operate dangerous machinery or do jobs that require you to be alert until you know how you are going to react to this drug.

☐ If this medicine causes dizziness, you should be careful going up and down stairs and you should not change positions too rapidly. Get out of bed slowly in the morning and dangle your feet over the edge of the bed for a few minutes before standing up. Sit down or lie down at the first sign of dizziness. Tell your doctor you have been dizzy. Avoid hot showers and baths because they could make you dizzy.

☐ If your mouth becomes dry, suck a hard sour candy (sugarless) or ice chips, or chew gum. It is especially important to brush your teeth regularly if you develop a dry mouth.

☐ If you do feel nauseated when you first start taking the medicine, it may help if you lie down for a few minutes.

☐ If you become constipated, try increasing the amount of bulk in your diet (for example, bran and salads), exercising more often, or drinking more water. Call your doctor if the constipation continues.

☐ Most people experience few or no side effects from their drugs. However, any medicine can sometimes cause unwanted effects. Call your doctor if you develop shortness of breath, a slow heart beat, unusual nervousness, stomach pain, or difficulty in urinating ("passing your water").

☐ Always tell your dentist, pharmacist, and other doctors who are treating you that you are taking this medicine.

* * * * *

Mephenytoin (*Oral Anticonvulsant*)
United States: Mesantoin
Canada: Mesantoin

☐ This medicine is used to help control convulsions and seizures. It is commonly used in the treatment of epilepsy.

☐ IMPORTANT: If you have ever had an allergic reaction to an anticonvulsant or seizure medicine, tell your doctor or pharmacist before you take any of this medicine.

HOW TO USE THIS MEDICINE

☐ Take this medicine with food if it upsets your stomach. Call your doctor if you continue to have stomach upset.

☐ It is very important that you take this medicine regularly and that you do not miss any doses. Try to take the medicine at the same time(s) every day. This is the only way that you can receive the full benefit of the medicine. If you forget to take this medicine, the amount of medicine in your blood will go down and you may have seizures.

SPECIAL INSTRUCTIONS

☐ If you forget to take a dose, take it as soon as possible. However, if it is almost time for your next dose, do not take the missed dose. Instead, continue with your regular dosing schedule. Do not double doses.

☐ Do not stop taking this medicine suddenly or change the amount you are taking without the approval of your doctor.

☐ Avoid swimming alone or taking part in high-risk sports in which a sudden seizure could cause injury.

☐ In some people, this drug may cause dizziness or drowsiness. Do not drive a car or operate dangerous machinery or do jobs that require you to be alert until you know how you are going to react to this drug. If you become dizzy, you should be careful going up and down stairs. Sit or lie down at the first sign of dizziness.

☐ If this medicine is for a child, do not let him (her) ride a bike or climb trees until you can determine how he (she) is going to react to the medicine. Children could hurt themselves if they participated in these activities if they were dizzy.

☐ Do not drink alcoholic beverages while taking this drug without the approval of your doctor.

☐ It is important that you obtain the advice of your doctor or pharmacist before taking pain relievers, nonprescription drugs, sleeping pills, tranquilizers, or medicines for depression while you are taking this drug.

☐ This medicine may cause your urine to turn pink or red-brown in color. This is not unusual.

☐ Women who are pregnant, breast-feeding, or planning to become pregnant should tell their doctor before taking this medicine.

☐ Most people experience few or no side effects from their drugs. However, any medicine can sometimes cause unwanted effects. Call your doctor if you develop a sore throat, fever or mouth sores, skin rash, persistent headache,

492

slurred speech, fast eye movements, joint pain, swollen glands, difficulty in walking, easy bruising or bleeding, or a yellow color to the skin or eyes.

☐ Do not go without this medicine between prescription refills. Call your pharmacist 2 or 3 days before you will run out of the medicine.

☐ Carry an identification card indicating that you are taking this medicine. Always tell your pharmacist, dentist, and other doctors who are treating you that you are taking this medicine.

*   *   *   *   *

Mephobarbital (*Oral Sedative-Anticonvulsant*)
United States: Mebaral
Canada: Mebaral

☐ This medicine is used to cause sleep and for certain types of nervous tension. It is also specially prescribed to help prevent seizures in some patients. Check with your doctor if you do not fully understand why you are taking it.

☐ IMPORTANT: If you have ever had an allergic reaction to a barbiturate medicine, tell your doctor or pharmacist before you take any of this medicine.

HOW TO USE THIS MEDICINE
☐ This medicine may be taken with food or a full glass of water.

SPECIAL INSTRUCTIONS
☐ Sleeping medicines are only useful for a short time. If used for too long, they lose their effectiveness. Do not take any more of this medicine than your doctor has prescribed and do not stop taking this medicine suddenly without the approval of your doctor.

☐ Women who are pregnant, breast-feeding, or planning to become pregnant should tell their doctor before taking this medicine.

☐ In some people, this drug may cause dizziness or drowsiness. Do not drive a car or operate dangerous machinery or do jobs that require you to be alert until you know how you are going to react to this drug.

☐ If you become dizzy, you should be careful going up and down stairs. Sit or lie down at the first sign of dizziness.

☐ Do not drink alcoholic beverages while taking this drug without the approval of your doctor.

☐ It is important that you obtain the advice of your doctor or pharmacist before taking ANY other medicines including pain relievers, sleeping pills, tranquilizers or medicines for depression, cough/cold medicines, or allergy medicines.

- ☐ If you are taking this medicine to help you sleep, take it about 20 minutes before you want to go to sleep. Go to bed after you have taken it. Do not smoke in bed after you have taken it.

- ☐ Do not store this medicine at the bedside and keep it out of the reach of children.

- ☐ Call your doctor immediately if you think you may be allergic to the medicine or if you develop a skin rash, hives, itching, swelling of the face, or difficulty in breathing. If you cannot reach your doctor, phone a hospital emergency department.

- ☐ Most people experience few or no side effects from their drugs. However, any medicine can sometimes cause unwanted effects. Call your doctor if you develop a sore throat, bothersome sleepiness or laziness during the day, nightmares, staggering walk, unusual nervousness, a yellow color to the skin or eyes, easy bruising, or slow heartbeats.

* * * * *

Meprednisone (*Oral Corticosteroid*)
United States: Betapar

- ☐ This medicine is similar to cortisone which is a hormone normally produced by the body. This medicine is used to help decrease inflammation which then relieves pain, redness, and swelling. It is used to treat certain kinds of arthritis and severe allergies or skin conditions.

HOW TO USE THIS MEDICINE
- ☐ Take this medicine with food or a glass of milk in order to help prevent stomach upset. Call your doctor if you develop stomach upset or stomach pain or heartburn (especially if it awakens you during the night). Do not try to treat this yourself.

- ☐ If your doctor has prescribed only ONE dose of this medicine every day, it is best to take it before 9 A.M. or with breakfast.

- ☐ If you forget to take a dose, take it as soon as possible. However, if it is almost time for your next dose, do not take the missed dose. Instead, continue with your regular dosing schedule.

SPECIAL INSTRUCTIONS
- ☐ Women who are pregnant, breast-feeding, or planning to become pregnant should tell their doctor before taking this medicine.

- ☐ It is best not to drink alcoholic beverages while you are taking this medicine because the combination can cause stomach problems.

- ☐ Do not take any more of this medicine than your doctor has prescribed and do not stop taking this medicine suddenly without the approval of your doctor. It may be necessary for your doctor to slowly reduce your dose since your body becomes used to this medicine and it might be harmful if you suddenly did not receive this medicine.

☐ Do not take aspirin or medicines containing aspirin without the approval of your doctor.

☐ While you are taking this medicine you may gain some weight. This could be due to an increase in your appetite or increased water in your system. Your doctor may prescribe a special diet to decrease the number of calories you eat and/or to lower the amount of sodium or increase the amount of potassium in your diet. Follow any diet that your doctor may order.

☐ You may find that you bruise more easily. Try to protect yourself from all injuries to prevent bruising.

☐ Diabetic patients should regularly check the sugar in their urine and report any unusual levels to their doctor.

☐ Carry an identification card indicating that you are taking this medicine. Always tell your pharmacist, dentist, and other doctors who are treating you that you are taking this medicine. If you have an acute infection, injury, operation, or dental surgery within 1 year of taking this medicine, it is important to tell your doctor.

☐ Most people experience few or no side effects from their drugs. However, any medicine can sometimes cause unwanted effects. Call your doctor if you develop stomach pain, sore throat, fever, swelling of the legs or ankles, a wound which does not heal, eye pain or blurred vision, frequent urination ("passing your water"), nightmares or depression, muscle cramps, red or black stools, puffing of the face, or menstrual problems.

* * * * *

Meprobamate (Oral Antianxiety Agent)

United States: Equanil, Meprospan, Miltown, Robamate, Saronil, SK-Bamate, Tranmep

Canada: Equanil, Lan-Dol, Meditran, Mep-E, Meprospan-400, Miltown, Neo-Tran, Novomepro, Quietal

☐ This medicine is used to help relieve the symptoms of anxiety and tension.

☐ IMPORTANT: If you have ever had an allergic reaction to a sleeping pill or a tranquilizer, tell your doctor or pharmacist before you take any of this medicine.

HOW TO USE THIS MEDICINE

☐ This medicine may be taken with food.

☐ This medicine must be swallowed whole. Do not crush, chew, or break it into pieces. (**United States:** Equanil Wyseals, Meprospan; **Canada:** Meprospan-400)

495

SPECIAL INSTRUCTIONS

☐ If you forget to take a dose, take it as soon as possible. However, if it is almost time for your next dose, do not take the missed dose. Instead, continue with your regular dosing schedule.

☐ Women who are pregnant, breast-feeding, or planning to become pregnant should tell their doctor before taking this medicine.

☐ Do not take any more of this medicine than your doctor has prescribed because the drug could become habit-forming. Do not stop taking this medicine suddenly without the approval of your doctor.

☐ In some people, this drug may cause dizziness or drowsiness. Do not drive a car or operate dangerous machinery or do jobs that require you to be alert until you know how you are going to react to this drug.

☐ If this medicine causes dizziness, you should be careful going up and down stairs and you should not change positions too rapidly. Get out of bed slowly in the morning and dangle your feet over the edge of the bed for a few minutes before standing up. Sit down or lie down at the first sign of dizziness. Tell your doctor you have been dizzy. Avoid hot showers and baths because they could make you dizzy.

☐ Do not drink alcoholic beverages while taking this drug without the approval of your doctor.

☐ It is important that you obtain the advice of your doctor or pharmacist before taking ANY other medicines including pain relievers, sleeping pills, other tranquilizers or medicines for depression, cough/cold or allergy medicines, or weight-reducing medicines.

☐ Call your doctor immediately if you think you may be allergic to the medicine or if you develop a skin rash, hives, itching, swelling of the face, or difficulty in breathing. If you cannot reach your doctor, phone a hospital emergency department.

☐ Most people experience few or no side effects from their drugs. However, any medicine can sometimes cause unwanted effects. Call your doctor if you develop a sore throat, fever or mouth sores, easy bruising or bleeding, palpitations or a slow heartbeat, nightmares, or unusual nervousness.

☐ Carry an identification card indicating that you are taking this medicine. Always tell your pharmacist, dentist, and other doctors who are treating you that you are taking this medicine.

* * * * *

Mercaptopurine (*Oral Antineoplastic*)
United States: Purinethol
Canada: Purinethol

☐ This medicine is used in certain medical conditions to help slow down the growth and reproduction of some of the body's cells.

496

☐ This drug is sometimes called 6-mercaptopurine; "6" is part of the name and has nothing to do with the dosage.

HOW TO USE THIS MEDICINE

☐ It is best to take this medicine on an empty stomach at least 1 hour before (or 2 hours after) eating food. Take it at the proper time even if you skip a meal.

☐ It is very important that you take this medicine exactly as your doctor has prescribed and that you do not miss any doses. Try to take this medicine at the same time every day.

☐ Even if you become nauseated or lose your appetite, do not stop taking the medicine but check with your doctor.

☐ If you miss a dose of this medicine, do not take the missed dose and do not double your next dose. Check with your doctor.

SPECIAL INSTRUCTIONS

☐ Always keep your doctor appointments so that your doctor can watch your progress.

☐ If your doctor has prescribed some other medicines for you, it is important that you take them in the right order and that you do not miss them.

☐ Men and women should take appropriate birth control measures to avoid conception while they are taking this medicine and for at least 2 months after the medicine has been stopped.

☐ Always tell your pharmacist, dentist, and any other doctors who are treating you that you are taking this medicine. This is especially important if you plan to have surgery or any vaccinations.

☐ This is a very strong medicine. In addition to its benefits, there may be some unwanted effects, even for a short time after you stop taking the medicine. Call your doctor if you develop unusual bruising or bleeding, black "tarry" stools, sore throat, fever, mouth sores or white creamy patches in the mouth, a skin rash, swelling of the legs or ankles, shortness of breath, a yellow color to the skin or eyes, stomach or joint pain, severe nausea, or vomiting.

*   *   *   *   *

Mesoridazine (Oral Antipsychotic)
United States: Serentil
Canada: Serentil

☐ This medicine is used to help treat certain types of emotional problems. This drug has several other uses and the reason it was prescribed depends upon your condition. Check with your doctor if you do not fully understand why you are taking it.

☐ IMPORTANT: If you have ever had an allergic reaction to a phenothiazine medicine, tell your doctor or pharmacist before you take any of this medicine.

497

HOW TO USE THIS MEDICINE

☐ This medicine may be taken with food or a full glass of water.

☐ If a dropper or a dispensing spoon is used to measure the dose and you do not fully understand how to use it, check with your pharmacist.

☐ Store the liquid medicine in a cool dark place and do not get the liquid on your skin or clothing.

☐ Do not take this medicine at the same time as antacids or diarrhea medicine. Try to space them at least 1 hour apart.

☐ The effect of the medicine may not be noticed immediately, but may take from 2 to 4 weeks. Be patient. Take the medicine regularly and try not to miss any doses.

☐ Do not stop taking this medicine suddenly without the approval of your doctor.

SPECIAL INSTRUCTIONS

☐ If you forget to take a dose, take it as soon as possible. However, if it is almost time for your next dose, do not take the missed dose. Instead, continue with your regular dosing schedule.

☐ Any medicine has a few unwanted side effects. Because this medicine takes a few weeks to work, the side effects show the doctor that the drug is being absorbed. Many of these side effects will go away as your body adjusts to the medicine.

☐ Women who are pregnant, breast-feeding, or planning to become pregnant should tell their doctor before taking this medicine.

☐ In some people, this drug may cause dizziness or drowsiness. Do not drive a car or operate dangerous machinery or do jobs that require you to be alert until you know how you are going to react to this drug.

☐ If this medicine causes dizziness, you should be careful going up and down stairs and you should not change positions too rapidly. Get out of bed slowly in the morning and dangle your feet over the edge of the bed for a few minutes before standing up. Sit down or lie down at the first sign of dizziness. Tell your doctor you have been dizzy. Avoid hot showers and baths because they could make you dizzy.

☐ Do not drink alcoholic beverages while taking this drug without the approval of your doctor.

☐ This medicine may make some people more sensitive to sunlight and sunlamps. When you begin taking this medicine, try to avoid getting too much sun until you see how you are going to react. If your skin does become more sensitive to sunlight, tell your doctor and try to stay out of direct sunlight. While in the sun, wear protective clothing and sunglasses. You may wish to ask your pharmacist about suitable sunscreen products. Check with your doctor if you become sunburned.

☐ If your mouth becomes dry, suck a hard sour candy (sugarless) or ice chips, or chew gum. It is especially important to brush your teeth regularly if you develop a dry mouth.

☐ It is important that you obtain the advice of your doctor or pharmacist before taking **any** other medicines including pain relievers, sleeping pills, other tranquilizers or medicines for depression, cough/cold or allergy medicines, weight-reducing medicines, or laxatives.

☐ This medicine may cause your urine to turn pink, red, or red-brown in color. This is not unusual.

☐ In hot weather or during exercise, be careful not to become overheated. You may be more sensitive to heat since this medicine may affect the body's ability to regulate temperature.

☐ If you become constipated, try increasing the amount of bulk in your diet (for example, bran and salads), exercising more often, or drinking more water. Call your doctor if the constipation continues.

☐ Call your doctor if you develop a sore throat, fever, mouth sores, skin rash, changes in eyesight, rapid heart rate, a yellow color in the eyes or skin, unusual weakness or unusual movements of the face, tongue or hands, or difficulty in urinating ("passing your water"). Also call your doctor if you become restless or unable to sit still or sleep.

☐ Carry an identification card indicating that you are taking this medicine. Always tell your pharmacist, and other doctors who are treating you that you are taking this medicine.

*　*　*　*　*

Metaproterenol (*See Orciprenaline*)

*　*　*　*　*

Metaxalone (*Oral Skeletal Muscle Relaxant*)
United States: Skelaxin
Canada: Skelaxin

☐ This medicine is used to relax muscles and helps to relieve muscle pain and stiffness.

☐ IMPORTANT: If you have ever had an allergic reaction to any medicines, tell your doctor or pharmacist before you take any of this medicine.

HOW TO USE THIS MEDICINE
☐ This medicine may be taken with food or a glass of water.

☐ If you forget to take a dose, take it as soon as possible. However, if it is almost time for your next dose, do not take the missed dose. Instead, continue with your regular dosing schedule.

SPECIAL INSTRUCTIONS

- [ ] Do not drink alcoholic beverages while taking this drug without the approval of your doctor.

- [ ] It is important that you obtain the advice of your doctor or pharmacist before taking ANY other medicines including pain relievers, sleeping pills, tranquilizers or medicine for depression, cough/cold medicines, or allergy medicines.

- [ ] In some people, this drug may cause dizziness or drowsiness. Do not drive a car or operate dangerous machinery or do jobs that require you to be alert until you know how you are going to react to this drug.

- [ ] If you become dizzy, you should be careful going up and down stairs. Sit or lie down at the first sign of dizziness.

- [ ] Most people experience few or no side effects from their drugs. However, any medicine can sometimes cause unwanted effects. Call your doctor if you develop a skin rash, dark-colored urine, a yellow color to the skin or eyes, or unusual tiredness.

*   *   *   *   *

Metformin HCl *(Oral Hypoglycemic)*
Canada: Glucophage

- [ ] This medicine is used in the treatment of diabetes. When you have diabetes, the body either is not producing enough insulin or is not able to use what is produced. Insulin is needed for the body's proper use of food, especially sugar. In a diabetic, the sugar in the blood can build up to dangerous levels and is excreted in the urine. Your doctor has prescribed this medicine to help keep your blood sugar at nearly normal levels.

HOW TO USE THIS MEDICINE

- [ ] This medicine may be taken with food to help prevent stomach upset.

- [ ] It is very important that you take this medicine exactly as your doctor has prescribed. Do not miss any doses. Try to take this medicine at the same time every day. Do not take extra tablets without your doctor's approval.

- [ ] Do not take this medicine at bedtime unless your doctor tells you to.

- [ ] If you forget to take a dose, take it as soon as possible. However, if it is almost time for your next dose, do not take the missed dose. Instead, continue with your regular dosing schedule.

SPECIAL INSTRUCTIONS

- [ ] Women who are pregnant, breast-feeding, or planning to become pregnant should tell their doctor before taking this medicine.

☐ Most people experience few or no side effects from their drugs. However, any medicine can sometimes cause unwanted effects. Call your doctor if you develop loss of appetite or unexplained weight loss, nausea or vomiting, unusual tiredness, stomach pain, or deep breathing.

GENERAL INSTRUCTIONS FOR DIABETIC PATIENTS

☐ Keep a regular schedule of daily activities. Eat, exercise, and take your insulin at approximately the same time every day.

☐ The diet that your doctor has prescribed has been carefully planned especially for you. It is to your advantage to follow it closely.

☐ Test your urine regularly for sugar and if your doctor recommends, test it for acetone.

☐ Learn the signs of hypoglycemia (low blood sugar). When this happens, your urine sugar will be negative. Hypoglycemia may occur if you delay or skip a meal, exercise too much, become sick or emotionally upset, take too much insulin, drink alcohol, or take certain drugs. If you develop sweating, drowsiness, unusual hunger, dizziness, nausea, nervousness, blurred vision, weakness, shaking, or trembling, eat or drink any of the following:
  • 2 sugar cubes or 2 teaspoons of sugar in water
  • 4 ounces orange juice
  • 4 ounces regular ginger ale, cola beverages, or any other sweetened carbonated beverage. Do NOT use low-calorie or diet beverages.
  • 2 to 3 teaspoons honey or corn syrup
  • 4 Lifesaver candies

Artificial sweeteners are of no use. Call your doctor if one of the above does not relieve your symptoms in about 15 minutes.

☐ Always carry sugar cubes or hard candy in case you have a hypoglycemic (low blood sugar) reaction.

☐ Before you purchase any nonprescription medicine (for example, cough and cold medicines), ask your pharmacist if the medicine is safe for diabetic patients to use. Some nonprescription medicines have very high sugar contents which could interfere with the control of your diabetes. Aspirin and medicines containing salicylates or vitamin C could affect your urine test results. Check with your pharmacist.

☐ Ask your doctor if it is safe for you to drink alcoholic beverages because the combination may cause low blood sugar as well as a pounding headache, flushing, upset stomach, dizziness, or sweating.

☐ Take special care of your feet.
  • Wash your feet daily and dry them well.
  • Check your feet daily for minor injuries. Bring these to the attention of your doctor immediately.
  • Wear clean shoes and stockings and choose shoes that fit well.
  • If you develop corns or calluses, soak your feet in lukewarm water for about 10 minutes. Then rub them off gently with a pumice stone.

501

Never use a knife to cut corns or calluses on your feet. Do NOT use commercial corn removers, or commercial arch supports.
- Soften dry skin by rubbing it with oil or lotion.
- Trim your toenails straight across with a file or a nail cutter. Do not cut your own toenails if your eyesight is poor.
- Do not wear garters or socks with tight elastic tops. Do NOT sit with your knees crossed.
- Do not warm your feet with a hot water bottle or a heating pad. Use loose bed socks instead. If your feet are cold under normal conditions, tell your doctor. Your circulation may be poor and your doctor can offer advice.
- Call your doctor if you injure your toes or feet. Cuts and scratches in the diabetic patient can become infected easily and take longer to heal. Do not apply iodine or strong antiseptics to the feet at any time.

☐ Call your doctor immediately if you develop any of the following symptoms of hyperglycemia (high blood sugar): high urine sugar, acetone in urine, drowsiness, hunger, unusual thirst, fast breathing, nausea, confusion, a flushed dry skin, increase in urination ("passing your water"), or a fruity odor to the breath. These symptoms may occur if you are taking too little insulin, miss a dose, overeat, or if you have a fever or infection.

☐ Call your doctor if you become sick and have a fever, an infection, nausea, or vomiting.

☐ Carry an identification card or wear a bracelet indicating that you are a diabetic and that you are taking this medicine. Always tell your pharmacist, dentist, and other doctors who are treating you that you are taking this medicine.

*   *   *   *   *

Methacycline HCl (Oral Antibiotic)
United States: Rondomycin

☐ This medicine is an antibiotic used to treat certain types of infections and to help control acne.

☐ IMPORTANT: If you have ever had an allergic reaction to tetracycline or any other antibiotic, tell your doctor or pharmacist before you take any of this medicine.

HOW TO USE THIS MEDICINE

☐ It is best to take this medicine on an empty stomach 1 hour before eating food or 2 hours after eating food. Take it at the proper time even if you skip a meal. If this medicine upsets your stomach, take it with some crackers (not with dairy products). Call your doctor if you continue to have stomach upset.

☐ Take this medicine with a full glass of water.

502

- ☐ Do not drink milk or eat cheese, cottage cheese, ice cream, or other dairy products 1 hour before or 2 hours after you have taken a dose of this medicine.

- ☐ For LIQUID MEDICINE (**United States:** Rondomycin Syrup)
  - Shake the bottle well before using so that you can measure an accurate dose.
  - Store the liquid medicine in the refrigerator. Do not freeze.

SPECIAL INSTRUCTIONS

- ☐ It is important that you take **all** of this medicine plus any refills that your doctor told you to take. Do not stop taking this medicine earlier than your doctor has recommended in spite of the fact that you may feel better. Otherwise, the infection may return.

- ☐ If you forget to take a dose, take it as soon as you remember and then continue with your regular schedule.

- ☐ Women who are pregnant, breast-feeding, or planning to become pregnant should tell their doctor before taking this medicine.

- ☐ Some antacids and some laxatives can make this medicine less effective if they are taken at the same time. If you must take them, they should be taken at least 2 to 3 hours after this medicine. If you have any questions, ask your pharmacist.

- ☐ If you must take iron products or vitamins containing iron, take them 2 hours before (or 3 hours after) this medicine.

- ☐ This medicine may make some people more sensitive to sunlight or sunlamps. When you begin taking this medicine, try to avoid getting too much sun until you see how you are going to react. If your skin does become more sensitive, try to stay out of direct sunlight. While in the sun, wear protective clothing and sunglasses. You may wish to ask your pharmacist about suitable sunscreen products. You may remain sensitive to sunlight and sunlamps for several weeks after you have stopped taking the drug. Check with your doctor if you become sunburned.

- ☐ Most people experience few or no side effects from their drugs. However, any medicine can sometimes cause unwanted effects. Call your doctor if you develop a dark-colored tongue, sore mouth, yellow-green stools or, in women, a vaginal discharge that was not present before you started taking this medicine.

- ☐ Store the medicine in a cool, dark place and keep tightly closed.

- ☐ If for some reason you cannot take all of the medicine, discard the unused portion by flushing it down the toilet. Do not save this medicine for future use. Outdated methacycline can be harmful.

*   *   *   *   *

Methadone HCl

United States: Dolophine, Methadone Diskets, Westadone
Canada: Methadone

☐ This medicine is used to help relieve pain. It is also used in some special treatment programs to help people who are dependent on heroin or other narcotics.

HOW TO USE THIS MEDICINE

☐ These tablets may be taken with food or a glass of water. (*United States:* Dolophine)

☐ These tablets must be dissolved in water or fruit juice before you take them. (*United States:* Methadone Diskets, Westadone)

☐ The liquid medicine may have to be mixed with water or juice before you take it. Your pharmacist will tell you how to take it.

☐ Do not take any more of this medicine than your doctor has prescribed. The drug could become habit-forming or you could take an overdose if you take it more often or longer than prescribed.

SPECIAL INSTRUCTIONS

☐ Women who are pregnant, breast-feeding, or planning to become pregnant should tell their doctor before taking this medicine.

☐ Do not drink alcoholic beverages while taking this drug without the approval of your doctor.

☐ It is important that you obtain the advice of your doctor or pharmacist before taking ANY other medicines including other pain relievers, sleeping pills, tranquilizers or medicines for depression, cough/cold or allergy medicines, or weight-reducing medicines.

☐ In some people, this drug may cause dizziness or drowsiness. Do not drive a car or operate dangerous machinery or do jobs that require you to be alert until you know how you are going to react to this drug.

☐ If you become dizzy, you should be careful going up and down stairs. Sit or lie down at the first sign of dizziness. Get up slowly if you have been lying or sitting down.

☐ If you do feel nauseated when you first start taking the medicine, it may help if you lie down for a few minutes.

☐ If you become constipated, try increasing the amount of bulk in your diet (for example, bran and salads), exercising more often, or drinking more water. Call your doctor if the constipation continues.

☐ Most people experience few or no side effects from their drugs. However, any medicine can sometimes cause unwanted effects. Call your doctor if you

develop shortness of breath, slow heartbeats, unusual nervousness, stomach pain, or difficulty in urinating ("passing your water").

☐ Always tell your dentist, pharmacist, and other doctors who are treating you that you are taking this medicine.

*   *   *   *   *

Methallenestril (Oral Estrogen)
Canada: Vallestril

☐ This medicine is a hormone. It has many uses and the reason it was prescribed depends on your condition. If you do not understand why you are taking it, check with your doctor.

HOW TO USE THIS MEDICINE
☐ The tablets may be taken after meals or with a snack if they upset your stomach.

SPECIAL INSTRUCTIONS
☐ Women who are pregnant, breast-feeding, or planning to become pregnant should tell their doctor before taking this medicine.

☐ It is recommended that you do not smoke while you are taking this medicine because smoking may increase the incidence of heart attacks.

☐ Diabetic patients should regularly check the sugar in their urine while they are taking this medicine.

☐ Contact your doctor if any of the following side effects occur:
- Severe or persistent headaches
- Vomiting, dizziness, or fainting
- Blurred vision or slurred speech
- Pain in the calves of the legs or numbness in an arm or leg
- Chest pain, shortness of breath, or coughing of blood
- Lumps in the breast
- Severe depression
- A yellow color to the skin or eyes or dark-colored urine
- Severe abdominal pain
- Vaginal bleeding

☐ Carry an identification card indicating that you are taking this medicine. Always tell your pharmacist, dentist, and other doctors who are treating you that you are taking this medicine.

*   *   *   *   *

Methamphetamine (*Oral Sympathomimetic*)
United States: Desoxyn, Methampex, Obedrin-LA

- ☐ This medicine has many uses and the reason it was prescribed depends upon your condition. If you do not fully understand why you are taking it, check with your doctor.

- ☐ IMPORTANT: If you have ever had an allergic reaction to an amphetamine medicine or any other medicine, tell your doctor or pharmacist before you take any of this medicine.

HOW TO USE THIS MEDICINE

- ☐ This medicine may be taken with food or a glass of water.

- ☐ Do not take the medicine late in the day or it may cause insomnia (difficulty in sleeping).

- ☐ This medicine must be swallowed whole. Do not crush, chew, or break it into pieces. (**United States:** Desoxyn Gradumets, Obedrin-LA)

SPECIAL INSTRUCTIONS

- ☐ If you forget to take a dose, take it as soon as possible. However, if it is almost time for your next dose, do not take the missed dose. Instead, continue with your regular dosing schedule.

- ☐ Women who are pregnant, breast-feeding, or planning to become pregnant should tell their doctor before taking this medicine.

- ☐ Do not take any more of this medicine than your doctor has prescribed and do not stop taking this medicine suddenly without the approval of your doctor.

- ☐ If your mouth becomes dry, suck a hard sour candy (sugarless) or ice chips, or chew gum. It is especially important to brush your teeth regularly if you develop a dry mouth.

- ☐ In some people, this drug may cause dizziness. Do not drive a car or operate dangerous machinery or do jobs that require you to be alert until you know how you are going to react to this drug. Therefore, you should be careful going up and down stairs. Sit or lie down at the first sign of dizziness.

- ☐ If this medicine is for a child, do not let him (her) ride a bike or climb trees until you can determine how he (she) is going to react to the medicine. Children could hurt themselves if they participated in these activities if they were dizzy.

- ☐ Do not treat yourself with baking soda or antacids without the approval of your doctor.

- ☐ Most people experience few or no side effects from their drugs. However, any medicine can sometimes cause unwanted effects. Call your doctor if you develop a skin rash; chest pain or palpitations; unusual movements of the head, arms, or legs; or unusual restlessness.

- Carry an identification card indicating that you are taking this medicine. Always tell your pharmacist, dentist, and other doctors who are treating you that you are taking this medicine.

* * * * *

Methandrostenolone (*Oral Anabolic Steroid*)
United States: Dianabol
Canada: Danabol

- This medicine is similar to a hormone which is normally produced by the body. This medicine has many uses and the reason it was prescribed depends upon your condition. If you do not understand why you are taking it, check with your doctor.

HOW TO USE THIS MEDICINE
- Take the drug after meals or with a snack if it upsets your stomach.
- It is very important that you take this drug as your doctor has prescribed.

SPECIAL INSTRUCTIONS
- Women who are pregnant, breast-feeding, or planning to become pregnant should tell their doctor before taking this medicine.
- Diabetic patients should regularly check the sugar in the urine and report any abnormal results to their doctor.
- Carry an identification card indicating that you are taking this medicine. Always tell your pharmacist, dentist, and other doctors who are treating you that you are taking this medicine.
- Most people experience few or no side effects from their drugs. However, any medicine can sometimes cause unwanted effects. Call your doctor if you develop swelling of the hands, legs, or ankles; sore throat and fever; acne; unusual restlessness; dark-colored urine; or a yellow color to the skin or eyes. Women should call their doctor if they develop menstrual problems, hoarseness or a deepening of the voice, baldness, or increased facial hair.

* * * * *

Methantheline Bromide (*Oral Anticholinergic*)
United States: Banthine

- This medicine is used to help relax muscles of the stomach, bowels, and bladder as well as to decrease the amount of acid formed in the stomach.
- IMPORTANT: If you have ever had an allergic reaction to atropine or bromides or any other drug used to relax the stomach or bowels, tell your doctor or pharmacist before you take any of this medicine.

507

HOW TO USE THIS MEDICINE

☐ Take this medicine approximately 30 minutes before a meal unless otherwise directed.

☐ If you miss a dose of this medicine, do not take the missed dose and do not double the next dose.

SPECIAL INSTRUCTIONS

☐ If your mouth becomes dry, suck a hard sour candy (sugarless) or ice chips, or chew gum. It is especially important to brush your teeth regularly if you develop a dry mouth.

☐ In some people, this drug may cause dizziness or drowsiness. Do not drive a car or operate dangerous machinery or do jobs that require you to be alert until you know how you are going to react to this drug.

☐ If you become dizzy, you should be careful going up and down stairs. Sit or lie down at the first sign of dizziness. Tell your doctor you have been dizzy.

☐ A desire to urinate ("pass your water") with an inability to do so is not an uncommon effect with this drug. Urinating each time before taking the drug may help relieve this problem. Call your doctor if it continues.

☐ You may become more sensitive to heat because your body may perspire less while you are taking this drug. Be careful not to become overheated during exercise or in hot weather.

☐ Do not take antacids within 1 hour of taking this medicine as they could make this medicine less effective.

☐ If you become constipated, try increasing the amount of bulk in your diet (for example, bran and salads), exercising more often, or drinking more water. Call your doctor if the constipation continues.

☐ If your eyes become more sensitive to sunlight, it may help to wear sunglasses.

☐ Most people experience few or no side effects from their drugs. However, any medicine can sometimes cause unwanted effects. Call your doctor if you develop a skin rash, diarrhea, unusual restlessness, flushing, or eye pain.

* * * * *

Methapyrilene HCl (*Oral Antihistamine*)
United States: Nytol, Relax-U-caps

☐ This medicine is used to help relieve the symptoms of certain types of allergic conditions, coughs and colds, and certain skin conditions.

HOW TO USE THIS MEDICINE

☐ This medicine may be taken with food or a glass of milk if it upsets your stomach.

508

SPECIAL INSTRUCTIONS

☐ If you forget to take a dose, take it as soon as possible. However, if it is almost time for your next dose, do not take the missed dose. Instead, continue with your regular dosing schedule.

☐ In some people, this drug may initially cause dizziness or drowsiness. Do not drive a car or operate dangerous machinery or do jobs that require you to be alert until you know how you are going to react to this drug. If you become dizzy, you should be careful going up and down stairs. Sit or lie down at the first sign of dizziness. Tell your doctor if it continues.

☐ Do not drink alcoholic beverages while taking this drug without the approval of your doctor.

☐ If your mouth becomes dry, suck a hard sour candy (sugarless) or ice chips, or chew gum. It is especially important to brush your teeth regularly if you develop a dry mouth.

☐ It is important that you obtain the advice of your doctor or pharmacist before taking pain relievers, nonprescription drugs, sleeping pills or tranquilizers, or other medicines for allergies.

☐ Do not take this medicine more often or longer than recommended by your doctor.

☐ Most people experience few or no side effects from their drugs. However, any medicine can sometimes cause unwanted effects. Call your doctor if you develop a skin rash, fast heartbeats, blurred vision, stomach pain, or difficulty in urinating ("passing your water").

* * * * *

Methaqualone (Oral Sedative-Hypnotic)
United States: Parest, Quaalude, Sopor

Canada: Mequelon, Rouqualone-"300," Sedalone, Triador, Tualone-300, Vitalone

☐ This medicine is used to cause sleep and for certain types of nervous tension.

HOW TO USE THIS MEDICINE
☐ This medicine may be taken with food or a glass of water.

SPECIAL INSTRUCTIONS
☐ Sleeping medicines are only useful for a short time. If used for too long, they lose their effectiveness. Do not take any more of this medicine than your doctor has prescribed and do not stop taking this medicine suddenly without the approval of your doctor. Do not smoke in bed after you have taken this medicine.

☐ Women who are pregnant, breast-feeding, or planning to become pregnant should tell their doctor before taking this medicine.

- [] In some people, this drug may cause dizziness or drowsiness. Do not drive a car or operate dangerous machinery or do jobs that require you to be alert until you know how you are going to react to this drug.

- [] If you become dizzy, you should be careful going up and down stairs. Sit or lie down at the first sign of dizziness.

- [] Do not drink alcoholic beverages while taking this drug without the approval of your doctor.

- [] It is important that you obtain the advice of your doctor or pharmacist before taking ANY other medicines including pain relievers, sleeping pills, tranquilizers or medicines for depression, cough/cold medicines, or allergy medicines.

- [] Call your doctor immediately if you think you may be allergic to the medicine or if you develop a skin rash, hives, itching, swelling of the face, or difficulty in breathing. If you cannot reach your doctor, phone a hospital emergency department.

- [] Most people experience few or no side effects from their drugs. However, any medicine can sometimes cause unwanted effects. Call your doctor if you develop a sore throat, fever or mouth sores, or unusual nervousness.

*   *   *   *   *

Metharbital (*Oral Sedative-Anticonvulsant*)
United States: Gemonil

- [] This medicine is used to cause sleep and for certain types of nervous tension. It is also specially prescribed to help prevent seizures in some patients. Check with your doctor if you do not fully understand why you are taking it.

- [] IMPORTANT: If you have ever had an allergic reaction to a barbiturate medicine, tell your doctor or pharmacist before you take any of this medicine.

HOW TO USE THIS MEDICINE
- [] This medicine may be taken with food or a full glass of water.

SPECIAL INSTRUCTIONS
- [] Sleeping medicines are only useful for a short time. If used for too long, they lose their effectiveness. Do not take any more of this medicine than your doctor has prescribed and do not stop taking this medicine suddenly without the approval of your doctor.

- [] Women who are pregnant, breast-feeding, or planning to become pregnant should tell their doctor before taking this medicine.

- [] In some people, this drug may cause dizziness or drowsiness. Do not drive a car or operate dangerous machinery or do jobs that require you to be alert until you know how you are going to react to this drug.

510

- [ ] If you become dizzy, you should be careful going up and down stairs. Sit or lie down at the first sign of dizziness.

- [ ] Do not drink alcoholic beverages while taking this drug without the approval of your doctor.

- [ ] It is important that you obtain the advice of your doctor or pharmacist before taking ANY other medicines including pain relievers, sleeping pills, tranquilizers or medicines for depression, cough/cold medicines, or allergy medicines.

- [ ] If you are taking this medicine to help you sleep, take it about 20 minutes before you want to go to sleep. Go to bed after you have taken it. Do not smoke in bed after you have taken it.

- [ ] Do not store this medicine at the bedside and keep it out of the reach of children.

- [ ] Call your doctor immediately if you think you may be allergic to the medicine or if you develop a skin rash, hives, itching, swelling of the face, or difficulty in breathing. If you cannot reach your doctor, phone a hospital emergency department.

- [ ] Most people experience few or no side effects from their drugs. However, any medicine can sometimes cause unwanted effects. Call your doctor if you develop a sore throat, bothersome sleepiness or laziness during the day, nightmares, a staggering walk, unusual nervousness, a yellow color to the skin or eyes, easy bruising or slow heartbeats.

* * * * *

Methazolamide (*Oral Carbonic Anhydrase Inhibitor*)
United States: Neptazane
Canada: Neptazane

- [ ] This medicine is used in the treatment of glaucoma.

- [ ] IMPORTANT: If you have ever had an allergic reaction to a sulfa drug, thiazide "water pill," or diabetes medicine that you take by mouth, tell your doctor or pharmacist before you take any of this medicine.

HOW TO USE THIS MEDICINE
- [ ] Take the medicine with food or a glass of water.

- [ ] If you forget a dose, take it as soon as possible. However, if it is almost time for your next dose, do not take the missed dose. Instead, continue with your regular dosing schedule.

SPECIAL INSTRUCTIONS
- [ ] In some people, this medicine will cause the body to lose a little potassium. Call your doctor if you develop any of the following: unusual thirst, leg

cramps, unusual weakness, tiredness, vomiting, confusion, or an increased pulse. Your doctor may want you to take some extra potassium or to eat certain foods that contain potassium.

☐ Women who are pregnant, breast-feeding, or planning to become pregnant should tell their doctor before taking this medicine.

☐ Most people experience few or no side effects from their drugs. However, any medicine can sometimes cause unwanted effects. Call your doctor if you develop a fever, numbness or tingling of the hands or feet, or eye pain.

* * * * *

Methdilazine HCl (Oral Antiallergic-Antipruritic)
United States: Tacaryl
Canada: Dilosyn

☐ This medicine is used to help relieve the symptoms of certain types of allergic conditions, coughs and colds, and certain skin conditions.

HOW TO USE THIS MEDICINE
☐ This medicine may be taken with food or a glass of milk if it upsets your stomach.

☐ Chew these tablets well before swallowing. (**United States:** Tacaryl Chewable Tablets)

SPECIAL INSTRUCTIONS
☐ If you forget to take a dose, take it as soon as possible. However, if it is almost time for your next dose, do not take the missed dose. Instead, continue with your regular dosing schedule.

☐ In some people, this drug may initially cause dizziness or drowsiness. Do not drive a car or operate dangerous machinery or do jobs that require you to be alert until you know how you are going to react to this drug. If you become dizzy, you should be careful going up and down stairs. Sit or lie down at the first sign of dizziness. Tell your doctor if it continues.

☐ Do not drink alcoholic beverages while taking this drug without the approval of your doctor.

☐ If your mouth becomes dry, suck a hard sour candy (sugarless) or ice chips, or chew gum. It is especially important to brush your teeth regularly if you develop a dry mouth.

☐ It is important that you obtain the advice of your doctor or pharmacist before taking pain relievers, nonprescription drugs, sleeping pills or tranquilizers, or other medicines for allergies.

☐ Do not take this medicine more often or longer than recommended by your doctor.

512

☐ Most people experience few or no side effects from their drugs. However, any medicine can sometimes cause unwanted effects. Call your doctor if you develop a skin rash, fast heartbeats, blurred vision, stomach pain, or difficulty in urinating ("passing your water").

*   *   *   *   *

Methenamine Mandelate (*Oral Urinary Anti-infective*)
United States: Mandelamine, Mandelets, Prov-U-Sep
Canada: Mandelamine, Methandine, Sterine

Methenamine Hippurate
United States: Hiprex, Urex
Canada: Hip-Rex

Methenamine Sulfosalicylate
United States: Hexalet

Methenamine Mandelate-Phenazopyridine
United States: Azo-Mandelamine
Canada: Azo-Mandelamine

☐ This medicine is used to treat urinary tract infections.

HOW TO USE THIS MEDICINE
☐ This medicine may be taken with food.

☐ Take the medicine with a glass of water and try to drink several additional glasses of water or other fluids every day unless otherwise directed.

☐ This medicine has a special coating and must be swallowed whole. Do not crush, chew, or break it into pieces. Do not take chipped tablets. (**United States:** Azo-Mandelamine, Mandelamine, Mandelets. **Canada:** Azo-Mandelamine, Mandelamine, Methandine, Sterine)

☐ Dissolve the contents of each package in 2 to 4 ounces of water and stir well. Drink immediately and be sure to take all of the liquid in order to get the full dose. (**United States:** Mandelamine Granules)

☐ For LIQUID MEDICINE
    • Shake the bottle well before using so that you can measure an accurate dose. (**United States** and **Canada:** Mandelamine Suspension)

SPECIAL INSTRUCTIONS
☐ It is important to take **all** of this medicine plus any refills that your doctor told you to take. Do not stop taking it earlier than your doctor has recommended

513

in spite of the fact that you may feel better. Otherwise, the infection may return.

□ If you forget to take a dose, take it as soon as you remember and then continue with your regular schedule.

□ For this drug to be effective, your urine must be acidic at all times. This is measured by testing the urine with a special type of paper. The 'pH' of the urine must be as low as 5.5. Check with your pharmacist on methods of testing the pH of the urine.

□ Unless you are on a special diet prescribed by your doctor, you should **avoid** the following foods which can make your urine less acidic and which would make the drug less effective: citrus fruits and fruit juices, milk and other dairy products, and peanuts. You should not take antacids without the approval of your doctor.

□ Your doctor may recommend that you eat some of the following foods to make the urine more acidic: cranberries and cranberry juice, plums, prunes, and high-protein foods.

□ This medicine may cause the urine to turn red-orange in color. This is not unusual. (**United States** and **Canada:** Azo-Mandelamine)

□ Most people experience few or no side effects from their drugs. However, any medicine can sometimes cause unwanted effects. Call your doctor if you develop a skin rash, lower back pain, or difficulty in urinating ("passing your water").

* * * * *

Methimazole (*Oral Antithyroid*)
United States: Tapazole
Canada: Tapazole

□ This medicine is used to treat an overactive thyroid gland and is also used before thyroid surgery.

HOW TO USE THIS MEDICINE
□ This medicine may be taken with meals or on an empty stomach. To make sure that you always get the same effect, always take it the same way.

□ If you miss a dose of this medicine, take it as soon as you remember.

SPECIAL INSTRUCTIONS
□ It is very important that you take this medicine exactly as your doctor has prescribed and that you do not miss any doses. Try to take this medicine at the same time every day. Do not take extra tablets without your doctor's approval. Do not stop taking this medicine without the approval of your doctor.

514

- Women who are pregnant, breast-feeding, or planning to become pregnant should tell their doctor before taking this medicine.

- Check with your doctor or pharmacist before taking any nonprescription drugs that contain iodides (for example, some cough, cold, or asthma products).

- Call your doctor immediately if you become sick or develop a fever, sore throat, skin abscess, or other symptoms of an infection.

- Most people experience few or no side effects from their drugs. However, any medicine can sometimes cause unwanted effects. Call your doctor if you develop a sore throat, fever or mouth sores, skin rash, dark-colored urine or a yellow color to the skin or eyes, easy bruising or bleeding, swelling of the legs, swollen glands, changes in urination ("passing your water"), fast heartbeats, or unusual tiredness.

* * * * *

Methixene HCl (*Oral Antispasmodic*)
United States: Trest

- This medicine is used to help relax muscles of the stomach and bowels as well as to decrease the amount of acid formed in the stomach.

- IMPORTANT: If you have ever had an allergic reaction to atropine or any other drug used to relax the stomach or bowels, tell your doctor or pharmacist before you take any of this medicine.

HOW TO USE THIS MEDICINE

- Take this medicine approximately 30 minutes before a meal unless otherwise directed.

- If you miss a dose of this medicine, do not take the missed dose and do not double the next dose.

SPECIAL INSTRUCTIONS

- If your mouth becomes dry, suck a hard sour candy (sugarless) or ice chips, or chew gum. It is especially important to brush your teeth regularly if you develop a dry mouth.

- In some people, this drug may cause dizziness or drowsiness. Do not drive a car or operate dangerous machinery or do jobs that require you to be alert until you know how you are going to react to this drug.

- If you become dizzy, you should be careful going up and down stairs. Sit or lie down at the first sign of dizziness. Tell your doctor you have been dizzy.

- A desire to urinate ("pass your water") with an inability to do so is not an uncommon effect with this drug. Urinating each time before taking the drug may help relieve this problem. Call your doctor if it continues.

515

☐ You may become more sensitive to heat because your body may perspire less while you are taking this drug. Be careful not to become overheated during exercise or in hot weather.

☐ Do not take antacids within 1 hour of taking this medicine as they could make this medicine less effective.

☐ If you become constipated, try increasing the amount of bulk in your diet (for example, bran and salads), exercising more often, or drinking more water. Call your doctor if the constipation continues.

☐ If your eyes become more sensitive to sunlight, it may help to wear sunglasses.

☐ Most people experience few or no side effects from their drugs. However, any medicine can sometimes cause unwanted effects. Call your doctor if you develop a skin rash, diarrhea, unusual restlessness, flushing, or eye pain.

*   *   *   *   *

Methocarbamol (*Oral Skeletal Muscle Relaxant*)

United States: Delaxin, Forbaxin, Metho-500, Robaxin, Spenaxin
Canada: Robaxin

☐ This medicine is used to relax muscles and helps to relieve muscle pain and stiffness.

☐ IMPORTANT: If you have ever had an allergic reaction to any medicines, tell your doctor or pharmacist before you take any of this medicine.

HOW TO USE THIS MEDICINE

☐ This medicine may be taken with food or a glass of water.

☐ If you forget to take a dose, take it as soon as possible. However, if it is almost time for your next dose, do not take the missed dose. Instead, continue with your regular dosing schedule.

SPECIAL INSTRUCTIONS

☐ Do not drink alcoholic beverages while taking this drug without the approval of your doctor.

☐ It is important that you obtain the advice of your doctor or pharmacist before taking ANY other medicines including pain relievers, sleeping pills, tranquilizers or medicine for depression, cough/cold medicines, or allergy medicines.

☐ In some people, this drug may cause dizziness or drowsiness. Do not drive a car or operate dangerous machinery or do jobs that require you to be alert until you know how you are going to react to this drug.

☐ If this medicine causes dizziness, you should be careful going up and down stairs and you should not change positions too rapidly. Get out of bed slowly

in the morning and dangle your feet over the edge of the bed for a few minutes before standing up. Sit down or lie down at the first sign of dizziness. Tell your doctor you have been dizzy. Avoid hot showers and baths because they could make you dizzy.

☐ Call your doctor immediately if you think you may be allergic to the medicine or if you develop a skin rash, hives, or itching. If you cannot reach your doctor, phone a hospital emergency department.

☐ Most people experience few or no side effects from their drugs. However, any medicine can sometimes cause unwanted effects. Call your doctor if you develop a skin rash, itching, nasal stuffiness, blurred vision, bloodshot eyes, or a fever.

*   *   *   *   *

Methocarbamol-ASA (*Oral Skeletal Muscle Relaxant*)
United States: Robaxisal
Canada: Robaxisal

Methocarbamol-ASA-Codeine Phosphate
Canada: Robaxisal C-1/4, Robaxisal C-1/8

☐ This medicine is used to relax muscles and helps to relieve muscle pain and stiffness.

☐ IMPORTANT: If you have ever had an allergic reaction to aspirin or any medicines, tell your doctor or pharmacist before you take any of this medicine.

HOW TO USE THIS MEDICINE
☐ This medicine may be taken with food or a glass of water.

☐ If you forget to take a dose, take it as soon as possible. However, if it is almost time for your next dose, do not take the missed dose. Instead, continue with your regular dosing schedule.

SPECIAL INSTRUCTIONS
☐ Do not drink alcoholic beverages while taking this drug without the approval of your doctor.

☐ Women who are pregnant, breast-feeding, or planning to become pregnant should tell their doctor before taking this medicine.

☐ It is important that you obtain the advice of your doctor or pharmacist before taking ANY other medicines including pain relievers, sleeping pills, tranquilizers or medicine for depression, cough/cold medicines, or allergy medicines.

- [ ] In some people, this drug may cause dizziness or drowsiness. Do not drive a car or operate dangerous machinery or do jobs that require you to be alert until you know how you are going to react to this drug.

- [ ] If this medicine causes dizziness, you should be careful going up and down stairs and you should not change positions too rapidly. Get out of bed slowly in the morning and dangle your feet over the edge of the bed for a few minutes before standing up. Sit down or lie down at the first sign of dizziness. Tell your doctor you have been dizzy. Avoid hot showers and baths because they could make you dizzy.

- [ ] Call your doctor immediately if you think you may be allergic to the medicine or if you develop a skin rash, hives, or itching. If you cannot reach your doctor, phone a hospital emergency department.

- [ ] Do not take this medicine if it smells strongly like vinegar since this means that the aspirin in the medicine is not fresh.

- [ ] Do not take any more of this medicine than your doctor has prescribed and do not stop taking this medicine suddenly without the approval of your doctor.

- [ ] Most people experience few or no side effects from their drugs. However, any medicine can sometimes cause unwanted effects. Call your doctor if you develop a skin rash, itching, nasal stuffiness, blurred vision, bloodshot eyes, or a fever. Also call your doctor if you develop "ringing" or "buzzing" of the ears, red or black stools, stomach pain, fast breathing, or confusion.

*   *   *   *   *

Methoserpidine-Hydrochlorothiazide (Oral Antihypertensive)
Canada: Decaserpyl Plus

- [ ] Hypertension (high blood pressure) is a long-term condition and it will probably be necessary for you to take the drug for a long time in spite of the fact that you feel better. It is very important that you take this medicine as your doctor has directed and that you do not miss any doses. Otherwise, you cannot expect the drug to keep your blood pressure down.

- [ ] IMPORTANT: If you have allergies, tell your doctor or pharmacist before you take any of this medicine.

HOW TO USE THIS MEDICINE
- [ ] Take this medicine with food, meals, or milk.
- [ ] Try to take the medicine at the same time(s) every day.

SPECIAL INSTRUCTIONS
- [ ] If you forget to take a dose, take it as soon as possible. However, if it is almost time for your next dose, do not take the missed dose. Instead, continue with your regular dosing schedule.

518

☐ Women who are pregnant, breast-feeding, or planning to become pregnant should tell their doctor before taking this medicine.

☐ This medicine normally causes your body to lose potassium. The body has warning signs to let you know if too much potassium is being lost. Call your doctor if you become unusually thirsty or if you develop leg cramps, unusual weakness, fatigue, vomiting, confusion, or an irregular pulse.

☐ If your doctor recommends that you eat foods which are high in potassium, one or more of the foods listed in Appendix A should be eaten daily. All of these foods are rich in potassium. CHANGE YOUR DIET ONLY IF YOUR DOCTOR TELLS YOU TO.

☐ This medicine may make some people more sensitive to sunlight and sun-lamps. When you begin taking this medicine, try to avoid getting too much sun until you see how you are going to react. If your skin does become more sensitive to sunlight, tell your doctor and try to stay out of direct sunlight. While in the sun, wear protective clothing and sunglasses. You may wish to ask your pharmacist about suitable sunscreen products. Check with your doctor if you become sunburned.

☐ In some people, this drug may cause dizziness or drowsiness. Do not drive a car or operate dangerous machinery or do jobs that require you to be alert until you know how you are going to react to this drug.

☐ This medicine may cause dizziness or fainting if you get up quickly from a lying or sitting position. Get up slowly, especially in the morning. It is advis-able to dangle your feet over the edge of the bed for a few minutes before standing up. Sit or lie down at the first sign of dizziness. Tell your doctor that you have been dizzy.

☐ In order to help prevent dizziness and fainting, it is also recommended that you avoid strenuous exercise, standing for long periods of time (especially in hot weather), and hot showers or hot baths.

☐ If you develop a stuffy nose, tell your doctor.

☐ Some nonprescription drugs can aggravate your condition. Do not take any of the following without the approval of your doctor or pharmacist: cough, cold, or sinus products; asthma or allergy products; or diet or weight-reduc-ing medicines.

☐ Most people experience few or no side effects from their drugs. However, any medicine can sometimes cause unwanted effects. Call your doctor if you develop severe diarrhea (loose bowel movements), stomach pain, a skin rash, nightmares, loss of appetite or depression, swelling of the legs or an-kles, sudden weight gain of 5 pounds or more, chest pains, difficulty in breathing. Also call your doctor if you develop sharp joint pain, easy bruising or bleeding, or a yellow color to the skin or eyes.

☐ Carry an identification card indicating that you are taking this medicine. Always tell your pharmacist, dentist, and other doctors who are treating you that you are taking this medicine.

☐ Do not stop taking this medicine without your doctor's approval and do not go without medicine between prescription refills. Call your pharmacist 2 or 3 days before you will run out of the medicine.

* * * * *

Methotrexate (*Oral Antineoplastic*)
United States: Methotrexate
Canada: Methotrexate

☐ This medicine is used in certain medical conditions to help slow down the growth and reproduction of some of the body's cells. It is also used in the treatment of psoriasis.

HOW TO USE THIS MEDICINE
☐ It is best to take this medicine on an empty stomach at least 1 hour before (or 2 hours after) eating food. Take it at the proper time even if you skip a meal.

☐ It is very important that you take this medicine exactly as your doctor has prescribed and that you do not miss any doses. Try to take this medicine at the same time every day.

☐ Even if you become nauseated or lose your appetite, do not stop taking the medicine but check with your doctor.

☐ If you miss a dose of this medicine, do not take the missed dose and do not double your next dose. Check with your doctor.

SPECIAL INSTRUCTIONS
☐ Always keep your doctor appointments so that your doctor can watch your progress.

☐ If your doctor has prescribed some other medicines for you, it is important that you take them in the right order and that you do not miss them.

☐ Unless otherwise directed, drink plenty of fluids (2 to 3 quarts daily) while you are taking this medicine. This will help your kidneys handle the medicine and help prevent bladder problems.

☐ This medicine may cause a temporary loss of hair. Brush your hair gently and no more often than necessary. After your treatment is finished, your hair should grow back in.

☐ Do not drink alcoholic beverages while you are taking this medicine because alcohol may increase the possibility of liver problems.

☐ This medicine may make some people more sensitive to sunlight and sunlamps. When you begin taking this medicine try to avoid getting to much sun until you see how you are going to react. If your skin does become more sensitive to sunlight, tell your doctor and try to stay out of direct sunlight. While in the sun, wear protective clothing and sunglasses. You may wish to

520

ask your pharmacist about suitable sunscreen products. Check with your doctor if you become sunburned.

- ☐ Do not take products containing aspirin or salicylates or vitamin preparations containing folic acid until you have checked with your doctor.

- ☐ Men and women should take appropriate birth control measures to avoid conception while taking this medicine and for at least 2 months after the medicine has been stopped.

- ☐ In some people, this drug may rarely cause dizziness or drowsiness or blurred vision. Do not drive a car or operate dangerous machinery or do jobs that require you to be alert until you know how you are going to react to this drug.

- ☐ Always tell your pharmacist, dentist, and any other doctors who are treating you that you are taking this medicine. This is especially important if you plan to have surgery or any vaccinations.

- ☐ This is a very strong medicine. In addition to its benefits, there may be some unwanted effects, even for a short time after you stop taking the medicine. Call your doctor if you develop unusual bruising or bleeding, sore throat, fever or mouth sores, a skin rash, swelling of the legs or ankles, shortness of breath, a yellow color to the skin or eyes, stomach, bone or joint pain, black "tarry" stools, diarrhea, or blood in the urine.

*　*　*　*　*

Methotrimeprazine (Oral Antipsychotic-Antianxiety)
Canada: Nozinan

- ☐ This medicine is used to treat certain types of mental and emotional problems.

- ☐ IMPORTANT: If you have ever had an allergic reaction to a phenothiazine medicine, tell your doctor or pharmacist before you take any of this medicine.

HOW TO USE THIS MEDICINE
- ☐ This medicine may be taken with food or a full glass of water.

- ☐ Do not take this medicine at the same time as antacids or diarrhea medicine. Try to space them at least 1 hour apart.

- ☐ The effect of the medicine may not be noticed immediately, but may take from 2 to 4 weeks. Be patient. Take the medicine regularly and try not to miss any doses.

- ☐ Do not stop taking this medicine suddenly without the approval of your doctor.

SPECIAL INSTRUCTIONS
- ☐ If you forget to take a dose, take it as soon as possible. However, if it is almost time for your next dose, do not take the missed dose. Instead, continue with your regular dosing schedule.

☐ Any medicine has a few unwanted side effects. Because this medicine takes a few weeks to work, the side effects show the doctor that the drug is being absorbed. Many of these side effects will go away as your body adjusts to the medicine.

☐ Women who are pregnant, breast-feeding, or planning to become pregnant should tell their doctor before taking this medicine.

☐ In some people, this drug may cause dizziness or drowsiness. Do not drive a car or operate dangerous machinery or do jobs that require you to be alert until you know how you are going to react to this drug.

☐ If this medicine causes dizziness, you should be careful going up and down stairs and you should not change positions too rapidly. Get out of bed slowly in the morning and dangle your feet over the edge of the bed for a few minutes before standing up. Sit down or lie down at the first sign of dizziness. Tell your doctor you have been dizzy. Avoid hot showers and baths because they could make you dizzy.

☐ Do not drink alcoholic beverages while taking this drug without the approval of your doctor.

☐ This medicine may make some people more sensitive to sunlight and sunlamps. When you begin taking this medicine, try to avoid getting too much sun until you see how you are going to react. If your skin does become more sensitive to sunlight, tell your doctor and try to stay out of direct sunlight. While in the sun, wear protective clothing and sunglasses. You may wish to ask your pharmacist about suitable sunscreen products. Check with your doctor if you become sunburned.

☐ If your mouth becomes dry, suck a hard sour candy (sugarless) or ice chips, or chew gum. It is especially important to brush your teeth regularly if you develop a dry mouth.

☐ It is important that you obtain the advice of your doctor or pharmacist before taking **any** other medicines including pain relievers, sleeping pills, other tranquilizers or medicines for depression, cough/cold or allergy medicines, weight-reducing medicines, or laxatives.

☐ This medicine may cause your urine to turn pink, red, or red-brown in color. This is not unusual.

☐ In hot weather or during exercise, be careful not to become overheated. You may be more sensitive to heat since this medicine may affect your body's ability to regulate temperature.

☐ If you become constipated, try increasing the amount of bulk in your diet (for example, bran and salads), exercising more often, or drinking more water. Call your doctor if the constipation continues.

☐ Call your doctor if you develop a sore throat; fever; mouth sores; skin rash; changes in eyesight; rapid heartrate; a yellow color in the eyes or skin; unusual weakness or unusual movements of the face, tongue, or hands; or

522

difficulty in urinating ("passing your water"). Also call your doctor if you become restless or unable to sit still or sleep.

☐ Carry an identification card indicating that you are taking this medicine. Always tell your pharmacist, dentist, and other doctors who are treating you that you are taking this medicine.

*   *   *   *   *

Methoxsalen (*Oral Melanin Repigmentation*)
United States: Oxsoralen
Canada: Oxsoralen

☐ This medicine is used to restore color to the skin or to promote tanning.

HOW TO USE THIS MEDICINE
☐ Take the capsules after meals or with milk to reduce stomach upset.

SPECIAL INSTRUCTIONS
☐ Persons sensitive to sunlight and tanning should not stay out in the sunlight longer than 30 minutes for the first 3 or 4 days after taking the medicine.

☐ If blistering or pain occurs while using this medicine, contact your doctor and do not stay out in the sun for such a long period of time.

*   *   *   *   *

Methoxsalen (*Topical Melanin Repigmentation*)
United States: Oxsoralen
Canada: Oxsoralen

☐ This medicine is used to restore color to the skin.

HOW TO USE THIS MEDICINE
☐ Apply the lotion exactly as your doctor has directed. Use only a small amount of the medicine on the spots to be treated. Apply as evenly as possible so that streaking will not result.

☐ Do not use the drug more frequently, in larger quantities, or for a longer period of time than prescribed by your doctor.

SPECIAL INSTRUCTIONS
☐ Protect the treated areas from exposure to ultraviolet light. The treated areas may be sensitive to sunlight for up to 2 months after use and you should wear protective clothing.

☐ Call your doctor if you develop swelling, blistering, redness, or pain around the treated areas.

*   *   *   *   *

523

Methscopolamine Bromide (*Oral Anticholinergic*)

United States: Pamine

Canada: Pamine

☐ This medicine is used to help relax muscles of the stomach, bowels, and bladder as well as to decrease the amount of acid formed in the stomach.

☐ IMPORTANT: If you have ever had an allergic reaction to atropine or bromides or any other drug used to relax the stomach or bowels, tell your doctor or pharmacist before you take any of this medicine.

HOW TO USE THIS MEDICINE

☐ Take this medicine approximately 30 minutes before a meal unless otherwise directed.

☐ If you miss a dose of this medicine, do not take the missed dose and do not double the next dose.

SPECIAL INSTRUCTIONS

☐ If your mouth becomes dry, suck a hard sour candy (sugarless) or ice chips, or chew gum. It is especially important to brush your teeth regularly if you develop a dry mouth.

☐ In some people, this drug may cause dizziness or drowsiness. Do not drive a car or operate dangerous machinery or do jobs that require you to be alert until you know how you are going to react to this drug.

☐ If you become dizzy, you should be careful going up and down stairs. Sit or lie down at the first sign of dizziness. Tell your doctor you have been dizzy.

☐ A desire to urinate ("pass your water") with an inability to do so is not an uncommon effect with this drug. Urinating each time before taking the drug may help relieve this problem. Call your doctor if it continues.

☐ You may become more sensitive to heat because your body may perspire less while you are taking this drug. Be careful not to become overheated during exercise or in hot weather.

☐ Do not take antacids within 1 hour of taking this medicine as they could make this medicine less effective.

☐ If you become constipated, try increasing the amount of bulk in your diet (for example, bran and salads), exercising more often, or drinking more water. Call your doctor if the constipation continues.

☐ If your eyes become more sensitive to sunlight, it may help to wear sunglasses.

☐ Most people experience few or no side effects from their drugs. However, any medicine can sometimes cause unwanted effects. Call your doctor if you develop a skin rash, diarrhea, unusual restlessness, flushing, or eye pain.

*   *   *   *   *

524

Methsuximide (*Oral Anticonvulsant*)
United States: Celontin
Canada: Celontin

☐ This medicine is used to help control convulsions and seizures. It is commonly used in the treatment of epilepsy.

☐ IMPORTANT: If you have ever had an allergic reaction to an anticonvulsant or seizure medicine, tell your doctor or pharmacist before you take any of this medicine.

HOW TO USE THIS MEDICINE

☐ Take this medicine with food if it upsets your stomach. Call your doctor if you continue to have stomach upset.

☐ It is very important that you take this medicine regularly and that you do not miss any doses. Try to take the medicine at the same time(s) every day. This is the only way that you can receive the full benefit of the medicine. If you forget to take this medicine, the amount of medicine in your blood will go down and you may have seizures.

SPECIAL INSTRUCTIONS

☐ If you forget to take a dose, take it as soon as possible. However, if it is almost time for your next dose, do not take the missed dose. Instead, continue with your regular dosing schedule. Do not double doses.

☐ Do not stop taking this medicine suddenly or change the amount you are taking without the approval of your doctor.

☐ Avoid swimming alone or taking part in high-risk sports in which a sudden seizure could cause injury.

☐ In some people, this drug may cause dizziness or drowsiness. Do not drive a car or operate dangerous machinery or do jobs that require you to be alert until you know how you are going to react to this drug. If you become dizzy, you should be careful going up and down stairs. Sit or lie down at the first sign of dizziness.

☐ If this medicine is for a child, do not let him (her) ride a bike or climb trees until you can determine how he (she) is going to react to the medicine. Children could hurt themselves if they participated in these activities if they were dizzy.

☐ Do not drink alcoholic beverages while taking this drug without the approval of your doctor.

☐ It is important that you obtain the advice of your doctor or pharmacist before taking pain relievers, nonprescription drugs, sleeping pills, tranquilizers, or medicines for depression while you are taking this drug.

☐ Women who are pregnant, breast-feeding, or planning to become pregnant should tell their doctor before taking this medicine.

☐ Most people experience few or no side effects from their drugs. However, any medicine can sometimes cause unwanted effects. Call your doctor if you develop a sore throat, fever or mouth sores, skin rash, swollen glands, easy bruising or bleeding, or if you become depressed.

☐ Do not go without this medicine between prescription refills. Call your pharmacist 2 or 3 days before you will run out of the medicine.

☐ Carry an identification card indicating that you are taking this medicine. Always tell your pharmacist, dentist, and other doctors who are treating you that you are taking this medicine.

*   *   *   *   *

Methychlothiazide (Oral Diuretic-Antihypertensive)
United States: Aquatensen, Enduron
Canada: Duretic

☐ This medicine is used to help rid the body of excess water and to decrease swelling. It is also used to treat high blood pressure. It is commonly called a "water pill."

☐ IMPORTANT: If you have ever had an allergic reaction to sulfa drugs or thiazide diuretics, tell your doctor or pharmacist before taking any of this medicine.

HOW TO USE THIS MEDICINE
☐ Take the medicine with food, meals, or milk.

☐ Try to take it at the same time(s) every day so that you have a constant level of the medicine in your body. Do not miss any doses. Otherwise, you cannot expect the drug to work as well.

☐ When you first start taking this medicine, you will probably urinate ("pass your water") more often and in larger amounts than usual. Therefore, if you are to take one dose every day, take it in the morning after breakfast. If you are to take more than one dose every day, take the last dose 6 hours before bedtime so that you will not have to get up during the night to go to the bathroom. This effect will usually lessen after you have taken the drug for awhile.

SPECIAL INSTRUCTIONS
☐ If you forget to take a dose, take it as soon as possible. However, if it is almost time for your next dose, do not take the missed dose. Instead, continue with your regular dosing schedule.

☐ Women who are pregnant, breast-feeding, or planning to become pregnant should tell their doctor before taking this medicine.

☐ This medicine normally causes your body to lose potassium. The body has warning signs to let you know if too much potassium is being lost. Call your

doctor if you become unusually thirsty or if you develop leg cramps, unusual weakness, fatigue, vomiting, confusion, or irregular pulse.

☐ If your doctor recommends that you eat foods which are high in potassium, one or more of the foods listed in Appendix A should be eaten daily. All of these foods are rich in potassium. Your goal should be to take in 1000 to 2000 mg. of potassium (approximately 25.6 to 51 mEq) each day. The calorie content and sodium content are included for your convenience in meal planning. CHANGE YOUR DIET ONLY IF YOUR DOCTOR TELLS YOU TO.

☐ If this medicine causes dizziness, you should be careful going up and down stairs and you should not change positions too rapidly. Get out of bed slowly in the morning and dangle your feet over the edge of the bed for a few minutes before standing up. Sit down or lie down at the first sign of dizziness. Tell your doctor you have been dizzy. Be careful drinking alcoholic beverages while taking this medicine because they could make the dizziness worse. Do not drive a car or operate dangerous machinery or do jobs that require you to be alert if you are dizzy.

☐ In order to help prevent dizziness and fainting, your doctor may also recommend that you avoid strenuous exercises, standing for long periods of time (especially in hot weather) or hot showers or hot baths.

☐ This medicine may make some people more sensitive to sunlight and sunlamps. When you begin taking this medicine, try to avoid getting too much sun until you see how you are going to react. If your skin does become more sensitive to sunlight, tell your doctor and try to stay out of direct sunlight. While in the sun, wear protective clothing and sunglasses. You may wish to ask your pharmacist about suitable sunscreen products. Check with your doctor if you become sunburned.

☐ Call your doctor immediately if you think you may be allergic to the medicine or if you develop a skin rash, hives, itching, swelling of the face, or difficulty in breathing. If you cannot reach your doctor, phone a hospital emergency department.

☐ Most people experience few or no side effects from their drugs. However, any medicine can sometimes cause unwanted effects. Call your doctor if you develop a sore throat, fever, sharp stomach pain, chest pain, sharp joint pain, easy bruising or bleeding, a yellow color to the skin or eyes, or a sudden weight gain of 5 pounds or more.

*　　*　　*　　*　　*

Methylcellulose Compounds (*Ocular Lubricant*)

United States: Adsorbotear, Bro-Lac, Isopto Alkaline, Isopto Plain, Isopto Tears, Lacril, Lyteers, Methulose, Tearisol, Tears Naturale, Ultratears, Visculose

Canada: Isopto Tears, Lacril, Lyteers, Tears Naturale

Polyvinyl Alcohol Solution

United States: Contique Artificial Tears, Liquifilm Tears
Canada: Liquifilm Tears

☐ This preparation is used to moisten and lubricate "dry" eyes.

HOW TO USE THIS MEDICINE
☐ For EYE DROPS

INSTILLATION OF EYE DROPS

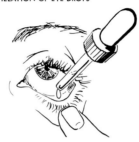

- The person administering the eye drops should wash his hands with soap and water.
- The eye drops must be kept clean. Do not touch the dropper against the face or anything else.
- Lie down or tilt your head backward and look at the ceiling.
- Gently pull down the lower lid of your eye to form a pouch.
- Hold the dropper in your other hand and approach the eye from the side. Place the dropper as close to the eye as possible without touching it.
- Place the prescribed number of drops into the pouch of the eye.
- Close your eyes. Do not rub them.
- Apply gentle pressure for a minute with your fingers to the bridge of the nose (inside corner of the eye) to prevent the eye drops from being drained from the eye.
- Blot excess solution around the eye with a tissue.

☐ If necessary, have someone else administer the eye drops for you.

☐ Do not use the eye drops if they have changed in color or have changed in any way since you purchased them.

☐ Keep the eye drop bottle tightly closed when not in use.

SPECIAL INSTRUCTIONS
☐ For external use only. Do not swallow.

*   *   *   *   *

528

Methyldopa (*Oral Antihypertensive*)

United States: Aldomet

Canada: Aldomet, Dopamet, Medimet-250, Novomedopa

☐ Hypertension (high blood pressure) is a long-term condition and it will probably be necessary for you to take the drug for a long time in spite of the fact that you feel better. It is very important that you take this medicine as your doctor has directed and that you do not miss any doses. Otherwise, you cannot expect the drug to keep your blood pressure down.

HOW TO USE THIS MEDICINE

☐ Try to take the medicine at the same time(s) every day.

SPECIAL INSTRUCTIONS

☐ If you forget to take a dose, take it as soon as possible. However, if it is almost time for your next dose, do not take the missed dose. Instead, continue with your regular dosing schedule.

☐ Drowsiness may occur during the first 2 or 3 days or after any increase in your dose and then usually disappears. Do not drive a car or operate dangerous machinery or do jobs that require you to be alert until you know how you are going to react to this drug.

☐ If this medicine causes dizziness, lie or sit down. Always get up slowly from lying or sitting positions. Call your doctor if the dizziness does not go away.

☐ Do not drink alcoholic beverages while taking this drug without the approval of your doctor.

☐ Some nonprescription drugs can aggravate your condition. Do not take any of the following products without the approval of your doctor or pharmacist: cough, cold, or sinus products; asthma or allergy products; or diet or weight-reducing medicines.

☐ Call your doctor if you develop an unexplained fever, especially during the first few weeks of taking this medicine.

☐ Most people experience few or no side effects from their drugs. However, any medicine can sometimes cause unwanted effects. Call your doctor if you develop unusual tiredness or weakness, swelling of the legs or ankles, sudden weight gain of 5 pounds or more, chest pains or difficulty in breathing, a sore throat, severe diarrhea (loose bowel movements) or stomach upset, easy bruising, or a yellow color to the skin or eyes.

☐ Carry an identification card indicating that you are taking this medicine. Always tell your pharmacist, dentist, and other doctors who are treating you that you are taking this medicine.

☐ Do not stop taking this medicine without your doctor's approval and do not go without medicine between prescription refills. Call your pharmacist 2 or 3 days before you will run out of the medicine.

*   *   *   *   *

Methyldopa-Chlorothiazide (*Oral Antihypertensive*)
United States: Aldoclor
Canada: Supres

Methyldopa-Hydrochlorothiazide
United States: Aldoril
Canada: Aldoril

☐ Hypertension (high blood pressure) is a long-term condition, and it will probably be necessary for you to take the drug for a long time in spite of the fact that you feel better. It is very important that you take this medicine as your doctor has directed and that you do not miss any doses. Otherwise, you cannot expect the drug to keep your blood pressure down.

☐ IMPORTANT: If you have ever had an allergic reaction to a sulfa drug or thiazide "water pill" or diabetes medicine that you take by mouth, tell your doctor or pharmacist before you take any of this medicine.

HOW TO USE THIS MEDICINE
☐ Take the medicine with food, meals, or milk.

☐ Try to take it at the same time(s) every day so that you have a constant level of the medicine in your body. Do not miss any doses. Otherwise, you cannot expect the drug to work as well.

SPECIAL INSTRUCTIONS
☐ If you forget to take a dose, take it as soon as possible. However, if it is almost time for your next dose, do not take the missed dose. Instead, continue with your regular dosing schedule.

☐ Women who are pregnant, breast-feeding, or planning to become pregnant should tell their doctor before taking this medicine.

☐ When you first start taking this medicine, you will probably urinate ("pass your water") more often and in larger amounts than usual. Therefore, if you are to take one dose every day, take it in the morning after breakfast. If you are to take more than one dose every day, take the last dose 4 to 6 hours before bedtime so that you will not have to get up during the night to go to the bathroom. This effect will usually lessen after you have taken the drug for awhile.

☐ Drowsiness may occur during the first 2 or 3 days or after any increase in your dose and then will usually disappear. Do not drive a car or operate dangerous machinery or do jobs that require you to be alert until you know how you are going to react to this drug.

☐ This medicine may make some people more sensitive to sunlight and sunlamps. When you begin taking this medicine, try to avoid getting too much sun until you see how you are going to react. If your skin does become more sensitive to sunlight, tell your doctor and try to stay out of direct sunlight. While in the sun, wear protective clothing and sunglasses. You may wish to ask your pharmacist about suitable sunscreen products. Check with your doctor if you become sunburned.

☐ This medicine normally causes you to lose some potassium. Depending upon your dose, your doctor may recommend that you eat foods rich in potassium (see Appendix A). Call your doctor if you develop any of the following warning signs that your body is low in potassium: unusual thirst, leg cramps, unusual weakness, fatigue, vomiting, confusion, or an irregular pulse.

☐ If this medicine causes dizziness, lie or sit down. Always get up slowly from lying or sitting positions. Call your doctor if the dizziness does not go away.

☐ Do not drink alcoholic beverages while taking this drug without the approval of your doctor.

☐ If your mouth becomes dry, suck a hard sour candy (sugarless) or ice chips, or chew gum. It is especially important to brush your teeth regularly if you develop a dry mouth.

☐ Some nonprescription drugs can aggravate your condition. Do not take any of the following products without the approval of your doctor or pharmacist: cough, cold, or sinus products; asthma or allergy products; or diet or weight-reducing medicines.

☐ Call your doctor if you develop a fever especially during the first few weeks of taking this medicine.

☐ Call your doctor immediately if you think you may be allergic to the medicine or if you develop a skin rash, hives, itching, swelling of the face, or difficulty in breathing. If you cannot reach your doctor, phone a hospital emergency department.

☐ Most people experience few or no side effects from their drugs. However, any medicine can sometimes cause unwanted effects. Call your doctor if you develop unusual tiredness or weakness, swelling of the legs or ankles, sudden weight gain of 5 pounds or more, chest pains or difficulty in breathing, a sore throat, severe diarrhea (loose bowel movements) or stomach upset, easy bruising, or a yellow color to the skin or eyes.

☐ Carry an identification card indicating that you are taking this medicine. Always tell your pharmacist, dentist, and other doctors who are treating you that you are taking this medicine.

☐ Do not stop taking this medicine without your doctor's approval and do not go without medicine between prescription refills. Call your pharmacist 2 or 3 days before you will run out of the medicine.

*   *   *   *   *

Methylphenidate HCl (*Oral CNS Stimulant*)
United States: Ritalin
Canada: Methidate, Ritalin

☐ This medicine has many uses and the reason it was prescribed depends upon your condition. Check with your doctor if you do not fully understand why you are taking it.

HOW TO USE THIS MEDICINE
☐ This medicine may be taken with food or a glass of water.

☐ Do not take the medicine late in the day (4 to 6 hours before bedtime) as it may cause insomnia (difficulty in sleeping).

SPECIAL INSTRUCTIONS
☐ If you forget to take a dose, take it as soon as possible. However, if it is almost time for your next dose, do not take the missed dose. Instead, continue with your regular dosing schedule.

☐ Do not take any more of this medicine than your doctor has prescribed and do not stop taking this medicine suddenly without the approval of your doctor.

☐ If your mouth becomes dry, suck a hard sour candy (sugarless) or ice chips, or chew gum. It is especially important to brush your teeth regularly if you develop a dry mouth.

☐ In some people, this drug may cause dizziness and drowsiness. Do not drive a car or operate dangerous machinery or do jobs that require you to be alert until you know how you are going to react to this drug. Therefore, you should be careful going up and down stairs. Sit or lie down at the first sign of dizziness.

☐ If this medicine is for a child, do not let him (her) ride a bike or climb trees until you can determine how he (she) is going to react to the medicine. Children could hurt themselves if they participated in these activities if they were dizzy.

☐ Most people experience few or no side effects from their drugs. However, any medicine can sometimes cause unwanted effects. Call your doctor if you develop a skin rash, sore throat, fever, chest pain or fast heartbeats, joint pain, unusual movements of the head, arms or legs, easy bruising, blurred vision, or unusual nervousness, or if you become depressed.

532

☐ Carry an identification card indicating that you are taking this medicine. Always tell your pharmacist, dentist, and other doctors who are treating you that you are taking this medicine.

* * * * *

Methylprednisolone (*Eye-Ear Corticosteroid*)
Canada: Medrol

☐ This medicine is used to help relieve the pain, redness, and swelling of certain types of eye and ear condtions.

HOW TO USE THIS MEDICINE

☐ For EYE DROPS

INSTILLATION OF EYE DROPS

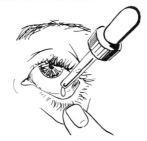

- The person administering the eye drops should wash his hands with soap and water.
- The eye drops must be kept clean. Do not touch the dropper against the face or anything else.
- Lie down or tilt your head backward and look at the ceiling.
- Gently pull down the lower lid of your eye to form a pouch.
- Hold the dropper in your other hand and approach the eye from the side. Place the dropper as close to the eye as possible without touching it.
- Place the prescribed number of drops into the pouch of the eye.
- Close your eyes. Do not rub them.
- Apply gentle pressure for a minute with your fingers to the bridge of the nose (inside corner of the eye) to prevent the eye drops from being drained from the eye.
- Blot excess solution around the eye with a tissue.
- If necessary, have someone else administer the eye drops for you.
- Do not use the eye drops if they have changed in color or have changed in any way since you purchased them.
- Keep the eye drop bottle tightly closed when not in use.

533

☐ For EYE OINTMENT

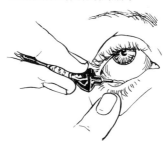

- The person administering the eye ointment should wash his hands with soap and water.
- The eye ointment must be kept clean. Do not touch the tube against the face or anything else.
- Lie down or tilt your head backward and look at the ceiling.
- Gently pull down the lower lid of your eye to form a pouch.
- Hold the tube in your other hand and place the tube as close as possible to the eye without touching it.
- Squeeze the prescribed amount of ointment (usually $\frac{1}{2}$ inch in adults) from the tube along the pouch.
- Close your eyes. Do not rub them.
- Wipe off any excess ointment around the eye with a tissue.
- Clean the tip of the ointment tube with a tissue.
- If necessary, have someone else administer the eye ointment for you.
- Keep the eye ointment tube tightly closed when not in use.

☐ For EAR DROPS

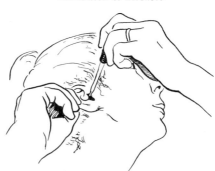

- Warm the ear drops to body temperature by holding the bottle in your hands for a few minutes. Do NOT heat the drops in hot water.
- The person administering the ear drops should wash his hands with soap and water.
- The ear drops must be kept clean. Do not touch the dropper against the ear or anything else.

- Tilt your head or lie on your side so that the ear to be treated is facing up.
- In ADULTS, hold the ear lobe up and back.
  In CHILDREN, hold the ear lobe down and back.
- Place the prescribed number of drops into the ear. Do not insert the dropper into the ear as it may cause injury.
- Remain in the same position for a short time (2 minutes) after you have administered the drops.
  - Dry the ear lobe if there are any drops on it.
- If necessary, have someone else administer the ear drops for you.
- Do not use the ear drops if they have changed in color or have changed in any way since you purchased them.
- Keep the bottle tightly closed when not in use.

☐ Ear drops after application of ear wick: (*Canada:* Medrol)
  - Warm the medicine to body temperature by holding it in your hands for a few minutes.
  - Tilt your head to the side or lie on your side so that the ear to be treated is uppermost.
  - Drop the prescribed amount of medicine into the ear canal.
  - Do not use the solution if it is discolored or if it appears to have changed in any way since you purchased it.

☐ Do not use this drug more frequently or in larger quantities than prescribed by your doctor.

SPECIAL INSTRUCTIONS

☐ This medicine should be used as long as prescribed by your doctor. Do not stop using it earlier than your doctor has recommended in spite of the fact that your symptoms seem to have improved.

☐ If you forget to use the medicine, use it as soon as possible. However, if it is almost time for your next dose, do not use the missed dose but continue with your regular schedule.

☐ Vision may be blurred for a few minutes after using the eye medicine.

☐ Do not drive a car or operate dangerous machinery or do jobs that require you to be alert until your vision has cleared.

☐ Do not use this medicine at the same time as any other eye medicine without the approval of your doctor. Some medicines cannot be mixed.

☐ Call your doctor if the condition for which you are using this medicine persists or becomes worse or if the medicine causes itching or burning for more than a few minutes after instillation.

☐ For external use only. Do not swallow.

* * * * *

Methylprednisolone (*Oral Corticosteroid*)
United States: Medrol
Canada: Medrol

☐ This medicine is similar to cortisone, which is a hormone normally produced by the body. This medicine is used to help decrease inflammation which then relieves pain, redness, and swelling. It is used in the treatment of certain kinds of arthritis, severe allergies, or skin conditions.

HOW TO USE THIS MEDICINE

☐ Take this medicine with food or a glass of milk in order to help prevent stomach upset. Call your doctor if you develop stomach upset or stomach pain or heartburn (especially if it awakens you during the night). Do not try to treat this yourself.

☐ If your doctor has prescribed only ONE dose of this medicine every day, it is best to take it before 9 A.M. or with breakfast.

☐ If you forget to take a dose, take it as soon as possible. However, if it is almost time for your next dose, do not take the missed dose. Instead, continue with your regular dosing schedule.

SPECIAL INSTRUCTIONS

☐ Women who are pregnant, breast-feeding, or planning to become pregnant should tell their doctor before taking this medicine.

☐ It is best not to drink alcoholic beverages while you are taking this medicine because the combination can cause stomach problems.

☐ Do not take any more of this medicine than your doctor has prescribed and do not stop taking this medicine suddenly without the approval of your doctor. It may be necessary for your doctor to slowly reduce your dose since your body becomes used to this medicine and it might be harmful if you suddenly did not receive this medicine.

☐ Do not take aspirin or medicines containing aspirin without the approval of your doctor.

☐ While you are taking this medicine you may gain some weight. This could be due to an increase in your appetite or an increase in the water in your system. Your doctor may prescribe a special diet to decrease the number of calories you eat and/or to lower the amount of sodium or increase the amount of potassium in your diet. Follow any diet that your doctor may order.

☐ You may find that you bruise more easily. Try to protect yourself from all injuries to prevent bruising.

☐ Diabetic patients should regularly check the sugar in their urine and report any unusual levels to their doctor.

☐ Carry an identification card indicating that you are taking this medicine.

Always tell your pharmacist, dentist, and other doctors who are treating you that you are taking this medicine. If you have an acute infection, injury, operation, or dental surgery within 1 year of taking this medicine, it is important to tell your doctor.

☐ Most people experience few or no side effects from their drugs. However, any medicine can sometimes cause unwanted effects. Call your doctor if you develop stomach pain, sore throat, fever, swelling of the legs or ankles, a wound which does not heal, eye pain or blurred vision, frequent urination ("passing your water"), nightmares or depression, muscle cramps, red or black stools, puffing of the face, or menstrual problems.

* * * * *

Methylprednisolone (*Topical Corticosteroid*)
United States: Medrol Acetate
Canada: Medrol Topical

Methylprednisolone-Sulfur
Canada: Medrol Acne Lotion

☐ This medicine is used to help relieve redness, swelling and itching, and inflammation of certain types of skin conditions.

HOW TO USE THIS MEDICINE
☐ For CREAM, OINTMENT, and LOTION
- Each time you apply the medicine, wash your hands and gently cleanse the skin area well with water unless otherwise directed by your doctor. Do not allow the skin to dry completely. Pat with a clean towel until slightly damp.
- Apply a small amount of the drug to the affected area and spread lightly. Only the medicine that is actually touching the skin will work. A thick layer is not more effective than a thin layer. Do not bandage unless directed by your doctor.

☐ For LIQUID MEDICINE
- Shake the liquid preparation well before using. (*Canada:* Medrol Acne Lotion)
- The liquid preparation may cause a slight temporary stinging sensation after it is applied.

☐ Do not use the drug more frequently or in larger quantities than prescribed by your doctor. Overuse of this medicine may cause you to absorb too much of the drug and increase the risk of side effects.

☐ Keep the medicine away from the eyes, nose, and mouth.

537

SPECIAL INSTRUCTIONS

☐ If you forget to apply the medicine, apply it as soon as possible. However, if it is almost time for your next dose, do not apply the missed dose but continue with your regular schedule.

☐ Do not use this medicine for any other skin problems without checking with your doctor.

☐ Do not apply cosmetics or lotions on top of the drug unless your doctor approves.

☐ Call your doctor if the condition for which this drug is being used persists or becomes worse or if you have a constant irritation such as itching or burning that was not present before you started using this medicine. Also call your doctor if you develop abnormal lines or thinning of the skin, especially under the arms or between the legs.

☐ Store in a cool place but do not freeze.

☐ For external use only. Do not swallow.

☐ Tell future doctors that you have used this medicine.

*   *   *   *   *

Methyltestosterone (*Oral Androgen*)

United States: Android, Metandren, Oreton Methyl, Testred, Virilon
Canada: Metandren

☐ This medicine is similar to a hormone which is normally produced by the body. This medicine has many uses and the reason it was prescribed depends upon your condition. If you do not understand why you are taking it, check with your doctor.

HOW TO USE THIS MEDICINE

☐ Take the drug after meals or with a snack if it upsets your stomach.

☐ It is very important that you take this drug as your doctor has prescribed.

☐ For BUCCAL TABLETS

• Place the tablet in the pouch of the cheek (between the outside of the teeth and the cheek) and let the tablet dissolve. DO NOT SWALLOW until the tablet has dissolved and the taste of the drug has disappeared. Avoid eating, drinking, or smoking immediately after taking the tablet. Change the place in the cheek where you place the tablet with each dose. (**United States:** Android, Metandren Linguets, Oreton Methyl Buccal Tablets; **Canada:** Metandren Linguets)

☐ This medicine must be swallowed whole. Do not crush, chew, or break it into pieces. (**United States:** Virilon)

538

SPECIAL INSTRUCTIONS

☐ Women who are pregnant, breast-feeding, or planning to become pregnant should tell their doctor before taking this medicine.

☐ Diabetic patients should regularly check the sugar in their urine and report any abnormal results to their doctor.

☐ Carry an identification card indicating that you are taking this medicine. Always tell your pharmacist, dentist, and other doctors who are treating you that you are taking this medicine.

☐ Most people experience few or no side effects from their drugs. However, any medicine can sometimes cause unwanted effects. Call your doctor if you develop swelling of the hands, legs, or ankles; sore throat and fever; acne; unusual restlessness; dark-colored urine; or a yellow color to the skin or eyes. Women should call their doctor if they develop menstrual problems, hoarseness or a deepening of the voice, baldness, or increased facial hair.

* * * * *

Methyprylon (Oral Hypnotic)
United States: Noludar
Canada: Noludar

☐ This medicine is used to cause sleep.

HOW TO USE THIS MEDICINE
☐ This medicine may be taken with food or a glass of water.

SPECIAL INSTRUCTIONS

☐ Sleeping medicines are only useful for a short time. If used for too long, they lose their effectiveness. Do not take any more of this medicine than your doctor has prescribed and do not stop taking this medicine suddenly without the approval of your doctor.

☐ Women who are breast-feeding should tell their doctor before taking this medicine.

☐ In some people, this drug may cause dizziness or drowsiness. Do not drive a car or operate dangerous machinery or do jobs that require you to be alert until you know how you are going to react to this drug.

☐ If you become dizzy, you should be careful going up and down stairs. Sit or lie down at the first sign of dizziness.

☐ Do not drink alcoholic beverages while taking this drug without the approval of your doctor.

☐ It is important that you obtain the advice of your doctor or pharmacist before taking ANY other medicines including pain relievers, sleeping pills, tranquilizers or medicines for depression, cough/cold medicines, or allergy medicines.

- ☐ Go to bed after you have taken this medicine. Do not smoke in bed after you have taken it.

- ☐ Most people experience few or no side effects from their drugs. However, any medicine can sometimes cause unwanted effects. Call your doctor if you develop a skin rash, mouth sores, easy bruising or bleeding, unusual nervousness, or bothersome sleepiness during the day.

* * * * *

Methysergide Bimaleate (*Oral Migraine Prophylaxis*)
United States: Sansert
Canada: Sansert

- ☐ This medicine is used to help prevent migraine headaches and certain types of throbbing headaches.

HOW TO USE THIS MEDICINE
- ☐ This medicine may be taken with food to help prevent stomach upset.

SPECIAL INSTRUCTIONS
- ☐ Do not take any more of this medicine than your doctor has prescribed and do not stop taking this medicine suddenly without the approval of your doctor.

- ☐ If you forget to take a dose, take it as soon as possible. However, if it is almost time for your next dose, do not take the missed dose. Instead, continue with your regular dosing schedule.

- ☐ In some people, this drug may cause dizziness or drowsiness. Do not drive a car or operate dangerous machinery or do jobs that require you to be alert until you know how you are going to react to this drug.

- ☐ If this medicine causes dizziness, you should be careful going up and down stairs and you should not change positions too rapidly. Get out of bed slowly in the morning and dangle your feet over the edge of the bed for a few minutes before standing up. Sit down or lie down at the first sign of dizziness. Tell your doctor you have been dizzy. Avoid hot showers and baths because they could make you dizzy.

- ☐ An increase in weight may occur. Follow any diet that your doctor may recommend.

- ☐ Most people experience few or no side effects from their drugs. However, any medicine can sometimes cause unwanted effects. Call your doctor if you develop cold, numb, or painful hands and feet; leg cramps when walking; chest pain; painful urination ("passing your water"); shortness of breath; unusual tiredness; backache; fever; or swelling of the legs or ankles.

* * * * *

Metoclopramide (*Oral Upper Gastrointestinal Tract Motility Modifier*)

Canada: Maxeran, Reglan

☐ This medicine is used to treat certain types of stomach disorders.

HOW TO USE THIS MEDICINE

☐ Take this medicine one half hour before meals.

☐ Do not use this medicine more often than recommended by your doctor.

SPECIAL INSTRUCTIONS

☐ While taking this medicine and for 2 weeks after your treatment ends, be careful about eating any of the following foods or beverages:

- Aged and natural cheeses (for example, cheddar, blue, Camembert, Stilton, Gruyère, Brie, Swiss, and Emmenthaler). In general, avoid food in which aging is used to increase the flavor. Cream cheese, processed cheese, and cottage cheese are safe to eat.
- Sour cream or yogurt.
- Wines, especially Chianti and other heavy red wines.
- Alcoholic beverages, including sherry and beer.
- Canned figs or raisins.
- Yeast extracts (such as Marmite or Bovril) or meat extracts.
- Chicken livers.
- Broad beans (also called fava beans).
- Fermented sausage (such as fermented bolognas and salamis, pepperoni, and summer sausage).
- Pickled or kippered herring.
- Meats prepared with tenderizers.
- Avocados, bananas.
- Soya sauce.
- Chocolate.
- Excessive amounts of caffeine (for example, coffee, tea, cola beverages).

☐ Women who are pregnant, breast-feeding, or planning to become pregnant should tell their doctor before taking this medicine.

☐ Do not drink alcoholic beverages while taking this drug without the approval of your doctor.

☐ In some people, this drug may cause dizziness or drowsiness. Do not drive a car or operate dangerous machinery or do jobs that require you to be alert until you know how you are going to react to this drug.

☐ If you become dizzy, you should be careful going up and down stairs. Sit or lie down at the first sign of dizziness.

☐ Several cold or hay fever remedies and nasal sprays can interact with this medicine and cause an unpleasant reaction. Consult with your pharmacist before purchasing any of these products. Do not take sleeping pills, pain relievers, tranquilizers, or medicines for depression without the permission of your doctor.

☐ This medicine can interact with other prescription medicines. If you visit another pharmacist, doctor, or dentist, it is important that you tell them you are taking this drug.

☐ Most people experience few or no side effects from their drugs. However, any medicine can sometimes cause unwanted effects. Call your doctor if you develop unusual movements of the face, tongue, hands, or eyes.

*　*　*　*　*

Metolazone (*Oral Diuretic-Antihypertensive*)
United States: Diulo, Zaroxolyn
Canada: Zaroxolyn

☐ This medicine is used to help rid the body of excess water and to decrease swelling. It is also used to treat high blood pressure. It is commonly called a "water pill."

☐ IMPORTANT: If you have ever had an allergic reaction to sulfa drugs or thiazide diuretics, tell your doctor or pharmacist before taking any of this medicine.

HOW TO USE THIS MEDICINE
☐ Take the medicine with food, meals, or milk.

☐ Try to take it at the same time(s) every day so that you have a constant level of the medicine in your body. Do not miss any doses. Otherwise, you cannot expect the drug to work as well.

☐ When you first start taking this medicine, you will probably urinate ("pass your water") more often and in larger amounts than usual. Therefore, if you are to take one dose every day, take it in the morning after breakfast. If you are to take more than one dose every day, take the last dose 6 hours before bedtime so that you will not have to get up during the night to go to the bathroom. This effect will usually lessen after you have taken the drug for awhile.

SPECIAL INSTRUCTIONS
☐ If you forget to take a dose, take it as soon as possible. However, if it is almost time for your next dose, do not take the missed dose. Instead, continue with your regular dosing schedule.

☐ Women who are pregnant, breast-feeding, or planning to become pregnant should tell their doctor before taking this medicine.

☐ This medicine normally causes your body to lose potassium. The body has warning signs to let you know if too much potassium is being lost. Call your

doctor if you become unusually thirsty or if you develop leg cramps, unusual weakness, fatigue, vomiting, confusion, or irregular pulse.

☐ If your doctor recommends that you eat foods which are high in potassium, one or more of the foods listed in Appendix A should be eaten daily. All of these foods are rich in potassium. Your goal should be to take in 1000 to 2000 mg. of potassium (approximately 25.6 to 51 mEq) each day. The calorie content and sodium content are included for your convenience in meal planning. CHANGE YOUR DIET ONLY IF YOUR DOCTOR TELLS YOU TO.

☐ If this medicine causes dizziness, you should be careful going up and down stairs and you should not change positions too rapidly. Get out of bed slowly in the morning and dangle your feet over the edge of the bed for a few minutes before standing up. Sit down or lie down at the first sign of dizziness. Tell your doctor you have been dizzy. Be careful drinking alcoholic beverages while taking this medicine because they could make the dizziness worse. Do not drive a car or operate dangerous machinery or do jobs that require you to be alert if you are dizzy.

☐ In order to help prevent dizziness and fainting, your doctor may also recommend that you avoid strenuous exercises, standing for long periods of time (especially in hot weather), or hot showers or hot baths.

☐ This medicine may make some people more sensitive to sunlight and sunlamps. When you begin taking this medicine, try to avoid getting too much sun until you see how you are going to react. If your skin does become more sensitive to sunlight, tell your doctor and try to stay out of direct sunlight. While in the sun, wear protective clothing and sunglasses. You may wish to ask your pharmacist about suitable sunscreen products. Check with your doctor if you become sunburned.

☐ Call your doctor immediately if you think you may be allergic to the medicine or if you develop a skin rash, hives, itching, swelling of the face, or difficulty in breathing. If you cannot reach your doctor, phone a hospital emergency department.

☐ Most people experience few or no side effects from their drugs. However, any medicine can sometimes cause unwanted effects. Call your doctor if you develop a sore throat, fever, sharp stomach pain, chest pain, sharp joint pain, easy bruising or bleeding, a yellow color to the skin or eyes, or a sudden weight gain of 5 pounds or more.

*   *   *   *   *

Metoprolol
United States: Lopressor
Canada: Betaloc, Lopressor

☐ This medicine is used to lower the blood pressure. It is sometimes prescribed to help relieve chest pain (angina).

543

☐ Hypertension (high blood pressure) is a long-term condition and it will probably be necessary for you to take the drug for a long time in spite of the fact that you feel better. It is very important that you take this medicine as your doctor has directed and that you do not miss any doses. Otherwise, you cannot expect the drug to keep your blood pressure down.

HOW TO USE THIS MEDICINE

☐ It is best to take this medicine with food.

☐ Try to take the medicine at the same time(s) every day.

SPECIAL INSTRUCTIONS

☐ If you forget to take a dose, take it as soon as possible. However, if it is almost time for your next dose, do not take the missed dose. Instead, continue with your regular dosing schedule.

☐ If you become dizzy, you should be careful going up and down stairs and you should not change positions too rapidly. Get out of bed slowly in the morning and dangle your feet over the edge of the bed for a few minutes before standing up. Sit or lie down at the first sign of dizziness. Tell your doctor you have been dizzy.

☐ In some people, this drug may cause blurred vision. Do not drive a car or operate dangerous machinery or do jobs that require you to be alert until you know how you are going to react to this drug.

☐ Follow any special diet that your doctor may have ordered. He may want you to limit the amount of salt in your food.

☐ Some nonprescription drugs can aggravate your condition. Do not take any of the following without the approval of your doctor or pharmacist: cough, cold, or sinus products; asthma or allergy products; or diet or weight-reducing medicine.

☐ If your mouth becomes dry, suck a hard sour candy (sugarless) or ice chips, or chew gum. It is especially important to brush your teeth regularly if you develop a dry mouth.

☐ Most people experience few or no side effects from their drugs. However, any medicine can sometimes cause unwanted effects. Call your doctor if you develop a sore throat, fever and mouth sores, swelling of the legs or ankles, sudden weight gain of 5 pounds or more, chest pains or difficulty in breathing, a skin rash, or diarrhea, or if your pulse becomes slower than normal (less than 60 beats per minute). Also call your doctor if you develop nightmares or headaches, or if you become depressed.

☐ Carry an identification card indicating that you are taking this medicine. Always tell your pharmacist, dentist, and other doctors who are treating you that you are taking this medicine.

544

☐ Do not stop taking this medicine without your doctor's approval and do not go without medicine between prescription refills. Call your pharmacist 2 or 3 days before you will run out of the medicine.

* * * * *

Metronidazole (*Oral Trichomonacide*)
United States: Flagyl
Canada: Flagyl, Neo-Tric, Novonidazol, Trikacide

☐ This medicine is used to treat certain types of infections.

HOW TO USE THIS MEDICINE
☐ Take the tablets with meals, food, or a glass of milk to help prevent stomach upset.

☐ It is very important that you take this medicine exactly as your doctor has prescribed and that you do not miss any doses. Try to take this medicine at the same time every day. Do not take extra tablets without your doctor's approval.

SPECIAL INSTRUCTIONS
☐ If you forget to take a dose, take it as soon as possible. However, if it is almost time for your next dose, do not take the missed dose. Instead, continue with your regular dosing schedule.

☐ Women who are pregnant, breast-feeding, or planning to become pregnant should tell their doctor before taking this medicine.

☐ Do not drink alcoholic beverages while taking this medicine because they could cause a very unpleasant reaction.

☐ This medicine may cause the urine to turn red-brown or darker in color. This is not unusual.

☐ If your mouth becomes dry, suck a hard sour candy (sugarless) or ice chips, or chew gum. It is especially important to brush your teeth regularly if you develop a dry mouth.

☐ Good personal hygiene is very important in order to keep the infection under control. Wash your hands before preparing or eating food and after urination and bowel movements.

☐ It is recommended that women not wear pantyhose or tight underwear or take bubble baths while using this medicine.

☐ Most people experience few or no side effects from their drugs. However, any medicine can sometimes cause unwanted effects. Call your doctor if you develop a sore throat, fever or mouth sores, a white coating on the tongue, numbness in the hands or feet, or trembling.

* * * * *

545

Metronidazole (*Vaginal Trichomonacide*)
Canada: Flagyl, Neo-Tric, Novonidazol, Trikacide

☐ This medicine is used to treat certain types of vaginal infections.

HOW TO USE THIS MEDICINE
☐ For VAGINAL INSERTS
- Remove the wrapper and dip the tablet into water quickly, just enough to moisten it.
- Put the tablet into the applicator.
- Insert the applicator into the vaginal canal and depress the plunger.
- Remove the applicator.
- Wash the applicator with warm water and soap after each use.

☐ For VAGINAL TABLETS
- This is *not* an oral medicine.
- Remove the wrapper and dip the tablet into water quickly, just enough to moisten it.
- Insert the wide end of the tablet high into the vagina.

☐ For VAGINAL CREAM
- Remove the cap from the tube of medicine.
- Screw the applicator to the tube. Apply a small amount of the cream to the outside of the applicator.
- Squeeze the tube until the applicator plunger is fully extended. The applicator will now be filled with medicine. If your doctor has ordered a smaller dose, use as he has directed.
- Unscrew the applicator by the cylinder and gently insert it into the vaginal canal as far as it will comfortably go.
- While still holding the cylinder, press the plunger gently to deposit the medicine.
- While keeping the plunger depressed, remove the applicator from the vagina.
- After *each* use, take the applicator apart by holding the cylinder of the plunger and turning the cap counterclockwise.
- Wash thoroughly with warm soap and water and rinse thoroughly.
- Reassemble by dropping the plunger back into the cylinder as far as it will go. Place the cap on the end of the plunger and turn until the cap is tight.

SPECIAL INSTRUCTIONS
☐ Do *not* drink alcoholic beverages while using this medicine.

☐ This medicine may cause the urine to be darker in color. This is not an unusual effect.

☐ It is important to use *all* of this medicine, plus any refills that your doctor told you to use. Do not stop using it earlier than your doctor has recommended

546

in spite of the fact that your symptoms seem to have improved. Otherwise, the infection may return.

☐ Do not use the drug more frequently or in larger quantities than prescribed by your doctor.

☐ If you forget to use the medicine, use it as soon as possible. However, if it is almost time for your next dose, do not use the missed dose but continue with your regular schedule.

☐ You may wish to wear a sanitary napkin to protect your clothing.

☐ Call your doctor if the condition for which this drug is being used persists or becomes worse or if you develop a constant irritation such as itching or burning that was not present before you started using this medicine. Also call your doctor if you develop a sore throat, fever or mouth sores, a white coating on the tongue, or numbness or pain in the hands or feet.

☐ For external use only. Do not swallow.

*   *   *   *   *

Metronidazole-Nystatin (*Vaginal Trichomonacide-Moniliacide*)
Canada: Flagylstatin

☐ This medicine is used to treat vaginal infections.

☐ This is not an oral medicine.

HOW TO USE THIS MEDICINE
☐ For VAGINAL SUPPOSITORIES
- Dip the tablet into water quickly (1 to 2 seconds) in order to moisten it.
- Put the tablet into the applicator.
- Insert the applicator into the vaginal canal and depress the plunger.
- Clean the applicator after each use.

SPECIAL INSTRUCTIONS
☐ It is important to use **all** of this medicine, plus any refills that your doctor told you to use. Use only as directed. Do not stop using it earlier than your doctor has recommended in spite of the fact that your symptoms seem to have improved. Otherwise, the infection may return.

☐ If you forget to apply the medicine, apply it as soon as possible. However, if it is almost time for your next dose, do not apply the missed dose but continue with your regular schedule.

☐ This medicine should be used continuously even during your menstrual period.

☐ Do not drink alcoholic beverages while you are using this medicine because the combination could cause a very unpleasant reaction.

☐ This medicine may cause your urine to be darker in color. This is not an unusual effect.

☐ Call your doctor if the condition for which this drug is being used persists or becomes worse or if you develop a constant irritation such as itching or burning that was not present before you started using this medicine. Also call your doctor if you develop a sore throat, fever or mouth sores, a white coating on the tongue, or numbness or pain in the hands or feet.

☐ For external use only. Do not swallow.

* * * * *

Miconazole Nitrate (*Topical Antifungal*)
United States: Micatin
Canada: Micatin

☐ This medicine is used to treat fungal infections of the skin.

HOW TO USE THIS MEDICINE

- Each time you apply the medicine, wash your hands and gently cleanse the skin area well with water unless otherwise directed by your doctor. Do not allow the skin to dry completely. Pat with a clean towel until almost dry.
- Apply a small amount of the drug to the affected area and spread lightly. Only the medicine that is actually touching the skin will work. A thick layer is not more effective than a thin layer. Do not bandage unless directed by your doctor.

☐ Do not use the drug more frequently or in larger quantities than prescribed by your doctor.

SPECIAL INSTRUCTIONS

☐ It is important to use **all** of this medicine, plus any refills that your doctor told you to use. Do not stop using it earlier than your doctor has recommended in spite of the fact that your symptoms seem to have improved. Otherwise, the infection may return.

☐ If you forget to apply the medicine, apply it as soon as possible. However, if it is almost time for your next dose, do not apply the missed dose but continue with your regular schedule.

☐ If you have a fungal infection of the feet, it is important to dry the feet (especially between the toes) well after washing.

☐ Do not apply cosmetics or lotions on top of the drug unless your doctor approves.

☐ Keep this preparation away from the eyes. If you should accidentally get some in your eyes, wash it away with water immediately.

☐ Call your doctor if the condition for which this drug is being used persists or becomes worse or if you develop a constant irritation such as itching or burning that was not present before you started using this medicine.

☐ For external use only. Do not swallow.

*   *   *   *   *

Miconazole Nitrate (*Vaginal Antifungal*)
United States: Monistat 7
Canada: Monistat, Monistat 7

☐ This medicine is used to treat fungal infections of the vagina.

HOW TO USE THIS MEDICINE
☐ For VAGINAL CREAM
  • Remove the cap from the tube of medicine.
  • Screw the applicator to the tube.
  • Squeeze the tube until the applicator plunger is fully extended (the applicator will now be filled with medicine). If your doctor has ordered a smaller dose, use as he has directed.
  • Unscrew the applicator by the cylinder. Apply a small amount of the cream to the applicator and gently insert it into the vaginal canal as far as it will comfortably go.
  • While still holding the cylinder, press the plunger gently to deposit the medicine.
  • While keeping the plunger depressed, remove the applicator from the vaginal canal.
  • After **each** use, take the applicator apart by holding the cylinder of the plunger and turning the cap counterclockwise.
  • Wash thoroughly with warm soap and water and rinse thoroughly.
  • Reassemble by dropping the plunger back into the cylinder as far as it will go. Place the cap on the end of the plunger and turn until the cap is tight.

☐ For VAGINAL SUPPOSITORIES
  • Remove the wrapper from the suppository.
  • Insert the wide end of the suppository into the vaginal canal.

☐ Do not use the drug more frequently or in larger quantities than prescribed by your doctor.

SPECIAL INSTRUCTIONS
☐ During therapy, your doctor may recommend that you abstain from sexual intercourse or that your partner use a condom.

☐ It is important to use **all** of this medicine, plus any refills that your doctor told you to use. Do not stop using it earlier than your doctor has recommended

in spite of the fact that your symptoms seem to have improved. Otherwise, the infection may return.

☐ If you forget to apply the medicine, apply it as soon as possible. However, if it is almost time for your next dose, do not apply the missed dose but continue with your regular schedule.

☐ Call your doctor if the condition for which this drug is being used persists or becomes worse or if you develop a constant irritation such as itching or burning that was not present before you started using this medicine.

☐ For external use only. Do not swallow.

*   *   *   *   *

Minocycline HCl (*Oral Antibiotic*)
United States: Minocin, Vectrin
Canada: Minocin, Ultramycin

☐ This medicine is an antibiotic used to treat certain types of infections.

☐ IMPORTANT: If you have ever had an allergic reaction to tetracycline or any other antibiotic, tell your doctor or pharmacist before you take any of this medicine.

HOW TO USE THIS MEDICINE
☐ This medicine may be taken with food if it upsets your stomach. Call your doctor if you continue to have stomach upset.

☐ Take the drug with a full glass of water.

SPECIAL INSTRUCTIONS
☐ It is important that you take **all** of this medicine plus any refills that your doctor told you to take. Do not stop taking this medicine earlier than your doctor has recommended in spite of the fact that you may feel better. Otherwise, the infection may return.

☐ If you forget to take a dose, take it as soon as you remember and then continue with your regular schedule.

☐ Women who are pregnant, breast-feeding, or planning to become pregnant should tell their doctor before taking this medicine.

☐ Some antacids and some laxatives can make this medicine less effective if they are taken at the same time. If you must take them, they should be taken at least 2 to 3 hours after this medicine. If you have any questions, ask your pharmacist.

☐ If you must take iron products or vitamins containing iron, take them 2 hours before (or 3 hours after) taking this medicine.

☐ In some people, this drug may cause dizziness. Do not drive a car or operate dangerous machinery or do jobs that require you to be alert until you know how you are going to react to this drug. Call your doctor if the dizziness does not disappear.

☐ Most people experience few or no side effects from their drugs. However, any medicine can sometimes cause unwanted effects. Call your doctor if you develop a dark-colored tongue, sore mouth, yellow-green stools or, in women, a vaginal discharge that was not present before you started taking this medicine.

☐ Store the medicine in a cool, dark place and keep tightly closed.

☐ If for some reason you cannot take all of the medicine, discard the unused portion by flushing it down the toilet. Do not save this medicine for future use. Outdated minocycline can be harmful.

* * * * *

Minoxidil (Oral Vasodilator)
United States: Loniten

☐ This medicine is used to lower the blood pressure.

☐ Hypertension (high blood pressure) is a long-term condition and it may be necessary for you to take the drug for a long time in spite of the fact that you feel better. It is very important that you take this medicine as your doctor has directed and that you do not miss any doses. Otherwise, you cannot expect the drug to keep your blood pressure down.

HOW TO USE THIS MEDICINE
☐ This medicine may be taken with water or food.

☐ Try to take the medicine at the same time(s) every day.

SPECIAL INSTRUCTIONS
☐ If you forget to take a dose, take it as soon as possible. However, if it is almost time for your next dose, do not take the missed dose. Instead, continue with your regular dosing schedule.

☐ Follow any special diet your doctor may have ordered. He may want you to limit the amount of salt in your food.

☐ Some nonprescription drugs can aggravate your condition. Do not take any of the following without the approval of your doctor or pharmacist: cough, cold, or sinus products; antacids; asthma or allergy products; or diet or weight-reducing medicines.

☐ Most people experience few or no side effects from their drugs. However, any medicine can sometimes cause unwanted effects. Call your doctor if you develop a skin rash, fainting, fast heartbeats, swelling of the legs or ankles, increased hair growth, sudden weight gain of 5 pounds or more, chest pains or difficulty in breathing, dizziness, or fainting.

- Carry an identification card indicating that you are taking this medicine. Always tell your pharmacist, dentist, and other doctors who are treating you that you are taking this medicine.

- Do not stop taking this medicine without your doctor's approval and do not go without medicine between prescription refills. Call your pharmacist 2 or 3 days before you will run out of the medicine.

* * * * *

Mitotane (*Oral Antineoplastic*)
United States: Lysodren
Canada: Lysodren

- This medicine is used to help control the activity of a part of the body called the adrenal cortex.

HOW TO USE THIS MEDICINE
- It is best to take this medicine 1 hour before breakfast or 2 hours after supper in order to help prevent nausea or vomiting.

- It is very important that you take this medicine exactly as your doctor has prescribed and that you do not miss any doses. Try to take this medicine at the same time every day.

- If you forget to take a dose, take it as soon as possible. However, if it is almost time for your next dose, do not take the missed dose. Instead, continue with your regular dosing schedule.

SPECIAL INSTRUCTIONS
- Always keep your doctor appointments so that your doctor can watch your progress.

- In some people, this drug may cause dizziness or drowsiness. Do not drive a car or operate dangerous machinery or do jobs that require you to be alert until you know how you are going to react to this drug. Tell your doctor you have been dizzy or drowsy.

- Always tell your pharmacist, dentist, and other doctors who are treating you that you are taking this drug.

- This is a very strong medicine. In addition to its benefits, there may be some unwanted effects, even for a short time after you stop taking the medicine. Call your doctor if you develop a fever, infection or injury, blurred or double vision, fainting spells, diarrhea, loss of appetite, or blood in the urine.

* * * * *

Molindone HCl (*Oral Tranquilizer*)
United States: Lidone, Moban

☐ This medicine is used to treat certain types of emotional conditions.

HOW TO USE THIS MEDICINE
☐ This medicine may be taken with food or a full glass of water.

SPECIAL INSTRUCTIONS
☐ If you forget to take a dose, take it as soon as possible. However, if it is almost time for your next dose, do not take the missed dose. Instead, continue with your regular dosing schedule.

☐ In some people, this drug may cause dizziness or drowsiness. Do not drive a car or operate dangerous machinery or do jobs that require you to be alert until you know how you are going to react to this drug.

☐ If you become dizzy, you should be careful going up and down stairs. Sit or lie down at the first sign of dizziness.

☐ If your mouth becomes dry, suck a hard sour candy (sugarless) or ice chips, or chew gum. It is especially important to brush your teeth regularly if you develop a dry mouth.

☐ Do not drink alcoholic beverages while taking this drug without the approval of your doctor.

☐ It is important that you obtain the advice of your doctor or pharmacist before taking ANY other medicines including pain relievers, sleeping pills, tranquilizers or medicines for depression, cough/cold or allergy medicines, or weight-reducing medicines.

☐ Do not take any more of this medicine than your doctor has prescribed and do not stop taking this medicine suddenly without the approval of your doctor.

☐ Most people experience few or no side effects from their drugs. However, any medicine can sometimes cause unwanted effects. Call your doctor if you develop a sore throat, fever, mouth sores, skin rash, a staggering walk, changes in eyesight, unusual movements of the hands, face, or tongue or difficulty in urinating ("passing your water").

*　*　*　*　*

Monobenzone (*Topical Depigmenting Agent*)
United States: Benoquin
Canada: Benoquin

☐ This medicine is used to reduce dark pigmentation or coloring of the skin.

HOW TO USE THIS MEDICINE

☐ For OINTMENT

- Cleanse the area well with water unless otherwise directed.
- Apply the medicine and spread lightly.

☐ Do not use the drug more frequently, in larger quantities, or for a longer period of time than prescribed by your doctor.

SPECIAL INSTRUCTIONS

☐ Keep this preparation away from the eyes. If you should accidentally get some in your eyes, wash it away with water immediately.

☐ Keep this medicine away from open cuts. It must not be applied to skin that is sensitive to sunburns, prickly heat, or hair removal creams.

☐ Discontinue using this ointment if a burning sensation or irritation of the skin occurs when you apply it.

☐ For external use only.

*　*　*　*　*

Morphine (Oral Analgesic)

United States: Morphine Sulfate Oral Solution
Canada: M.O.S.

☐ This medicine is used to help relieve pain.

HOW TO USE THIS MEDICINE

☐ This medicine may be taken with food or a glass of water.

☐ For LIQUID MEDICINE

- Mix the dose of medicine with a half glass of water just before you take it unless otherwise directed. This will help prevent the medicine from numbing your mouth and throat.

☐ Do not take any more of this medicine than your doctor has prescribed. The drug could become habit-forming or you could take an overdose if you take it more often or longer than prescribed.

☐ Do not wait to take this medicine until the pain becomes severe. This medicine works best if you take it at the beginning of the pain. Call your doctor if you feel you need it more often than he prescribed.

SPECIAL INSTRUCTIONS

☐ Women who are pregnant, breast-feeding, or planning to become pregnant should tell their doctor before taking this medicine.

☐ Do not drink alcoholic beverages while taking this drug without the approval of your doctor.

- [ ] It is important that you obtain the advice of your doctor or pharmacist before taking ANY other medicines including other pain relievers, sleeping pills, tranquilizers or medicines for depression, cough/cold or allergy medicines, or weight-reducing medicines.

- [ ] In some people, this drug may cause dizziness or drowsiness. Do not drive a car or operate dangerous machinery or do jobs that require you to be alert until you know how you are going to react to this drug.

- [ ] If this medicine causes dizziness, you should be careful going up and down stairs and you should not change positions too rapidly. Get out of bed slowly in the morning and dangle your feet over the edge of the bed for a few minutes before standing up. Sit down or lie down at the first sign of dizziness. Tell your doctor you have been dizzy. Avoid hot showers and baths because they could make you dizzy.

- [ ] If your mouth becomes dry, suck a hard sour candy (sugarless) or ice chips or chew gum. It is especially important to brush your teeth regularly if you develop a dry mouth.

- [ ] If you do feel nauseated when you first start taking the medicine, it may help if you lie down for a few minutes.

- [ ] If you become constipated, try increasing the amount of bulk in your diet (for example, bran and salads), exercising more often, or drinking more water. Call your doctor if the constipation continues.

- [ ] Most people experience few or no side effects from their drugs. However, any medicine can sometimes cause unwanted effects. Call your doctor if you develop shortness of breath, slow heartbeats, unusual nervousness, stomach pain, or difficulty in urinating ("passing your water").

- [ ] Always tell your dentist, pharmacist, and other doctors who are treating you that you are taking this medicine.

*　*　*　*　*

Nadolol (Oral Antianginal-Antihypertensive)
United States: Corgard
Canada: Corgard

- [ ] This medicine is used to help relieve chest pain (angina), and it is sometimes used to treat high blood pressure.

- [ ] IMPORTANT: If you have a history of allergies, tell your doctor or pharmacist before taking any of this medicine.

- [ ] It may be necessary for you to take this medicine for a long time in spite of the fact that you may feel better. It is very important that you take the medicine as your doctor has prescribed and that you do not miss any doses. Otherwise, you cannot expect the drug to work for you.

HOW TO USE THIS MEDICINE

☐ This medicine may be taken with food or a glass of water.

☐ Try to take the medicine at the same time(s) every day.

SPECIAL INSTRUCTIONS

☐ If you forget to take a dose, take it as soon as possible. However, if your next dose is within 8 hours, do not take the missed dose. Instead continue with your regular dosing schedule.

☐ In some people, this drug may cause dizziness or drowsiness. Do not drive a car or operate dangerous machinery or do jobs that require you to be alert until you know how you are going to react to this drug. Sit down or lie down at the first sign of dizziness. Tell your doctor you have been dizzy.

☐ In order to help prevent dizziness and fainting, your doctor may also recommend that you avoid strenuous exercises, standing for long periods of time (especially in hot weather), or hot showers or hot baths.

☐ If your mouth becomes dry, suck a hard sour candy (sugarless) or ice chips, or chew gum. It is especially important to brush your teeth regularly if you develop a dry mouth.

☐ Some nonprescription drugs can aggravate your condition. Do not take any of the following without the approval of your doctor or pharmacist: cough, cold, or sinus products; asthma or allergy products; or diet or weight-reducing medicines.

☐ Most people experience few or no side effects from their drugs. However, any medicine can sometimes cause unwanted effects. Call your doctor if you develop a skin rash, shortness of breath, fever or sore throat, easy bruising, swelling of the hands or feet, sudden weight gain, earache, or mouth sores.

☐ It is recommended that patients receiving this drug stop smoking.

☐ Carry an identification card indicating that you are taking this medicine. Always tell your pharmacist, dentist, and other doctors who are treating you that you are taking this medicine.

☐ Do not stop taking this medicine without your doctor's approval and do not go without medicine between prescription refills. Call your pharmacist 2 or 3 days before you will run out of the medicine.

*   *   *   *   *

Nafcillin (*Oral Antibiotic*)
United States: Unipen

☐ This medicine is an antibiotic used to treat certain types of infections.

☐ IMPORTANT: If you have ever had an allergic reaction to penicillin or any other antibiotic, tell your doctor or pharmacist before you take any of this medicine.

556

HOW TO USE THIS MEDICINE

☐ It is best to take this medicine on an empty stomach 1 hour before (or 2 hours after) meals or food unless otherwise directed by your doctor. Take it at the proper time even if you skip a meal.

☐ Take this medicine with a full glass of water.

☐ For LIQUID MEDICINE (**United States:** Unipen Oral Solution)
- Store the liquid medicine in the refrigerator. Do not freeze.
- Do not take the medicine after the discard date on the bottle. Throw away any unused medicine after that date.

SPECIAL INSTRUCTIONS

☐ It is important to take **all** of this medicine plus any refills that your doctor told you to take. Do not stop taking this medicine earlier than your doctor has recommended in spite of the fact that you may feel better. Otherwise, the infection may return.

☐ If you forget to take a dose, take it as soon as you remember and then continue with your regular schedule.

☐ Most people experience few or no side effects from their drugs. However, any medicine can sometimes cause unwanted effects. Call your doctor if you develop a dark-colored tongue, yellow-green stools or, in women, a vaginal discharge that was not present before you started taking this medicine.

☐ This medicine sometimes causes diarrhea (loose bowel movements). Call your doctor if the diarrhea becomes severe or lasts for more than 2 days.

☐ Call your doctor immediately if you think you may be allergic to the medicine or if you develop a skin rash, hives, itching, swelling of the face, or difficulty in breathing. If you cannot reach your doctor, phone a hospital emergency department.

☐ If for some reason you cannot take all of the medicine, throw away the unused portion by flushing it down the toilet. Do not take or save old medicine.

*   *   *   *   *

Nalidixic Acid (*Oral Antibiotic*)
United States: NegGram
Canada: NegGram

☐ This medicine is used to treat urinary tract infections.

HOW TO USE THIS MEDICINE

☐ It is best to take this medicine on an empty stomach 1 hour before (or 2 hours after) meals or food. However, if the medicine upsets your stomach, it may be taken with food or milk.

☐ Take the medicine with a full glass of water.

- [ ] For LIQUID MEDICINE
    - Shake the bottle well before using so that you can measure an accurate dose. (*United States* and *Canada:* NegGram Suspension)

SPECIAL INSTRUCTIONS

- [ ] It is important to take *all* of this medicine plus any refills that your doctor told you to take. Do not stop taking it earlier than your doctor has recommended in spite of the fact that you may feel better. Otherwise, the infection may return.

- [ ] If you forget to take a dose, take it as soon as you remember and then continue with your regular schedule.

- [ ] Women who are pregnant, breast-feeding, or planning to become pregnant should tell their doctor before taking this medicine.

- [ ] This medicine may make some people more sensitive to sunlight and sunlamps. When you begin taking this medicine, try to avoid getting too much sun until you see how you are going to react. If your skin does become more sensitive to sunlight, tell your doctor and try to stay out of direct sunlight. While in the sun, wear protective clothing and sunglasses. You may wish to ask your pharmacist about suitable sunscreen products. Check with your doctor if you become sunburned.

- [ ] In some people, this drug may cause dizziness, drowsiness, or blurred vision. Do not drive a car or operate dangerous machinery or do jobs that require you to be alert until you know how you are going to react to this drug.

- [ ] Most people experience few or no side effects from their drugs. However, any medicine can sometimes cause unwanted effects. Call your doctor if you develop blurred vision, fever, sore throat, stomach pain, easy bruising, a yellow color to the skin or eyes, or a skin rash.

* * * * *

Naphazoline HCl (*Ophthalmic Decongestant*)

United States: Albalon Liquifilm, Clear Eyes, Naphcon, Naphcon Forte, Vasocon

Canada: Albalon Liquifilm, Degest-2, Naphcon Forte, Optozoline, Vasacon Regular

Naphazoline HCl-Antazoline Phosphate

United States: Albalon-A, Vasocon A

Canada: Albalon-A, Vasocon-A

- [ ] This medicine is used to treat eye conditions and helps relieve burning, itching, or smarting of the eye.

HOW TO USE THIS MEDICINE
- [ ] For EYE DROPS

INSTILLATION OF EYE DROPS

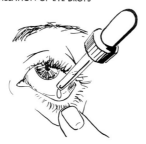

- The person administering the eye drops should wash his hands with soap and water.
- The eye drops must be kept clean. Do not touch the dropper against the face or anything else.
- Lie down or tilt your head backward and look at the ceiling.
- Gently pull down the lower lid of your eye to form a pouch.
- Hold the dropper in your other hand and approach the eye from the side. Place the dropper as close to the eye as possible without touching it.
- Place the prescribed number of drops into the pouch of the eye.
- Close your eyes. Do not rub them.
- Apply gentle pressure for a minute with your fingers to the bridge of the nose (inside corner of the eye) to prevent the eye drops from being drained from the eye.
- Blot excess solution around the eye with a tissue.

- [ ] If necessary, have someone else administer the eye drops for you.

- [ ] Do not use the eye drops if they have changed in color or have changed in any way since you purchased them.

- [ ] Keep the eye drop bottle tightly closed when not in use.

- [ ] Do not use the drug more frequently or in larger quantities than prescribed by your doctor.

SPECIAL INSTRUCTIONS
- [ ] Vision may be blurred for a few minutes after using the eye medicine. Do not drive a car or operate dangerous machinery or do jobs that require you to be alert until your vision has cleared.

- [ ] If you forget to use the medicine, use it as soon as possible. However, if it is almost time for your next dose, do not use the missed dose but continue with your regular schedule.

- [ ] Do not use this medicine at the same time as any other eye medicine without the approval of your doctor. Some medicines cannot be mixed.

559

☐ Check with your doctor if you develop a headache which does not go away as your body adjusts to the medicine.

☐ Contact your doctor if the condition for which you are using this medicine does not improve or if the eye becomes irritated by it for more than a few minutes. Many eye medicines sting for a short time immediately after use. Also call your doctor if you develop fast heartbeats, trembling, or excessive sweating.

☐ Store the solution in a cool dark place as it is sensitive to heat and light.

☐ For external use only. Do not swallow.

* * * * *

Naphazoline HCl (*Nasal Decongestant*)
United States: Privine
Canada: Privine, Rhino-Mex-N

Naphazoline HCl-Antazoline
Canada: Antistine-Privine

☐ This medicine is used to help reduce nasal stuffiness.

HOW TO USE THIS MEDICINE
☐ For NASAL SPRAY
- Blow your nose gently.
- Sit upright with your head slightly back.
- Place the atomizer at the entrance of the nostril and close the other nostril by pressing your finger on the side.
- Squeeze the atomizer the prescribed number of times.
- Repeat for the other nostril if necessary.

☐ For NOSE DROPS

INSTILLATION OF NOSE DROPS

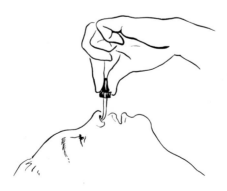

- Blow your nose gently before administration of drops.
- Sit in a chair and tilt your head backward, or lie down on a bed with your head extending over the edge of the bed, or lie down and place a pillow under your shoulders so that your head is tipped backward.
- Insert the dropper into your nostril about one third inch and drop the prescribed number of drops into the nose.
- Try not to touch the inside of the nose with the dropper as it will probably make you sneeze and will contaminate the dropper.
- Remain in the same position for at least 5 minutes.
- For children: Let the child's head hang over the edge of table, bed, or mother's lap and follow the same procedure.

SPECIAL INSTRUCTIONS

☐ Do not use this medicine more often or longer than recommended by your doctor. If used for too long, this medicine may actually cause a type of congestion.

☐ Call your doctor if the nasal stuffiness persists after using this medicine for 5 days.

☐ Rinse the dropper in hot water after each use.

☐ If you forget to use the medicine, use it as soon as possible. However, if it is almost time for your next dose, do not use the missed dose but continue with your regular schedule.

☐ Do not use this medicine at the same time as any other nasal medicine without the approval of your doctor. Some medicines cannot be mixed.

☐ Contact your doctor if the condition for which you are using this medicine does not improve. Also call your doctor if you develop fast heartbeats, headache, dizziness, trembling, blurred vision, or drowsiness.

☐ Check with your doctor if you develop a stinging sensation which does not go away after your body adjusts to the medicine.

☐ For external use only. Do not swallow.

*   *   *   *   *

Naproxen (*Oral Anti-inflammatory-Analgesic*)
United States: Naprosyn
Canada: Naprosyn

☐ This medicine is used to help relieve pain, redness, stiffness, and swelling in certain kinds of arthritis.

☐ IMPORTANT: If you have ever had an allergic reaction to aspirin or any other medicine for arthritis, tell your doctor or pharmacist before you take any of this medicine.

561

□ It is very important that you take this medicine regularly and that you DO NOT MISS ANY DOSES. If you miss a dose, the level of the medicine in your body will fall and the drug will not be as effective. Only if the level of the drug is high enough can it decrease the inflammation and swelling in your joints and help prevent further damage.

□ The full benefit of this medicine may not be noticed immediately but may take from a few days to 3 weeks.

HOW TO USE THIS MEDICINE

□ It is best to take this medicine on an empty stomach at least 1 hour before (or 2 hours after) food unless otherwise directed. If you develop stomach upset, take the medicine with food or immediately after meals. Call your doctor if you continue to have stomach upset.

SPECIAL INSTRUCTIONS

□ In some people, this drug may cause dizziness or drowsiness. Do not drive a car or operate dangerous machinery or do jobs that require you to be alert until you know how you are going to react to this drug.

□ If you become dizzy, you should be careful going up and down stairs. Sit or lie down at the first sign of dizziness.

□ If you forget to take a dose, take it as soon as possible. However, if it is almost time for your next dose, do not take the missed dose. Instead, continue with your regular dosing schedule.

□ While you are taking this medicine, do not drink alcoholic beverages or take aspirin without the permission of your doctor. It is usually safe to take acetaminophen for the occasional headache. Check with your pharmacist.

□ Call your doctor immediately if you think you may be allergic to the medicine or if you develop a skin rash, hives, itching, swelling of the face, or difficulty in breathing. If you cannot reach your doctor, phone a hospital emergency department.

□ Most people experience few or no side effects from their drugs. However, any medicine can sometimes cause unwanted effects. Call your doctor if you develop a skin rash, sore throat or fever, "ringing" or "buzzing" in the ears, fast heartbeats, swelling of the legs or ankles or sudden weight gain, blurred vision or changes in your eyesight, red or black stools, severe stomach pain, easy bruising or bleeding, or a yellow color to the skin or eyes.

□ Carry an identification card indicating that you are taking this medicine. Always tell your pharmacist, dentist, and other doctors who are treating you that you are taking this medicine.

*   *   *   *   *

Natamycin (*Ophthalmic Antifungal*)

United States: Natamycin Ophthalmic

☐ This medicine is used to treat certain types of fungal infections of the eye.

HOW TO USE THIS MEDICINE

☐ For EYE DROPS

INSTILLATION OF EYE DROPS

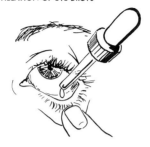

- The person administering the eye drops should wash his hands with soap and water.
- The eye drops must be kept clean. Do not touch the dropper against the face or anything else.
- Lie down or tilt your head backward and look at the ceiling.
- Shake the bottle well before using.
- Gently pull down the lower lid of your eye to form a pouch.
- Hold the dropper in your other hand and approach the eye from the side. Place the dropper as close to the eye as possible without touching it.
- Place the prescribed number of drops into the pouch of the eye.
- Close your eyes. Do not rub them.
- Apply gentle pressure for a minute with your fingers to the bridge of the nose (inside corner of the eye) to prevent the eye drops from being drained from the eye.
- Blot excess solution around the eye with a tissue.

☐ If necessary, have someone else administer the eye drops for you.

☐ Do not use the eye drops if they have changed in color or have changed in any way since you purchased them.

☐ Keep the eye drop bottle tightly closed when not in use.

☐ Do not use the drug more frequently or in larger quantities than prescribed by your doctor.

SPECIAL INSTRUCTIONS

☐ Vision may be blurred for a few minutes after using the eye medicine. Do not drive a car or operate dangerous machinery or do jobs that require you to be alert until your vision has cleared.

☐ It is important to use **all** of this medicine, plus any refills that your doctor told you to use. Do not stop using it earlier than your doctor has recommended in spite of the fact that your symptoms seem to have improved. Otherwise, the infection may return.

☐ If you forget to use the medicine, use it as soon as possible. However, if it is almost time for your next dose, do not use the missed dose but continue with your regular schedule.

☐ Do not use this medicine at the same time as any other eye medicine without the approval of your doctor. Some medicines cannot be mixed.

☐ Contact your doctor if the condition for which you are using this medicine does not improve or if the eye becomes irritated by it for more than a few minutes. Many eye medicines sting for a short time immediately after use.

☐ For external use only. Do not swallow.

* * * * *

Neomycin Sulfate (*Oral Antibiotic*)
United States: Mycifradin Sulfate, Neobiotic
Canada: Mycifradin

☐ This medicine is used to treat certain types of infections and bowel or liver conditions.

☐ IMPORTANT: If you have ever had an allergic reaction to any antibiotics, tell your doctor or pharmacist before you take any of this medicine.

HOW TO USE THIS MEDICINE
☐ This medicine may be taken either with meals or on an empty stomach.

SPECIAL INSTRUCTIONS
☐ It is important to take **all** of this medicine plus any refills that your doctor told you to take. Do not stop taking it earlier than your doctor has recommended in spite of the fact that you may feel better. Otherwise, the infection may return.

☐ If you forget to take a dose, take it as soon as you remember and then continue with your regular schedule.

☐ Most people experience few or no side effects from their drugs. However, any medicine can sometimes cause unwanted effects. Call your doctor if you develop "ringing" or "buzzing" in the ears or difficulty hearing, or dizziness, or if you become very thirsty or urinate ("pass your water") less frequently or in smaller amounts than normal.

☐ Call your doctor immediately if you think you may be allergic to the medicine or if you develop a skin rash, hives, itching, swelling of the face, or difficulty

in breathing. If you cannot reach your doctor, phone a hospital emergency department.

☐ If for some reason you cannot take all of the medicine, throw away the unused portion by flushing it down the toilet. Do not take or save old medicine.

* * * * *

Neomycin Sulfate (*Ophthalmic Antibiotic*)
United States: Myciguent
Canada: Myciguent

☐ This medicine is an antibiotic used to treat certain types of eye infections.

☐ IMPORTANT: If you have ever had an allergic reaction to neomycin or any antibiotic medicine, tell your doctor or pharmacist before you use any of this drug.

HOW TO USE THIS MEDICINE
☐ For EYE OINTMENT

INSTILLATION OF EYE OINTMENT

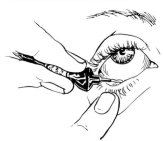

- The person administering the eye ointment should wash his hands with soap and water.
- The eye ointment must be kept clean. Do not touch the tube against the face or anything else.
- Lie down or tilt your head backward and look at the ceiling.
- Gently pull down the lower lid of your eye to form a pouch.
- Hold the tube in your other hand and place the tube as close as possible to the eye without touching it.
- Squeeze the prescribed amount of ointment (usually one half inch in adults) from the tube along the pouch.
- Close your eyes. Do not rub them.
- Wipe off any excess ointment around the eye with a tissue.
- Clean the tip of the ointment tube with a tissue.

☐ If necessary, have someone else administer the eye ointment for you.

☐ Keep the eye ointment tube tightly closed when not in use.

SPECIAL INSTRUCTIONS

☐ Vision may be blurred for a few minutes after using the eye medicine. Do not drive a car or operate dangerous machinery or do jobs that require you to be alert until your vision has cleared.

☐ Eye medicines should be used as prescribed by your doctor. Often eye infections clear rapidly after a few days of use of the medicine, but not always completely. It is important to use **all** of this medicine, plus any refills that you doctor told you to use. Do not stop using it earlier than your doctor has recommended in spite of the fact that your symptoms seem to have improved. Otherwise, the infection may return.

☐ If you forget to use the medicine, use it as soon as possible. However, if it is almost time for your next dose, do not use the missed dose but continue with your regular schedule.

☐ Do not use this medicine at the same time as any other eye medicine without the approval of your doctor. Some medicines cannot be mixed.

☐ Contact your doctor if the condition for which you are using this medicine does not improve or if the eye becomes irritated by it for more than a few minutes. Many eye medicines sting for a short time immediately after use.

☐ For external use only. Do not swallow.

* * * * *

Neomycin Sulfate (*Topical Antibiotic*)
United States: Myciguent
Canada: Herisan Antibiotic, Myciguent

☐ This medicine is an antibiotic used to treat infections of the skin.

☐ IMPORTANT: If you have ever had an allergic reaction to neomycin or any antibiotic medicine, tell your doctor or pharmacist before you use any of this drug.

HOW TO USE THIS MEDICINE

☐ • Each time you apply the medicine, wash your hands and gently cleanse the skin area well with water unless otherwise directed by your doctor. Do not allow the skin to dry completely. Pat with a clean towel until almost dry.
  • Apply a small amount of the drug to the affected area and spread lightly. Only the medicine that is actually touching the skin will work. A thick layer is not more effective than a thin layer. Do not bandage unless directed by your doctor.

☐ Do not use the drug more frequently or in larger quantities than prescribed by your doctor.

566

SPECIAL INSTRUCTIONS

☐ It is important to use **all** of this medicine, plus any refills that your doctor told you to use. Do not stop using it earlier than your doctor has recommended in spite of the fact that your symptoms seem to have improved. Otherwise, the infection may return.

☐ If you forget to apply the medicine, apply it as soon as possible. However, if it is almost time for your next dose, do not apply the missed dose but continue with your regular schedule.

☐ Do not apply cosmetics or lotions on top of the drug unless your doctor approves.

☐ Keep this preparation away from the eyes. If you should accidentally get some in your eyes, wash it away with water immediately.

☐ Call your doctor if the condition for which this drug is being used persists or becomes worse or if you develop a constant irritation such as itching or burning that was not present before you started using this medicine. Also call your doctor if you develop a rash, redness, swelling, or trouble with your hearing.

☐ Store in a cool place.

☐ For external use only. Do not swallow.

*   *   *   *   *

Neomycin-Bacitracin-Polymyxin B Sulfate (*Topical Antibiotic*)

United States: Neosporin, Neo-Polycin, Mycitracin
Canada: Neo-Polycin, Neosporin

☐ This medicine is an antibiotic used to treat infections of the skin.

☐ IMPORTANT: If you have ever had an allergic reaction to neomycin or any antibiotic medicine, tell your doctor or pharmacist before you use any of this drug.

HOW TO USE THIS MEDICINE

☐ For CREAM or OINTMENT

- Each time you apply the medicine, wash your hands and gently cleanse the skin area well with water unless otherwise directed by your doctor. Do not allow the skin to dry completely. Pat with a clean towel until almost dry.
- Apply a small amount of the drug to the affected area and spread lightly. Only the medicine that is actually touching the skin will work. A thick layer is not more effective than a thin layer. Do not bandage unless directed by your doctor.

567

☐ For AEROSOL

- Shake the container well each time before using.
- Cleanse the affected area well with water unless otherwise directed by your doctor.
- Hold the container straight up and about 6 to 8 inches away from the skin.
- Spray the affected area for 1 to 3 seconds.
- Shake the container well between sprays.
- Do not spray into the eyes, nose, or mouth and try to avoid inhaling the vapors.
- Do not smoke while using this spray or use near an open flame, fire, or heat. Do not use the spray near food.
- Do not place the aerosol container in hot water or near radiators, stoves, or other sources of heat. Do not puncture or incinerate the container (even when empty). Do not store at temperatures greater than 120°F (49°C).

☐ For POWDER

- Cleanse the affected area well with water unless otherwise directed by your doctor.
- Sprinkle the powder on the affected area.

☐ Do not use the drug more frequently or in larger quantities than prescribed by your doctor.

SPECIAL INSTRUCTIONS

☐ It is important to use **all** of this medicine, plus any refills that your doctor told you to use. Do not stop using it earlier than your doctor has recommended in spite of the fact that your symptoms seem to have improved. Otherwise, the infection may return.

☐ If you forget to apply the medicine, apply it as soon as possible. However, if it is almost time for your next dose, do not apply the missed dose but continue with your regular schedule.

☐ Do not apply cosmetics or lotions on top of the drug unless your doctor approves.

☐ Keep this preparation away from the eyes. If you should accidentally get some in your eyes, wash it away with water immediately.

☐ Call your doctor if the condition for which this drug is being used persists or becomes worse or if you develop a constant irritation such as itching or burning that was not present before you started using this medicine. Also call your doctor if you develop a rash, redness, swelling, or trouble with your hearing.

☐ For external use only. Do not swallow.

*   *   *   *   *

Neomycin-Steroid Combinations (*Eye/Ear Antibiotic-Corticosteroid*)

United States: Cortisporin, Maxitrol, Neo-Cortef, Neo-Decadron, Neo-Deltef, Neo-Delta-Cortef, Neo-Hydeltrasol, Neo-Medrol, Neosone

Canada: Adrenomyxin, Cortisporin, Maxitrol, Neo-Cortef, Neo-Decadron, Neo-Medrol

☐ This medicine is used to help relieve the pain, redness, and swelling of certain types of eye and ear conditions.

☐ IMPORTANT: If you have ever had an allergic reaction to a neomycin or any antibiotic medicine, tell your doctor or pharmacist before you use any of this drug.

HOW TO USE THIS MEDICINE

☐ Shake the drops well before using.

☐ For EAR DROPS

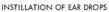

INSTILLATION OF EAR DROPS

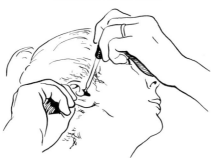

- Warm the ear drops to body temperature by holding the bottle in your hands for a few minutes. Do NOT heat the drops in hot water.
- The person administering the ear drops should wash his hands with soap and water.
- The ear drops must be kept clean. Do not touch the dropper against the ear or anything else.
- Tilt your head or lie on your side so that the ear to be treated is facing up.
- In ADULTS, hold the ear lobe up and back.
  In CHILDREN, hold the ear lobe down and back.
- Place the prescribed number of drops into the ear. Do not insert the dropper into the ear as it may cause injury.
- Remain in the same position for a short time (2 minutes) after you have administered the drops.
- Dry the ear lobe if there are any drops on it.
- If necessary, have someone else administer the ear drops for you.
- Do not use the ear drops if they have changed in color or have changed in any way since being purchased.
- Keep the bottle tightly closed when not in use.

569

□ EAR DROPS AFTER APPLICATION OF EAR WICK:

- Warm the medicine to body temperature by holding it in your hands for a few minutes.
- Tilt your head to the side so that the ear to be treated is uppermost.
- Drop the prescribed amount of medicine into the ear canal.
- Do not use the solution if it is discolored or if it appears to have changed in any way since you purchased it.

□ For EYE OINTMENT

INSTILLATION OF EYE OINTMENT

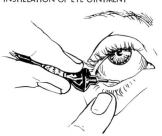

- The person administering the eye ointment should wash his hands with soap and water.
- The eye ointment must be kept clean. Do not touch the tube against the face or anything else.
- Lie down or tilt your head backward and look at the ceiling.
- Gently pull down the lower lid of your eye to form a pouch.
- Hold the tube in your other hand and place the tube as close as possible to the eye without touching it.
- Squeeze the prescribed amount of ointment (usually one half inch in adults) from the tube along the pouch.
- Close your eyes. Do not rub them.
- Wipe off any excess ointment around the eye with a tissue.
- Clean the tip of the ointment tube with a tissue.
- If necessary, have someone else administer the eye ointment for you.
- Keep the eye ointment tube tightly closed when not in use.

□ For EYE DROPS

INSTILLATION OF EYE DROPS

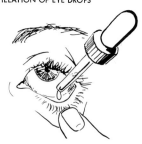

- The person administering the eye drops should wash his hands with soap and water.

570

- The eye drops must be kept clean. Do not touch the dropper against the face or anything else.
- Lie down or tilt your head backward and look at the ceiling.
- Gently pull down the lower lid of your eye to form a pouch.
- Hold the dropper in your other hand and approach the eye from the side. Place the dropper as close to the eye as possible without touching it.
- Place the prescribed number of drops into the pouch of the eye.
- Close your eyes. Do not rub them.
- Apply gentle pressure for a minute with your fingers to the bridge of the nose (inside corner of the eye) to prevent the eye drops from being drained from the eye.
  - Blot excess solution around the eye with a tissue.
- If necessary, have someone else administer the eye drops for you.
- Do not use the eye drops if they have changed in color or have changed in any way since you purchased them.
- Keep the eye drop bottle tightly closed when not in use.

☐ Do not use this drug more frequently or in larger quantities than prescribed by your doctor.

SPECIAL INSTRUCTIONS

☐ This medicine should be used as long as prescribed by your doctor. Do not stop using it earlier than your doctor has recommended in spite of the fact that your symptoms seem to have improved.

☐ If you forget to use the medicine, use it as soon as possible. However, if it is almost time for your next dose, do not use the missed dose but continue with your regular schedule.

☐ Vision may be blurred for a few minutes after using the eye medicine. Do not drive a car or operate dangerous machinery or do jobs that require you to be alert until your vision has cleared.

☐ Do not use this medicine at the same time as any other eye or ear medicine without the approval of your doctor. Some medicines cannot be mixed.

☐ Call your doctor if the condition for which you are using this medicine persists or becomes worse or if the medicine causes itching or burning for more than a few minutes after instillation.

☐ For external use only. Do not swallow.

* * * * *

Neomycin-Steroid Combinations (*Topical Antibiotic-Corticosteroid*)

United States: Cordran-N, Cortisporin, Neo-Cort Dome, Neo-Cortef, Neo-Hytone, Neo-Decadron, Neo-Medrol, Neo-Synalar

Canada: Cortisporin, Neo-Cortef, Neo-Medrol, Neo-Synalar

- ☐ This medicine is used to help relieve redness, swelling, itching, and inflammation of certain types of skin conditions.

- ☐ IMPORTANT: If you have ever had an allergic reaction to neomycin or any antibiotic medicine, tell your doctor or pharmacist before you use any of this drug.

HOW TO USE THIS MEDICINE
- ☐ For CREAM
  - Each time you apply the medicine, wash your hands and gently cleanse the skin area well with water unless otherwise directed by your doctor. Do not allow the skin to dry completely. Pat with a clean towel until slightly damp.
  - Apply a small amount of the drug to the affected area and spread lightly. Only the medicine that is actually touching the skin will work. A thick layer is not more effective than a thin layer. Do not bandage unless directed by your doctor.

- ☐ Do not use the drug more frequently or in larger quantities than prescribed by your doctor. Overuse of this medicine may cause you to absorb too much of the drug and increase the risk of side effects.

- ☐ Keep the medicine away from the eyes, nose, and mouth.

SPECIAL INSTRUCTIONS
- ☐ If you forget to apply the medicine, apply it as soon as possible. However, if it is almost time for your next dose, do not apply the missed dose but continue with your regular schedule.

- ☐ Do not use this medicine for any other skin problems without checking with your doctor.

- ☐ Do not apply cosmetics or lotions on top of the drug unless your doctor approves.

- ☐ Call your doctor if the condition for which this drug is being used persists or becomes worse or if you develop a constant irritation such as itching or burning that was not present before you started using this medicine. Also call your doctor if you develop abnormal lines or thinning of the skin, especially under the arms or between the legs.

- ☐ Store in a cool place but do not freeze.

- ☐ For external use only. Do not swallow.

- ☐ Tell future doctors that you have used this medicine.

* * * * *

Neomycin Sulfate-Sodium Propionate (*Otitis Therapy*)
United States: Otobiotic

☐ This medicine is used to treat certain types of ear infections.

☐ IMPORTANT: If you have ever had an allergic reaction to neomycin or any antibiotic medicine, tell your doctor or pharmacist before you use any of this drug.

HOW TO USE THIS MEDICINE

☐ Do not use this drug more frequently or in larger quantities than prescribed by your doctor.

☐ For EAR DROPS

INSTILLATION OF EAR DROPS

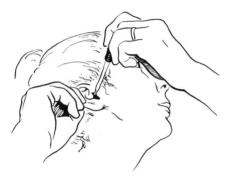

- Warm the ear drops to body temperature by holding the bottle in your hands for a few minutes. Do NOT heat the drops in hot water.
- The person administering the ear drops should wash his hands with soap and water.
- The ear drops must be kept clean. Do not touch the dropper against the ear or anything else.
- Tilt your head or lie on your side so that the ear to be treated is facing up.
- In ADULTS, hold the ear lobe up and back.
  In CHILDREN, hold the ear lobe down and back.
- Place the prescribed number of drops into the ear. Do not insert the dropper into the ear as it may cause injury.
- Remain in the same position for a short time (2 minutes) after you have administered the drops.
- Dry the ear lobe if there are any drops on it.
- If necessary, have someone else administer the ear drops for you.
- Do not use the ear drops if they have changed in color or have changed in any way since you purchased them.
- Keep the bottle tightly closed when not in use.

☐ EAR DROPS AFTER ADMINISTRATION OF EAR WICK:
- Warm the medicine to body temperature by holding it in your hands for a few minutes.
- Tilt your head to the side or lie on your side so that the ear to be treated is uppermost.
- Drop the prescribed amount of medicine into the ear canal on top of the ear wick.
- Do not use the solution if it is discolored or if it appears to have changed in any way since being dispensed.

SPECIAL INSTRUCTIONS

☐ It is important to use **all** of this medicine, plus any refills that your doctor told you to use. Do not stop using it earlier than your doctor has recommended in spite of the fact that your symptoms seem to have improved. Otherwise, the infection may return.

☐ If you forget to use the medicine, use it as soon as possible. However, if it is almost time for your next dose, do not use the missed dose but continue with your regular schedule.

☐ Do not use this medicine at the same time as any other ear medicine without the approval of your doctor. Some medicines cannot be mixed.

☐ Consult your doctor if the condition for which this medicine is being used persists or becomes worse, or if the medicine causes an irritation such as itching or burning for more than just a few minutes after use.

☐ Store in a cool place.

☐ For external use only. Do not swallow.

* * * * *

Neostigmine (*Oral Parasympathomimetic*)
United States: Prostigmin Bromide
Canada: Prostigmin

☐ This medicine has many uses and the reason it was prescribed depends upon your condition. If you do not understand why you are taking it, check with your doctor.

HOW TO USE THIS MEDICINE
☐ This medicine may be taken with food or a glass of water.

SPECIAL INSTRUCTIONS
☐ If you forget to take a dose, take it as soon as possible. However, if it is almost time for your next dose, do not take the missed dose. Instead, continue with your regular dosing schedule.

- [ ] In some people, this drug may cause "double vision." Do not drive a car or operate dangerous machinery or do jobs that require you to be alert until you know how you are going to react to this drug.

- [ ] It is important that you obtain the advice of your doctor or pharmacist before taking pain relievers, nonprescription drugs, sleeping pills or tranquilizers, or medicines for depression while you are taking this drug.

- [ ] It is a good idea to keep a diary of "peaks and valleys" of your muscle strength. This will help your doctor in designing your treatment.

- [ ] Most people experience few or no side effects from their drugs. However, any medicine can sometimes cause unwanted effects. Call your doctor if you develop slow or fast heartbeats, changes in vision, muscle cramps, nausea, vomiting or diarrhea, difficulty in breathing, fainting spells or dizziness, convulsions, or unusual sweating, or if you urinate ("pass your water") more frequently than usual.

* * * * *

Nicotinic Acid (Niacin) (*Oral Vitamin*)

United States: Nicobid, Nicocap, Nico-400, Nicolar, Nico-Span, SK-Niacin, Tega-Span, Wampocap

- [ ] This medicine has many uses and the reason it was prescribed depends upon your condition. Be sure you understand why you are taking it.

HOW TO USE THIS MEDICINE
- [ ] Take this medicine with food or after meals to help prevent stomach upset.

- [ ] This medicine must be swallowed whole. Do not crush, chew, or break it into pieces. (*United States:* Nicobid, Nico-400, Nico-Span, Tega-Span)

SPECIAL INSTRUCTIONS
- [ ] After taking this medicine, you may feel a warm tingling and itching sensation of the skin. This is a normal effect of the drug.

- [ ] If you forget to take a dose, take it as soon as possible. However, if it is almost time for your next dose, do not take the missed dose. Instead, continue with your regular dosing schedule.

- [ ] It is very important to follow any diet that your doctor may also prescribe for you.

- [ ] In some people, this drug may cause dizziness. Do not drive a car or operate dangerous machinery or do jobs that require you to be alert until you know how you are going to react to this drug. If you become dizzy, you should be careful going up and down stairs. Sit or lie down at the first sign of dizziness.

- [ ] Do not take any more of this medicine than your doctor has prescribed and do not stop taking this medicine suddenly without the approval of the doctor.

☐ Most people experience few or no side effects from their drugs. However, any medicine can sometimes cause unwanted effects. Call your doctor if you develop a rapid pulse, chest pain, fainting spells, dark-colored urine or a yellow color to the skin or eyes, sharp stomach pain, blurred vision, or sharp joint pain (especially in the large toe).

* * * * *

Nicotinyl Alcohol Tartrate (*Oral Peripheral Vasodilator*)
United States: Roniacol, Speniacol
Canada: Roniacol Supraspan

☐ This medicine is used to improve the circulation of blood in the body.

HOW TO USE THIS MEDICINE

☐ For ORAL and LIQUID MEDICINE
- This medicine may be taken with food or on an empty stomach.
- If you forget to take a dose, take it as soon as possible. However, if it is almost time for your next dose, do not take the missed dose. Instead, continue with your regular dosing schedule.

☐ For SUSTAINED RELEASE MEDICINE
- This medicine may be taken with food or on an empty stomach.
- Swallow the tablets whole. Do not crush, chew, or break them into pieces. (**United States:** Roniacol Timespan, Speniacol Timed Release; **Canada:** Roniacol Supraspan)
- If you forget to take a dose, take it as soon as possible. However, if your next dose is within 6 hours, do not take the missed dose but continue with your regular schedule.

SPECIAL INSTRUCTIONS

☐ This medicine commonly produces flushing of the face and a feeling of warmth. This is normal and you should not become concerned.

☐ If this medicine causes dizziness, you should be careful going up and down stairs and you should not change positions too rapidly. Get out of bed slowly in the morning and dangle your feet over the edge of the bed for a few minutes before standing up. Sit down or lie down at the first sign of dizziness. Tell your doctor you have been dizzy. Do not drive a car or operate dangerous machinery if you are dizzy. Avoid hot showers and baths because they could make you dizzy.

☐ The activity of this drug is improved if you keep warm. Avoid getting cold or exposing yourself to a cold environment.

☐ Some nonprescription drugs can aggravate your condition. Do not take any of the following without the approval of your doctor or pharmacist: cough, cold, or sinus products; asthma or allergy products; or diet or weight-reducing medicines.

☐ Do not drink alcoholic beverages while taking this drug without the approval of your doctor.

☐ Most people experience few or no side effects from their drugs. However, any medicine can sometimes cause unwanted effects. Call your doctor if you develop a skin rash, fainting spells, nausea, vomiting or stomach pain, a yellow color to the skin or eyes, or dark-colored urine.

* * * * *

Nitrazine Paper* (*pH Indicator*)
United States: Nitrazine Paper
Canada: Nitrazine Paper

☐ This preparation is used to test the pH (acidity/alkalinity) of the urine.

☐ Testing procedure:
1. Dip the paper into the urine; shake off excess fluid and read immediately.
2. Subtract 0.2 pH units from the reading obtained.
3. Do **not** dilute the urine before the test.

* * * * *

Nitrofurantoin (*Oral Urinary Antibacterial*)
United States: Cyantin, Furalan, Furadantin, Macrodantin, Sarodant
Canada: Furatine, Macrodantin, Nephronex, Nifuran, Novofuran

☐ This medicine is used to treat urinary tract infections.

☐ IMPORTANT: If you have ever had an allergic reaction to furazolidone or nitrofurazone or any other antibiotic, tell your doctor or pharmacist before you take any of this medicine.

HOW TO USE THIS MEDICINE
☐ It is best to take this medicine with food or milk.

☐ Swallow the tablets and capsules whole. Do not crush, chew, or break them into pieces.

☐ For LIQUID MEDICINE (**United States:** Furadantin Suspension; **Canada:** Furatine, Novofuran Suspensions)
- Shake the bottle well before using so that you can measure an accurate dose.
- The liquid may be mixed with water, milk, or fruit juices just before taking.
- Use a straw or rinse your mouth with water after swallowing the liquid preparation because this will help prevent any staining of the teeth.

*Nitrazine Paper (Package Insert), E. R. Squibb & Sons, Inc., New York

577

SPECIAL INSTRUCTIONS

☐ It is important to take **all** of this medicine plus any refills that your doctor told you to take. Do not stop taking it earlier than your doctor has recommended in spite of the fact that you may feel better. Otherwise, the infection may return.

☐ If you forget to take a dose, take it as soon as you remember and then continue with your regular schedule.

☐ This medicine may cause your urine to turn brown in color. This is not an unusual effect.

☐ Women who are pregnant, breast-feeding, or planning to become pregnant should tell their doctor before taking this medicine.

☐ Most people experience few or no side effects from their drugs. However, any medicine can sometimes cause unwanted effects. Call your doctor if you develop fever, cough, difficulty in breathing, chest pain, chills, numbness or tingling, or a yellow color to the skin or eyes.

* * * * *

Nitrofurazone (*Topical Antibacterial*)
United States: Furacin
Canada: Furacin Soluble Dressing

☐ This medicine is an antibiotic used to treat certain types of infections of the skin.

HOW TO USE THIS MEDICINE

☐ Instructions for use:
  - Cleanse the affected area well with soap and water.
  - Apply cream directly to the area, or place on gauze and then apply to the affected area.

SPECIAL INSTRUCTIONS

☐ If you forget to apply the medicine, apply it as soon as possible. However, if it is almost time for your next dose, do not apply the missed dose but continue with your regular schedule.

☐ Do not apply cosmetics or lotions on top of the drug unless your doctor approves.

☐ Keep this preparation away from the eyes. If you should accidentally get some in your eyes, wash it away with water immediately.

☐ Call your doctor if the condition for which this drug is being used persists or becomes worse or if you develop a constant irritation such as itching or burning that was not present before you started using this medicine.

☐ For external use only. Do not swallow.

* * * * *

578

Nitroglycerin *(Sublingual Coronary Vasodilator)*

United States: Nitroglycerin, Nitrostat

Canada: Nitrostabilin, Nitrostat

☐ This medicine is used to help relieve and sometimes prevent a type of chest pain called angina.

☐ Carry this medicine with you all the time.

HOW TO USE THIS MEDICINE

☐ This medicine should be used at the FIRST sign of an attack of angina. Do not wait until severe pain develops. Sit down or lie down as soon as you feel an attack of angina coming on.

☐ Then place a tablet UNDER YOUR TONGUE or in the pouch of your cheek until it is completely dissolved. Do NOT swallow or chew the tablet.

☐ Try not to swallow until the drug is dissolved and do not rinse the mouth for a few minutes. Do not eat, drink, or smoke while the tablet is dissolving.

☐ If your angina is not relieved within 5 minutes, you may dissolve a second tablet under your tongue. If the angina continues for another 5 minutes, you may dissolve a third tablet. If this does not relieve your chest pains, call your doctor immediately or go to the nearest hospital emergency department.

☐ Try to relax and remain calm. If you become dizzy or feel faint, breathe deeply and bend forward with your head between your knees. Always get up slowly after you have been sitting or lying down.

HOW TO STORE THIS MEDICINE

☐ This medicine must be fresh in order to work. It must be stored in the following way:

- Keep the tablets in the brown glass container supplied by your pharmacist and keep the container tightly closed.
- Remove the cotton that comes in the bottle and do not put labels, other drugs, or any other material into the bottle.
- Store the medicine in a cool, dry place. Do NOT store it in the refrigerator or the bathroom medicine cabinet because the moisture in these areas could spoil the tablets.
- Transfer the number of tablets you usually use in one week to a glass container (available from your pharmacist) or an empty nitroglycerin container. Do not carry this container close to your body, but keep it in a cool place such as your purse or coat pocket. At the end of the week, discard the remaining tablets in this container and obtain a fresh supply from your original bottle.
- As soon as you remove a tablet, reclose the lid tightly.

☐ Take only fresh tablets and test your tablets at least once a month. A fresh, potent tablet will produce a tingling or burning sensation when you place it under your tongue. If this does not occur, call your doctor or pharmacist to obtain a new supply.

579

☐ Inform the members of your family of the place where you store your nitro-glycerin.

SPECIAL INSTRUCTIONS

☐ After using this medicine, you may get a headache or flushing which will usually disappear within a few minutes. These are common side effects. If the headaches are severe or do not go away, tell your doctor.

☐ Do not drink alcoholic beverages too soon after taking this medicine as they may make the dizziness or fainting worse.

☐ Some nonprescription drugs can aggravate your heart condition. Do not take any of the following without the approval of your doctor or pharmacist: cough, cold, or sinus products; asthma or allergy products, or diet or weight-reducing medicines.

☐ You may help prevent angina by taking a tablet 5 to 10 minutes before activities you know are likely to trigger attacks, such as strenuous exercise, emotional stress, a heavy meal, high altitudes, or exposure to cold. Let your doctor know what things usually cause your angina so that he can advise you about preventing attacks.

☐ Cigarette smoking can aggravate angina and is a special risk for people who have heart conditions.

☐ Most people experience few or no side effects from their drugs. However, any medicine can sometimes cause unwanted effects. Call your doctor if you develop a skin rash, blurred vision, or dry mouth, or if your chest pain is not relieved after you have taken the number of tablets that your doctor has prescribed.

☐ Carry an identification card indicating that you are taking this medicine. Always tell your pharmacist, dentist, and other doctors who are treating you that you are taking this medicine.

* * * * *

Nitroglycerin (*Oral Sustained-Release Coronary Vasodilator*)
United States: Cardabid, Nitroglycerin Sustained Release, Nitrobon, Nitrospan, Ro-Nitro
Canada: Nitrong, Nitrostablin

☐ This medicine is used to help prevent angina (chest pain) attacks. It will not relieve an angina attack because it works too slowly.

HOW TO USE THIS MEDICINE

☐ It is best to take this medicine on an empty stomach 1 hour before (or 2 hours after) eating food. Take it with a full glass of water.

☐ This medicine must be swallowed whole. Do not crush, chew, or break it into pieces.

☐ Store in a cool, dry place but not in the refrigerator.

SPECIAL INSTRUCTIONS

☐ If you forget to take a dose, take it as soon as possible unless your next dose is within 6 hours. Instead, continue with your regular dosing schedule.

☐ Take the medicine regularly as your doctor prescribed. Do not stop taking it suddenly or it could cause an angina attack.

☐ If you become dizzy or feel faint, breathe deeply and bend forward with your head between your knees. Always get up slowly after you have been sitting or lying down. Get out of bed slowly in the morning and dangle your feet over the edge of the bed for a few minutes before standing up. Do not drive a car or operate dangerous machinery or do jobs that require you to be alert if you are dizzy.

☐ Do not drink alcoholic beverages while you are taking this medicine as they may make the dizziness and fainting worse.

☐ Some nonprescription drugs can aggravate your heart condition. Do not take any of the following without the approval of your doctor or pharmacist: cough, cold, or sinus products; asthma or allergy products; or diet or weight-reducing medicines.

☐ When you first start taking this medicine, you may get a headache or flushing. These are common side effects and will usually disappear after you have taken the drug a few times. If the headaches do not go away or are severe, check with your doctor.

☐ Cigarette smoking can aggravate angina and is a special risk for people who have angina.

☐ Most people experience few or no side effects from their drugs. However, any medicine can sometimes cause unwanted effects. Call your doctor if you develop a skin rash, blurred vision, dry mouth, nausea or vomiting, dizziness or fainting, or rapid pulse, or if your chest pain is not relieved.

☐ Carry an identification card indicating that you are taking this medicine. Always tell your pharmacist, dentist, and other doctors who are treating you that you are taking this medicine.

* * * * *

Nitroglycerin (*Topical Vasodilator*)
United States: Nitrol
Canada: Nitrol

☐ This medicine is used to help prevent angina (chest pain) attacks. It will not relieve an angina attack because it works too slowly.

581

HOW TO USE THIS MEDICINE

☐ Remove any old ointment before applying a new dose.

☐ This ointment must be carefully measured using the dose-measuring papers that come with it.

☐ Squeeze the prescribed amount of ointment onto the paper and use the paper, NOT THE FINGERS, to spread the ointment on the skin.

☐ Apply the thin layer of ointment to non-hairy skin such as the chest, stomach, front of the thighs, or forearm. Do not use the same spot all the time but rotate to different areas.

☐ DO NOT RUB OR MASSAGE the ointment into the skin. Just spread it in a thin, even layer approximately the size of the dose-measuring papers.

NITROL® OINTMENT
(NITROGLYCERIN OINTMENT 2%)
APPLI-RULER™

the applicator that
measures the dose

KREMERS-URBAN COMPANY
MILWAUKEE, WISCONSIN 53201

☐ If your doctor wants you to cover the ointment with transparent kitchen wrap, be sure you understand the correct method. Do not cover the area unless your doctor directs you to do so.

SPECIAL INSTRUCTIONS

☐ Use the ointment as your doctor has prescribed. Do not stop using it suddenly without your doctor's approval or it could cause an angina attack.

☐ If you become dizzy or feel faint, breathe deeply and bend forward with your head between your knees. Always get up slowly after you have been sitting or lying down. Get out of bed slowly in the morning and dangle your feet over the edge of the bed for a few minutes before standing up. Do not drive a car or operate dangerous machinery or do jobs that require you to be alert if you are dizzy.

☐ Do not drink alcoholic beverages while you are taking this medicine because they may make the dizziness and fainting worse.

☐ Some nonprescription drugs can aggravate your heart condition. Do not

582

take any of the following without the approval of your doctor or pharmacist: cough, cold, or sinus products; asthma or allergy products; or diet or weight-reducing medicines.

☐ When you first start using this medicine, you will probably get a headache or flushing. These are common side effects and will usually disappear after you have used the drug a few times. If the headaches do not go away or are severe, check with your doctor.

☐ Cigarette smoking can aggravate angina and is a special risk for people who have angina.

☐ Most people experience few or no side effects from their drugs. However, any medicine can sometimes cause unwanted effects. Call your doctor if you develop a skin rash, blurred vision, dry mouth, nausea and vomiting, dizziness, fainting, severe headache, or rapid pulse, or if your chest pain is not relieved.

☐ Carry an identification card indicating that you are taking this medicine. Always tell your pharmacist, dentist, and other doctors who are treating you that you are taking this medicine.

☐ Store the ointment in a cool place and keep tightly closed.

*   *   *   *   *

Nonoxynol-9 Compounds (*Vaginal Contraceptive*)
United States: Conceptrol Cream, Delfen, Ortho-Creme
Canada: Delfen, Emko Contraceptive Foam, Ortho-Creme

☐ This medicine is used as a birth control measure.

HOW TO USE THIS MEDICINE
☐ Insertion of the medicine should be made just before intercourse (sex). One applicator full is adequate only for one time. An additional applicator full is required each time intercourse is repeated.

☐ Always wait 6 to 8 hours after intercourse before douching; otherwise, the effectiveness of the medicine will be lost.

☐ Instructions for use: (**Canada:** Emko Contraceptive Foam)
  • Shake the container well.
  • Fill the applicator by placing it on the white button at the top of the container and push down slowly. The container must **not** be upside down or on its side while filling the applicator.
  • Place the applicator deep into the vaginal canal and expel the foam by pushing the plunger back into applicator.
  • Remove the applicator from the vaginal canal.
  • After each use, wash the applicator with warm water and soap and rinse thoroughly.

☐ Instructions for use: (**United States** and **Canada:** Delfen Cream)*
- Remove the cap from the tube of medicine, and attach the applicator by turning clockwise.

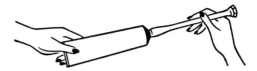

- Squeeze the tube of medicine from the bottom, forcing the cream into the cylinder until the plunger is pushed out as far as it will go and the cylinder is completely filled. Always roll the tube from the bottom, to reduce wastage. After each use replace the cap on the tube.

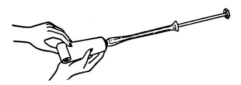

- Remove the filled applicator from the tube by turning counterclockwise.
- Hold the filled applicator by the cylinder and gently insert the cylinder well into the vaginal canal. (Insertion is easier when lying on the back with knees bent.)

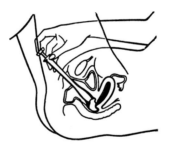

- Depress the plunger to deposit the cream into the vagina.
- With the plunger still depressed, remove the applicator, holding it by the cylinder.

☐ Instructions for use: (**United States** and **Canada:** Delfen Foam)
- Shake the container well before using.
- Place the container on a level surface and remove the cap.
- Place the applicator over the top of the vial and gently tilt the applicator to one side. The foam will rise slowly to fill the applicator.

*Delfen (Package Insert), Ortho Pharmaceuticals (Canada) Ltd., Don Mills, Ontario.

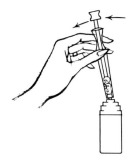

- To stop the flow of foam when the applicator is filled, return the applicator to the upright position.
- Remove the applicator from the vial.
- Hold the filled applicator by the cylinder and gently insert well into the vagina. (Insertion is easier when lying on the back with knees bent.)

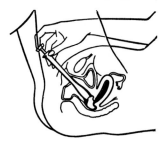

- Press the plunger in to deposit the foam in the vaginal canal.
- With the plunger still depressed, remove the applicator. (Note: When you hear a sputtering sound and the applicator fills very slowly with the foam, this means the container is nearly empty. Purchase a new supply.)
- After each use the applicator should be taken apart for cleaning. Hold the plunger with one hand and turn the cap counterclockwise with the other hand. When the cap is removed, the plunger will drop out of the cylinder. Wash all parts thoroughly with soap and warm water. Rinse well and reassemble the applicator.

SPECIAL INSTRUCTIONS

☐ Consult your doctor and discontinue use of this medicine if an irritation should develop.

☐ Avoid keeping the tube of cream in a cold place.

☐ Do not place the aerosol foam in hot water or near radiators, stoves, or other sources of heat. Do not puncture or incinerate the container (even when empty). Do not store at temperatures greater than 120°F (49°C). (**United States:** Delfen Foam; **Canada:** Delfen Aerosol, Emko Contraceptive Foam)

* * * * *

585

Norethandrolone (*Oral Anabolic Steroid*)
Canada: Nilevar

☐ This medicine is a hormone and is used to treat menstrual problems.

HOW TO USE THIS MEDICINE
☐ The tablets may be taken after meals or with a snack if they upset your stomach.

SPECIAL INSTRUCTIONS
☐ It is recommended that you do not smoke while you are taking this medicine because smoking may increase the incidence of heart attacks.

☐ Women who are pregnant, breast-feeding, or planning to become pregnant should tell their doctor before taking this medicine.

☐ Diabetic patients should regularly check the sugar in their urine while they are taking this medicine.

☐ Contact your doctor if any of the following side effects occur:
- Severe or persistent headaches
- Vomiting, dizziness, or fainting
- Blurred vision or slurred speech
- Pain in the calves of the legs or numbness in an arm or leg
- Chest pain, shortness of breath, or coughing of blood
- Lumps in the breast
- Severe depression
- A yellow color to the skin or eyes or dark-colored urine
- Severe abdominal pain
- Breakthrough vaginal bleeding

☐ Carry an identification card indicating that you are taking this medicine. Always tell your pharmacist, dentist, and other doctors who are treating you that you are taking this medicine.

*   *   *   *   *

Norethindrone (*Oral Progestogen*)
United States: Norlutate, Norlutin
Canada: Norlutate, Norlutin

☐ This medicine is a hormone and is used to treat menstrual problems.

HOW TO USE THIS MEDICINE
☐ The tablets may be taken after meals or with a snack if they upset your stomach.

SPECIAL INSTRUCTIONS
☐ It is recommended that you do not smoke while you are taking this medicine because smoking may increase the incidence of heart attacks.

- ☐ Women who are pregnant, breast-feeding, or planning to become pregnant should tell their doctor before taking this medicine.

- ☐ Diabetic patients should regularly check the sugar in their urine while they are taking this medicine.

- ☐ Contact your doctor if any of the following side effects occur:
  - Severe or persistent headaches
  - Vomiting, dizziness, or fainting
  - Blurred vision or slurred speech
  - Pain in the calves of the legs or numbness in an arm or leg
  - Chest pain, shortness of breath, or coughing of blood
  - Lumps in the breast
  - Severe depression
  - A yellow color to the skin or dark-colored urine
  - Severe abdominal pain
  - Breakthrough vaginal bleeding

- ☐ Carry an identification card indicating that you are taking this medicine. Always tell your pharmacist, dentist, and other doctors who are treating you that you are taking this medicine.

$$* \quad * \quad * \quad * \quad *$$

Nortriptyline HCl (*Oral Antidepressant*)
United States: Aventyl
Canada: Aventyl

- ☐ This medicine is used to help relieve the symptoms of depression. It is important that you take the medicine regularly and that you do not miss any doses. The full effect of the medicine will not be noticed immediately, but may take from a few days to several weeks. Early signs of improvement are increased appetite, better sleep, increased energy, and later improved mood. DO NOT STOP TAKING the medicine when you first feel better or you may feel worse in 3 or 4 days.

HOW TO USE THIS MEDICINE
- ☐ This medicine may be taken with food unless otherwise directed.

SPECIAL INSTRUCTIONS
- ☐ If you forget to take a dose, take it as soon as possible. However, if it is almost time for your next dose, do not take the missed dose. Instead, continue with your regular dosing schedule.

- ☐ Any medicine has a few unwanted side effects. Because this medicine takes a few weeks to work, the side effects are the only thing that tell the doctor that the drug is being absorbed. Most of these side effects will go away as your body adjusts to the medicine.

- ☐ Women who are pregnant, breast-feeding, or planning to become pregnant should tell their doctor before taking this medicine.

- [ ] In some people, this drug may cause dizziness or drowsiness. Do not drive a car or operate dangerous machinery or do jobs that require you to be alert until you know how you are going to react to this drug.

- [ ] If this medicine causes dizziness, you should be careful going up and down stairs and you should not change positions too quickly. Get out of bed slowly in the morning and dangle your feet over the edge of the bed for a few minutes before standing up. Sit or lie down at the first sign of dizziness. Tell your doctor you have been dizzy and he may adjust your dose.

- [ ] Do not drink alcoholic beverages while taking this drug without the approval of your doctor.

- [ ] It is important that you obtain the advice of your doctor or pharmacist before taking any other medicines, including pain relievers, sleeping pills, tranquilizers, other medicines for depression, cough/cold or allergy medicines, or weight-reducing medicine.

- [ ] If your mouth becomes dry, suck a hard sour candy (sugarless) or ice chips, or chew gum. It is especially important to brush your teeth regularly if you develop a dry mouth.

- [ ] If you become constipated, try increasing the amount of bulk in your diet (for example, bran and salads), exercising more often, or drinking water.

- [ ] Call your doctor if you develop a sore throat, fever, mouth sores, eye pain or blurred vision, difficulty in urinating ("passing your water"), fast heartbeats, or a skin rash.

- [ ] Do not stop taking this medicine suddenly without your doctor's approval. When your doctor tells you to stop this medicine, you must follow these precautions for 1 week since some of the medicine will still be in your body.

- [ ] Carry an identification card indicating that you are taking this medicine. Always tell your dentist, pharmacist, and other doctors who are treating you that you are taking this medicine.

* * * * *

Noscapine (*Oral Antitussive*)
United States: Tusscapine
Canada: Noscatuss

- [ ] This medicine is used to help relieve dry irritating coughs.

HOW TO USE THIS MEDICINE
- [ ] Shake the bottle well before using so that you can measure an accurate dose. (**Canada:** Noscatuss Suspension)

- [ ] Chew the tablets completely before swallowing: (**United States:** Tusscapine Chewable)

588

- [ ] Do not dilute the syrup. The soothing effect will be enhanced if you do not drink liquids immediately after taking the medicine.

SPECIAL INSTRUCTIONS

- [ ] In some people, this drug may cause dizziness or drowsiness. Do not drive a car or operate dangerous machinery or do jobs that require you to be alert until you know how you are going to react to this drug.

- [ ] If you become dizzy, you should be careful going up and down stairs. Sit or lie down at the first sign of dizziness.

- [ ] Call your doctor if the cough lasts longer than 1 week or if you develop a fever, skin rash, or persistent headache.

- [ ] Do not use this medicine for more than 1 week without the advice of your doctor.

*   *   *   *   *

Nylidrin HCl (*Oral Peripheral Vasodilator*)
United States: Arlidin, Circlidrin, Rolidrin
Canada: Arlidin, Pervadil

- [ ] This medicine increases the blood flow to the hands, legs, head, and feet and improves the circulation.

HOW TO USE THIS MEDICINE

- [ ] This medicine may be taken with food or on an empty stomach.

SPECIAL INSTRUCTIONS

- [ ] If you forget to take a dose, take it as soon as possible. However, if your next dose is within 2 hours, do not take the missed dose but continue with your regular schedule.

- [ ] Women who are pregnant, breast-feeding, or planning to become pregnant should tell their doctor before taking this medicine.

- [ ] If this medicine causes dizziness, you should be careful going up and down stairs and you should not change positions too rapidly. Get out of bed slowly in the morning and dangle your feet over the edge of the bed for a few minutes before standing up. Sit down or lie down at the first sign of dizziness. Tell your doctor you have been dizzy. Do not drive a car or operate dangerous machinery if you are dizzy. Avoid hot showers and baths because they could make you dizzy.

- [ ] Some nonprescription drugs can aggravate your condition. Do not take any of the following without the approval of your doctor or pharmacist: cough/cold or sinus products; asthma or allergy products; or diet or weight-reducing medicines.

- ☐ Do not drink alcoholic beverages while taking this drug without the approval of your doctor.

- ☐ The activity of this drug is improved if you keep warm. Avoid getting cold or exposing yourself to a cold environment.

- ☐ Most people experience few or no side effects from their drugs. However, any medicine can sometimes cause unwanted effects. Call your doctor if you develop a skin rash, fainting spells, flushing of the face, a rapid pulse, chest pain, or sharp stomach pain.

*   *   *   *   *

Nystatin (*Oral Antifungal-Antibiotic*)
United States: Mycostatin, Nilstat
Canada: Mycostatin, Nadostine, Nilstat

- ☐ This medicine is used to treat certain types of fungal infections.

HOW TO USE THIS MEDICINE
- ☐ If you are taking the liquid form of this medicine for an infection of the mouth, clear the mouth of any food particles. Place one half of the dose in each side of the mouth and then swish the liquid around the mouth for a few minutes. Brush your teeth or rinse your mouth after each meal and floss the teeth daily.

- ☐ This medicine may be dropped directly on the tongue from the dropper, or it may be mixed with milk, lukewarm formula, other nonacid liquids or foods, honey, jelly, or peanut butter. (*Canada:* Mycostatin Suspension, Nadostine Oral Suspension, Nilstat Drops)

- ☐ Shake well before using in order to get an accurate dose. (*United States:* Mycostatin and Nilstat Suspensions; *Canada:* Mycostatin, Nadostine, Nilstat Suspensions)

SPECIAL INSTRUCTIONS
- ☐ It is important to take *all* of this medicine plus any refills that your doctor told you to take. Do not stop taking it earlier than your doctor has recommended in spite of the fact that you may feel better. Otherwise, the infection may return.

- ☐ If you forget to take a dose, take it as soon as possible. However, if it is almost time for your next dose, do not take the missed dose. Instead, continue with your regular dosing schedule.

- ☐ Most people experience few or no side effects from their drugs. However, any medicine can sometimes cause unwanted effects. Call your doctor if you develop vomiting or severe diarrhea.

*   *   *   *   *

Nystatin (*Topical Antifungal-Antibiotic*)

United States: Candex, Mycostatin, Nilstat

Canada: Mycostatin, Nadostine, Viaderm-N

☐ This medicine is used to treat fungal infections of the skin.

HOW TO USE THIS MEDICINE

☐ • Each time you apply the medicine, wash your hands and gently cleanse the skin area well with water unless otherwise directed by your doctor. Do not allow the skin to dry completely. Pat with a clean towel until almost dry.
  • Apply a small amount of the drug to the affected area and spread lightly. Only the medicine that is actually touching the skin will work. A thick layer is not more effective than a thin layer. Do not bandage unless directed by your doctor.

☐ Do not use the drug more frequently or in larger quantities than prescribed by your doctor.

SPECIAL INSTRUCTIONS

☐ It is important to use *all* of this medicine, plus any refills that your doctor told you to use. Do not stop using it earlier than your doctor has recommended in spite of the fact that your symptoms seem to have improved. Otherwise, the infection may return.

☐ If you forget to apply the medicine, apply it as soon as possible. However, if it is almost time for your next dose, do not apply the missed dose but continue with your regular schedule.

☐ If you have a fungal infection of the feet, it is important to dry the feet (especially between the toes) well after washing.

☐ Do not apply cosmetics or lotions on top of the drug unless your doctor approves.

☐ Keep this preparation away from the eyes. If you should accidentally get some in your eyes, wash it away with water immediately.

☐ Call your doctor if the condition for which this drug is being used persists or becomes worse or if you develop a constant irritation such as itching or burning that was not present before you started using this medicine.

☐ For external use only. Do not swallow.

* * * * *

Nystatin (*Vaginal Antifungal-Antibiotic*)

United States: Korostatin, Mycostatin, Nilstat, O-V Statin

Canada: Mycostatin, Nadostine, Nilstat

☐ This medicine is used to treat fungal infections of the vagina.

591

HOW TO USE THIS MEDICINE

☐ For VAGINAL TABLETS

- This is not an oral medicine.
- Remove the wrapper from the tablet.
- Put the tablet into the applicator.
- Insert the applicator into the vaginal canal and depress the plunger.
- Clean the applicator after each use.

☐ For VAGINAL CREAM*

- Loading the applicator: Remove the cap from the tube and place the threaded tip (open end) of the applicator over the mouth of the tube. Twist the applicator gently until it is firmly attached to the tube. Holding tube and applicator upright, squeeze the tube from the bottom and fill the applicator until the plunger is fully extended. Remove the applicator from the tube.

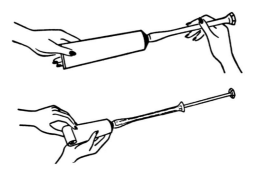

- Inserting the applicator: For proper insertion, you should be lying on your back, knees drawn up as illustrated. Pointing the applicator slightly downward, insert it deeply into the vagina as far as it will comfortably go without using force. Press the plunger all the way and empty the cream into the vagina. Withdraw the applicator from the vagina.

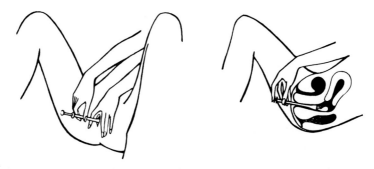

*Mycostatin Vaginal Cream (Package Insert), E. R. Squibb & Sons Ltd., Montreal, Quebec.

- Cleaning the applicator: Separate the plunger from the barrel by pulling it all the way out. Wash both sections thoroughly under a stream of water, allowing the water to flow through the barrel. Sterilization of the applicator is unnecessary and extremely hot water should not be used because it may soften the plastic applicator. Dry the applicator and store it in a clean place.
- Caution: During pregnancy, the applicator should be used only on the advice of a doctor.

SPECIAL INSTRUCTIONS

☐ The vaginal medicine should be used continuously even during the menstrual period.

☐ Continue using this medicine for the prescribed length of time in spite of the fact that the symptoms of your infection may have disappeared.

☐ If you forget to apply the medicine, apply it as soon as possible. However, if it is almost time for your next dose, do not apply the missed dose but continue with your regular dosing schedule.

☐ You may wish to wear a sanitary napkin to protect your clothing.

☐ Call your doctor if the condition for which this drug is being used persists or becomes worse or if you develop a constant irritation such as itching or burning that was not present before you started using this medicine.

☐ For external use only. Do not swallow.

* * * * *

Nystatin-Clioquinol (*Topical Antifungal Agent*)
United States: Nystaform
Canada: Nystaform

☐ This medicine is used to treat fungal infections of the skin.

HOW TO USE THIS MEDICINE

☐ Instructions for use:
- Cleanse the affected area well with water unless otherwise directed by your doctor.
- Apply the medicine and spread lightly.

SPECIAL INSTRUCTIONS

☐ Keep this medicine away from the eyes.

☐ This medicine may stain bed linen, clothing, and hair; therefore you should protect these from the medicine by wearing protective underclothing and using old bed linen.

593

□ Consult your doctor if the condition for which this medicine is being used persists or becomes worse, or if the medicine causes an irritation such as itching or burning.

□ Keep this medicine in a cool place, but do not freeze.

□ For external use only. Do not swallow.

*　*　*　*　*

Oatmeal Compound (*Topical Emollient Antipruritic*)
United States: Aveeno Preparations
Canada: Aveeno Preparations

□ These medicines are used to help relieve dry, itchy skin.

HOW TO USE THIS MEDICINE
□ Use in the same manner as regular soap. (**United States** and **Canada:** Aveeno Bar, Aveeno Oilated Bar)

□ This preparation should be used in the bath water, mixed with water or applied directly to the skin. (**United States** and **Canada:** Aveeno Colloidal Oatmeal, Aveeno Oilated)

SPECIAL INSTRUCTIONS
□ Consult your doctor if the condition for which this medicine is being used persists or becomes worse, or if the medicine causes an irritation such as itching or burning.

□ For external use only.

*　*　*　*　*

Orciprenaline Sulfate (*Oral Bronchodilator*)
United States: Alupent, Metaprel
Canada: Alupent

□ This medicine is used to help open the bronchioles (air passages in the lungs) to make breathing easier.

□ IMPORTANT: If you have ever had an allergic reaction to any cough/cold, allergy, heart, or weight-reducing medicines, tell your doctor or pharmacist before you take any of this medicine.

HOW TO USE THIS MEDICINE
□ This medicine may be taken with food or a glass of water.

SPECIAL INSTRUCTIONS

☐ Do not change the dose of your regular asthma or bronchitis medicines except on the advice of your doctor.

☐ Call your doctor if the medicine does not relieve your breathing problems, or if your sputum turns yellow or green in color.

☐ Most people experience few or no side effects from their drugs. However, any medicine can sometimes cause unwanted effects. Call your doctor if you develop chest pain, headaches, sweating, palpitations, or dizziness.

* * * * *

Orciprenaline Sulfate (*Inhalation Bronchodilator*)
United States: Alupent, Metaprel
Canada: Alupent

☐ This medicine is used to help open the bronchioles (air passages in the lungs) to make breathing easier.

☐ IMPORTANT: If you have ever had an allergic reaction to any cough/cold, allergy, heart or weight-reducing medicines, tell your doctor or pharmacist before you take any of this medicine.

HOW TO USE THIS MEDICINE

☐ Instructions for use:
- Remove the protective plastic cap from the mouthpiece.
- *Shake well.*
- Hold the apparatus so that the metal canister is upside down.
- Breathe out as completely as possible.
- Place the mouthpiece well into your mouth, closing your lips over it.

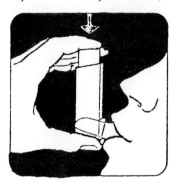

- Breathe in deeply through the mouth and at the same time firmly press the canister down into the mouth piece. This releases the medicine. (Repeat only as directed by your doctor.)

595

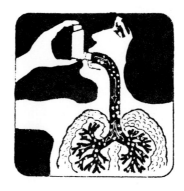

- Hold your breath for a few seconds, then remove the mouthpiece and breathe out slowly through your nose.

☐ Do not inhale the medicine more often than directed by your doctor. If difficulty in breathing persists or if relief is not obtained with your usual dosage, consult your doctor immediately. As a general rule, you should not exceed a total of 12 inhalations in 24 hours.

☐ If troubled with sputum, try to clear your chest as completely as possible before inhalation of the medicine. This will facilitate the passage of the drug more deeply into the lungs, which in turn will allow more thorough clearing of mucus during subsequent coughing.

☐ Care of mouthpiece:
  - The mouthpiece must be kept clean. Remove the metal vial and rinse the mouthpiece in warm running water. Dry and replace.

SPECIAL INSTRUCTIONS

☐ Do not change the dose of your regular asthma or bronchitis medicines except on the advice of your doctor.

☐ Store the container in a cool place. Do not place the container in hot water or near radiators, stoves, or other sources of heat. Do not puncture, burn, or incinerate the container (even when it is empty).

☐ Call your doctor if the medicine does not relieve your breathing problems, or if your sputum turns yellow or green in color.

☐ Most people experience few or no side effects from their drugs. However, any medicine can sometimes cause unwanted effects. Call your doctor if you develop chest pain, headaches, sweating, palpitations, or dizziness.

*   *   *   *   *

Orphenadrine HCl (*Oral Antiparkinsonian Agent*)
United States: Disipal
Canada: Disipal

596

Orphenadrine Citrate (*Oral Skeletal Muscle Relaxant*)
United States: Marflex, Norflex
Canada: Norflex

☐ This medicine is used to help improve muscle control and relieve muscle spasm.

HOW TO USE THIS MEDICINE
☐ This medicine may be taken with food or a glass of water.

SPECIAL INSTRUCTIONS
☐ If you forget to take a dose, take it as soon as possible. However, if it is almost time for your next dose, do not take the missed dose. Instead, continue with your regular dosing schedule.

☐ Do not drink alcoholic beverages while taking this drug without the approval of your doctor.

☐ It is important that you obtain the advice of your doctor or pharmacist before taking pain relievers, nonprescription drugs, sleeping pills, tranquilizers, or medicines for depression while you are taking this drug.

☐ In some people, this drug may cause dizziness or drowsiness. Do not drive a car or operate dangerous machinery or do jobs that require you to be alert until you know how you are going to react to this drug.

☐ If you become dizzy, you should be careful going up and down stairs. Sit or lie down at the first sign of dizziness. Tell your doctor you have been dizzy.

☐ If your mouth becomes dry, suck a hard sour candy (sugarless) or ice chips, or chew gum. It is especially important to brush your teeth regularly if you develop a dry mouth.

☐ If you become constipated, try increasing the amount of bulk in your diet (for example, bran and salads), exercising more often, or drinking more water. Call your doctor if the constipation continues.

☐ If you have difficulty urinating ("passing your water"), it may help if you urinate before taking this drug. Call your doctor if the problem continues.

☐ Most people experience few or no side effects from their drugs. However, any medicine can sometimes cause unwanted effects. Call your doctor if you develop a skin rash, unusual restlessness, flushing, eye pain, or fast heartbeats.

*   *   *   *   *

Orphenadrine Citrate-ASA-Caffeine (*Oral Skeletal Muscle Relaxant*)
Canada: Norgesic

Orphenadrine Citrate-ASA-Caffeine-Phenacetin (*Oral Skeletal Muscle Relaxant*)

United States: Norgesic, Norgesic Forte

☐ This medicine is used to help relieve pain and muscle spasm.

☐ IMPORTANT: If you have ever had an allergic reaction to aspirin or phenacetin medicine, tell your doctor or pharmacist before you take any of this medicine.

HOW TO USE THIS MEDICINE

☐ This medicine may be taken with food or a glass of water.

☐ Do not take this medicine if it smells like vinegar since this means that the aspirin in the medicine is not fresh.

SPECIAL INSTRUCTIONS

☐ If you forget to take a dose, take it as soon as possible. However, if it is almost time for your next dose, do not take the missed dose. Instead, continue with your regular dosing schedule.

☐ Women who are pregnant, breast-feeding, or planning to become pregnant should tell their doctor before taking this medicine.

☐ Do not drink alcoholic beverages while taking this drug without the approval of your doctor.

☐ It is important that you obtain the advice of your doctor or pharmacist before taking pain relievers, nonprescription drugs, sleeping pills, tranquilizers, or medicines for depression while you are taking this drug.

☐ In some people, this drug may cause dizziness or drowsiness. Do not drive a car or operate dangerous machinery or do jobs that require you to be alert until you know how you are going to react to this drug.

☐ If you become dizzy, you should be careful going up and down stairs. Sit or lie down at the first sign of dizziness. Tell your doctor if you have been dizzy.

☐ If your mouth becomes dry, suck a hard sour candy (sugarless) or ice chips, or chew gum. It is especially important to brush your teeth regularly if you develop a dry mouth.

☐ If you become constipated, try increasing the amount of bulk in your diet (for example, bran and salads), exercising more often, or drinking more water. Call your doctor if the constipation continues.

☐ If you have difficulty urinating ("passing your water"), it may help if you urinate before taking the drug. Call your doctor if the problem continues.

☐ Most people experience few or no side effects from their drugs. However, any medicine can sometimes cause unwanted effects. Call your doctor if you develop a skin rash, unusual restlessness, flushing, eye pain, or fast heartbeats. Also call your doctor if you develop "ringing" or "buzzing" in the ears, stomach pain, red or black stools, or swelling of the legs or ankles.

*   *   *   *   *

Oxacillin (*Oral Antibiotic*)
United States: Bactocill, Prostaphlin
Canada: Prostaphlin

☐ This medicine is an antibiotic used to treat certain types of infections.

☐ IMPORTANT: If you have ever had an allergic reaction to penicillin or any other antibiotics, tell your doctor or pharmacist before you take any of this medicine.

HOW TO USE THIS MEDICINE
☐ It is best to take this medicine on an empty stomach 1 hour before (or 2 hours after) meals or food unless otherwise directed by your doctor. Take it at the proper time even if you skip a meal.

☐ Take this medicine with a full glass of water.

☐ For LIQUID MEDICINE (**United States** and **Canada:** Prostaphlin Oral Solution)
- Store the liquid medicine in the refrigerator. Do not freeze.
- Do not take the medicine after the discard date on the bottle. Throw away any unused medicine after that date.

SPECIAL INSTRUCTIONS
☐ It is important to take **all** of this medicine plus any refills that your doctor told you to take. Do not stop taking this medicine earlier than your doctor has recommended in spite of the fact that you may feel better. Otherwise, the infection may return.

☐ If you forget to take a dose, take it as soon as you remember and then continue with your regular schedule.

☐ Most people experience few or no side effects from their drugs. However, any medicine can sometimes cause unwanted effects. Call your doctor if you develop a dark-colored tongue, yellow-green stools or, in women, a vaginal discharge that was not present before you started taking this medicine.

☐ This medicine sometimes causes diarrhea (loose bowel movements). Call your doctor if the diarrhea becomes severe or lasts for more than 2 days.

☐ Call your doctor immediately if you think you may be allergic to the medicine or if you develop a skin rash, hives, itching, swelling of the face, or difficulty in breathing. If you cannot reach your doctor, phone a hospital emergency department.

□ If for some reason you cannot take all of the medicine, throw away the unused portion by flushing it down the toilet. Do not take or save old medicine.

*   *   *   *   *

Oxandrolone (*Oral Anabolic Steroid*)
United States: Anavar

□ This medicine is similar to a hormone which is normally produced by the body. This medicine has many uses and the reason it was prescribed depends upon your condition. If you do not understand why you are taking it, check with your doctor.

HOW TO USE THIS MEDICINE
□ Take the drug after meals or with a snack if it upsets your stomach.

□ It is very important that you take this drug as your doctor has prescribed.

SPECIAL INSTRUCTIONS
□ Women who are pregnant, breast-feeding, or planning to become pregnant should tell their doctor before taking this medicine.

□ Diabetic patients should regularly check the sugar in the urine and report any abnormal results to their doctor.

□ Carry an identification card indicating that you are taking this medicine. Always tell your pharmacist, dentist, and other doctors who are treating you that you are taking this medicine.

□ Most people experience few or no side effects from their drugs. However, any medicine can sometimes cause unwanted effects. Call your doctor if you develop swelling of the hands, legs, or ankles; sore throat and fever; acne; unusual restlessness; dark-colored urine; or a yellow color to the skin or eyes. Women should call their doctor if they develop menstrual problems, hoarseness or a deepening of the voice, baldness, or increased facial hair.

*   *   *   *   *

Oxazepam (*Oral Antianxiety Agent*)
United States: Serax
Canada: Serax

□ This medicine is used to help relieve anxiety and tension. It is also used to help relax muscles as well as to treat some other conditions. Check with your doctor if you do not fully understand why you are taking it.

□ IMPORTANT: If you have ever had an allergic reaction to a benzodiazepine medicine, tell your doctor or pharmacist before you take any of this medicine.

600

HOW TO USE THIS MEDICINE

☐ This medicine may be taken with food or a full glass of water.

SPECIAL INSTRUCTIONS

☐ If you forget to take a dose, take it as soon as possible. However, if it is almost time for your next dose, do not take the missed dose. Instead, continue with your regular dosing schedule.

☐ Women who are pregnant, breast-feeding, or planning to become pregnant should tell their doctor before taking this medicine.

☐ In some people, this drug may cause dizziness or drowsiness. Do not drive a car or operate dangerous machinery or do jobs that require you to be alert until you know how you are going to react to this drug.

☐ If you become dizzy, you should be careful going up and down stairs. Sit or lie down at the first sign of dizziness.

☐ Do not drink alcoholic beverages while taking this drug without the approval of your doctor.

☐ It is important that you obtain the advice of your doctor or pharmacist before taking ANY other medicines including pain relievers, sleeping pills, tranquilizers or medicines for depression, cough/cold or allergy medicines, or weight-reducing medicines.

☐ Do not take any more of this medicine than your doctor has prescribed because the drug could become habit-forming. Do not stop taking this medicine suddenly without the approval of your doctor.

☐ Most people experience few or no side effects from their drugs. However, any medicine can sometimes cause unwanted effects. Call your doctor if you develop a sore throat, fever, mouth sores, a staggering walk, a yellow color to the skin or eyes, slow heartbeats, shortness of breath, unusual tiredness, nervousness, or stomach pain.

* * * * *

Oxolinic Acid (*Oral Antibiotic*)
United States: Utibid

☐ This medicine is used to treat infections of the urinary tract.

HOW TO USE THIS MEDICINE

☐ Take this medicine with food or a glass of water.

☐ If you forget to take a dose, take it as soon as you remember and then continue with your regular schedule.

SPECIAL INSTRUCTIONS

☐ Women who are pregnant, breast-feeding, or planning to become pregnant should tell their doctor before taking this medicine.

601

- [ ] In some people, this drug may cause dizziness or drowsiness. Do not drive a car or operate dangerous machinery or do jobs that require you to be alert until you know how you are going to react to this drug.

- [ ] Most people experience few or no side effects from their drugs. However, any medicine can sometimes cause unwanted effects. Call your doctor if you develop a skin rash, stomach pain, vomiting, unusual weakness, swelling of the hands or feet, fast heartbeats, or unusual nervousness.

* * * * *

Oxtriphylline (*Oral Bronchodilator*)
United States: Choledyl
Canada: Choledyl, Theophylline Choline

Oxtriphylline-Guaifenesin
Canada: Choledyl Expectorant

- [ ] This medicine is used to help open up the bronchioles (air passages in the lungs) to make breathing easier.

- [ ] IMPORTANT: If you have ever had an allergic reaction to caffeine or any medicine for lung conditions, tell your doctor or pharmacist before you take any of this medicine.

HOW TO USE THIS MEDICINE
- [ ] It is best to take this medicine on an empty stomach with a glass of water. However, if it upsets your stomach, it may be taken with a glass of milk or a snack. Call your doctor if the stomach upset continues.

- [ ] It is very important that you take this medicine exactly as your doctor has prescribed and that you do not miss any doses. Try to take this medicine at the same time every day. Do not take extra tablets without your doctor's approval.

SPECIAL INSTRUCTIONS
- [ ] Do not alter the dose of any other asthma or bronchitis medicines except on the advice of your doctor.

- [ ] Women who are breast-feeding should tell their doctor before taking this medicine.

- [ ] If you forget to take a dose, take it as soon as possible. However, if it is almost time for your next dose, do not take the missed dose. Instead, continue with your regular dosing schedule.

- [ ] In some people, this drug may cause dizziness or drowsiness. Do not drive a car or operate dangerous machinery or do jobs that require you to be alert until you know how you are going to react to this drug.

- [ ] If you become dizzy, you should be careful going up and down stairs. Sit or lie down at the first sign of dizziness.

- [ ] It is important that you obtain the advice of your doctor or pharmacist before taking ANY other medicines including pain relievers, sleeping pills, tranquilizers or medicines for depression, cough/cold or allergy medicines, or weight-reducing medicines.

- [ ] Do not smoke while you are on this medicine because smoking can make the drug less effective.

- [ ] Avoid drinking large amounts of coffee, tea, cocoa, or cola drinks because you could be more sensitive to the caffeine in these beverages.

- [ ] Most people experience few or no side effects from their drugs. However, any medicine can sometimes cause unwanted effects. Call your doctor if you develop a skin rash, vomiting, stomach pain or red or black stools, fast heartbeats, confusion, unusual tiredness, restlessness, or thirst, or increased urination ("passing your water").

* * * * *

Oxybutynin Chloride (*Oral Antispasmodic*)
United States: Ditropan

- [ ] This medicine is used to help relieve muscle spasm of the urinary tract and difficult urination.

HOW TO USE THIS MEDICINE
- [ ] It is best to take this medicine on an empty stomach with a glass of water. However, if it upsets your stomach, it may be taken with a glass of milk or a snack. Call your doctor if the stomach upset continues.

SPECIAL INSTRUCTIONS
- [ ] If you forget to take a dose, take it as soon as possible. However, if it is almost time for your next dose, do not take the missed dose. Instead, continue with your regular dosing schedule.

- [ ] In some people, this drug may cause dizziness, drowsiness, or blurred vision. Do not drive a car or operate dangerous machinery or do jobs that require you to be alert until you know how you are going to react to this drug.

- [ ] If you become dizzy, you should be careful going up and down stairs. Sit or lie down at the first sign of dizziness.

- [ ] It is important that you obtain the advice of your doctor or pharmacist before taking ANY other medicines including pain relievers, sleeping pills, tranquilizers or medicines for depression, cough/cold or allergy medicines, or weight-reducing medicines.

- [ ] If your mouth becomes dry, suck a hard sour candy (sugarless) or ice chips, or chew gum. It is especially important to brush your teeth regularly if you develop a dry mouth.

- [ ] You may become sensitive to heat while you are taking this medicine. Be careful not to get overheated during exercise or in hot weather in order to prevent fever and possible heat stroke.

- [ ] Most people experience few or no side effects from their drugs. However, any medicine can sometimes cause unwanted effects. Call your doctor if you develop eye pain or changes in vision, a skin rash, fast heartbeats or chest pain, sore throat, fever or confusion, diarrhea, or severe constipation.

*   *   *   *   *

Oxycodone-Acetaminophen (*Oral Analgesic*)
United States: Percocet-5

Oxycodone-Acetaminophen-Caffeine
Canada: Percocet, Percocet-Demi

- [ ] This medicine is used to help relieve pain.

- [ ] IMPORTANT: If you have a stomach ulcer or if you have ever had an allergic reaction to acetaminophen, phenacetin, caffeine, or a pain reliever, tell your doctor or pharmacist before you take any of this medicine.

HOW TO USE THIS MEDICINE
- [ ] This medicine may be taken with food or a glass of water.

- [ ] Do not take any more of this medicine than your doctor has prescribed. The drug could become habit-forming or you could take an overdose if you take it more often or longer than prescribed.

- [ ] Do not wait to take this medicine until the pain becomes severe. This medicine works best if you take it at the beginning of the pain. Call your doctor if you feel you need it more often than he prescribed.

SPECIAL INSTRUCTIONS
- [ ] Do not drink alcoholic beverages while taking this drug without the approval of your doctor.

- [ ] It is important that you obtain the advice of your doctor or pharmacist before taking ANY other medicines including other pain relievers, sleeping pills, tranquilizers or medicines for depression, cough/cold or allergy medicines, or weight-reducing medicines.

- [ ] In some people, this drug may cause dizziness or drowsiness. Do not drive a car or operate dangerous machinery or do jobs that require you to be alert until you know how you are going to react to this drug.

- [ ] If this medicine causes dizziness, you should be careful going up and down stairs and you should not change positions too rapidly. Get out of bed slowly

in the morning and dangle your feet over the edge of the bed for a few minutes before standing up. Sit down or lie down at the first sign of dizziness. Tell your doctor you have been dizzy. Avoid hot showers and baths because they could make you dizzy.

☐ If you do feel nauseated when you first start taking the medicine, it may help if you lie down for a few minutes.

☐ If you become constipated, try increasing the amount of bulk in your diet (for example, bran and salads), exercising more often, or drinking more water. Call your doctor if the constipation continues.

☐ Most people experience few or no side effects from their drugs. However, any medicine can sometimes cause unwanted effects. Call your doctor if you develop a skin rash, shortness of breath, slow heartbeats, a sore throat or fever, easy bruising or bleeding, a yellow color to the skin or eyes, difficulty urinating ("passing your water"), or stomach pain.

☐ Always tell your dentist, pharmacist, and other doctors who are treating you that you are taking this medicine.

*　*　*　*　*

Oxycodone-ASA-Caffeine (Oral Analgesic)
Canada: Percodan, Percodan-Demi

Oxycodone-ASA-Caffeine-Phenacetin
United States: Percodan, Percodan-Demi

☐ This medicine is used to help relieve pain.

☐ IMPORTANT: If you have ever had an allergic reaction to aspirin, caffeine or a pain reliever, or if you have a stomach ulcer, tell your doctor or pharmacist before you take any of this medicine.

HOW TO USE THIS MEDICINE
☐ This medicine may be taken with food or a glass of water.

☐ Do not take any more of this medicine than your doctor has prescribed. The drug could become habit-forming or you could take an overdose if you take it more often or longer than prescribed.

☐ Do not wait to take this medicine until the pain becomes severe. This medicine works best if you take it at the beginning of the pain. Call your doctor if you feel you need it more often than he prescribed.

☐ Do not take this medicine for longer than 10 days without consulting your doctor. (**United States:** Pecodan, Percodan-Demi)

☐ Do not take this medicine if it smells strongly like vinegar since this means that the aspirin in the medicine is not fresh.

SPECIAL INSTRUCTIONS

- ☐ Women who are pregnant, breast-feeding, or planning to become pregnant should tell their doctor before taking this medicine.

- ☐ Do not drink alcoholic beverages while taking this drug without the approval of your doctor.

- ☐ It is important that you obtain the advice of your doctor or pharmacist before taking ANY other medicines including other pain relievers, sleeping pills, tranquilizers or medicines for depression, cough/cold or allergy medicines, or weight-reducing medicines.

- ☐ In some people, this drug may cause dizziness or drowsiness. Do not drive a car or operate dangerous machinery or do jobs that require you to be alert until you know how you are going to react to this drug.

- ☐ If this medicine causes dizziness, you should be careful going up and down stairs and you should not change positions too rapidly. Get out of bed slowly in the morning and dangle your feet over the edge of the bed for a few minutes before standing up. Sit down or lie down at the first sign of dizziness. Tell your doctor you have been dizzy. Avoid hot showers and baths because they could make you dizzy.

- ☐ If you do feel nauseated when you first start taking the medicine, it may help if you lie down for a few minutes.

- ☐ If you become constipated, try increasing the amount of bulk in your diet (for example, bran and salads), exercising more often, or drinking more water. Call your doctor if the constipation continues.

- ☐ Call your doctor immediately if you think you may be allergic to the medicine or if you develop a skin rash, hives, itching, swelling of the face, or difficulty in breathing. If you cannot reach your doctor, phone a hospital emergency department.

- ☐ Most people experience few or no side effects from their drugs. However, any medicine can sometimes cause unwanted effects. Call your doctor if you develop "ringing" or "buzzing" in the ears, red or black stools, a slow heartbeat, stomach pain, difficulty in urinating ("passing your water"), unusual weakness, or swelling of the legs and ankles.

- ☐ Always tell your dentist, pharmacist, and other doctors who are treating you that you are taking this medicine.

*   *   *   *   *

Oxymetazoline HCl (*Nasal Decongestant*)

United States: Afrin, Duration, St. Joseph Decongestant for Children
Canada: Nafrine

- ☐ This medicine is used to help relieve nasal stuffiness.

HOW TO USE THIS MEDICINE

☐ For NASAL SPRAY
- Blow nose gently.
- Sit upright with your head slightly back.
- Place the atomizer at the entrance of the nostril and close the other nostril by pressing your finger on the side.
- Squeeze the atomizer the prescribed number of times.
- Repeat for the other nostril if necessary.

☐ For NOSE DROPS

INSTILLATION OF NOSE DROPS

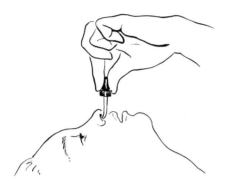

- Blow your nose gently before administration of drops.
- Sit in a chair and tilt your head backward, or lie down on a bed with your head extending over the edge of the bed, or lie down and place a pillow under your shoulders so that your head is tipped backward.
- Insert the dropper into the nostril about $\frac{1}{3}$ inch and drop the prescribed number of drops into the nose.
- Try not to touch the inside of the nose with the dropper as it will probably make you sneeze and will contaminate the dropper.
- Remain in the same position for at least 5 minutes.

SPECIAL INSTRUCTIONS

☐ Do not use this medicine more often or longer than recommended by your doctor. If used for too long, this medicine may actually cause a type of congestion.

☐ Rinse the dropper in hot water after each use.

☐ If you forget to use the medicine, use it as soon as possible. However, if it is almost time for your next dose, do not use the missed dose but continue with your regular schedule.

☐ Do not use this medicine at the same time as any other nasal medicine without the approval of your doctor. Some medicines cannot be mixed.

☐ Contact your doctor if the condition for which you are using this medicine does not improve. Also call your doctor if you develop fast heartbeats, head-ache, dizziness, trembling, blurred vision, or drowsiness.

☐ Check with your doctor if you develop a stinging sensation which does not go away as your body adjusts to the medicine.

☐ For external use only. Do not swallow.

* * * * *

Oxymetholone (*Oral Anabolic Steroid*)
United States: Androyd, Anadrol-50
Canada: Adroyd, Anapolon 50

☐ This medicine is similar to a hormone which is normally produced by the body. This medicine has many uses and the reason it was prescribed depends upon your condition. If you do not understand why you are taking it, check with your doctor.

HOW TO USE THIS MEDICINE
☐ Take this drug after meals or with a snack if it upsets your stomach.

☐ It is very important that you take this drug as your doctor has prescribed.

SPECIAL INSTRUCTIONS
☐ Women who are pregnant, breast-feeding, or planning to become pregnant should tell their doctor before taking this medicine.

☐ Diabetic patients should regularly check the sugar in the urine and report any abnormal results to their doctor.

☐ Carry an identification card indicating that you are taking this medicine. Always tell your pharmacist, dentist, and other doctors who are treating you that you are taking this medicine.

☐ Most people experience few or no side effects from their drugs. However, any medicine can sometimes cause unwanted effects. Call your doctor if you develop swelling of the hands, legs, or ankles; sore throat and fever; acne; unusual restlessness; dark-colored urine; or a yellow color to the skin or eyes. Women should call their doctor if they develop menstrual problems, hoarseness or a deepening of the voice, baldness, or increased facial hair.

* * * * *

Oxymorphone HCl (*Rectal Analgesic*)
United States: Numorphan
Canada: Numorphan

☐ This medicine is used to help relieve pain.

608

HOW TO USE THIS MEDICINE

☐ Administration of SUPPOSITORIES

- Remove the wrapper from the suppository.
- Lie on your side and raise your knee to your chest.
- Insert the suppository with the tapered (pointed) end first into the rectum.
- Remain lying down for a few minutes so that the suppository will dissolve in the rectum.
- Try to avoid having a bowel movement for at least one hour so that the drug will have time to work.

☐ Do not use any more of this medicine than your doctor has prescribed and do not stop using this medicine suddenly without the approval of your doctor.

☐ Do not wait to take this medicine until the pain becomes severe. This medicine works best if you take it at the beginning of the pain. Call your doctor if you feel you need it more often than he prescribed.

SPECIAL INSTRUCTIONS

☐ Do not drink alcoholic beverages while taking this drug without the approval of your doctor.

☐ It is important that you obtain the advice of your doctor or pharmacist before taking ANY other medicines including other pain relievers, sleeping pills, tranquilizers or medicines for depression, cough/cold or allergy medicines, or weight-reducing medicines.

☐ In some people, this drug may cause dizziness or drowsiness. Do not drive a car or operate dangerous machinery or do jobs that require you to be alert until you know how you are going to react to this drug.

☐ If you become dizzy, you should be careful going up and down stairs. Sit or lie down at the first sign of dizziness. Get up slowly if you have been lying or sitting down.

☐ If you do feel nauseated when you first start taking this medicine, it may help if you lie down for awhile.

☐ If you become constipated, try increasing the amount of bulk in your diet (for example, bran and salads), exercising more often, or drinking more water. Call your doctor if the constipation continues.

☐ Most people experience few or no side effects from their drugs. However, any medicine can sometimes cause unwanted effects. Call your doctor if you develop shortness of breath, slow heartbeats, unusual nervousness, stomach pain, or difficulty in urinating ("passing your water").

☐ Always tell your dentist, pharmacist, and other doctors who are treating you that you are taking this medicine.

* * * * *

Oxyphenbutazone (*Oral Antiarthritic-Anti-inflammatory*)
United States: Oxalid, Tandearil
Canada: Tandearil

Oxyphenbutazone-Antacid
Canada: Alka-Tandearil

☐ This medicine is used to help relieve pain, redness, stiffness, and swelling in certain kinds of arthritis and other medical conditions.

☐ IMPORTANT: If you have ever had an allergic reaction to aspirin or any other medicine for arthritis, tell your doctor or pharmacist before you take any of this medicine.

☐ Do not use this medicine more often or longer than recommended by your doctor. If you do not feel better after 1 week, call your doctor.

HOW TO USE THIS MEDICINE
☐ Always take this medicine with food or a glass of milk or immediately after meals to help prevent stomach upset.

SPECIAL INSTRUCTIONS
☐ Women who are pregnant, breast-feeding, or planning to become pregnant should tell their doctor before taking this medicine.

☐ In some people, this drug may cause drowsiness. Do not drive a car or operate dangerous machinery or do jobs that require you to be alert until you know how you are going to react to this drug.

☐ If you forget to take a dose, take it as soon as possible. However, if it is almost time for your next dose, do not take the missed dose. Instead, continue with your regular dosing schedule.

☐ Do not take antacids containing large amounts of sodium while you are taking this medicine. Check with your pharmacist.

☐ While you are taking this medicine, do not drink alcoholic beverages or take aspirin without the permission of your doctor. It is usually safe to take acetaminophen for the occasional headache. Check with your pharmacist.

☐ Call your doctor immediately if you think you may be allergic to the medicine or if you develop a skin rash, hives, itching, swelling of the face, or difficulty in breathing. If you cannot reach your doctor, phone a hospital emergency department.

☐ Most people experience few or no side effects from their drugs. However, any medicine can sometimes cause unwanted effects. Call your doctor if you develop a skin rash, sore throat, fever or mouth sores, swollen glands, any loss of hearing, blurred vision or changes in eyesight, easy bruising, red or black stools or pink urine, stomach pain, vomiting, swelling of the legs or

610

ankles or a sudden weight gain, a yellow color to the skin or eyes, difficulty in urinating ("passing your water"), or unusual tiredness.

☐ Carry an identification card indicating that you are taking this medicine. Always tell your pharmacist, dentist, and other doctors who are treating you that you are taking this medicine.

* * * * *

Oxyphencyclimine HCl (*Oral Anticholinergic*)
United States: Daricon

☐ This medicine is used to help relax muscles of the stomach and bowels and to decrease the amount of acid formed in the stomach.

☐ IMPORTANT: If you have ever had an allergic reaction to atropine or any other drug used to relax the stomach or bowels, tell your doctor or pharmacist before you take any of this medicine.

HOW TO USE THIS MEDICINE
☐ Take this medicine approximately 30 minutes before a meal unless otherwise directed.

☐ If you miss a dose of this medicine, do not take the missed dose and do not double the next dose.

SPECIAL INSTRUCTIONS
☐ If your mouth becomes dry, suck a hard sour candy (sugarless) or ice chips, or chew gum. It is especially important to brush your teeth regularly if you develop a dry mouth.

☐ In some people, this drug may cause dizziness or drowsiness. Do not drive a car or operate dangerous machinery or do jobs that require you to be alert until you know how you are going to react to this drug.

☐ If you become dizzy, you should be careful going up and down stairs. Sit or lie down at the first sign of dizziness. Tell your doctor you have been dizzy.

☐ A desire to urinate ("pass your water") with an inability to do so is not an uncommon effect with this drug. Urinating each time before taking the drug may help relieve this problem. Call your doctor if it continues.

☐ You may become more sensitive to heat because your body may perspire less while you are taking this drug. Be careful not to become overheated during exercise or in hot weather.

☐ Do not take antacids within 1 hour of taking this medicine because they could make this medicine less effective.

☐ If you become constipated, try increasing the amount of bulk in your diet (for example, bran and salads), exercising more often, or drinking more water. Call your doctor if the constipation continues.

- [ ] If your eyes become more sensitive to sunlight, it may help to wear sunglasses.

- [ ] Most people experience few or no side effects from their drugs. However, any medicine can sometimes cause unwanted effects. Call your doctor if you develop a skin rash, diarrhea, unusual restlessness, flushing, or eye pain.

*　*　*　*　*

Oxphenonium Bromide (*Oral Antispasmodic*)
United States: Antrenyl

- [ ] This medicine is used to help relax muscles of the stomach and bowels and to decrease the amount of acid formed in the stomach.

- [ ] IMPORTANT: If you have ever had an allergic reaction to atropine or bromides or any other drug used to relax the stomach or bowels, tell your doctor or pharmacist before you take any of this medicine.

HOW TO USE THIS MEDICINE
- [ ] Take this medicine approximately 30 minutes before a meal unless otherwise directed.

- [ ] If you miss a dose of this medicine, do not take the missed dose and do not double the next dose.

SPECIAL INSTRUCTIONS
- [ ] If your mouth becomes dry, suck a hard sour candy (sugarless) or ice chips, or chew gum. It is especially important to brush your teeth regularly if you develop a dry mouth.

- [ ] In some people, this drug may cause dizziness or drowsiness. Do not drive a car or operate dangerous machinery or do jobs that require you to be alert until you know how you are going to react to this drug.

- [ ] If you become dizzy, you should be careful going up and down stairs. Sit or lie down at the first sign of dizziness. Tell your doctor you have been dizzy.

- [ ] A desire to urinate ("pass your water") with an inability to do so is not an uncommon effect with this drug. Urinating each time before taking the drug may help relieve this problem. Call your doctor if it continues.

- [ ] You may become more sensitive to heat because your body may perspire less while you are taking this drug. Be careful not to become overheated during exercise or in hot weather.

- [ ] Do not take antacids within 1 hour of taking this medicine because they could make this medicine less effective.

- [ ] If you become constipated, try increasing the amount of bulk in your diet (for example, bran and salads), exercising more often, or drinking more water. Call your doctor if the constipation continues.

612

- ☐ If your eyes become more sensitive to sunlight, it may help to wear sunglasses.

- ☐ Most people experience few or no side effects from their drugs. However, any medicine can sometimes cause unwanted effects. Call your doctor if you develop a skin rash, diarrhea, unusual restlessness, flushing, or eye pain.

*   *   *   *   *

Oxytetracycline (Oral Antibiotic)
United States: Oxlopar, Oxy-Tetrachel, Terramycin, Tetramine
Canada: Terramycin

- ☐ This medicine is an antibiotic used to treat certain types of infections and to help control acne.

- ☐ IMPORTANT: If you have ever had an allergic reaction to tetracycline or any other antibiotic, tell your doctor or pharmacist before you take any of this medicine.

HOW TO USE THIS MEDICINE
- ☐ It is best to take this medicine on an empty stomach 1 hour before eating food or 2 hours after eating food. Take it at the proper time even if you skip a meal. If this medicine upsets your stomach, take it with some crackers (not with dairy products). Call your doctor if you continue to have stomach upset.

- ☐ Take this medicine with a full glass of water.

- ☐ Do not drink milk or eat cheese, cottage cheese, ice cream, or other dairy products 1 hour before or 2 hours after you have taken a dose of this medicine.

- ☐ For LIQUID MEDICINE
    - Shake the bottle well before using so that you can measure an accurate dose. (**United States** and **Canada:** Terramycin Syrup)

SPECIAL INSTRUCTIONS
- ☐ It is important that you take **all** of this medicine plus any refills that your doctor told you to take. Do not stop taking this medicine earlier than your doctor has recommended in spite of the fact that you may feel better. Otherwise, the infection may return.

- ☐ If you forget to take a dose, take it as soon as you remember and then continue with your regular schedule.

- ☐ Women who are pregnant, breast-feeding, or planning to become pregnant should tell their doctor before taking this medicine.

- ☐ Some antacids and some laxatives can make this medicine less effective if they are taken at the same time. If you must take them, they should be taken at least 2 to 3 hours after this medicine. If you have any questions, ask your pharmacist.

☐ If you must take iron products or vitamins containing iron, take them 2 hours before (or 3 hours after) this medicine.

☐ This medicine may make some people more sensitive to sunlight or sun-lamps. When you begin taking this medicine, try to avoid getting too much sun until you see how you are going to react. If your skin does become more sensitive, try to stay out of direct sunlight. While in the sun, wear protective clothing and sunglasses. You may wish to ask your pharmacist about suitable sunscreen products. You may remain sensitive to sunlight or sunlamps for several weeks after you have stopped taking the drug. Check with your doctor if you become sunburned.

☐ Most people experience few or no side effects from their drugs. However, any medicine can sometimes cause unwanted effects. Call your doctor if you develop a dark-colored tongue, sore mouth, yellow-green stools or, in women, a vaginal discharge that was not present before you started taking this medicine.

☐ Store the medicine in a cool, dark place and keep tightly closed.

☐ If for some reason you cannot take all of the medicine, discard the unused portion by flushing it down the toilet. Do not save this medicine for future use. Outdated oxytetracycline can be harmful.

* * * * *

Oxytetracycline-Polymyxin B *(Ophthalmic Antibiotic)*
United States: Terramycin with Polymyxin B
Canada: Terramycin

☐ This medicine is used to treat certain types of eye infections.

☐ IMPORTANT: If you have ever had an allergic reaction to neomycin, tetracy-cline, or any antibiotic medicines, tell your doctor or pharmacist before you use any of this drug.

HOW TO USE THIS MEDICINE
☐ For EYE OINTMENT

INSTILLATION OF EYE OINTMENT

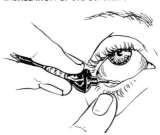

- The person administering the eye ointment should wash his hands with soap and water.
- The eye ointment must be kept clean. Do not touch the tube against the face or anything else.
- Lie down or tilt your head backward and look at the ceiling.
- Gently pull down the lower lid of your eye to form a pouch.
- Hold the tube in your other hand and place the tube as close as possible to the eye without touching it.
- Squeeze the prescribed amount of ointment (usually one-half inch in adults) from the tube along the pouch.
- Close your eyes. Do not rub them.
- Wipe off any excess ointment around the eye with a tissue.
- Clean the tip of the ointment tube with a tissue.

☐ If necessary, have someone else administer the eye ointment for you.

☐ Keep the eye ointment tube tightly closed when not in use.

☐ Do not use the drug more frequently or in larger quantities than prescribed by your doctor.

SPECIAL INSTRUCTIONS

☐ Vision may be blurred for a few minutes after using the eye medicine. Do not drive a car or operate dangerous machinery or do jobs that require you to be alert until your vision is cleared.

☐ Eye medicines should be used as prescribed by your doctor. Often eye infections clear rapidly after a few days of use of the medicine, but not always completely. It is important to use *all* of this medicine, plus any refills that your doctor told you to use. Do not stop using it earlier than your doctor has recommended in spite of the fact that your symptoms seem to have improved. Otherwise, the infection may return.

☐ If you forget to use the medicine, use it as soon as possible. However, if it is almost time for your next dose, do not use the missed dose, but continue with your regular schedule.

☐ Do not use this medicine at the same time as any other eye medicine without the approval of your doctor. Some medicines cannot be mixed.

☐ Contact your doctor if the condition for which you are using this medicine does not improve or if the eye becomes irritated by it for more than a few minutes. Many eye medicines sting for a short time immediately after use.

☐ Store the ointment in a cool place.

☐ For external use only. Do not swallow.

*   *   *   *   *

Pancreatin (*Oral Digestant*)
United States: Elzyme 303, Pancreatin, Panteric, Viokase
Canada: Panteric, Viokase

☐ This medicine is used in certain conditions to aid digestion.

HOW TO USE THIS MEDICINE
☐ Take this medicine with meals unless otherwise directed.

☐ Take the tablets 1 hour after meals. (**Canada:** Panteric Tablets)

☐ This medicine has a special coating and must be swallowed whole. Do not crush, chew, or break it into pieces. (**United States:** Elzyme 303, Pancreatin Triple Strength Enseals, Panteric Triple Strength Filmseals; **Canada:** Panteric Tablets)

SPECIAL INSTRUCTIONS
☐ If you miss a dose of this medicine, do not take the missed dose and do not double your next dose.

☐ It is important that you follow the diet your doctor has prescribed.

☐ Call your doctor immediately if you think you may be allergic to the medicine or if you develop a skin rash, hives, itching, swelling of the face, or difficulty in breathing. If you cannot reach your doctor, phone a hospital emergency department.

☐ Most people experience few or no side effects from their drugs. However, any medicine can sometimes cause unwanted effects. Call your doctor if you develop nausea or diarrhea.

* * * * *

Pancrelipase (*Oral Enzyme-Digestant*)
United States: Cotazyme, Ilozyme
Canada: Accelerase, Cotazym

☐ This medicine is used in certain conditions to aid digestion.

HOW TO USE THIS MEDICINE
☐ Take this medicine before eating or with food unless otherwise prescribed.

SPECIAL INSTRUCTIONS
☐ If you miss a dose of this medicine, do not take the missed dose and do double your next dose.

☐ It is important that you follow the diet that your doctor has prescribed.

☐ Call your doctor immediately if you think you may be allergic to the medicine or if you develop a skin rash, hives, itching, swelling of the face, or difficulty in breathing. If you cannot reach your doctor, phone a hospital emergency department.

☐ Most people experience few or no side effects from their drugs. However, any medicine can sometimes cause unwanted effects. Call your doctor if you develop nausea or diarrhea.

*   *   *   *   *

Para-Aminosalicylic Acid (*Oral Tuberculosis Therapy*)
Canada: Nemasol

Para-Aminosalicylate Sodium
United States: Pamisyl Sodium, Parasal Sodium, Pasdium, Teebacin

Para-Aminosalicylic Acid-Isoniazid
United States: Di-Isopacin, Double Isopacin
Canada: Inapasade-SQ

☐ This medicine is use to prevent or help the body overcome tuberculosis. Because tuberculosis (TB) heals very slowly, it may be necessary for you to take this medicine for a long time.

☐ It is very important that you keep taking this medicine for the full length of time that your doctor has prescribed. Do not stop taking this medicine earlier than your doctor has recommended in spite of the fact that you may feel better. DO NOT MISS ANY DOSES and DO NOT RUN OUT OF THIS MEDICINE.

☐ The most important thing you can do to protect others from catching your TB is to take your medicine regularly and to cover your coughs and sneezes with a double-ply tissue. This will reduce the spray of germs into the air. Covering your mouth with the bare hand does no good.

HOW TO USE THIS MEDICINE
☐ This medicine may be taken with food if it upsets your stomach. Call your doctor if you continue to have stomach upset.

☐ Swallow the contents of the packet with a beverage after eating some food. Do not dissolve the granules in water or chew them. (**Canada:** Inapasade-SQ)

SPECIAL INSTRUCTIONS
☐ If you forget to take a dose, take it as soon as you can remember and then continue with your regular schedule. However, if it is almost time for your next dose, do not take the dose you forgot.

☐ Women who are pregnant, breast-feeding, or planning to become pregnant should tell their doctor before taking this medicine.

617

- Call your doctor immediately if you think you may be allergic to the medicine or if you develop a skin rash, hives, itching, swelling of the face, or difficulty in breathing. If you cannot reach your doctor, phone a hospital emergency department.

- Most people experience few or no side effects from their drugs. However, any medicine can sometimes cause unwanted effects. Call your doctor if you develop a sore throat, fever, mouth sores, tingling or numbness in the hands and feet, dark-colored urine or a yellow color in the skin or eyes, or unusual tiredness or weakness.

- Store the medicine in a cool, dark, dry place. Do not take the powder if it turns brown or purple in color.

*   *   *   *   *

Paramethadione (*Oral Anticonvulsant*)
United States: Paradione
Canada: Paradione

- This medicine is used to help control convulsions and seizures. It is commonly used in the treatment of epilepsy.

- IMPORTANT: If you have ever had an allergic reaction to an anticonvulsant or seizure medicine, tell your doctor or pharmacist before you take any of this medicine.

HOW TO USE THIS MEDICINE

- Take this medicine with food if it upsets your stomach. Call your doctor if you continue to have stomach upset.

- If a dropper or a dispensing spoon is used to measure the dose and you do not fully understand how to use it, check with your pharmacist. (**United States:** Paradione Solution)

- It is very important that you take this medicine regularly and that you do not miss any doses. Try to take the medicine at the same time(s) every day. This is the only way that you can receive the full benefit of the medicine. If you forget to take this medicine, the amount of medicine in your blood will go down and you may have seizures.

SPECIAL INSTRUCTIONS

- If you forget to take a dose, take it as soon as possible. However, if it is almost time for your next dose, do not take the missed dose. Instead, continue with your regular dosing schedule. Do not double doses.

- Do not stop taking this medicine suddenly or change the amount you are taking without the approval of your doctor.

- Avoid swimming alone or taking part in high-risk sports in which a sudden seizure could cause injury.

618

- [ ] In some people, this drug may cause dizziness or drowsiness. Do not drive a car or operate dangerous machinery or do jobs that require you to be alert until you know how you are going to react to this drug. If you become dizzy, you should be careful going up and down stairs. Sit or lie down at the first sign of dizziness.

- [ ] If this medicine is for a child, do not let him (her) ride a bike or climb trees until you can determine how he (she) is going to react to the medicine. Children could hurt themselves if they participated in these activities when they were dizzy.

- [ ] Do not drink alcoholic beverages while taking this drug without the approval of your doctor.

- [ ] It is important that you obtain the advice of your doctor or pharmacist before taking pain relievers, nonprescription drugs, sleeping pills, tranquilizers, or medicines for depression while you are taking this drug.

- [ ] This medicine may cause your eyes to become more sensitive to sunlight and changes in brightness of light. Wearing sunglasses during the day may help. Be careful driving a car at night if you find the bright lights of cars irritating to your eyes.

- [ ] Women who are pregnant, breast-feeding, or planning to become pregnant should tell their doctor before taking this medicine.

- [ ] Most people experience few or no side effects from their drugs. However, any medicine can sometimes cause unwanted effects. Call your doctor if you develop a sore throat, fever or mouth sores, skin rash, swelling of the hands, legs or face, joint pain, easy bruising or bleeding, yellow color to the skin or eyes, dark-colored urine, or swollen glands.

- [ ] Do not go without this medicine between prescription refills. Call your pharmacist 2 or 3 days before you will run out of the medicine.

- [ ] Carry an identification card indicating that you are taking this medicine. Always tell your pharmacist, dentist, and other doctors who are treating you that you are taking this medicine.

*   *   *   *   *

Parathamethasone Acetate (Oral Corticosteroid)
United States: Haldrone

- [ ] This medicine is similar to cortisone, which is a hormone normally produced by the body. This medicine is used to help decrease inflammation which then relieves pain, redness, and swelling. It is used in the treatment of certain kinds of arthritis as well as severe allergies or skin conditions.

HOW TO USE THIS MEDICINE
- [ ] Take this medicine with food or a glass of milk in order to help prevent stomach upset. Call your doctor if you develop stomach upset or stomach

pain or heartburn (especially if it awakens you during the night). Do not try to treat this yourself.

- [ ] If your doctor has prescribed only ONE dose of this medicine every day, it is best to take it before 9 A.M. or with breakfast.

- [ ] If you forget to take a dose, take it as soon as possible. However, if it is almost time for your next dose, do not take the missed dose. Instead, continue with your regular dosing schedule.

SPECIAL INSTRUCTIONS

- [ ] Women who are pregnant, breast-feeding, or planning to become pregnant should tell their doctor before taking this medicine.

- [ ] It is best not to drink alcoholic beverages while you are taking this medicine because the combination can cause stomach problems.

- [ ] Do not take any more of this medicine than your doctor has prescribed and do not stop taking this medicine suddenly without the approval of your doctor. It may be necessary for your doctor to slowly reduce your dose since your body becomes used to this medicine and it might be harmful if you suddenly did not receive this medicine.

- [ ] Do not take aspirin or medicines containing aspirin without the approval of your doctor.

- [ ] While you are taking this medicine you may gain some weight. This could be due to an increase in your appetite or increased water in your system. Your doctor may prescribe a special diet to decrease the number of calories you eat and/or to lower the amount of sodium or increase the amount of potassium in your diet. Follow any diet that your doctor may order.

- [ ] You may find that you bruise more easily. Try to protect yourself from all injuries to prevent bruising.

- [ ] Diabetic patients should regularly check the sugar in their urine and report any unusual levels to their doctor.

- [ ] Carry an identification card indicating that you are taking this medicine. Always tell your pharmacist, dentist, and other doctors who are treating you that you are taking this medicine. If you have an acute infection, injury, operation, or dental surgery within 1 year of taking this medicine, it is important to tell your doctor.

- [ ] Most people experience few or no side effects from their drugs. However, any medicine can sometimes cause unwanted effects. Call your doctor if you develop stomach pain, sore throat, fever, swelling of the legs or ankles, a wound which does not heal, eye pain or blurred vision, frequent urination ("passing your water"), nightmares or depression, muscle cramps, red or black stools, puffing of the face, or menstrual problems.

* * * * *

Pargyline HCl (*Oral Antihypertensive*)
United States: Eutonyl

☐ Hypertension (high blood pressure) is a long-term condition, and it will probably be necessary for you to take the drug for a long time in spite of the fact that you feel better. It is very important that you take this medicine as your doctor has directed and that you do not miss any doses. Otherwise, you cannot expect the drug to keep your blood pressure down.

HOW TO USE THIS MEDICINE

☐ It is best to take this medicine with a glass of water.

☐ While taking this medicine and for at least 2 weeks after your treatment ends, you must be very careful about your diet. You must not eat any of the following foods or beverages because you could experience a very unpleasant reaction (severe headache, nausea, vomiting, and chest pains):

- Aged and natural cheeses (for example, cheddar, blue, Camembert, Stilton, Gruyère, Brie, Swiss, and Emmenthaler). In general, avoid food in which aging is used to increase the flavor. Cream cheese, processed cheese, and cottage cheese are safe to eat.
- Sour cream or yogurt.
- Wines, especially Chianti and other heavy red wines.
- Alcoholic beverages, including sherry and beer.
- Canned figs or raisins.
- Yeast extracts (such as Marmite or Bovril) or meat extracts.
- Chicken livers.
- Broad beans (also called fava beans).
- Fermented sausage (such as fermented bolognas and salamis, pepperoni, and summer sausage).
- Pickled or kippered herring.
- Meats prepared with tenderizers.
- Avocados, bananas.
- Soya sauce.
- Chocolate.
- Excessive amounts of caffeine (for example, coffee, tea, cola beverages).

SPECIAL INSTRUCTIONS

☐ If you forget to take a dose, take it as soon as possible. However, if your next dose is within 2 hours, do not take the missed dose but continue with your regular schedule.

☐ Any medicine has a few unwanted side effects. Because this medicine takes a few weeks to work, the side effects are the only thing that tell the doctor that the drug is being absorbed. Most of these side effects will go away as your body adjusts to the medicine.

☐ In some people, this drug may cause dizziness or drowsiness. Do not drive a car or operate dangerous machinery or do jobs that require you to be alert until you know how you are going to react to this drug.

☐ If this medicine causes dizziness, you should be careful going up and down stairs and you should not change positions too quickly. Get out of bed slowly in the morning and dangle your feet over the edge of the bed for a few minutes before standing up. Sit or lie down at the first sign of dizziness. Tell your doctor you have been dizzy.

☐ It is important that you obtain the advice of your doctor or pharmacist before taking any other medicines, including pain relievers, sleeping pills, tranquilizers, other medicines for depression, cough/cold or allergy medicines, or weight-reducing medicine.

☐ If your mouth becomes dry, suck a hard sour candy (sugarless) or ice chips, or chew gum. It is especially important to brush your teeth regularly if you develop a dry mouth.

☐ This medicine may make some people more sensitive to sunlight and sunlamps. When you begin taking this medicine, try to avoid getting too much sun until you see how you are going to react. If your skin does become more sensitive to sunlight, tell your doctor and try to stay out of direct sunlight. While in the sun, wear protective clothing and sunglasses. You may wish to ask your pharmacist about suitable sunscreen products. Check with your doctor if you become sunburned.

☐ If you become constipated, try increasing the amount of bulk in your diet (for example, bran, salads), exercising more often, or drinking more water.

☐ Call your doctor immediately if you develop frequent or severe headaches, chest pains, rapid heartrate, nausea, or vomiting. If you cannot reach your doctor call a hospital emergency department.

☐ Most people experience few or no side effects from their drugs. However, any medicine can sometimes cause unwanted effects. Call your doctor if you develop a skin rash, fever, fainting, difficulty in urinating ("passing your water"), swelling of the legs and ankles, eye pain, or changes in your ability to see red and green colors.

☐ Do not stop taking this medicine suddenly without your doctor's approval. Have your prescriptions refilled before you are completely out of this medicine so that you will not miss any doses. When your doctor tells you to stop this medicine, you must follow the precautions about diet and other medicines for 2 weeks since some of the medicine will still be in your body.

☐ Carry an identification card indicating that you are taking this medicine. Always tell your pharmacist, dentist, and other doctors who are treating you that you are taking this medicine.

* * * * *

Pemoline (*Oral Cerebral Stimulant*)
United States: Cylert

☐ This medicine is used in the treatment of behavioral problems in children.

622

HOW TO USE THIS MEDICINE

☐ This medicine should be taken in the morning.

☐ These tablets should be chewed well before swallowing. (**United States:** Cylert Chewable)

SPECIAL INSTRUCTIONS

☐ If the child forgets to take a dose, he should take it as soon as possible. However, if it is almost time for the next dose, he should not take the missed dose. Instead, the regular dosing schedule should be continued.

☐ The child should not take any more of this medicine than your doctor has prescribed and he should not stop taking this medicine suddenly without the approval of your doctor.

☐ It is recommended that you do not let the child ride a bike or climb trees until you can determine how he is going to react to the medicine. Children could hurt themselves if they participated in these activities when they were dizzy.

☐ Most people experience few or no side effects from their drugs. However, any medicine can sometimes cause unwanted effects. Call your doctor if your child develops a skin rash; unusual movements of the head, arms, or legs; fast heartbeats; unusual nervousness; fast eye movements; weight loss; or a yellow color to the skin or eyes.

☐ The child should carry an identification card indicating that he is taking this medicine. Always tell your pharmacist, dentist, and other doctors who are treating your child that he is taking this medicine.

* * * * *

Penicillamine (Oral Chelating Agent)
United States: Cuprimine
Canada: Cuprimine

☐ This medicine has many uses and the reason it was prescribed depends upon your condition. If you do not fully understand why you are taking it, check with your doctor.

☐ IMPORTANT: If you have ever had an allergic reaction to a penicillin medicine, tell your doctor or pharmacist before you take any of this medicine.

HOW TO USE THIS MEDICINE

☐ Take this medicine on an empty stomach 1 hour before or 2 hours after meals.

☐ If you forget to take a dose, take it as soon as possible. However, if it is almost time for your next dose, do not take the missed dose. Instead, continue with your regular dosing schedule.

SPECIAL INSTRUCTIONS

☐ Women who are pregnant, breast-feeding, or planning to become pregnant should tell their doctor before taking this medicine.

☐ If you are taking this medicine to prevent kidney stones, you should drink 2 glasses of water at bedtime and another 2 glasses of water during the night.

☐ Depending on your condition, your doctor may prescribe a special diet. If you must limit the amount of copper in your diet, do not eat the following foods: chocolate, nuts, shellfish, mushrooms, enriched cereals, molasses, liver, or broccoli.

☐ Do not take any more of this medicine than your doctor has prescribed and do not stop taking this medicine suddenly without the approval of your doctor.

☐ Do not take iron or vitamins containing iron within 2 hours of taking this medicine. Do not take iron or mineral supplements without the advice of your doctor.

☐ Most people experience few or no side effects from their drugs. However, any medicine can sometimes cause unwanted effects. Call your doctor if you develop a skin rash, blisters, fever, loss of taste, sore throat or mouth sores, joint pain, unusual bruising or bleeding, blood in the urine, or swollen glands. Also call your doctor if you develop a yellow color to the skin or eyes, dark-colored urine, weakness, eye pain, changes in vision, or difficulty in breathing.

* * * * *

Penicillin G Ammonium (*Oral Antibiotic*)
Canada: P.G.A.

Penicillin G Potassium
United States: Genecillin-400, G-Recillin, G-Recillin-T, K-Cillin, K-Pen, Palocillin, Pentids, Pfizerpen G, SK-Penicillin G, Sugracillin
Canada: Falapen, Megacillin, Novopen, P-50

Penicillin G Benzathine
United States: Bicillin
Canada: Megacillin Suspension

☐ This medicine is an antibiotic used to treat certain types of infections.

☐ IMPORTANT: If you have ever had an allergic reaction to penicillin or any other antibiotic, tell your doctor or pharmacist before you take any of this medicine.

624

HOW TO USE THIS MEDICINE

☐ It is best to take this medicine on an empty stomach 1 hour before (or 2 hours after) meals or food unless otherwise directed. Take it at the proper time even if you skip a meal.

☐ Take the tablets or capsules with a full glass of water. Do not take it with acidic fruit juices such as grapefruit or orange juice.

☐ For LIQUID MEDICINE
   • If you were prescribed a suspension, shake the bottle well before using so that you can measure an accurate dose. (**Canada:** Megacillin, Novopen Suspensions)
   • If a dropper is used to measure the dose and you do not fully understand how to use it, check with your pharmacist.
   • Store the bottle of medicine in a refrigerator unless otherwise directed. Do not freeze.
   • If there is a discard date on the bottle, throw away any unused medicine after that date.

☐ This tablet has a special coating and must be swallowed whole. Do not crush, chew, or break it into pieces. It is recommended that milk or antacids not be taken at the same time as this medicine. (**Canada:** Falapen)

SPECIAL INSTRUCTIONS

☐ It is important to take **all** of this medicine plus any refills that your doctor told you to take. Do not stop taking this medicine earlier than your doctor has recommended in spite of the fact that you may feel better. Otherwise, the infection may return.

☐ If you forget to take a dose, take it as soon as you remember and then continue with your regular schedule.

☐ Women who are breast-feeding should tell their doctor before taking this medicine.

☐ Most people experience few or no side effects from their drugs. However, any medicine can sometimes cause unwanted effects. Contact your doctor if you develop a dark-colored tongue, yellow-green stools or, in women, a vaginal discharge that was not present before you started taking the medicine.

☐ Call your doctor immediately if you think you may be allergic to the medicine or if you develop a skin rash, hives, itching, swelling of the face, or difficulty in breathing. If you cannot reach your doctor, phone a hospital emergency department.

☐ If for some reason you cannot take all of the medicine, throw away the unused portion by flushing it down the toilet. Do not take or save old medicine.

* * * * *

625

Penicillin V (Phenoxymethyl Penicillin) (*Oral Antibiotic*)

United States: V-Cillin Drops
Canada: Pen-Vee, 'PVF'

Penicillin V Potassium (Phenoxymethyl Penicillin Potassium)

United States: Betapen VK, Compocillin-VK, Deltapen-VK, Leder-cillin VK, Penapar VK, Pen-Vee K, Pfizerpen VK, Redpen-VK, Robicillin VK, SK-Penicillin VK, Uticillin VK, V-Cillin K, Veetids
Canada: Ledercillin-VK, Nadopen-V, Novopen-V, Penbec-V, Pen-Vee K, 'PVF' K, VC-K 500, V-Cillin K

☐ This medicine is an antibiotic used to treat certain types of infections.

☐ IMPORTANT: If you have ever had an allergic reaction to penicillin or any other antibiotic, tell your doctor or pharmacist before you take any of this medicine.

HOW TO USE THIS MEDICINE

☐ It is best to take this medicine on an empty stomach 1 hour before (or 2 hours after) meals or food unless otherwise directed by your doctor. Take it at the proper time even if you skip a meal.

☐ Take the tablets or capsules with a full glass of water.

☐ For LIQUID MEDICINE
  • If you were prescribed a SUSPENSION, shake the bottle well before using so that you can measure an accurate dose. (**United States:** V-Cillin Drops, V-Cillin K Oral; **Canada:** Novopen-V-500, Pen-Vee, 'PVF' Suspensions)
  • If a dropper is used to measure the dose and you do not fully understand how to use it, check with your pharmacist (**United States:** V-Cillin Drops)
  • Store the bottle of medicine in a refrigerator unless otherwise directed. Do not freeze. (**United States:** V-Cillin K Solution; **Canada:** V-Cillin K, VC-K-500 Solutions)
  • If there is a discard date on the bottle, throw away any unused medicine after that date.

SPECIAL INSTRUCTIONS

☐ It is important to take *all* of this medicine plus any refills that your doctor told you to take. Do not stop taking this medicine earlier than your doctor has recommended in spite of the fact that you may feel better. Otherwise, the infection may return.

☐ If you forget to take a dose, take it as soon as you remember and then continue with your regular schedule.

- ☐ Women who are breast-feeding should tell their doctor before taking this medicine.

- ☐ Most people experience few or no side effects from their drugs. However, any medicine may sometimes cause unwanted effects. Call your doctor if you develop a dark-colored tongue, yellow-green stools or, in women, a vaginal discharge that was not present before you started taking the medicine.

- ☐ Call your doctor immediately if you think you may be allergic to the medicine or if you develop a skin rash, hives, itching, swelling of the face, or difficulty in breathing. If you cannot reach your doctor, phone a hospital emergency department.

- ☐ If for some reason you cannot take all of the medicine, throw away the unused portion by flushing it down the toilet. Do not take or save old medicine.

* * * * *

Pentaerythritol Tetranitrate (*Oral Coronary Vasodilator*)
United States: Angitrate, Antora, Duotrate Plateau Cap, Neo-Corovas, Pentritol Pentryate, Peritrate, Tranite, Vaso-80 Unicelles
Canada: Peritrate

Pentaerythritol Tetranitrate-Butabarbital
United States: Covap

Pentaerythritol Tetranitrate-Chlordiazepoxide
Canada: Pentrium

Pentaerythritol Tetranitrate-Meprobamate
United States: Equanitrate, Miltrate
Canada: Equanitrate

Pentaerythritol Tetranitrate-Phenobarbital
United States: Pennpheno, Pentylan with Phenobarbital, Peritrate with Phenobarbital, Quintrate PB
Canada: Peritrate with Phenobarbital

- ☐ This medicine is used to help prevent angina attacks and must be taken regularly as your doctor has prescribed. Do not miss any doses. It will not relieve an angina attack that has already started because it works too slowly.

HOW TO USE THIS MEDICINE
- ☐ It is best to take this medicine on an empty stomach 1 hour before (or 2 hours after) eating food.

627

□ For SUSTAINED RELEASE MEDICINE
  • Swallow this medicine whole. Do not crush, chew, or break it into pieces. (*United States:* Antora, Duotrate Plateau Caps, Peritrate Sustained Action, Pentryate Timed, Pentryate Stronger Timed, Tranite D-Lay, Vaso-80 Unicelles; *Canada:* Peritrate SA, Peritrate with Phenobarbital SA)
  • If you do forget to take a dose, take it as soon as possible. However, if your next dose is within 6 hours, do not take the missed dose but continue with your regular schedule.

□ For ORAL TABLETS
  • If you forget to take a dose, take it as soon as possible. However, if your next dose is within 2 hours, do not take the missed dose but continue with your regular schedule.

HOW TO STORE THIS MEDICINE

□ Store in a cool, dry place, but not in the bathroom medicine cabinet or refrigerator because these areas are humid.

SPECIAL INSTRUCTIONS

□ If you become dizzy or feel faint, breathe deeply and bend forward with your head between your knees. Always get up slowly after you have been sitting or lying down. Get out of bed slowly in the morning and dangle your feet over the edge of the bed for a few minutes before standing up. Do not drive a car or operate dangerous machinery or do jobs that require you to be alert if you are dizzy or drowsy.

□ Do not drink alcoholic beverages while you are taking this medicine as they may make the dizziness and fainting worse.

□ Some nonprescription drugs can aggravate your heart condition. Do not take any of the following without the approval of your doctor or pharmacist: cough, cold, or sinus products; asthma or allergy products; or diet or weight-reducing medicines.

□ Check with your doctor before you take any other drugs such as sleeping pills, tranquilizers, pain relievers, medicine for seizures, or allergies. Used together, they could make you very drowsy. (*United States:* Covap, Equanitrate, Miltrate, Pennpheno, Pentylan with Phenobarbital, Peritrate with Phenobarbital, Quintrate PB; *Canada:* Equanitrate, Pentrium, Peritrate with Phenobarb)

□ When you first start taking this medicine, you may get a headache or flushing. This is a common side effect and will usually disappear after you have taken the drug a few times. If the headaches do not go away or are severe, call your doctor.

□ Cigarette smoking can aggravate angina and is a special risk for people who have angina.

628

☐ Most people experience few or no side effects from their drugs. However, any medicine can sometimes cause unwanted effects. Call your doctor if you develop a skin rash, fainting spells, nausea or vomiting, or a rapid pulse, or if your chest pain is not relieved.

☐ Do not stop taking the medicine suddenly or it could cause an angina attack.

☐ Call your doctor if you develop a sore throat or fever, easy bruising, shortness of breath or difficulty in breathing, or changes in your vision. (**United States:** Equanitrate, Miltrate; **Canada:** Equanitrate, Pentrium)

☐ Carry an identification card indicating that you are taking this medicine. Always tell your pharmacist, dentist, and other doctors who are treating you that you are taking this medicine.

*   *   *   *   *

Pentazocine (*Oral Analgesic*)
United States: Talwin
Canada: Talwin

Pentazocine-ASA-Caffeine
Canada: Talwin Compound

☐ This medicine is used to help relieve pain.

☐ IMPORTANT: If you have ever had an allergic reaction to aspirin, caffeine, or a pain reliever, or if you have a stomach ulcer, tell your doctor or pharmacist before you take any of this medicine.

HOW TO USE THIS MEDICINE
☐ This medicine may be taken with food or a glass of water.

☐ Do not take any more of this medicine than your doctor has prescribed. The drug could become habit-forming or you could take an overdose if you take it more often or longer than prescribed.

☐ Do not wait to take this medicine until the pain becomes severe. This medicine works best if you take it at the beginning of the pain. Call your doctor if you feel you need it more often than he prescribed.

☐ Do not take this medicine if it smells strongly like vinegar since this means that the aspirin in the medicine is not fresh.

SPECIAL INSTRUCTIONS
☐ Women who are pregnant, breast-feeding, or planning to become pregnant should tell their doctor before taking this medicine.

☐ Do not drink alcoholic beverages while taking this drug without the approval of your doctor.

- ☐ It is important that you obtain the advice of your doctor or pharmacist before taking ANY other medicines including other pain relievers, sleeping pills, tranquilizers or medicines for depression, cough/cold or allergy medicines, or weight-reducing medicines.

- ☐ In some people, this drug may cause dizziness or drowsiness. Do not drive a car or operate dangerous machinery or do jobs that require you to be alert until you know how you are going to react to this drug.

- ☐ If you become dizzy, you should be careful going up and down stairs. Sit or lie down at the first sign of dizziness. Get up slowly if you have been lying or sitting down.

- ☐ If you do feel nauseated when you first start taking the medicine, it may help if you lie down for a few minutes.

- ☐ If you become constipated, try increasing the amount of bulk in your diet (for example, bran and salads), exercising more often, or drinking more water. Call your doctor if the constipation continues.

- ☐ Most people experience few or no side effects from their drugs. However, any medicine can sometimes cause unwanted effects. Call your doctor if you develop a skin rash, shortness of breath, difficulty in urinating ("passing your water"), stomach pain, nightmares, confusion, a change in your mood, or depression.

- ☐ Also call your doctor if you develop "ringing" or "buzzing" in the ears, or red or black stools. (**Canada:** Talwin Compound)

- ☐ Always tell your dentist, pharmacist, and other doctors who are treating you that you are taking this medicine.

*　*　*　*　*

Pentobarbital Sodium (*Oral Sedative-Hypnotic*)
United States: Nembutal Sodium
Canada: Ibatal, Nembutal, Pentogen

- ☐ This medicine is used to cause sleep.

- ☐ IMPORTANT: If you have ever had an allergic reaction to a barbiturate medicine, tell your doctor or pharmacist before you take any of this medicine.

HOW TO USE THIS MEDICINE
- ☐ This medicine may be taken with food or a full glass of water.

SPECIAL INSTRUCTIONS
- ☐ Sleeping medicines are only useful for a short time. If used for too long, they lose their effectiveness. Do not take any more of this medicine than your doctor has prescribed and do not stop taking this medicine suddenly without the approval of your doctor.

- [ ] Women who are pregnant, breast-feeding, or planning to become pregnant should tell their doctor before taking this medicine.

- [ ] In some people, this drug may cause dizziness or drowsiness. Do not drive a car or operate dangerous machinery or do jobs that require you to be alert until you know how you are going to react to this drug.

- [ ] If you become dizzy, you should be careful going up and down stairs. Sit or lie down at the first sign of dizziness.

- [ ] Do not drink alcoholic beverages while taking this drug without the approval of your doctor.

- [ ] It is important that you obtain the advice of your doctor or pharmacist before taking ANY other medicines including pain relievers, sleeping pills, tranquilizers or medicines for depression, cough/cold or allergy medicines, or blood-thinning medicines.

- [ ] Since you are taking this medicine to help you sleep, take it about 20 minutes before you want to go to sleep. Go to bed after you have taken it. Do not smoke in bed after you have taken it.

- [ ] Do not store this medicine at the bedside and keep it out of the reach of children.

- [ ] Call your doctor immediately if you think you may be allergic to the medicine or if you develop a skin rash, hives, itching, swelling of the face, or difficulty in breathing. If you cannot reach your doctor, phone a hospital emergency department.

- [ ] Most people experience few or no side effects from their drugs. However, any medicine can sometimes cause unwanted effects. Call your doctor if you develop a sore throat, bothersome sleepiness or laziness during the day, nightmares, staggering walk, unusual nervousness, a yellow color to the skin or eyes, easy bruising, or slow heartbeats.

* * * * *

Pentobarbital Sodium *(Rectal Sedative-Hypnotic)*
United States: Nembutal Sodium Suppositories
Canada: Nembutal, Nova-Rectal

- [ ] This medicine is used to cause sleep.

- [ ] IMPORTANT: If you have ever had an allergic reaction to a barbiturate medicine, tell your doctor or pharmacist before you take any of this medicine.

HOW TO USE THIS MEDICINE
- [ ] Administration of SUPPOSITORIES
    - Remove the wrapper from the suppository.
    - Lie on your side and raise your knee to your chest.

631

- Insert the suppository with the tapered (pointed) end first into the rectum.
- Remain lying down for a few minutes so that the suppository will dissolve in the rectum.
- Try to avoid having a bowel movement for at least one hour so that the drug will have time to work.

☐ Store these suppositories in a cool place. (**United States:** Nembutal Sodium Suppositories; **Canada:** Nembutal Suppositories)

☐ Store these suppositories in the refrigerator. (**Canada:** Nova-Rectal)

SPECIAL INSTRUCTIONS

☐ Sleeping medicines are only useful for a short time. If used for too long, they lose their effectiveness. Do not use any more of this medicine than your doctor has prescribed, and do not stop using this medicine suddenly without the approval of your doctor.

☐ Women who are pregnant, breast-feeding, or planning to become pregnant should tell their doctor before taking this medicine.

☐ In some people, this drug may cause dizziness or drowsiness. Do not drive a car or operate dangerous machinery or do jobs that require you to be alert until you know how you are going to react to this drug.

☐ If you become dizzy, you should be careful going up and down stairs. Sit or lie down at the first sign of dizziness.

☐ Do not drink alcoholic beverages while taking this drug without the approval of your doctor.

☐ It is important that you obtain the advice of your doctor or pharmacist before taking ANY other medicines including pain relievers, sleeping pills, tranquilizers or medicines for depression, cough/cold or allergy medicines, or blood-thinning medicines.

☐ Since you are using this medicine to help you sleep, use it about 20 minutes before you want to go to sleep. Go to bed after you have used it. Do not smoke in bed after you have used it.

☐ Do not store this medicine at the bedside, and keep it out of the reach of children.

☐ Call your doctor immediately if you think you may be allergic to the medicine or if you develop a skin rash, hives, itching, swelling of the face, or difficulty in breathing. If you cannot reach your doctor, phone a hospital emergency department.

☐ Most people experience few or no side effects from their drugs. However, any medicine can sometimes cause unwanted effects. Call your doctor if you develop a sore throat, bothersome sleepiness or laziness during the day, nightmares, a staggering walk, unusual nervousness, a yellow color to the skin or eyes, easy bruising, or slow heartbeats.

* * * * *

Pentylenetetrazol (*Oral Analeptic*)
United States: Metrazol, Nelex-100, Nioric

☐ This medicine will help make you feel more alert.

HOW TO USE THIS MEDICINE
☐ Take the medicine with food or a full glass of water.

☐ Do not take more of this medicine than your doctor has recommended.

SPECIAL INSTRUCTIONS
☐ If you forget to take a dose, take it as soon as possible. However, if it is almost time for your next dose, do not take the missed dose. Instead, continue with your regular dosing schedule.

☐ Most people experience few or no side effects from their drugs. However, any medicine can sometimes cause unwanted effects. Call your doctor if you develop dizziness or a slow heartbeat.

* * * * *

Pericyazine (*Oral Antipsychotic*)
Canada: Neuleptil

☐ This medicine is used to help relieve the symptoms of anxiety and tension and certain types of emotional problems. This drug has several other uses and the reason it was prescribed depends upon your condition. Check with your doctor if you do not fully understand why you are taking it.

☐ IMPORTANT: If you have ever had an allergic reaction to a tranquilizer, tell your doctor or pharmacist before you take any of this medicine.

HOW TO USE THIS MEDICINE
☐ This medicine may be taken with food or a full glass of water.

☐ Do not take this medicine at the same time as antacids or diarrhea medicine. Try to space them at least 1 hour apart.

☐ If a dropper is used to measure the dose and you do not fully understand how to use it, check with your pharmacist.

☐ Store the liquid medicines in a cool, dark place and do not get the liquid on your skin or clothing.

☐ The full benefit of the medicine will not be noticed immediately, but may take from 4 to 8 weeks. Be patient. Take the medicine regularly and try not to miss any doses.

☐ Do not stop taking this medicine suddenly without the approval of your doctor.

SPECIAL INSTRUCTIONS

☐ If you forget to take a dose, take it as soon as possible. However, if it is almost time for your next dose, do not take the missed dose. Instead, continue with your regular dosing schedule.

☐ Any medicine has a few unwanted side effects. Because this medicine takes a few weeks to work, the side effects show the doctor that the drug is being absorbed. Many of these side effects will go away as your body adjusts to the medicine.

☐ In some people, this drug may cause dizziness or drowsiness. Do not drive a car or operate dangerous machinery or do jobs that require you to be alert until you know how you are going to react to this drug.

☐ If this medicine causes dizziness, you should be careful going up and down stairs and you should not change positions too rapidly. Get out of bed slowly in the morning and dangle your feet over the edge of the bed for a few minutes before standing up. Sit down or lie down at the first sign of dizziness. Tell your doctor you have been dizzy. Avoid hot showers and baths because they could make you dizzy.

☐ Do not drink alcoholic beverages while taking this drug without the approval of your doctor.

☐ This medicine may make some people more sensitive to sunlight and sunlamps. When you begin taking this medicine, try to avoid getting too much sun until you see how you are going to react. If your skin does become more sensitive to sunlight, tell your doctor and try to stay out of direct sunlight. While in the sun, wear protective clothing and sunglasses. You may wish to ask your pharmacist about suitable sunscreen products. Check with your doctor if you become sunburned.

☐ If your mouth becomes dry, suck a hard sour candy (sugarless) or ice chips, or chew gum. It is especially important to brush your teeth regularly if you develop a dry mouth.

☐ It is important that you obtain the advice of your doctor or pharmacist before taking **any** other medicines including pain relievers, sleeping pills, other tranquilizers or medicines for depression, cough/cold or allergy medicines, weight-reducing medicines, or laxatives.

☐ This medicine may cause your urine to turn pink or red in color. This is not unusual.

☐ In hot weather or during exercise, be careful not to become overheated. You may be more sensitive to heat because this medicine often makes people perspire less.

☐ Call your doctor if you develop a sore throat, fever, mouth sores, skin rash, changes in eyesight, rapid heartrate, a yellow color in the eyes or skin, unusual weakness or unusual movements of the face, tongue or hands, or difficulty in urinating ("passing your water").

634

☐ Stop taking the medicine and call your doctor if you become restless or unable to sit still or sleep.

☐ Carry an identification card indicating that you are taking this medicine. Always tell your pharmacist, dentist, and other doctors who are treating you that you are taking this medicine.

*   *   *   *   *

Perphenazine (*Oral Antipsychotic-Antiemetic-Antianxiety*)
United States: Trilafon
Canada: Phenazine, Trilafon

☐ This medicine is used to treat certain types of mental and emotional problems. This drug has several other uses and the reason it was prescribed depends upon your condition. Check with your doctor if you do not fully understand why you are taking it.

☐ IMPORTANT: If you have ever had an allergic reaction to a phenothiazine medicine, tell your doctor or pharmacist before you take any of this medicine.

HOW TO USE THIS MEDICINE
☐ This medicine may be taken with food or a full glass of water.

☐ These tablets must be swallowed whole. Do not crush, chew, or break them into pieces. (**United States:** Trilafon Repetabs)

☐ If a dropper or a dispensing spoon is used to measure the dose and you do not fully understand how to use it, check with your pharmacist.

☐ Store the liquid medicine in a cool dark place and do not get the liquid on your skin or clothing.

☐ Do not take this medicine at the same time as antacids or diarrhea medicine. Try to space them at least 1 hour apart.

☐ The effect of the medicine may not be noticed immediately but may take from 2 to 4 weeks. Be patient. Take the medicine regularly and try not to miss any doses.

☐ Do not stop taking this medicine suddenly without the approval of your doctor.

SPECIAL INSTRUCTIONS
☐ If you forget to take a dose, take it as soon as possible. However, if it is almost time for your next dose, do not take the missed dose. Instead, continue with your regular dosing schedule.

☐ Any medicine has a few unwanted side effects. Because this medicine takes a few weeks to work, the side effects show the doctor that the drug is being absorbed. Many of these side effects will go away as your body adjusts to the medicine.

☐ Women who are pregnant, breast-feeding, or planning to become pregnant should tell their doctor before taking this medicine.

☐ In some people, this drug may cause dizziness or drowsiness. Do not drive a car or operate dangerous machinery or do jobs that require you to be alert until you know how you are going to react to this drug.

☐ If this medicine causes dizziness, you should be careful going up and down stairs and you should not change positions too rapidly. Get out of bed slowly in the morning and dangle your feet over the edge of the bed for a few minutes before standing up. Sit down or lie down at the first sign of dizziness. Tell your doctor you have been dizzy. Avoid hot showers and baths because they could make you dizzy.

☐ Do not drink alcoholic beverages while taking this drug without the approval of your doctor.

☐ This medicine may make some people more sensitive to sunlight and sunlamps. When you begin taking this medicine, try to avoid getting too much sun until you see how you are going to react. If your skin does become more sensitive to sunlight, tell your doctor and try to stay out of direct sunlight. While in the sun, wear protective clothing and sunglasses. You may wish to ask your pharmacist about suitable sunscreen products. Check with your doctor if you become sunburned.

☐ If your mouth becomes dry, suck a hard sour candy (sugarless) or ice chips, or chew gum. It is especially important to brush your teeth regularly if you develop a dry mouth.

☐ It is important that you obtain the advice of your doctor or pharmacist before taking **any** other medicines including pain relievers, sleeping pills, other tranquilizers or medicines for depression, cough/cold or allergy medicines, weight-reducing medicines, or laxatives.

☐ This medicine may cause your urine to turn pink, red, or red-brown in color. This is not unusual.

☐ In hot weather or during exercise, be careful not to become overheated. You may be more sensitive to heat since this medicine may affect your body's ability to regulate temperature.

☐ If you become constipated, try increasing the amount of bulk in your diet (for example, bran and salads), exercising more often, and drinking more water. Call your doctor if the constipation continues.

☐ Call your doctor if you develop a sore throat, fever, mouth sores, skin rash, changes in eyesight, rapid heartrate, a yellow color to the eyes or skin, unusual weakness or unusual movements of the face, tongue or hands, or difficulty in urinating ("passing your water"). Also call your doctor if you become restless or unable to sit still or sleep.

☐ Carry an identification card indicating that you are taking this medicine. Always tell your pharmacist, dentist, and other doctors who are treating you that you are taking this medicine.

*   *   *   *   *

Perphenazine-Amitriptyline (*Oral Antidepressant-Antipsychotic-Antianxiety*)
United States: Etrafon-A, Etrafon Forte, Triavil
Canada: Etrafon, Triavil

☐ This medicine is used to help relieve the symptoms of anxiety and depression and certain types of emotional conditions. It is important that you take the medicine regularly and that you do not miss any doses. The full effect of the medicine will not be noticed immediately but may take from a few days to several weeks. Early signs of improvement are increased appetite, better sleep, increased energy, and later improved mood. DO NOT STOP TAKING the medicine when you first feel better or you may feel worse in 3 or 4 days.

☐ IMPORTANT: If you have ever had an allergic reaction to a tranquilizer, tell your doctor or pharmacist before you take any of this medicine.

HOW TO USE THIS MEDICINE
☐ This medicine may be taken with food or a full glass of water.

☐ Do not take this medicine at the same time as antacids or diarrhea medicine. Try to space them at least 1 hour apart.

SPECIAL INSTRUCTIONS
☐ If you forget to take a dose, take it as soon as possible. However, if it is almost time for your next dose, do not take the missed dose. Instead, continue with your regular dosing schedule.

☐ Any medicine has a few unwanted side effects. Because this medicine takes a few weeks to work, the side effects are the only thing that tell the doctor that the drug is being absorbed. Most of these side effects will go away as your body adjusts to the medicine.

☐ Women who are pregnant, breast-feeding, or planning to become pregnant should tell their doctor before taking this medicine.

☐ This medicine may cause your urine to turn pink or red in color. This is not unusual.

☐ In hot weather or during exercise, be careful not to become overheated. You may be more sensitive to heat because this medicine often makes people perspire less.

☐ In some people, this drug may cause dizziness or drowsiness. Do not drive a

car or operate dangerous machinery or do jobs that require you to be alert until you know how you are going to react to this drug.

☐ If this medicine causes dizziness, you should be careful going up and down stairs and you should not change positions too quickly. Get out of bed slowly in the morning and dangle your feet over the edge of the bed for a few minutes before standing up. Sit or lie down at the first sign of dizziness. Tell your doctor you have been dizzy and he may adjust your dose.

☐ Do not drink alcoholic beverages while taking this drug without the approval of your doctor.

☐ It is important that you obtain the advice of your doctor or pharmacist before taking any other medicines, including pain relievers, sleeping pills, tranquilizers, other medicines for depression, cough/cold or allergy medicines, or weight-reducing medicine.

☐ If your mouth becomes dry, suck a hard sour candy (sugarless) or ice chips, or chew gum. It is especially important to brush your teeth regularly if you develop a dry mouth.

☐ This medicine may make some people more sensitive to sunlight and sunlamps. When you begin taking this medicine, try to avoid getting too much sun until you see how you are going to react. If your skin does become more sensitive to sunlight, tell your doctor and try to stay out of direct sunlight. While in the sun, wear protective clothing and sunglasses. You may wish to ask your pharmacist about suitable sunscreen products. Check with your doctor if you become sunburned.

☐ If you become constipated, try increasing the amount of bulk in your diet (for example, bran and salads), exercising more often, or drinking more water.

☐ Stop taking the medicine and call your doctor if you become restless or unable to sit still or sleep.

☐ Call your doctor if you develop a sore throat, fever, mouth sores, eye pain or blurred vision, difficulty in urinating ("passing your water"), fast heartbeats, dark yellow-colored urine or a yellow color to the skin or eyes, a skin rash or nightmares, or unusual movements of the face, tongue, or hands.

☐ Do not stop taking this medicine suddenly without your doctor's approval. When your doctor tells you to stop this medicine, you must follow these precautions for 2 weeks since some of the medicine will still be in your body.

☐ Carry an identification card indicating that you are taking this medicine. Always tell your pharmacist, dentist, and other doctors who are treating you that you are taking this medicine.

* * * * *

Pethidine HCl (*See Meperidine HCl*)

* * * * *

Phenacemide (*Oral Anticonvulsant*)
United States: Phenurone

- [ ] This medicine is used to help control convulsions and seizures. It is commonly used in the treatment of epilepsy.

- [ ] IMPORTANT: If you have ever had an allergic reaction to an anticonvulsant or seizure medicine, tell your doctor or pharmacist before you take any of this medicine.

HOW TO USE THIS MEDICINE

- [ ] Take this medicine with food if it upsets your stomach. Call your doctor if you continue to have stomach upset.

- [ ] It is very important that you take this medicine regularly and that you do not miss any doses. Try to take the medicine at the same time(s) every day. This is the only way that you can receive the full benefit of the medicine. If you forget to take this medicine, the amount of medicine in your blood will go down and you may have seizures.

SPECIAL INSTRUCTIONS

- [ ] If you forget to take a dose, take it as soon as possible. However, if it is almost time for your next dose, do not take the missed dose. Instead, continue with your regular dosing schedule. Do not double doses.

- [ ] Do not stop taking this medicine suddenly or change the amount you are taking without the approval of your doctor.

- [ ] Avoid swimming alone or taking part in high-risk sports in which a sudden seizure could cause injury.

- [ ] In some people, this drug may cause dizziness or drowsiness. Do not drive a car or operate dangerous machinery or do jobs that require you to be alert until you know how you are going to react to this drug. If you become dizzy, you should be careful going up and down stairs. Sit or lie down at the first sign of dizziness.

- [ ] If this medicine is for a child, do not let him (her) ride a bike or climb trees until you can determine how he (she) is going to react to the medicine. Children could hurt themselves if they participated in these activities when they were dizzy.

- [ ] Do not drink alcoholic beverages while taking this drug without the approval of your doctor.

- [ ] It is important that you obtain the advice of your doctor or pharmacist before taking pain relievers, nonprescription drugs, sleeping pills, tranquilizers, or medicines for depression while you are taking this drug.

- [ ] Women who are pregnant, breast-feeding, or planning to become pregnant should tell their doctor before taking this medicine.

□ Most people experience few or no side effects from their drugs. However, any medicine can sometimes cause unwanted effects. Call your doctor if you develop a sore throat, fever or mouth sores, skin rash, dark-colored urine, a yellow color to the skin and eyes, easy bruising or bleeding, lower back pain, severe headaches, or nightmares, or if you become depressed.

□ Do not go without this medicine between prescription refills. Call your pharmacist 2 or 3 days before you will run out of the medicine.

□ Carry an identification card indicating that you are taking this medicine. Always tell your pharmacist, dentist, and other doctors who are treating you that you are taking this medicine.

* * * * *

Phenazopyridine (Oral Urinary Analgesic)
United States: Azo-Standard, Di-Azo, Pyridium, Urodine
Canada: Phenazo, Pyridium

□ This medicine is used to help relieve pain associated with infections of the urinary tract.

HOW TO USE THIS MEDICINE
□ It is best to take this medicine with meals.

SPECIAL INSTRUCTIONS
□ If you forget to take a dose, take it as soon as you remember and then continue with your regular schedule.

□ This medicine may cause your urine to turn orange-red in color. This is not an unusual effect. Protect your undergarments while you are taking this medicine as your urine could cause staining.

□ Most people experience few or no side effects from their drugs. However, any medicine can sometimes cause unwanted effects. Call your doctor if you develop a skin rash or a yellow color to your skin or eyes.

□ If for some reason you cannot take all of the medicine, throw away the unused portion by flushing it down the toilet. Do not take or save old medicine.

* * * * *

Phendimetrazine Tartrate (Oral Anorexiant)
United States: Adphen, Anorex, Aptrol, Bacarate, Bontril PDM, Ex-Obese, Limit, Obepar, Obeval, Phendimead, Ropledge, Trimstat, Trimtabs

□ This medicine is used to help reduce the appetite in weight reduction programs. It can help you develop new eating habits and is only useful for a short time. Do not take any more of this medicine than your doctor has

640

prescribed and do not stop taking this medicine suddenly without the approval of your doctor.

HOW TO USE THIS MEDICINE

☐ This medicine may be taken with a glass of water.

☐ Do not take the medicine late in the day or it may cause insomnia (difficulty in sleeping).

SPECIAL INSTRUCTIONS

☐ If you forget to take a dose, take it as soon as possible. However, if it is almost time for your next dose, do not take the missed dose. Instead, continue with your regular dosing schedule.

☐ It is very important that you follow the diet prescribed by your doctor.

☐ If your mouth becomes dry, suck a hard sour candy (sugarless) or ice chips, or chew gum. It is especially important to brush your teeth regularly if you develop a dry mouth.

☐ In some people, this drug may cause dizziness. Do not drive a car or operate dangerous machinery or do jobs that require you to be alert until you know how you are going to react to this drug. Therefore, you should be careful going up and down stairs. Sit or lie down at the first sign of dizziness.

☐ Most people experience few or no side effects from their drugs. However, any medicine can sometimes cause unwanted effects. Call your doctor if you develop a skin rash, sore throat, fever, mouth sores, unusual nervousness, difficulty in urinating ("passing your water"), or palpitations, or if you become depressed.

☐ Carry an identification card indicating that you are taking this medicine. Always tell your pharmacist, dentist, and other doctors who are treating you that you are taking this medicine.

* * * * *

Phenelzine Sulfate (*Oral Antidepressant*)
United States: Nardil
Canada: Nardil

☐ This medicine is used to help relieve the symptoms of depression. It is important that you take the medicine regularly and that you do not miss any doses. The full effect of the medicine will not be noticed immediately but may take from a few days to several weeks. Early signs of improvement are increased appetite, better sleep, increased energy and, later, improved mood. DO NOT STOP TAKING the medicine when you first feel better or you may feel worse in 3 or 4 days.

HOW TO USE THIS MEDICINE

☐ It is best to take this medicine with a glass of water.

☐ While taking this medicine and for at least 2 weeks after your treatment ends, you must be very careful about your diet. You must not eat any of the following foods or beverages because you could experience a very unpleasant reaction (severe headache, nausea, vomiting, and chest pains):

- Aged and natural cheeses (for example, cheddar, blue, Camembert, Stilton, Gruyère, Brie, Swiss, and Emmenthaler). In general, avoid foods in which aging is used to increase the flavor. Cream cheese, processed cheese, and cottage cheese are safe to eat.
- Sour cream or yogurt.
- Wines, especially Chianti and other heavy red wines.
- Alcoholic beverages, including sherry and beer.
- Canned figs or raisins.
- Yeast extracts (such as Marmite or Bovril) or meat extracts.
- Chicken livers.
- Broad beans (also called fava beans).
- Fermented sausage (such as fermented bolognas and salamis, pepperoni, and summer sausage).
- Pickled or kippered herring.
- Meats prepared with tenderizers.
- Avocados, bananas.
- Soya sauce.
- Chocolate.
- Excessive amounts of caffeine (for example, coffee, tea, cola beverages).

SPECIAL INSTRUCTIONS

☐ If you forget to take a dose, take it as soon as possible. However, if your next dose is within 2 hours, do not take the missed dose but continue with your regular schedule.

☐ Any medicine has a few unwanted side effects. Because this medicine takes a few weeks to work, the side effects are the only thing that tell the doctor that the drug is being absorbed. Most of these side effects will go away as your body adjusts to the medicine.

☐ In some people, this drug may cause dizziness or drowsiness. Do not drive a car or operate dangerous machinery or do jobs that require you to be alert until you know how you are going to react to this drug.

☐ If this medicine causes dizziness, you should be careful going up and down stairs and you should not change positions too quickly. Get out of bed slowly in the morning and dangle your feet over the edge of the bed for a few minutes before standing up. Sit or lie down at the first sign of dizziness. Tell your doctor you have been dizzy.

☐ It is important that you obtain the advice of your doctor or pharmacist before taking any other medicines, including pain relievers, sleeping pills, tranquiliz-

642

ers, other medicines for depression, cough/cold or allergy medicines, or weight-reducing medicine.

☐ If your mouth becomes dry, suck a hard sour candy (sugarless) or ice chips, or chew gum. It is especially important to brush your teeth regularly if you develop a dry mouth.

☐ This medicine may make some people more sensitive to sunlight and sunlamps. When you begin taking this medicine, try to avoid getting too much sun until you see how you are going to react. If your skin does become more sensitive to sunlight, tell your doctor and try to stay out of direct sunlight. While in the sun, wear protective clothing and sunglasses. You may wish to ask your pharmacist about suitable sunscreen products. Check with your doctor if you become sunburned.

☐ If you become constipated, try increasing the amount of bulk in your diet (for example, bran and salads), exercising more often, or drinking more water.

☐ Call your doctor immediately if you develop frequent or severe headaches, chest pains, rapid heartrate, nausea, or vomiting. If you cannot reach your doctor call a hospital emergency department.

☐ Most people experience few or no side effects from their drugs. However, any medicine can sometimes cause unwanted effects. Call your doctor if you develop a skin rash, fever, fainting, difficulty in urinating ("passing your water"), swelling of the legs and ankles, eye pain, or changes in ability to see red and green colors.

☐ Do not stop taking this medicine suddenly without your doctor's approval. Have your prescriptions refilled before you are completely out of this medicine so that you will not miss any doses. When your doctor tells you to stop this medicine, you must follow these precautions for 2 weeks since some of the medicine will still be in your body.

☐ Carry an identification card indicating that you are taking this medicine. Always tell your pharmacist, dentist, and other doctors who are treating you that you are taking this medicine.

* * * * *

Phenindione (*Oral Anticoagulant*)
United States: Hedulin
Canada: Danilone

☐ This medicine is used to help prevent harmful blood clots from forming. It is commonly called a "blood thinner."

HOW TO USE THIS MEDICINE
☐ Take this medicine **exactly** as your doctor has prescribed. Try to take the medicine at the same time every day and do not miss any doses. Do not take

extra tablets without your doctor's approval because overtreatment will cause bleeding.

☐ Regular blood tests, called "prothrombin times,'" are necessary in order for your doctor to prescribe the correct dose for you. Your dose may change from time to time depending on these tests.

☐ It is best to take this medicine with a glass of water. Do not take it with food or other drugs unless otherwise directed.

☐ If you forget to take a dose, take it as soon as possible. However, if it is almost time for your next dose, do not take the missed dose. Instead, continue with your regular dosing schedule. Record the date of the missed dose so that you can tell your doctor the next time you see him for a blood test. Call your doctor if you miss more than 1 dose.

SPECIAL INSTRUCTIONS

☐ Do not take any other drugs or stop taking any drugs you are currently taking without first consulting with your doctor. This even includes many products that you can buy without a prescription such as pain relievers and antacids. Always check with your pharmacist before you take or buy ANY nonprescription products.

☐ Do not take aspirin or medicines containing aspirin or salicylates. It is usually safe to take acetaminophen as a substitute for aspirin for occasional headaches and pain. Check with your pharmacist.

☐ It is best to avoid alcoholic beverages while you are taking this medicine because the combination may cause undesirable side effects. Ask your doctor if he feels it is safe for you to have an occasional drink.

☐ Do not eat unusually large amounts of leafy, green vegetables or change your diet without telling your doctor.

☐ If you have a tendency to cut yourself while shaving, you may wish to use an electric razor to avoid possible bleeding.

☐ Try to avoid contact sports or activities in which you could become injured because they could result in internal bleeding.

☐ This medicine may cause the urine to turn orange in color. This is not an unusual effect, but tell your doctor so that he can check to make sure you do not have any blood in your urine.

☐ If your body gets more medicine than it needs, bleeding may occur. Call your doctor if you notice any of the following signs of bleeding which you cannot explain or are unusual for you: nosebleeds, bruising or heavy menstrual bleeding, bleeding from the gums after brushing the teeth, heavy bleeding from cuts, red or black stools, red or dark brown urine, vomiting blood, or coughing up blood. Your doctor will do some blood tests and adjust your dose.

☐ Women who are pregnant, breast-feeding, or planning to become pregnant should tell their doctor before taking this medicine.

☐ Most people experience few or no side effects from their drugs. However, any medicine can sometimes cause unwanted effects. Call your doctor if you develop stomach or back pain, unusual headaches, changes in eyesight, constipation or diarrhea, dizziness, a skin rash, sore throat, fever, mouth sores, a yellow color to the skin or eyes, unusual tiredness, or blurred vision.

☐ Carry an identification card indicating that you are taking this medicine. Always tell your pharmacist, dentist, and other doctors who are treating you that you are taking this medicine.

☐ Do not go without this medicine between prescription refills. Call your pharmacist 2 or 3 days before you will run out of the medicine.

☐ After you stop taking the medicine, it will take your body some time to return to normal. Your doctor or pharmacist will tell you how long you must follow these instructions AFTER you have stopped taking this medicine.

* * * * *

Phenmetrazine HCl (*Oral Sympathomimetic*)
United States: Preludin

☐ This medicine is used to help reduce the appetite in weight reduction programs. It can help you develop new eating habits and is only useful for a short time.

☐ Do not take any more of this medicine than your doctor has prescribed and do not stop taking this medicine suddenly without the approval of your doctor.

HOW TO USE THIS MEDICINE
☐ This medicine may be taken with food or a glass of water.

☐ Do not take the medicine late in the day or it may cause insomnia (difficulty in sleeping).

☐ Take this medicine 1 hour before meals or before eating. (**United States:** Preludin)

☐ Take this medicine on arising. (**United States:** Preludin Endurets)

☐ This medicine must be swallowed whole. Do not crush, chew, or break it into pieces. (**United States:** Preludin Sustained Release)

SPECIAL INSTRUCTIONS
☐ If you forget to take a dose, take it as soon as possible. However, if it is almost time for your next dose, do not take the missed dose. Instead, continue with your regular dosing schedule.

☐ Women who are pregnant, breast-feeding, or planning to become pregnant should tell their doctor before taking this medicine.

☐ It is very important that you follow the diet prescribed by your doctor.

- ☐ If your mouth becomes dry, suck a hard sour candy (sugarless) or ice chips, or chew gum. It is especially important to brush your teeth regularly if you develop a dry mouth.

- ☐ In some people, this drug may cause dizziness. Do not drive a car or operate dangerous machinery or do jobs that require you to be alert until you know how you are going to react to this drug. Therefore, you should be careful going up and down stairs. Sit or lie down at the first sign of dizziness.

- ☐ Most people experience few or no side effects from their drugs. However, any medicine can sometimes cause unwanted effects. Call your doctor if you develop a skin rash, sore throat, fever, mouth sores, unusual nervousness, difficulty in urinating ("passing your water"), palpitations, or depression.

- ☐ Carry an identification card indicating that you are taking this medicine. Always tell your pharmacist, dentist, and other doctors who are treating you that you are taking this medicine.

* * * * *

Phenobarbital (*Oral Sedative-Antianxiety-Anticonvulsant*)
United States: Luminal, PBR/12, SK-Phenobarbital, Solfoton
Canada: Gardenal, Luminal, Nova-Pheno

- ☐ This medicine is used to cause sleep and for certain types of nervous tension. It is also specially prescribed to help prevent seizures in some patients. Check with your doctor if you do not fully understand why you are taking it.

- ☐ IMPORTANT: If you have ever had an allergic reaction to a barbiturate medicine, tell your doctor or pharmacist before you take any of this medicine.

HOW TO USE THIS MEDICINE
- ☐ This medicine may be taken with food or a full glass of water.

- ☐ This medicine must be swallowed whole. Do not crush, chew, or break it into pieces. (*United States:* PBR/12)

SPECIAL INSTRUCTIONS
- ☐ Sleeping medicines are only useful for a short time. If used for too long, they lose their effectiveness. Do not take any more of this medicine than your doctor has prescribed and do not stop taking this medicine suddenly without the approval of your doctor.

- ☐ Women who are pregnant, breast-feeding, or planning to become pregnant should tell their doctor before taking this medicine.

- ☐ In some people, this drug may cause dizziness or drowsiness. Do not drive a car or operate dangerous machinery or do jobs that require you to be alert until you know how you are going to react to this drug.

646

- ☐ If you become dizzy, you should be careful going up and down stairs. Sit or lie down at the first sign of dizziness.

- ☐ Do not drink alcoholic beverages while taking this drug without the approval of your doctor.

- ☐ It is important that you obtain the advice of your doctor or pharmacist before taking ANY other medicines including pain relievers, sleeping pills, tranquilizers or medicines for depression, cough/cold medicines, or allergy medicines.

- ☐ If you are taking this medicine to help you sleep, take it about 20 minutes before you want to go to sleep. Go to bed after you have taken it. Do not smoke in bed after you have taken it.

- ☐ Do not store this medicine at the bedside and keep it out of the reach of children.

- ☐ Call your doctor immediately if you think you may be allergic to the medicine or if you develop a skin rash, hives, itching, swelling of the face, or difficulty in breathing. If you cannot reach your doctor, phone a hospital emergency department.

- ☐ Most people experience few or no side effects from their drugs. However, any medicine can sometimes cause unwanted effects. Call your doctor if you develop a sore throat, bothersome sleepiness or laziness during the day, nightmares, a staggering walk, unusual nervousness, a yellow color to the skin or eyes, easy bruising, or slow heartbeats.

*   *   *   *   *

Phenoxybenzamine (Oral Sympatholytic)
United States: Dibenzyline

- ☐ This medicine is used in the treatment of pheochromocytoma and to improve the circulation in certain conditions.

HOW TO USE THIS MEDICINE
- ☐ This medicine may be taken with food or a glass of water.

SPECIAL INSTRUCTIONS
- ☐ If you forget to take a dose, take it as soon as possible. However, if it is almost time for your next dose, do not take the missed dose. Instead, continue with your regular dosing schedule.

- ☐ You may not feel the full benefit of this medicine until after 2 weeks of therapy. After you stop taking the medicine, it is important that you continue to follow these instructions for several days.

- ☐ Do not drink alcoholic beverages while taking this drug without the approval of the doctor.

☐ If this medicine causes dizziness, you should be careful going up and down stairs and you should not change positions too rapidly. Get out of bed slowly in the morning and dangle your feet over the edge of the bed for a few minutes before standing up. Sit down or lie down at the first sign of dizziness. Tell your doctor you have been dizzy. Do not drive a car or operate dangerous machinery if you are dizzy. Avoid hot showers and baths because they could make you dizzy.

☐ Check with your doctor if you develop fast heartbeats or dizziness which do not go away as your body adjusts to the medicine.

☐ Most people experience few or no side effects from their drugs. However, any medicine can sometimes cause unwanted effects. Call your doctor if you develop vomiting or unusual tiredness.

*　*　*　*　*

Phenprocoumon (Oral Anticoagulant)
United States: Liquamar
Canada: Marcumar

☐ This medicine is used to help prevent harmful blood clots from forming. It is commonly called a "blood thinner."

HOW TO USE THIS MEDICINE
☐ Take this medicine **exactly** as your doctor has prescribed. Try to take the medicine at the same time every day and do not miss any doses. Do not take extra tablets without your doctor's approval because overtreatment will cause bleeding.

☐ Regular blood tests, called "prothrombin times," are necessary in order for your doctor to prescribe the correct dose for you. Your dose may change from time to time depending on these tests.

☐ It is best to take this medicine with a glass of water. Do not take it with food or other drugs unless otherwise directed.

☐ If you forget to take a dose, take it as soon as possible. However, if it is almost time for your next dose, do not take the missed dose. Instead, continue with your regular dosing schedule. Record the date of the missed dose so that you can tell your doctor the next time you see him for a blood test. Call your doctor if you miss more than 1 dose.

SPECIAL INSTRUCTIONS
☐ Do not take any other drugs or stop taking any drugs you are currently taking without first consulting with your doctor. This even includes many products that you can buy without a prescription such as pain relievers and antacids. Always check with your pharmacist before you take or buy ANY nonprescription products.

☐ Do not take aspirin or medicines containing aspirin or salicylates. It is usu-

648

ally safe to take acetaminophen as a substitute for aspirin for occasional headaches and pain. Check with your pharmacist.

☐ It is best to avoid alcoholic beverages while you are taking this medicine because the combination may cause undesirable side effects. Ask your doctor if he feels it is safe for you to have an occasional drink.

☐ Do not eat unusually large amounts of leafy, green vegetables or change your diet without telling your doctor.

☐ If you have a tendency to cut yourself while shaving, you may wish to use an electric razor to avoid possible bleeding.

☐ Try to avoid contact sports or activities in which you could become injured because they could result in internal bleeding.

☐ If your body gets more medicine than it needs, bleeding may occur. Call your doctor if you notice any of the following signs of bleeding which you cannot explain or are unusual for you: nosebleeds, bruising or heavy menstrual bleeding, bleeding from the gums after brushing the teeth, heavy bleeding from cuts, red or black stools, red or dark brown urine, vomiting blood, or coughing up blood. Your doctor will do some blood tests and adjust your dose.

☐ Women who are pregnant, breast-feeding, or planning to become pregnant should tell their doctor before taking this medicine.

☐ Most people experience few or no side effects from their drugs. However, any medicine can sometimes cause unwanted effects. Call your doctor if you develop stomach or back pain, unusual headaches, changes in eyesight, constipation or diarrhea, dizziness, a skin rash, sore throat, fever, mouth sores, a yellow color to the skin or eyes, or unusual tiredness.

☐ Carry an identification card indicating that you are taking this medicine. Always tell your pharmacist, dentist, and other doctors who are treating you that you are taking this medicine.

☐ Do not go without this medicine between prescription refills. Call your pharmacist 2 or 3 days before you will run out of the medicine.

☐ After you stop taking the medicine, it will take your body some time to return to normal. Your doctor or pharmacist will tell you how long you must follow these instructions AFTER you have stopped taking this medicine.

* * * * *

Phensuximide (Oral Anticonvulsant)
United States: Milontin
Canada: Milontin

☐ This medicine is used to help control convulsions and seizures. It is commonly used in the treatment of epilepsy.

649

☐ IMPORTANT: If you have ever had an allergic reaction to an anticonvulsant or seizure medicine, tell your doctor or pharmacist before you take any of this medicine.

HOW TO USE THIS MEDICINE

☐ Take this medicine with food if it upsets your stomach. Call your doctor if you continue to have stomach upset.

☐ For LIQUID MEDICINE
  • Shake the bottle well before using so that you can measure an accurate dose. (**United States** and **Canada:** Milontin Suspension)

☐ It is very important that you take this medicine regularly and that you do not miss any doses. Try to take the medicine at the same time(s) every day. This is the only way that you can receive the full benefit of the medicine. If you forget to take this medicine, the amount of medicine in your blood will go down and you may have seizures.

SPECIAL INSTRUCTIONS

☐ If you forget to take a dose, take it as soon as possible. However, if it is almost time for your next dose, do not take the missed dose. Instead, continue with your regular dosing schedule. Do not double doses.

☐ Do not stop taking this medicine suddenly or change the amount you are taking without the approval of your doctor.

☐ Avoid swimming alone or taking part in high-risk sports in which a sudden seizure could cause injury.

☐ In some people, this drug may cause dizziness or drowsiness. Do not drive a car or operate dangerous machinery or do jobs that require you to be alert until you know how you are going to react to this drug. If you become dizzy, you should be careful going up and down stairs. Sit or lie down at the first sign of dizziness.

☐ If this medicine is for a child, do not let him (her) ride a bike or climb trees until you can determine how he (she) is going to react to the medicine. Children could hurt themselves if they participated in these activities when they were dizzy.

☐ Do not drink alcoholic beverages while taking this drug without the approval of your doctor.

☐ It is important that you obtain the advice of your doctor or pharmacist before taking pain relievers, nonprescription drugs, sleeping pills, tranquilizers, or medicines for depression while you are taking this drug.

☐ Women who are pregnant, breast-feeding, or planning to become pregnant should tell their doctor before taking this medicine.

☐ Most people experience few or no side effects from their drugs. However, any medicine can sometimes cause unwanted effects. Call your doctor if you

develop a sore throat, fever or mouth sores, skin rash, swollen glands, easy bruising or bleeding, or depression.

☐ Do not go without this medicine between prescription refills. Call your pharmacist 2 or 3 days before you will run out of the medicine.

☐ Carry an identification card indicating that you are taking this medicine. Always tell your pharmacist, dentist, and other doctors who are treating you that you are taking this medicine.

*   *   *   *   *

Phentermine HCl (*Oral Anorexiant*)

United States: Adipex 8, Ionamin, Obesamead, Parmine, Phentrol, Rolaphent

Canada: Ionamin

☐ This medicine is used to help reduce the appetite in weight reduction programs. It can help you develop new eating habits and is only useful for a short time. Do not take any more of this medicine than your doctor has prescribed and do not stop taking this medicine suddenly without the approval of your doctor.

HOW TO USE THIS MEDICINE

☐ This medicine may be taken with a glass of water.

☐ Do not take the medicine late in the day or it may cause insomnia (difficulty in sleeping).

☐ This medicine must be swallowed whole. Do not crush, chew, or break it into pieces. (**United States:** Ionamin, Obesamead, Parmine, Phentrol No. 4 and No. 5, Rolaphent-15, Rolaphent-30; **Canada:** Ionamin)

SPECIAL INSTRUCTIONS

☐ If you forget to take a dose, take it as soon as possible. However, if it is almost time for your next dose, do not take the missed dose. Instead, continue with your regular dosing schedule.

☐ It is very important that you follow the diet prescribed by your doctor.

☐ If your mouth becomes dry, suck a hard sour candy (sugarless) or ice chips, or chew gum. It is especially important to brush your teeth regularly if you develop a dry mouth.

☐ In some people, this drug may cause dizziness. Do not drive a car or operate dangerous machinery or do jobs that require you to be alert until you know how you are going to react to this drug. Therefore, you should be careful going up and down stairs. Sit or lie down at the first sign of dizziness.

☐ Most people experience few or no side effects from their drugs. However, any medicine can sometimes cause unwanted effects. Call your doctor if you

651

develop a skin rash, sore throat, fever, mouth sores, unusual nervousness, difficulty in urinating ("passing your water"), palpitations, or depression.

☐ Carry an identification card indicating that you are taking this medicine. Always tell your pharmacist, dentist, and other doctors who are treating you that you are taking this medicine.

*　*　*　*　*

Phenylbutazone (Oral Antiarthritic–Anti-inflammatory)
United States: Azolid, Butazolidin

Canada: Algoverine, Anevral, Butagesic, Butalgan, Butazolidin, Intrabutazone, Malgesic, Nadozone, Neo-Zoline, Novobutazone, Phenbutazone

Phenylbutazone-Antacids (Oral Anti-inflammatory–Antiarthritic)
United States: Azolid-A, Butazolidin Alka

Canada: Alka Butazolidin, Alkabutazone, Anevral, Buffazone, Butagesic-B, Butone, Malgesic-Alk

☐ This medicine is used to help relieve pain, redness, stiffness, and swelling in certain kinds of arthritis and other medical conditions.

☐ IMPORTANT: If you have ever had an allergic reaction to aspirin or any other medicine for arthritis, tell your doctor or pharmacist before you take any of this medicine.

☐ Do not use this medicine more often or longer than recommended by your doctor. If you do not feel better after 1 week, call your doctor.

HOW TO USE THIS MEDICINE
☐ The following medicine has a special coating and must be swallowed whole. Do not crush, chew, or break it into pieces. Do not take chipped tablets. (**Canada:** Intrabutazone, Nadozone)

☐ The following medicine must be swallowed whole. Do not crush, chew, or break it into pieces. (**Canada:** Alka Butazolidin)

☐ Always take this medicine with food or a glass of milk or immediately after meals to help prevent stomach upset.

SPECIAL INSTRUCTIONS
☐ Women who are pregnant, breast-feeding, or planning to become pregnant should tell their doctor before taking this medicine.

652

☐ In some people, this drug may cause drowsiness. Do not drive a car or operate dangerous machinery or do jobs that require you to be alert until you know how you are going to react to this drug.

☐ If you forget to take a dose, take it as soon as possible. However, if it is almost time for your next dose, do not take the missed dose. Instead, continue with your regular dosing schedule.

☐ Do not take antacids containing large amounts of sodium while you are taking this medicine. Check with your pharmacist.

☐ While you are taking this medicine, do not drink alcoholic beverages or take aspirin without the permission of your doctor. It is usually safe to take acetaminophen for the ocasional headache. Check with your pharmacist.

☐ Call your doctor immediately if you think you may be allergic to the medicine or if you develop a skin rash, hives, itching, swelling of the face, or difficulty in breathing. If you cannot reach your doctor, phone a hospital emergency department.

☐ Most people experience few or no side effects from their drugs. However, any medicine can sometimes cause unwanted effects. Call your doctor if you develop a skin rash, sore throat, fever or mouth sores, swollen glands, any loss of hearing, blurred vision or changes in eyesight, easy bruising, red or black stools or pink urine, stomach pain, vomiting, swelling of the legs or ankles or a sudden weight gain, a yellow color to the skin or eyes, difficulty in urinating ("passing your water"), or unusual tiredness.

☐ Carry an identification card indicating that you are taking this medicine. Always tell your dentist, pharmacist, and other doctors who are treating you that you are taking this medicine.

*   *   *   *   *

Phenylephrine HCl (*Ophthalmic Decongestant*)
United States: Efricel, Isopto Frin, Neo-Synephrine, Prefrin, Tear-Efrin

Canada: Isopto Frin, Neo-Synephrine, Optocrymal, Prefrin Liquifilm

Phenylephrine-Pyrilamine
United States: Prefrin-A
Canada: Prefrin-A

☐ This medicine is used to treat eye conditions to help relieve burning, itching, or smarting of the eye.

HOW TO USE THIS MEDICINE
☐ For EYE DROPS

INSTILLATION OF EYE DROPS

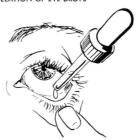

- The person administering the eye drops should wash his hands with soap and water.
- The eye drops must be kept clean. Do not touch the dropper against the face or anything else.
- Lie down or tilt your head backward and look at the ceiling.
- Gently pull down the lower lid of your eye to form a pouch.
- Hold the dropper in your other hand and approach the eye from the side. Place the dropper as close to the eye as possible without touching it.
- Place the prescribed number of drops into the pouch of the eye.
- Close your eyes. Do not rub them.
- Apply gentle pressure for a minute with your fingers to the bridge of the nose (inside corner of the eye) to prevent the eye drops from being drained from the eye.
- Blot excess solution around the eye with a tissue.

☐ If necessary, have someone else administer the eye drops for you.

☐ Do not use the eye drops if they have changed in color or have changed in any way since being purchased.

☐ Keep the eye drop bottle tightly closed when not in use.

☐ Do not use the drug more frequently or in larger quantities than prescribed by your doctor.

SPECIAL INSTRUCTIONS
☐ Vision may be blurred for a few minutes after using the eye medicine. Do not drive a car or operate dangerous machinery or do jobs that require you to be alert until your vision has cleared.

☐ If you forget to use the medicine, use it as soon as possible. However, if it is almost time for your next dose, do not use the missed dose but continue with your regular schedule.

☐ Do not use this medicine at the same time as any other eye medicine without the approval of your doctor. Some medicines cannot be mixed.

- ☐ Check with your doctor if you develop a headache which does not go away as your body adjusts to the medicine.
- ☐ Contact your doctor if the condition for which you are using this medicine does not improve or if the eye becomes irritated by it for more than a few minutes. Many eye medicines sting for a short time immediately after use. Also call your doctor if you develop fast heartbeats, trembling, or excessive sweating.
- ☐ Store the solution in a cool dark place as it is sensitive to heat and light.
- ☐ For external use only. Do not swallow.

* * * * *

Phenylephrine HCl (*Nasal Decongestant*)

United States: Alconefrin, Biomydrin, Coricidin Nasal Mist, Coryban D, Isophrin Nasal, Neo-Synephrine, Vacon

Canada: Neo-Synephrine

- ☐ This medicine is used to help relieve nasal stuffiness.

HOW TO USE THIS MEDICINE
- ☐ For NASAL SPRAY
  - Blow your nose gently.
  - Sit upright with your head slightly back.
  - Place the atomizer at the entrance of the nostril and close the other nostril by pressing your finger on the side.
  - Squeeze the atomizer the prescribed number of times.
  - Repeat for the other nostril if necessary.

- ☐ For NASAL JELLY
  - Blow your nose gently.
  - Place a small pea-sized portion of jelly at one nostril.
  - Breathe in strongly with mouth closed and finger closing other nostril, until jelly enters the nose.

- ☐ For NOSE DROPS

INSTILLATION OF NOSE DROPS

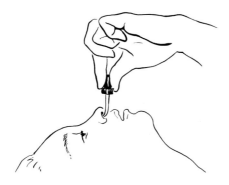

- Blow your nose gently before administration of drops.
- Sit in a chair and tilt your head backward or lie down on a bed with your head extending over the edge of the bed or lie down and place a pillow under your shoulders so that your head is tipped backward.
- Insert dropper into nostril about $\frac{1}{3}$ inch and drop the prescribed number of drops into the nose.
- Try not to touch the inside of the nose with the dropper as it will probably make you sneeze and will contaminate the dropper.
- Remain in the same position for at least 5 minutes.
- For children: Let the head hang over the edge of a table, bed, or mother's lap and follow the same procedure.

SPECIAL INSTRUCTIONS

☐ Do not use this medicine more often or longer than recommended by your doctor. If used for too long, this medicine may actually cause a type of congestion.

☐ Rinse the dropper in hot water after each use.

☐ If you forget to use the medicine, use it as soon as possible. However, if it is almost time for your next dose, do not use the missed dose but continue with your regular schedule.

☐ Do not use this medicine at the same time as any other nasal medicine without the approval of your doctor. Some medicines cannot be mixed.

☐ Contact your doctor if the condition for which you are using this medicine does not improve. Also call your doctor if you develop fast heartbeats, headache, dizziness, trembling, blurred vision, or drowsiness.

☐ Check with your doctor if you develop a stinging sensation which does not go away as your body adjusts to the medicine.

☐ For external use only. Do not swallow.

* * * * *

Phenylephrine HCl-Sulfacetamide (*Ophthalmic Antibacterial-Decongestant*)
United States: Vasosulf
Canada: Vasosulf

☐ This medicine is used to treat and help prevent eye infections.

☐ IMPORTANT: If you have ever had an allergic reaction to sulfa or sulfonamide medicines, tell your doctor or pharmacist before you use any of this drug.

656

HOW TO USE THIS MEDICINE
☐ For EYE DROPS

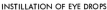

INSTILLATION OF EYE DROPS

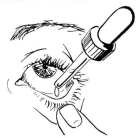

- The person administering the eye drops should wash his hands with soap and water.
- The eye drops must be kept clean. Do not touch the dropper against the face or anything else.
- Lie down or tilt your head backward and look at the ceiling.
- Gently pull down the lower lid of your eye to form a pouch.
- Hold the dropper in your other hand and approach the eye from the side. Place the dropper as close to the eye as possible without touching it.
- Place the prescribed number of drops into the pouch of the eye.
- Close your eyes. Do not rub them.
- Apply gentle pressure for a minute with your fingers to the bridge of the nose (inside corner of the eye) to prevent the eye drops from being drained from the eye.
- Blot excess solution around the eye with a tissue.

☐ If necessary, have someone else administer the eye drops for you.

☐ Do not use the eye drops if they have changed in color or have changed in any way since being purchased.

☐ Keep the eye drop bottle tightly closed when not in use.

☐ Do not use the drug more frequently or in larger quantities than prescribed by your doctor.

SPECIAL INSTRUCTIONS

☐ Vision may be blurred for a few minutes after using the eye medicine. Do not drive a car or operate dangerous machinery or do jobs that require you to be alert until your vision has cleared.

☐ If you forget to use the medicine, use it as soon as possible. However, if it is almost time for your next dose, do not use the missed dose but continue with your regular schedule.

☐ It is important to use *all* of this medicine, plus any refills that your doctor told you to use. Do not stop using it earlier than your doctor has recommended

657

in spite of the fact that your symptoms seem to have improved. Otherwise, the infection may return.

☐ Do not use this medicine at the same time as any other eye medicine without the approval of your doctor. Some medicines cannot be mixed.

☐ Contact your doctor if the condition for which you are using this medicine does not improve or if the eye becomes irritated by it for more than a few minutes. Many eye medicines sting for a short time immediately after use. Also call your doctor if you develop fast heartbeats, trembling, or excessive sweating.

☐ Store the solution tightly capped in a cool dark place as it is sensitive to heat and light.

☐ For external use only. Do not swallow.

* * * * *

Phenytoin (*Oral Anticonvulsant*)
United States: Dilantin
Canada: Dilantin

☐ This medicine is used to help control convulsions and seizures. It is commonly used in the treatment of epilepsy.

☐ IMPORTANT: If you have ever had an allergic reaction to an anticonvulsant or seizure medicine, tell your doctor or pharmacist before you take any of this medicine.

HOW TO USE THIS MEDICINE
☐ Take this medicine with food if it upsets your stomach. Call your doctor if you continue to have stomach upset.

☐ The following medicine should be chewed well before swallowing. (**United States:** Dilantin Infatabs)

☐ For LIQUID MEDICINE
  • Shake the bottle well before using so that you can measure an accurate dose. (**United States** and **Canada:** Dilantin Suspension)

☐ It is very important that you take this medicine regularly and that you do not miss any doses. Try to take the medicine at the same time(s) every day. This is the only way that you can receive the full benefit of the medicine. If you forget to take this medicine, the amount of medicine in your blood will go down and you may have seizures.

SPECIAL INSTRUCTIONS
☐ If you forget to take a dose, take it as soon as possible. However, if it is almost time for your next dose, do not take the missed dose. Instead, continue with your regular dosing schedule. Do not double doses.

658

☐ Do not stop taking this medicine suddenly or change the amount you are taking without the approval of your doctor.

☐ Avoid swimming alone or taking part in high-risk sports in which a sudden seizure could cause injury.

☐ In some people, this drug may cause dizziness. Do not drive a car or operate dangerous machinery or do jobs that require you to be alert until you know how you are going to react to this drug. If you become dizzy, you should be careful going up and down stairs. Sit or lie down at the first sign of dizziness.

☐ If this medicine is for a child, do not let him (her) ride a bike or climb trees until you can determine how he (she) is going to react to the medicine. Children could hurt themselves if they participated in these activities when they were dizzy.

☐ Do not drink alcoholic beverages while taking this drug without the approval of your doctor.

☐ It is important that you obtain the advice of your doctor or pharmacist before taking pain relievers, nonprescription drugs, sleeping pills, tranquilizers, or medicines for depression while you are taking this drug.

☐ While taking this medicine, brush your teeth and massage your gums regularly with a soft toothbrush. Also use dental floss daily. The next time you visit your dentist, tell him you are taking this medicine. Call your doctor if your gums become red, tender, or swollen.

☐ This medicine may cause your urine to turn pink or red-brown in color. This is not unusual.

☐ Women who are pregnant, breast-feeding, or planning to become pregnant should tell their doctor before taking this medicine.

☐ Most people experience few or no side effects from their drugs. However, any medicine can sometimes cause unwanted effects. Call your doctor if you develop a sore throat, fever or mouth sores, skin rash, persistent headache, slurred speech, fast eye movements, joint pain, swollen glands, difficulty in walking, easy bruising or bleeding, or a yellow color to the skin or eyes.

☐ Do not go without this medicine between prescription refills. Call your pharmacist 2 or 3 days before you will run out of the medicine.

☐ Carry an identification card indicating that you are taking this medicine. Always tell your pharmacist, dentist, and other doctors who are treating you that you are taking this medicine.

☐ Do not change brands of this drug after you have had your dosage stabilized.

*   *   *   *   *

Phosphate Preparations (*Rectal Laxative*)
United States: Fleet Enema, Saf-Tip Phosphate Enema
Canada: Fleet Enema, Travad Enema

- ☐ This medicine is a laxative used to treat constipation or to empty the bowels before certain types of hospital procedures.

HOW TO USE THIS MEDICINE
- ☐ Administration of ENEMA
  - Lie on your left side and raise your knee to your chest.
  - Remove the protective cap from the prelubricated rectal tube.
  - Insert the tip of the tube gently into the rectum and slowly squeeze the bottle until the desired amount has been given.
  - Withdraw the enema tip from the rectum.
  - Stay in this position until you feel the urge to empty your bowels. This usually occurs in 2 to 5 minutes.
  - Empty the bowels completely so that the solution does not remain in the body.

- ☐ Do not swallow this medicine.

SPECIAL INSTRUCTIONS
- ☐ Do not use this medicine more often or longer than your doctor has prescribed as your bowels may become dependent upon it. If you feel you require this medicine every day and cannot have a bowel movement without it, call your doctor.

- ☐ Unless otherwise directed, you should try increasing the amount of bulk foods in your diet (for example, bran, fresh fruits, and salads), exercising more often, and drinking 6 to 8 glasses of water every day.

- ☐ Do not use this medicine if you have any stomach pain, nausea, or vomiting.

- ☐ Call your doctor if your constipation is not relieved or if you develop rectal bleeding, muscle cramps, unusual weakness, or dizziness.

*   *   *   *   *

Phthalylsulfathiazole (*Oral Antibacterial*)
United States: Sulfathalidine
Canada: Sulfathalidine

- ☐ This medicine is used to treat conditions of the intestine.

- ☐ IMPORTANT: If you have ever had an allergic reaction to sulfa drugs, thiazide "water pills," diabetes medicine that you take by mouth, or glaucoma

660

medicine that you take by mouth, tell your doctor or pharmacist before you take any of this medicine.

HOW TO USE THIS MEDICINE
☐ Take the medicine with a glass of water unless otherwise directed.

SPECIAL INSTRUCTIONS
☐ Do not take mineral oil while you are taking this medicine.

☐ If you forget to take a dose, take it as soon as you remember and then continue with your regular schedule.

☐ Women who are pregnant, breast-feeding, or planning to become pregnant should tell their doctor before taking this medicine.

☐ Most people experience few or no side effects from their drugs. However, any medicine can sometimes cause unwanted effects. Call your doctor if you develop a sore throat, fever, mouth sores, easy bruising, a yellow color to the skin and eyes, constant headache, or troublesome diarrhea.

☐ Call your doctor immediately if you think you may be allergic to the medicine or if you develop a skin rash, hives, itching, swelling of the face, or difficulty in breathing. If you cannot reach your doctor, phone a hospital emergency department.

☐ If for some reason you cannot take all of the medicine, throw away the unused portion by flushing it down the toilet. Do not take or save old medicine.

* * * * *

Pilocarpine HCl (*Ophthalmic Miotic*)
United States: Almocarpine, Mi-Pilo, Isopto Carpine, Pilocar, Pilocel
Canada: Adsorbocarpine, Isopto Carpine, Miocarpine, Optopilo

Pilocarpine Nitrate
United States: P.V. Carpine
Canada: P.V. Carpine Liquifilm

Pilocarpine HCl-Epinephrine
United States: P_1E_1, P_2E_1, P_3E_1, P_4E_1, P_6E_1, E-Carpine, E-Pilo
Canada: E-Carpine, E-Pilo

☐ This medicine is used in the treatment of glaucoma and other eye conditions.

HOW TO USE THIS MEDICINE
☐ For EYE DROPS

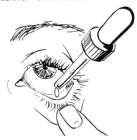

- The person administering the eye drops should wash his hands with soap and water.
- The eye drops must be kept clean. Do not touch the dropper against the face or anything else.
- Lie down or tilt your head backward and look at the ceiling.
- Gently pull down the lower lid of your eye to form a pouch.
- Hold the dropper in your other hand and approach the eye from the side. Place the dropper as close to the eye as possible without touching it.
- Place the prescribed number of drops into the pouch of the eye.
- Close your eyes. Do not rub them.
- Apply gentle pressure for a minute with your fingers to the bridge of the nose (inside corner of the nose) to prevent the eye drops from being drained from the eye.
- Blot excess solution around the eye with a tissue.
- Wash your hands after you have instilled the drops.

☐ If necessary, have someone else administer the eye drops for you.

☐ Do not use the eye drops if they have changed in color or have changed in any way since you purchased them.

☐ Keep the eye drop bottle tightly closed when not in use.

☐ Do not use the drug more frequently or in larger quantities than prescribed by your doctor.

SPECIAL INSTRUCTIONS
☐ Vision may be blurred for a few minutes after using the eye medicine. Do not drive a car or operate dangerous machinery or do jobs that require you to be alert until your vision has cleared.

☐ During the first few days of using the eye drops, you may experience aching in the eyes and head. This is not unusual and should disappear. Call your doctor if the pain persists.

662

☐ If you forget to use the medicine, use it as soon as possible. However, if it is almost time for your next dose, do not use the missed dose but continue with your regular schedule.

☐ Do not use this medicine at the same time as any other eye medicine without the approval of your doctor. Some medicines cannot be mixed.

☐ Contact your doctor if the condition for which you are using this medicine does not improve or if the eye becomes irritated by it for more than a few minutes. Many eye medicines sting for a short time immediately after use. Also call your doctor if you develop excessive sweating, flushing, stomach cramps, diarrhea (loose bowel movements), difficulty in breathing, or difficulty in urinating ("passing your water").

☐ Always tell any future doctors who are treating you that you have used this medicine.

☐ Store the eye drops in a dark place because the medicine is sensitive to light.

☐ For external use only. Do not swallow.

* * * * *

Pimozide (Oral Antipsychotic)
Canada: Orap

☐ This medicine is used to treat certain types of emotional conditions.

HOW TO USE THIS MEDICINE
☐ This medicine may be taken with food or a full glass of water.

SPECIAL INSTRUCTIONS
☐ If you forget to take a dose, take it as soon as possible. However, if it is almost time for your next dose, do not take the missed dose. Instead, continue with your regular dosing schedule.

☐ Women who are pregnant, breast-feeding, or planning to become pregnant should tell their doctor before taking this medicine.

☐ In some people, this drug may cause drowsiness which will usually go away after you have taken the medicine for a while. Do not drive a car or operate dangerous machinery or do jobs that require you to be alert until you know how you are going to react.

☐ If this medicine causes dizziness, you should be careful going up and down stairs and you should not change positions too rapidly. Get out of bed slowly in the morning and dangle your feet over the edge of the bed for a few minutes before standing up. Sit down or lie down at the first sign of dizziness. Tell your doctor you have been dizzy. Do not drive a car or operate dangerous machinery if you are dizzy. Avoid hot showers and baths because they could make you dizzy.

- ☐ If your mouth becomes dry, suck a hard sour candy (sugarless) or ice chips, or chew gum. It is especially important to brush your teeth regularly if you develop a dry mouth.

- ☐ Do not drink alcoholic beverages while taking this drug without the approval of your doctor.

- ☐ It is important that you obtain the advice of your doctor or pharmacist before taking **any** other medicines including pain relievers, sleeping pills, other tranquilizers or medicines for depression, cough/cold or allergy medicines or weight-reducing medicines.

- ☐ Do not take any more of this medicine than your doctor has prescribed, and do not stop taking this medicine suddenly without the approval of your doctor.

- ☐ Most people experience few or no side effects from their drugs. However, any medicine can sometimes cause unwanted effects. Call your doctor if you develop a sore throat, fever or mouth sores, fast heartbeats, stomach cramps or severe constipation, a yellow color to the skin or eyes, dark-colored urine, difficulty in urinating (passing your water), or unusual movements of the hands, face, or tongue.

*   *   *   *   *

Pindolol (*Oral Antihypertensive*)
Canada: Visken

- ☐ This medicine is used to lower the blood pressure.

- ☐ Hypertension (high blood pressure) is a long-term condition, and it will probably be necessary for you to take the drug for a long time in spite of the fact that you feel better. It is very important that you take this medicine as your doctor has directed and that you do not miss any doses. Otherwise, you cannot expect the drug to keep your blood pressure down.

- ☐ IMPORTANT: If you have a history of allergies, tell your doctor or pharmacist before you take any of this medicine.

HOW TO USE THIS MEDICINE
- ☐ Take this medicine with some food unless otherwise directed.

- ☐ Try to take the medicine at the same time(s) every day.

SPECIAL INSTRUCTIONS
- ☐ If you forget to take a dose, take it as soon as possible. However, if it is almost time for your next dose, do not take the missed dose. Instead, continue with your regular dosing schedule.

- ☐ Follow any special diet that your doctor may have ordered.

- [ ] In some people, this drug may cause dizziness or drowsiness. Do not drive a car or operate dangerous machinery or do jobs that require you to be alert until you know how you are going to react to this drug.

- [ ] If this medicine causes dizziness, you should be careful going up and down stairs and you should not change positions too rapidly. Get out of bed slowly in the morning and dangle your feet over the edge of the bed for a few minutes before standing up. Sit down or lie down at the first sign of dizziness. Tell your doctor you have been dizzy. Avoid hot showers and baths because they could make you dizzy.

- [ ] In order to help prevent dizziness and fainting, your doctor may also recommend that you avoid strenuous exercises, standing for long periods of time (especially in hot weather), or hot showers or hot baths.

- [ ] Some nonprescription drugs can aggravate your condition. Do not take any of the following without the approval of your doctor or pharmacist: cough, cold, or sinus products; asthma or allergy products; or diet or weight-reducing medicines.

- [ ] If your mouth becomes dry, suck a hard sour candy (sugarless) or ice chips, or chew gum. It is especially important to brush your teeth regularly if you develop a dry mouth.

- [ ] Most people experience few or no side effects from their drugs. However, any medicine can sometimes cause unwanted effects. Call your doctor if you develop a skin rash, mouth sores, swelling of the legs or ankles, sudden weight gain of 5 pounds or more, chest pains, earache, difficulty in breathing, or a slow heartbeat. Also call your doctor if you develop nightmares or headaches, or if you become depressed.

- [ ] Carry an identification card indicating that you are taking this medicine. Always tell your pharmacist, dentist, and other doctors who are treating you that you are taking this medicine.

- [ ] Do not stop taking this medicine without your doctor's approval, and do not go without medicine between prescription refills. Call your pharmacist 2 or 3 days before you will run out of the medicine.

*   *   *   *   *

Piperacetazine (Oral Antipsychotic)
United States: Quide
Canada: Quide

- [ ] This medicine is used to treat certain types of mental and emotional problems. Check with your doctor if you do not fully understand why you are taking it.

- [ ] IMPORTANT: If you have ever had an allergic reaction to a phenothiazine medicine, tell your doctor or pharmacist before you take any of this medicine.

665

HOW TO USE THIS MEDICINE

☐ This medicine may be taken with food or a full glass of water.

☐ Do not take this medicine at the same time as antacids or diarrhea medicine. Try to space them at least 1 hour apart.

☐ The effect of the medicine may not be noticed immediately but may take from 2 to 4 weeks. Be patient. Take the medicine regularly and try not to miss any doses.

☐ Do not stop taking this medicine suddenly without the approval of your doctor.

SPECIAL INSTRUCTIONS

☐ If you forget to take a dose, take it as soon as possible. However, if it is almost time for your next dose, do not take the missed dose. Instead, continue with your regular dosing schedule.

☐ Any medicine has a few unwanted side effects. Because this medicine takes a few weeks to work, the side effects show the doctor that the drug is being absorbed. Many of these side effects will go away as your body adjusts to the medicine.

☐ Women who are pregnant, breast-feeding, or planning to become pregnant should tell their doctor before taking this medicine.

☐ In some people, this drug may cause dizziness or drowsiness. Do not drive a car or operate dangerous machinery or do jobs that require you to be alert until you know how you are going to react to this drug.

☐ If this medicine causes dizziness, you should be careful going up and down stairs and you should not change positions too rapidly. Get out of bed slowly in the morning and dangle your feet over the edge of the bed for a few minutes before standing up. Sit down or lie down at the first sign of dizziness. Tell your doctor you have been dizzy. Avoid hot showers and baths because they could make you dizzy.

☐ Do not drink alcoholic beverages while taking this drug without the approval of your doctor.

☐ This medicine may make some people more sensitive to sunlight and sunlamps. When you begin taking this medicine, try to avoid getting too much sun until you see how you are going to react. If your skin does become more sensitive to sunlight, tell your doctor and try to stay out of direct sunlight. While in the sun, wear protective clothing and sunglasses. You may wish to ask your pharmacist about suitable sunscreen products. Check with your doctor if you become sunburned.

☐ If your mouth becomes dry, suck a hard sour candy (sugarless) or ice chips, or chew gum. It is especially important to brush your teeth regularly if you develop a dry mouth.

☐ It is important that you obtain the advice of your doctor or pharmacist before taking **any** other medicines including pain relievers, sleeping pills, other tranquilizers or medicines for depression, cough/cold or allergy medicines, weight-reducing medicines, or laxatives.

☐ This medicine may cause your urine to turn pink, red, or red-brown in color. This is not unusual.

☐ In hot weather or during exercise, be careful not to become overheated. You may be more sensitive to heat since this medicine may affect your body's ability to regulate temperature.

☐ If you become constipated, try increasing the amount of bulk in your diet (for example, bran and salads), exercising more often, or drinking more water. Call your doctor if the constipation continues.

☐ Call your doctor if you develop a sore throat, fever, mouth sores, skin rash, changes in eyesight, rapid heartrate, a yellow color to the eyes or skin, unusual weakness, difficulty in urinating ("passing your water"), or unusual movements of the face, tongue, or hands. Also call your doctor if you become restless or unable to sit still or sleep.

☐ Carry an identification card indicating that you are taking this medicine. Always tell your dentist, pharmacist, and other doctors who are treating you that you are taking this medicine.

*　*　*　*　*

Piperazine Adipate (*Oral Anthelmintic*)
Canada: Entacyl

Piperazine Citrate
United States: Antepar, Multifuge, Vermizine
Canada: Antepar

☐ This medicine is used to treat worm infections.

HOW TO USE THIS MEDICINE
☐ Dissolve the granules in 2 oz. of water, milk, or fruit juices. (**Canada:** Entacyl)

☐ Shake the liquid preparation well before swallowing in order to get an accurate dose. (**Canada:** Entacyl Suspensions)

☐ Take the medicine with a glass of water.

SPECIAL INSTRUCTIONS
☐ Do not take any more of this medicine than your doctor has prescribed, but it is important that you do not miss any doses. Otherwise, the infection will not be eliminated.

- [ ] It is not necessary to take a laxative or change your diet unless your doctor recommends that you do so.

- [ ] Most people experience few or no side effects from their drugs. However, any medicine can sometimes cause unwanted effects. Call your doctor if you develop a skin rash or easy bruising, fever, stomach cramps or joint pain, dizziness, blurred vision, trembling, or numbness of the hands and feet.

GENERAL INSTRUCTIONS

- [ ] Good personal hygiene is very important to prevent reinfection.

- [ ] It is recommended that you have a shower every morning in order to remove any eggs in the anal area that have appeared during the night.

- [ ] Wash your hands frequently, especially before handling food or anything that will be put into the mouth. Wash your hands after urination and bowel movements.

- [ ] Keep your nails short and clean and avoid biting them. Do not put your fingers in your mouth or nose.

- [ ] On the day of therapy, change the bed linen, underwear, and nightclothes. Wash or dry-clean them immediately.

- [ ] Do not scratch the affected area.

- [ ] Disinfect the toilet seat and bathtub daily.

*   *   *   *   *

Piperazine Estrone Sulfate (*Oral Estrogen*)
United States: Ogen
Canada: Ogen

This medicine is a hormone and is used to help relieve the symptoms of menopause or is used if the ovaries are not functioning correctly.

HOW TO USE THIS MEDICINE

- [ ] Take the medicine with a glass of water. Try not to miss any doses.

SPECIAL INSTRUCTIONS

- [ ] Women who are pregnant, breast-feeding, or planning to become pregnant should tell their doctor before taking this medicine.

- [ ] It is recommended that you do not smoke while you are taking this medicine because smoking may increase the incidence of heart attacks.

- [ ] Contact your doctor if any of the following side effects occur:
  - Severe or persistent headaches
  - Vomiting, dizziness, or fainting
  - Blurred vision or slurred speech

668

- Pain in the calves of the legs or numbness in an arm or leg
- Chest pain, shortness of breath, or coughing up of blood
- Lumps in the breast
- Severe depression
- A yellow color to the skin or eyes or dark-colored urine
- Severe abdominal pain
- Vaginal bleeding

☐ Carry an identification card indicating that you are taking this medicine. Always tell your pharmacist, dentist, and other doctors who are treating you that you are taking this medicine.

*   *   *   *   *

Piprobroman (*Oral Antineoplastic*)
United States: Vercyte
Canada: Vercyte

☐ This medicine is used in certain medical conditions to help slow down the growth and reproduction of some of the body's cells.

HOW TO USE THIS MEDICINE

☐ It is best to take this medicine 1 hour before breakfast or 2 hours after supper in order to help prevent nausea or vomiting.

☐ It is very important that you take this medicine exactly as your doctor has prescribed and that you do not miss any doses. Try to take this medicine at the same time every day.

☐ Even if you become nauseated or lose your appetite, do not stop taking the medicine but check with your doctor.

☐ If you miss a dose of this medicine, do not take the missed dose and do not double your next dose. Check with your doctor.

SPECIAL INSTRUCTIONS

☐ Always keep your doctor appointments so that your doctor can watch your progress.

☐ If your doctor has prescribed some other medicines for you, it is important that you take them in the right order and that you do not miss them.

☐ Always tell your pharmacist, dentist, and any other doctors who are treating you that you are taking this medicine. This is especially important if you plan to have surgery or any vaccinations.

☐ Men and women should take appropriate birth control measures to avoid conception while taking this medicine.

☐ This is a very strong medicine. In addition to its benefits, there may be some unwanted effects, even for a short time after you stop taking the medicine.

Call your doctor if you develop unusual bruising or bleeding, black tarry stools, sore throat, fever, stomach cramps or severe diarrhea, or a persistent skin rash.

* * * * *

Pizotyline (*Oral Vascular Headache Therapy*)
Canada: Sandomigran

☐ This medicine is used to treat migraine headaches and certain types of vascular headaches.

HOW TO USE THIS MEDICINE
☐ Take the medicine with a glass of water.

☐ If you forget to take a dose, take it as soon as possible. However, if it is almost time for your next dose, do not take the missed dose. Instead, continue with your regular dosing schedule.

SPECIAL INSTRUCTIONS
☐ In some people, this drug may cause dizziness or drowsiness. Do not drive a car or operate dangerous machinery or do jobs that require you to be alert until you know how you are going to react to this drug.

☐ If you become dizzy, you should be careful going up and down stairs. Sit or lie down at the first sign of dizziness.

☐ If your mouth becomes dry, suck a hard sour candy (sugarless) or ice chips, or chew gum. It is especially important to brush your teeth regularly if you develop a dry mouth.

☐ Do not drink alcoholic beverages while taking this drug without the approval of your doctor.

☐ It is important that you obtain the advice of your doctor before taking pain relievers, nonprescription drugs, sleeping pills, tranquilizers, or medicines for depression while you are taking this drug.

☐ Most people experience few or no side effects from their drugs. However, any medicine can sometimes cause unwanted effects. Call your doctor if you develop eye pain, sudden weight gain, difficulty in urinating ("passing your water"), or fast heartbeats.

☐ Do not take any more of this medicine than your doctor has prescribed, and do not stop taking this medicine suddenly without the approval of your doctor.

* * * * *

Polymyxin-Bacitracin (*Topical Antibiotic*)
United States: Polysporin Ointment
Canada: Polysporin Ointment

Polymyxin-Gramicidin
Canada: Polysporin Cream

☐ This medicine is an antibiotic used to treat infections of the skin.

HOW TO USE THIS MEDICINE
- Each time you apply the medicine, wash your hands and gently cleanse the skin area well with water unless otherwise directed by your doctor. Do not allow the skin to dry completely. Pat with a clean towel until almost dry.
- Apply a small amount of the drug to the affected area and spread lightly. Only the medicine that is actually touching the skin will work. A thick layer is not more effective than a thin layer. Do not bandage unless directed by your doctor.

☐ Do not use the drug more frequently or in larger quantities than prescribed by your doctor.

SPECIAL INSTRUCTIONS
☐ It is important to use **all** of this medicine, plus any refills that your doctor told you to use. Do not stop using it earlier than your doctor has recommended in spite of the fact that your symptoms seem to have improved. Otherwise, the infection may return.

☐ If you forget to apply the medicine, apply it as soon as possible. However, if it is almost time for your next dose, do not apply the missed dose but continue with your regular schedule.

☐ Do not apply cosmetics or lotions on top of the drug unless your doctor approves.

☐ Keep this preparation away from the eyes. If you should accidentally get some in your eyes, wash it away with water immediately.

☐ Call your doctor if the condition for which this drug is being used persists or becomes worse or if you develop a constant irritation such as itching or burning that was not present before you started using this medicine.

☐ For external use only. Do not swallow.

* * * * *

Polymyxin B-Gramicidin (*Eye-Ear Antibiotic*)
Canada: Polysporin Eye/Ear Drops

671

Polymyxin B–Neomycin–Combinations
United States: Mycitracin, Neo-Polycin, Neosporin, Neotal, Poly-spectrin Ophthalmic Ointment, Pyocidin

Canada: Neosporin Eye and Ear Solution

Polymyxin B Sulfate
United States: Aerosporin Sterile, Aerosporin Otic Solution

Canada: Aerosporin

☐ This medicine is an antibiotic used to treat certain types of eye and ear infections.

☐ IMPORTANT: If you have ever had an allergic reaction to neomycin or any antibiotic medicines, tell your doctor or pharmacist before you use any of this drug.

HOW TO USE THIS MEDICINE
☐ For EYE DROPS

INSTILLATION OF EYE DROPS

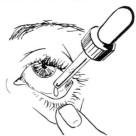

- The person administering the eye drops should wash his hands with soap and water.
- The eye drops must be kept clean. Do not touch the dropper against the face or anything else.
- Lie down or tilt your head backward and look at the ceiling.
- Gently pull down the lower lid of your eye to form a pouch.
- Hold the dropper in your other hand and approach the eye from the side. Place the dropper as close to the eye as possible without touching it.
- Place the prescribed number of drops into the pouch of the eye.
- Close your eyes. Do not rub them.
- Apply gentle pressure for a minute with your fingers to the bridge of the nose (inside corner of the eye) to prevent the eye drops from being drained from the eye.
- Blot excess solution around the eye with a tissue.
- If necessary, have someone else administer the eye drops for you.
- Do not use the eye drops if they have changed in color or have changed in any way since you purchased them.
- Keep the eye drop bottle tightly closed when not in use.

672

☐ For EYE OINTMENT

INSTILLATION OF EYE OINTMENT

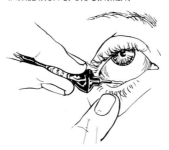

- The person administering the eye ointment should wash his hands with soap and water.
- The eye ointment must be kept clean. Do not touch the tube against the face or anything else.
- Lie down or tilt your head backward and look at the ceiling.
- Gently pull down the lower lid of your eye to form a pouch.
- Hold the tube in your other hand and place the tube as close as possible to the eye without touching it.
- Squeeze the prescribed amount of ointment (usually $\frac{1}{2}$ inch in adults) from the tube along the pouch.
- Close your eyes. Do not rub them.
- Wipe off any excess ointment around the eye with a tissue.
- Clean the tip of the ointment tube with a tissue.
- If necessary, have someone else administer the eye ointment for you.
- Keep the eye ointment tube tightly closed when not in use.

☐ For EAR DROPS

INSTILLATION OF EAR DROPS

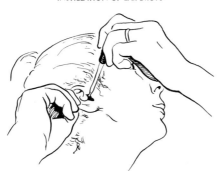

- Warm the ear drops to body temperature by holding the bottle in your hands for a few minutes. Do NOT heat the drops in hot water.
- The person administering the ear drops should wash his hands with soap and water.

673

- The ear drops must be kept clean. Do not touch the dropper against the ear or anything else.
- Tilt your head or lie on your side so that the ear to be treated is facing up.
- In ADULTS, hold the ear lobe up and back.
  In CHILDREN, hold the ear lobe down and back.
- Place the prescribed number of drops into the ear. Do not insert the dropper into the ear as it may cause injury.
- Remain in the same position for a short time (2 minutes) after you have administered the drops.
  - Dry the ear lobe if there are any drops on it.
- If necessary, have someone else administer the ear drops for you.
- Do not use the ear drops if they have changed in color or have changed in any way since you purchased them.
- Keep the bottle tightly closed when not in use.

SPECIAL INSTRUCTIONS

☐ Vision may be blurred for a few minutes after using the eye medicine. Do not drive a car or operate dangerous machinery or do jobs that require you to be alert until your vision has cleared.

☐ It is important to use *all* of this medicine, plus any refills that your doctor told you to use. Do not stop using it earlier than your doctor has recommended in spite of the fact that your symptoms seem to have improved. Otherwise, the infection may return.

☐ If you forget to use the medicine, use it as soon as possible. However, if it is almost time for your next dose, do not use the missed dose but continue with your regular schedule.

☐ Do not use this medicine at the same time as any other eye or ear medicine without the approval of your doctor. Some medicines cannot be mixed.

☐ Call your doctor if the condition for which you are using this medicine persists or becomes worse or if the medicine causes itching or burning for more than a few minutes after instillation.

☐ For external use only. Do not swallow.

*   *   *   *   *

Polythiazide (*Oral Diuretic-Antihypertensive*)
United States: Renese
Canada: Renese

☐ This medicine is used to help rid the body of excess water and to decrease swelling. It is also used to treat high blood pressure. It is commonly called a "water pill."

674

☐ IMPORTANT: If you have ever had an allergic reaction to sulfa drugs or thiazide diuretics, tell your doctor or pharmacist before taking any of this medicine.

HOW TO USE THIS MEDICINE

☐ Take the medicine with food, meals, or milk.

☐ Try to take it at the same time(s) every day so that you have a constant level of the medicine in your body. Do not miss any doses. Otherwise, you cannot expect the drug to work as well.

☐ When you first start taking this medicine, you will probably urinate ("pass your water") more often and in larger amounts than usual. Therefore, if you are to take one dose every day, take it in the morning after breakfast. If you are to take more than one dose every day, take the last dose 6 hours before bedtime so that you will not have to get up during the night to go to the bathroom. This effect will usually lessen after you have taken the drug for awhile.

SPECIAL INSTRUCTIONS

☐ If you forget to take a dose, take it as soon as possible. However, if it is almost time for your next dose, do not take the missed dose. Instead, continue with your regular dosing schedule.

☐ Women who are pregnant, breast-feeding, or planning to become pregnant should tell their doctor before taking this medicine.

☐ This medicine normally causes your body to lose potassium. The body has warning signs to let you know if too much potassium is being lost. Call your doctor if you become unusually thirsty or if you develop leg cramps, unusual weakness, fatigue, vomiting, confusion, or irregular pulse.

☐ If your doctor recommends that you eat foods which are high in potassium, one or more of the foods listed in Appendix A should be eaten daily. All of these foods are rich in potassium. Your goal should be to take in 1000 to 2000 mg. of potassium (approximately 25.6 to 51 mEq) each day. The calorie content and sodium content are included for your convenience in meal planning. CHANGE YOUR DIET ONLY IF YOUR DOCTOR TELLS YOU TO.

☐ If this medicine causes dizziness, you should be careful going up and down stairs and you should not change positions too rapidly. Get out of bed slowly in the morning and dangle your feet over the edge of the bed for a few minutes before standing up. Sit down or lie down at the first sign of dizziness. Tell your doctor you have been dizzy. Be careful drinking alcoholic beverages while taking this medicine because they could make the dizziness worse. Do not drive a car or operate dangerous machinery or do jobs that require you to be alert if you are dizzy.

☐ In order to help prevent dizziness and fainting, your doctor may also recom-

675

mend that you avoid strenuous exercises, standing for long periods of time (especially in hot weather), or hot showers or hot baths.

☐ This medicine may make some people more sensitive to sunlight and sun-lamps. When you begin taking this medicine, try to avoid getting too much sun until you see how you are going to react. If your skin does become more sensitive to sunlight, tell your doctor and try to stay out of direct sunlight. While in the sun, wear protective clothing and sunglasses. You may wish to ask your pharmacist about suitable sunscreen products. Check with your doctor if you become sunburned.

☐ Call your doctor immediately if you think you may be allergic to the medicine or if you develop a skin rash, hives, itching, swelling of the face, or difficulty in breathing. If you cannot reach your doctor, phone a hospital emergency department.

☐ Most people experience few or no side effects from their drugs. However, any medicine can sometimes cause unwanted effects. Call your doctor if you develop a sore throat, fever, sharp stomach pain, chest pain, sharp joint pain, easy bruising or bleeding, a yellow color to the skin or eyes, or a sudden weight gain of 5 pounds or more.

*   *   *   *   *

Potassium Chloride (*Oral Potassium Supplement*)

United States: K-10, Kaochlor Concentrate, Kaochlor 10%, Kaochlor S-F, Kato Powder, Kay Ciel, KEFF, Klor, Klor-Con, K-Lor Powder, K-Lyte, K-Lyte/CL, Kolyum Liquid, Klorvess, Kaochlor Eff, Pan-Cloride, Rum-K.

Canada: Kaochlor, Kaochlor-20 Concentrate, Kay Ciel Elixir, K-Lyte, K-Lyte/CL, Slow-K

Potassium Gluconate

United States: Kaon, Kao-Nor, Kaylixir

Canada: Kaon, Potassium Rougier

☐ This medicine is a potassium supplement.

HOW TO USE THIS MEDICINE

☐ Take this medicine immediately after meals or with some food to help pre-vent stomach upset.

☐ For LIQUID MEDICINE
  • Dilute the medicine with a glass of water, orange juice, or tomato juice. Do not use tomato juice if you are on a low-salt diet.
  • Dissolve the medicine in a glass of water. Let the bubbles subside before swallowing the solution. Sip slowly over a period of 5 to 10

676

minutes. (**United States:** K-Lyte, K-Lyte/CL, Kaochlor Eff, KEFF, Klorvess; **Canada:** K-Lyte)

- This medicine must be swallowed whole. Do not crush, chew, or break it into pieces. (**United States** and **Canada:** Slow-K)

SPECIAL INSTRUCTIONS

☐ If you forget to take a dose, take it as soon as possible. However, if your next dose is within 2 hours, do not take the missed dose but continue with your regular schedule.

☐ It is very important that you take this medicine exactly as your doctor has prescribed and that you do not miss any doses. Try to take this medicine at the same time every day. Do not take extra tablets without your doctor's approval.

☐ Do not use salt substitutes or low-salt foods without the permission of your doctor. These products may contain potassium.

☐ Do not take laxatives without the permission of your doctor.

☐ Most people experience few or no side effects from their drugs. However, any medicine can sometimes cause unwanted effects. Call your doctor if you develop severe stomach pain, black stools, a feeling of heaviness in the legs, tingling of the hands or feet, unusual weakness, or irregular heartbeats.

*   *   *   *   *

Povidone-Iodine (*Topical Antiseptic*)

United States: Betadine, Efodine, Isodine, Pharmadine
Canada: Betadine, Bridine, Proviodine

☐ This medicine is an antiseptic used for:
1. AEROSOL SPRAY: skin infections or minor wounds and burns
2. SHAMPOO: dandruff, itching, or scaling of the scalp
3. SKIN CLEANSER: various skin infections
4. SOLUTION: infections

☐ IMPORTANT: If you have ever had an allergic reaction to iodine medicine, tell your doctor or pharmacist before you use any of this drug.

HOW TO USE THIS MEDICINE

☐ For AEROSOL SPRAY
- Cleanse the affected area well with water. Spray the area thoroughly as needed.
- Do not place the medicine container in hot water or near radiators, stoves, or other sources of heat. Do not puncture or incinerate the container (even when empty). Do not store at temperatures greater than 120°F (49°C).

677

☐ For MOUTHWASH
- Gargle for 30 seconds with the mouthwash full strength or dilute as recommended by your doctor or dentist. Do *not* swallow.

☐ For SHAMPOO
- Apply 2 teaspoonfuls of shampoo to hair and scalp, using warm water to form lather. Rinse and repeat, massaging gently into the scalp. Allow lather to remain on your scalp for at least 5 minutes. Work up lather again, then rinse thoroughly. Repeat treatment twice a week for 6 to 8 weeks; then once a week or as directed by your doctor.

☐ For SKIN CLEANSER
- Wet the skin and apply a sufficient amount of liquid to cover the affected areas. Massage for 5 minutes, add a little water, and continue to work up a lather; then rinse thoroughly.

SPECIAL INSTRUCTIONS

☐ If this medicine should stain **synthetic fabrics,** these stains can be removed by washing and rinsing in dilute ammonia. If it should stain **starched linens,** these stains can be removed by washing in soap and water.

☐ Call your doctor if the condition for which this drug is being used persists or becomes worse or if you develop a constant irritation such as itching or burning that was not present before you started using this medicine.

☐ Keep this preparation away from the eyes. If you should accidentally get some in your eyes, wash it away with water immediately.

☐ For external use only. Do not swallow.

* * * * *

Povidone-Iodine (*Vaginal Antiseptic*)
United States: Betadine
Canada: Betadine, Bridine, Proviodine

☐ This medicine is an antiseptic used to treat vaginal infections.

☐ IMPORTANT: If you have ever had an allergic reaction to iodine medicine, tell your doctor or pharmacist before you use any of this drug.

HOW TO USE THIS MEDICINE

☐ For VAGINAL DOUCHE
- Prepare the solution as directed by your doctor.
- Transfer the solution into the bulb of the syringe or douching bag, which has been hung 3 or 4 feet above the level of the toilet seat or bathtub.
- Lie in the bathtub with hips elevated, or sit on the toilet seat, and insert the nozzle into the vaginal canal.

- Squeeze the bulb of the syringe slowly and steadily or turn the stopcock to permit the fluid to flow into the vaginal canal.

☐ For VAGINAL GEL
- Remove the cap from the tube of medicine.
- Screw the applicator to the tube.
- Squeeze the tube until the applicator plunger is fully extended. (The applicator will now be filled with medicine.)
- Unscrew the applicator from the tube of medicine.
- Hold the applicator by the cylinder and gently insert it into the vaginal canal, as far as it will comfortably go.
- While still holding the cylinder, press the plunger gently to deposit the medicine.
- While keeping the plunger depressed, remove the applicator from the vaginal canal.
- After *each* use, take the applicator apart. Wash with warm water and soap and rinse thoroughly. Reassemble the applicator.

☐ For VAGINAL SUPPOSITORIES
- Remove the wrapper from the suppository. Dip the suppository in water quickly just to moisten it.
- Gently insert the smaller end into the applicator.
- In a reclining position, with knees bent, insert the applicator into the vaginal canal and deposit the suppository by pressing the plunger into the applicator tube.
- Remove the applicator from the vaginal canal.
- After each use, take the applicator apart and wash thoroughly with warm water and soap. Rinse well and reassemble the applicator.

SPECIAL INSTRUCTIONS

☐ ***Caution:*** The vaginal products should not be used if pregnancy is desired. If you have used a vaginal contraceptive (for example, foam or cream), do not douche or use a Betadine suppository for at least 6 hours after intercourse.

☐ If this medicine should stain ***synthetic fabrics,*** these stains can be removed by washing and rinsing in dilute ammonia. If this medicine should stain ***starched linens,*** these stains can be removed by washing in soap and water.

☐ Store at room temperature. (***Canada:*** Betadine Vaginal Suppositories)

☐ Call your doctor if the condition for which this drug is being used persists or becomes worse or if you develop a constant irritation such as itching or burning that was not present before you started using this medicine.

☐ Keep this preparation away from the eyes. If you should accidentally get some in your eyes, wash it away with water immediately.

* * * * *

Pramoxine HCl (*Rectal Topical Anesthetic*)
Canada: Tronothane

☐ This medicine is used to help relieve pain and itching of certain rectal skin conditions.

HOW TO USE THIS MEDICINE
☐ For RECTAL OINTMENT
- Lie on your side and raise your knee to your chest.
- Gently insert the tip or rubber tubing attached to the ointment tube into the rectum.
- Squeeze the prescribed amount of ointment from the tube.
- Withdraw the rectal tip from the rectum.
- Try to avoid having a bowel movement for at least 1 hour so that the drug can be effective.
- Clean the tip of the tubing with warm water and soap after each use.

☐ Do not use the drug more frequently, in larger quantities, or for a longer period of time than prescribed by your doctor.

SPECIAL INSTRUCTIONS
☐ Call your doctor if the condition for which this drug is being used persists or becomes worse or if you have a constant irritation such as itching or burning that was not present before you started using this medicine. Also call your doctor if you develop new rectal bleeding.

☐ For external use only. Do not swallow.

* * * * *

Pramoxine HCl (*Topical Anesthetic*)
United States: Tronothane
Canada: Tronothane

☐ This medicine is used to help relieve pain and itching of the skin.

HOW TO USE THIS MEDICINE
☐ For CREAM and JELLY
- Each time you apply the medicine, wash your hands and gently cleanse the skin area well with water unless otherwise directed by your doctor. Do not allow the skin to dry completely. Pat with a clean towel until almost dry.
- Apply a small amount of the drug to the affected area and spread lightly. Only the medicine that is actually touching the skin will work. A thick layer is not more effective than a thin layer. Do not bandage unless directed by your doctor.

680

☐ Do not use the drug more frequently, in larger quantities, or for a longer period of time than prescribed by your doctor.

SPECIAL INSTRUCTIONS

☐ If you have a severe sunburn, you should consult with your doctor before using this medicine.

☐ Call your doctor if the condition for which this drug is being used persists or becomes worse or if you have a constant irritation such as itching or burning that was not present before you started using this medicine.

☐ For external use only. Do not swallow.

* * * * *

Prazepam (*Oral Anxiolytic-Sedative*)
United States: Verstran

☐ This medicine is used to help relieve anxiety as well as to treat some other conditions. Check with your doctor if you do not fully understand why you are taking it.

☐ IMPORTANT: If you have ever had an allergic reaction to a benzodiazepine medicine, tell your doctor or pharmacist before you take any of this medicine.

HOW TO USE THIS MEDICINE

☐ This medicine may be taken with food or a full glass of water.

SPECIAL INSTRUCTIONS

☐ If you forget to take a dose, take it as soon as possible. However, if it is almost time for your next dose, do not take the missed dose. Instead, continue with your regular dosing schedule.

☐ Women who are pregnant, breast-feeding, or planning to become pregnant should tell their doctor before taking this medicine.

☐ In some people, this drug may cause dizziness or drowsiness. Do not drive a car or operate dangeous machinery or do jobs that require you to be alert until you know how you are going to react to this drug.

☐ If you become dizzy, you should be careful going up and down stairs. Sit or lie down at the first sign of dizziness.

☐ Do not drink alcoholic beverages while taking this drug without the approval of your doctor.

☐ It is important that you obtain the advice of your doctor or pharmacist before taking ANY other medicines including pain relievers, sleeping pills, tranquilizers or medicines for depression, cough/cold or allergy medicines, or weight-reducing medicines.

☐ Do not take any more of this medicine than your doctor has prescribed. The drug could become habit-forming. Do not stop taking this medicine suddenly without the approval of your doctor.

☐ Most people experience few or no side effects from their drugs. However, any medicine can sometimes cause unwanted effects. Call your doctor if you develop a sore throat, fever, mouth sores, a staggering walk, a yellow color to the skin or eyes, slow heartbeats or shortness of breath, unusual tiredness or nervousness, or stomach pain.

* * * * *

Prazosin (*Oral Antihypertensive*)
United States: Minipress
Canada: Minipress

☐ This medicine is used to lower the blood pressure.

☐ Hypertension (high blood pressure) is a long-term condition, and it will probably be necessary for you to take the drug for a long time in spite of the fact that you feel better. It is very important that you take this medicine as your doctor has directed and that you do not miss any doses. Otherwise, you cannot expect the drug to keep your blood pressure down.

HOW TO USE THIS MEDICINE
☐ Take the very first dose of this medicine at bedtime.

☐ Try to take the medicine at the same time(s) every day.

SPECIAL INSTRUCTIONS
☐ If you forget to take a dose, take it as soon as possible. However, if it is almost time for your next dose, do not take the missed dose. Instead, continue with your regular dosing schedule.

☐ Women who are pregnant, breast-feeding, or planning to become pregnant should tell their doctor before taking this medicine.

☐ In some people, this medicine may cause dizziness, drowsiness, or headache (especially during the first few days of therapy). Do not drive a car or operate dangerous machinery or do jobs that require you to be alert until you know how you are going to react to this drug.

☐ If you become dizzy, you should be careful going up and down stairs and you should not change positions too rapidly. Get out of bed slowly in the morning and dangle your feet over the edge of the bed for a few minutes before standing up. Sit or lie down at the first sign of dizziness. Tell your doctor you have been dizzy. He may also want you to avoid strenuous exercises, standing for long periods of time (especially in hot weather), hot showers, and hot baths.

- [ ] Follow any special diet your doctor may have ordered. He may want you to limit the amount of salt in your food.

- [ ] If your mouth becomes dry, suck a hard sour candy (sugarless) or ice chips, or chew gum. It is especially important to brush your teeth regularly if you develop a dry mouth.

- [ ] Some nonprescription drugs can aggravate your condition. Do not take any of the following without the approval of your doctor or pharmacist: cough, cold, or sinus products; asthma or allergy products; or diet or weight-reducing medicines.

- [ ] Most people experience few or no side effects from their drugs. However, any medicine can sometimes cause unwanted effects. Call your doctor if you develop a skin rash, fainting, fast heartbeats, swelling of the legs or ankles, sudden weight gain of 5 pounds or more, chest pains, or difficulty in breathing.

- [ ] Carry an identification card indicating that you are taking this medicine. Always tell your pharmacist, dentist, and other doctors who are treating you that you are taking this medicine.

- [ ] Do not stop taking this medicine without your doctor's approval and do not go without medicine between prescription refills. Call your pharmacist 2 or 3 days before you will run out of the medicine.

*   *   *   *   *

Prednisolone (*Ophthalmic Corticosteroid*)

United States: Econopred, Hydeltrasol, Hydrocortone, Inflamase, Metreton, Pred Forte, Pred Mild, Predulose

Canada: Inflamase, Pred Forte, Pred Mild, Prednicon

- [ ] This medicine is used to help relieve the pain, redness, and itching of certain types of eye conditions.

HOW TO USE THIS MEDICINE
- [ ] For EYE DROPS

INSTILLATION OF EYE DROPS

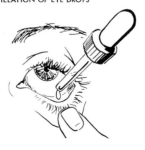

- The person administering the eye drops should wash his hands with soap and water.
- The eye drops must be kept clean. Do not touch the dropper against the face or anything else.
- Lie down or tilt your head backward and look at the ceiling.
- Shake the bottle well before using. (**United States:** Econopred, Hydrocortone, Pred Forte, Pred Mild, Predulose; **Canada:** Pred Forte, Pred Mild, Prednicon)
- Gently pull down the lower lid of your eye to form a pouch.
- Hold the dropper in your other hand and approach the eye from the side. Place the dropper as close to the eye as possible without touching it.
- Place the prescribed number of drops into the pouch of the eye.
- Close your eyes. Do not rub them.
- Apply gentle pressure for a minute with your fingers to the bridge of the nose (inside corner of the eye) to prevent the eye drops from being drained from the eye.
- Blot excess solution around the eye with a tissue.

☐ If necessary, have someone else administer the eye drops for you.

☐ Do not use the eye drops if they have changed in color or have changed in any way since you purchased them.

☐ Keep the eye drop bottle tightly closed when not in use.

SPECIAL INSTRUCTIONS

☐ This medicine should be used as long as prescribed by your doctor. Do not stop using it earlier than your doctor has recommended in spite of the fact that your symptoms seem to have improved.

☐ If you forget to use the medicine, use it as soon as possible. However, if it is almost time for your next dose, do not use the missed dose but continue with your regular schedule.

☐ Do not use this medicine at the same time as any other eye medicine without the approval of your doctor. Some medicines cannot be mixed.

☐ Contact your doctor if the condition for which you are using this medicine does not improve or if the eye becomes irritated by it for more than a few minutes. Many eye medicines sting for a short time immediately after use.

☐ For external use only. Do not swallow.

☐ Store in a cool dark place.

*　*　*　*　*

684

Prednisolone (*Oral Corticosteroid*)

United States: Delta-Cortef, Fernisolone-P, Predoxine, Sterane
Canada: Delta-Cortef

☐ This medicine is similar to cortisone which is a hormone normally produced by the body. This medicine is used to help decrease inflammation; this then relieves pain, redness, and swelling. It is used in the treatment of certain kinds of arthritis, severe allergies, or skin conditions.

HOW TO USE THIS MEDICINE

☐ Take this medicine with food or a glass of milk in order to help prevent stomach upset. Call your doctor if you develop stomach upset or stomach pain or heartburn (especially if it awakens you during the night). Do not try to treat this yourself.

☐ If your doctor has prescribed only ONE dose of this medicine every day, it is best to take it before 9 A.M. or with breakfast.

☐ If you forget to take a dose, take it as soon as possible. However, if it is almost time for your next dose, do not take the missed dose. Instead, continue with your regular dosing schedule.

SPECIAL INSTRUCTIONS

☐ Women who are pregnant, breast-feeding, or planning to become pregnant should tell their doctor before taking this medicine.

☐ It is best not to drink alcoholic beverages while you are taking this medicine because the combination can cause stomach problems.

☐ Do not take any more of this medicine than your doctor has prescribed and do not stop taking this medicine suddenly without the approval of your doctor. It may be necessary for your doctor to slowly reduce your dose since your body becomes used to this medicine and it might be harmful if you suddenly did not receive this medicine.

☐ Do not take aspirin or medicines containing aspirin without the approval of your doctor.

☐ While you are taking this medicine you may gain some weight. This could be due to an increase in your appetite or to increased water in your system. Your doctor may prescribe a special diet to decrease the number of calories you eat and/or to lower the amount of sodium or to increase the amount of potassium in your diet. Follow any diet that your doctor may order.

☐ You may find that you bruise more easily. Try to protect yourself from all injuries to prevent bruising.

☐ Diabetic patients should regularly check the sugar in their urine and report any unusual levels to their doctor.

☐ Carry an identification card indicating that you are taking this medicine. Always tell your pharmacist, dentist, and other doctors who are treating you that you are taking this medicine. If you have an acute infection, an injury, an operation, or dental surgery within 1 year of taking this medicine, it is important to tell your doctor.

☐ Most people experience few or no side effects from their drugs. However, any medicine can sometimes cause unwanted effects. Call your doctor if you develop stomach pain, sore throat, fever, swelling of the legs or ankles, a wound which does not heal, eye pain or blurred vision, frequent urination ("passing your water"), nightmares or depression, muscle cramps, red or black stools, puffing of the face, or menstrual problems.

* * * * *

Prednisolone (*Topical Corticosteroid*)
United States: Meti-Derm

☐ This medicine is used to help relieve redness, swelling, itching, and inflammation of certain types of skin conditions.

HOW TO USE THIS MEDICINE
☐ For CREAM and OINTMENT
- Each time you apply the medicine, wash your hands and gently cleanse the skin area well with water unless otherwise directed by your doctor. Do not allow the skin to dry completely. Pat with a clean towel until almost dry.
- Apply a small amount of the drug to the affected area and spread lightly. Only the medicine that is actually touching the skin will work. A thick layer is not more effective than a thin layer. Do not bandage unless directed by your doctor.

☐ For AEROSOL
- Shake the container well each time before using.
- Cleanse the affected area well with water unless otherwise directed by your doctor.
- Hold the container straight up and about 6 to 8 inches away from the skin.
- Spray the affected area for 1 to 3 seconds.
- Shake the container well between sprays.
- Do not spray into the eyes, nose, or mouth and try to avoid inhaling the vapors.
- Do not smoke while using this spray or use near an open flame, fire, or heat. Do not use the spray near food.

☐ Do not use the drug more frequently or in larger quantities than prescribed by your doctor. Overuse of this medicine may cause you to absorb too much of the drug and increase the risk of side effects.

☐ Keep the medicine away from the eyes, nose, and mouth.

686

SPECIAL INSTRUCTIONS

☐ If you forget to apply the medicine, apply it as soon as possible. However, if it is almost time for your next dose, do not apply the missed dose but continue with your regular schedule.

☐ Do not use this medicine for any other skin problems without checking with your doctor.

☐ Do not apply cosmetics or lotions on top of the drug unless your doctor approves.

☐ Call your doctor if the condition for which this drug is being used persists or becomes worse or if you have a constant irritation such as itching or burning that was not present before you started using this medicine. Also call your doctor if you develop abnormal lines or thinning of the skin, especially under the arms or between the legs.

☐ Store in a cool place but do not freeze.

☐ For external use only. Do not swallow.

☐ Do not place the aerosol container in hot water or near radiators, stoves, or other sources of heat. Do not puncture or incinerate the container (even when empty). Do not store at temperatures greater than 120°F (49°C).

☐ Tell future doctors that you have used this medicine.

* * * * *

Prednisolone-Sulfacetamide (*Ophthalmic Anti-inflammatory–Anti-infective*)

United States: Blephamide Ophthalmic, Blephamide S.O.P., Cetapred, Isopto-Cetapred, Metimyd, Optimyd

Canada: Blephamide Ointment, Isopto-Cetapred, Metimyd

☐ This medicine is used to help relieve the pain, redness, and itching of certain types of eye infections.

HOW TO USE THIS MEDICINE

☐ For EYE OINTMENT

INSTILLATION OF EYE OINTMENT

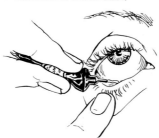

- The person administering the eye ointment should wash his hands with soap and water.
- The eye ointment must be kept clean. Do not touch the tube against the face or anything else.
- Lie down or tilt your head backward and look at the ceiling.
- Gently pull down the lower lid of your eye to form a pouch.
- Hold the tube in your other hand and place the tube as close as possible to the eye without touching it.
- Squeeze the prescribed amount of ointment (usually $\frac{1}{2}$ inch in adults) from the tube along the pouch.
- Close your eyes. Do not rub them.
- Wipe off any excess ointment around the eye with a tissue.
- Clean the tip of the ointment tube with a tissue.

☐ If necessary, have someone else administer the eye ointment for you.

☐ Keep the eye ointment tube tightly closed when not in use.

☐ Do not use this drug more frequently or in larger quantities than prescribed by your doctor.

SPECIAL INSTRUCTIONS

☐ It is important to use **all** of this medicine, plus any refills that your doctor told you to use. Do not stop using it earlier than your doctor has recommended in spite of the fact that your symptoms seem to have improved. Otherwise, the infection may return.

☐ If you forget to apply the medicine, apply it as soon as possible. However, if it is almost time for your next dose, do not apply the missed dose but continue with your regular schedule.

☐ Do not use this medicine at the same time as any other eye medicine without the approval of your doctor. Some medicines cannot be mixed.

☐ Vision may be blurred for a few minutes after using the eye medicine. Do not drive a car or operate dangerous machinery or do jobs that require you to be alert until your vision has cleared.

☐ Contact your doctor if the condition for which you are using this medicine does not improve or if the eye becomes irritated by it for more than a few minutes. Many eye medicines sting for a short time immediately after use.

☐ For external use only. Do not swallow.

*   *   *   *   *

Prednisolone-Sulfacetamide-Phenylephrine Compound
(Ophthalmic Antibacterial-Anti-inflammatory)

United States: Blephamide Liquifilm

Canada: Blephamide Liquifilm

☐ This medicine is used to treat eye conditions.

688

HOW TO USE THIS MEDICINE

☐ Do *not* use if the solution is discolored.

☐ Instructions for use (*in the eye and on the lid*):

- Cleanse the eyelids and eyelashes with a tissue if necessary. Wash your hands carefully.
- Open the eye and tilt your head backward.
- Gently pull down the lower lid to form a pouch.
- Approach the eye from the side and hold the dropper near the lid, but *do not* touch eyelids and/or eyelashes.
- Allow the prescribed number of drops to fall into the pouch.
- Close the eye and spread the excess medicine present after closing the eye over the full length of the upper and lower lids.
- Do *not* wipe any of the medicine off the lids. It will dry completely in 4 or 5 minutes to a clear film that remains on the lid for several hours.
- The medicine should be washed off the lids once or twice a day. It should be reapplied after each washing.

☐ Instructions for use (*on the lid*):

- Wash your hands carefully. With your head tilted back and eye *closed,* drop the medicine onto the lid, preferably at the corner of the eye close to the nose.
- Spread the medicine over the full length of the upper and lower lids.
- Do not wipe away any medicine; it will dry in 4 or 5 minutes to a clear invisible film that will remain on the lids for several hours.
- The medicine should be washed off the lids once or twice a day. However, it should be reapplied after washing.

☐ Do not use this drug more frequently or in larger quantities than prescribed by your doctor.

SPECIAL INSTRUCTIONS

☐ This medicine should be used as long as prescribed by your doctor. Do not stop using it earlier than your doctor has recommended in spite of the fact that your symptoms seem to have improved.

☐ If you forget to use the medicine, use it as soon as possible. However, if it is almost time for your next dose, do not use the missed dose but continue with your regular schedule.

☐ Do not use this medicine at the same time as any other eye medicine without the approval of your doctor. Some medicines cannot be mixed.

☐ Contact your doctor if the condition for which you are using this medicine does not improve or if the eye becomes irritated by it for more than a few minutes. Many eye medicines sting for a short time immediately after use.

☐ For external use only. Do not swallow.

* * * * *

Prednisone *(Oral Corticosteroid)*

United States: Deltasone, Meticorten, Orasone, Paracort, SK-Prednisone

Canada: Colisone, Deltasone, Paracort, Winpred

☐ This medicine is similar to cortisone which is a hormone normally produced by the body. This medicine is used to help decrease inflammation; this then relieves pain, redness, and swelling. It is used in the treatment of certain kinds of arthritis, severe allergies, or skin conditions.

HOW TO USE THIS MEDICINE

☐ Take this medicine with food or a glass of milk in order to help prevent stomach upset. Call your doctor if you develop stomach upset, stomach pain, or heartburn (especially if it awakens you during the night). Do not try to treat this yourself.

☐ If your doctor has prescribed only ONE dose of this medicine every day, it is best to take it before 9 A.M. or with breakfast.

☐ If you forget to take a dose, take it as soon as possible. However, if it is almost time for your next dose, do not take the missed dose. Instead, continue with your regular dosing schedule.

SPECIAL INSTRUCTIONS

☐ Women who are pregnant, breast-feeding, or planning to become pregnant should tell their doctor before taking this medicine.

☐ It is best not to drink alcoholic beverages while you are taking this medicine because the combination can cause stomach problems.

☐ Do not take any more of this medicine than your doctor has prescribed and do not stop taking this medicine suddenly without the approval of your doctor. It may be necessary for your doctor to slowly reduce your dose since your body becomes used to this medicine. It might be harmful if you suddenly did not receive this medicine.

☐ Do not take aspirin or medicines containing aspirin without the approval of your doctor.

☐ While you are taking this medicine you may gain some weight. This could be due to an increase in your appetite or to increased water in your system. Your doctor may prescribe a special diet to decrease the number of calories you eat, and/or to lower the amount of sodium, or to increase the amount of potassium in your diet. Follow any diet that your doctor may order.

☐ You may find that you bruise more easily. Try to protect yourself from all injuries to prevent bruising.

☐ Diabetic patients should regularly check the sugar in their urine and report any unusual levels to their doctor.

☐ Carry an identification card indicating that you are taking this medicine.

Always tell your pharmacist, dentist, and other doctors who are treating you that you are taking this medicine. If you have an acute infection, an injury, an operation, or dental surgery within 1 year of taking this medicine, it is important to tell your doctor.

☐ Most people experience few or no side effects from their drugs. However, any medicine can sometimes cause unwanted effects. Call your doctor if you develop stomach pain, sore throat, fever, swelling of the legs or ankles, a wound which does not heal, eye pain or blurred vision, frequent urination ("passing your water"), nightmares or depression, muscle cramps, red or black stools, puffing of the face, or menstrual problems.

*   *   *   *   *

Primaquine
United States: Primaquine Phosphate

☐ This medicine is an antimalarial used to treat and help prevent malaria.

HOW TO USE THIS MEDICINE
☐ Take this medicine immediately before or after meals or with food in order to help prevent stomach upset.

☐ It is very important that you take this medicine exactly as your doctor has prescribed and that you do not miss any doses. Try to take this medicine at the same time every day. Do not take extra tablets without your doctor's approval. Take the medicine for the full treatment.

SPECIAL INSTRUCTIONS
☐ If you forget to take a dose, take it as soon as possible. However, if it is almost time for your next dose, do not take the missed dose. Instead, continue with your regular dosing schedule.

☐ Women who are pregnant, breast-feeding, or planning to become pregnant should tell their doctor before taking this medicine.

☐ Most people experience few or no side effects from their drugs. However, any medicine can sometimes cause unwanted effects. Call your doctor if you develop reddening or darkening of the urine, fever, chills, stomach pain or chest pain, difficulty in breathing, unusual tiredness, or a decrease in the amount of urine you pass.

*   *   *   *   *

Primidone (Oral Anticonvulsant)
United States: Mysoline, Ro-Primidone
Canada: Mysoline, Sertan

☐ This medicine is used to help control convulsions and seizures. It is commonly used in the treatment of epilepsy.

☐ IMPORTANT: If you have ever had an allergic reaction to a barbiturate medicine, tell your doctor or pharmacist before you take any of this medicine.

HOW TO USE THIS MEDICINE

☐ Take this medicine with food or a full glass of water.

☐ For LIQUID MEDICINE
  • Shake the bottle well before using so that you can measure an accurate dose. (**United States** and **Canada:** Mysoline Suspension)

☐ It is very important that you take this medicine regularly and that you do not miss any dose. Try to take the medicine at the same time(s) every day. This is the only way that you can receive the full benefit of the medicine. If you forget to take this medicine, the amount of medicine in your blood will go down and you may have seizures.

SPECIAL INSTRUCTIONS

☐ If you forget to take a dose and remember it within 1 hour of the missed dose, take it and continue with your regular dosing schedule. Otherwise, do not take the missed dose at all.

☐ In some people, this drug may cause dizziness or drowsiness. Do not drive a car or operate dangerous machinery or do jobs that require you to be alert until you know how you are going to react to this drug.

☐ If you become dizzy, you should be careful going up and down stairs. Sit or lie down at the first sign of dizziness.

☐ If this medicine is for a child, do not let him (her) ride a bike or climb trees until you can determine how he (she) is going to react to the medicine. Children could hurt themselves if they participated in these activities when they were dizzy.

☐ Do not drink alcoholic beverages while taking this drug without the approval of your doctor.

☐ It is important that you obtain the advice of your doctor or pharmacist before taking ANY other medicines including pain relievers, sleeping pills, tranquilizers or medicines for depression, cough/cold medicines, or allergy medicines.

☐ Avoid swimming alone or taking part in high-risk sports in which a sudden seizure could cause injury.

☐ Women who are pregnant, breast-feeding, or planning to become pregnant should tell their doctor before taking this medicine.

☐ Call your doctor immediately if you think you may be allergic to the medicine or if you develop a skin rash, hives, itching, swelling of the face, or difficulty in breathing. If you cannot reach your doctor, phone a hospital emergency department.

- Most people experience few or no side effects from their drugs. However, any medicine can sometimes cause unwanted effects. Call your doctor if you develop a sore throat, nightmares, staggering walk, unusual nervousness or restlessness, or changes in vision.

- Do not stop taking this medicine suddenly without the approval of your doctor. Do not go without this medicine between prescription refills. Call your pharmacist 2 or 3 days before you will run out of the medicine.

- Carry an identification card indicating that you are taking this medicine. Always tell your pharmacist, dentist, and other doctors who are treating you that you are taking this medicine.

* * * * *

Probenecid (*Oral Uricosuric*)
United States: Benemid, Ro-Benecid
Canada: Benemid, Benuryl

- This medicine is used in the treatment of gout and other conditions in which the body has high levels of uric acid. It is sometimes used to make certain types of antibiotics more effective.

HOW TO USE THIS MEDICINE
- It is best to take this medicine with food or a glass of milk to help prevent stomach upset. Call your doctor if you continue to have stomach upset.

SPECIAL INSTRUCTIONS
- If you forget to take a dose, take it as soon as possible. However, if it is almost time for your next dose, do not take the missed dose. Instead, continue with your regular dosing schedule.

- It is very important that you take this medicine exactly as your doctor has prescribed and that you do not miss any doses. Otherwise, you cannot expect the medicine to help you.

- Try to drink at least 8 to 10 glasses of water or other liquids every day while you are taking this medicine unless otherwise directed.

- Do not take vitamin C, aspirin or salicylates, or alcohol while you are taking this medicine without the approval of your doctor.

- Call your doctor immediately if you think you may be allergic to the medicine or if you develop a skin rash, hives, itching, swelling of the face, or difficulty in breathing. If you cannot reach your doctor, phone a hospital emergency department.

- Most people experience few or no side effects from their drugs. However, any medicine can sometimes cause unwanted effects. Call your doctor if you develop a sore throat and fever, easy bruising or bleeding, blood in the urine, lower back pain, pain when you urinate ("pass your water"), dizziness, unusual tiredness, or weakness.

*　*　*　*　*

Probucol (*Oral Antilipemic*)
United States: Lorelco
Canada: Lorelco

☐ This medicine is used in certain types of conditions to lower the amount of cholesterol and triglycerides (fatty substances) in the blood.

HOW TO USE THIS MEDICINE
☐ Take this medicine with food or after meals.

SPECIAL INSTRUCTIONS
☐ If you forget to take a dose, take it as soon as possible. However, if it is almost time for your next dose, do not take the missed dose. Instead, continue with your regular dosing schedule.

☐ Women who are pregnant, breast-feeding, or planning to become pregnant should tell their doctor before taking this medicine.

☐ It is very important to follow any diet that your doctor may also prescribe for you. The cholesterol content of some common foods is listed in Appendix B.

☐ In some people, this drug may cause dizziness. Do not drive a car or operate dangerous machinery or do jobs that require you to be alert until you know how you are going to react to this drug. If you become dizzy, you should be careful going up and down stairs. Sit or lie down at the first sign of dizziness.

☐ In some people, this drug may cause diarrhea (loose bowel movements) which will usually disappear within a few days. Check with your doctor if the diarrhea continues.

☐ Do not take any more of this medicine than your doctor has prescribed and do not stop taking this medicine suddenly without the approval of your doctor.

☐ Most people experience few or no side effects from their drugs. However, any medicine can sometimes cause unwanted effects. Call your doctor if you develop a skin rash, rapid pulse, chest pain, fainting spells, easy bruising, sharp stomach pain, or tingling or numbness in your fingers or toes.

*　*　*　*　*

694

Procainamide HCl (*Oral Cardiac Arrhythmia Therapy*)

United States: Pronestyl, Sub-Quin
Canada: Pronestyl

☐ This medicine is used to help make the heart beat at a regular and normal rate.

☐ IMPORTANT: If you have ever had an allergic reaction to procainamide, procaine, any other drug spelled with "caine," or any local anesthetic or "freezing," tell your doctor or pharmacist before you take any of this medicine.

HOW TO USE THIS MEDICINE

☐ It is best to take this medicine on an empty stomach 1 hour before (or 2 hours after) eating food. However, if it upsets your stomach, take it with some food or milk.

SPECIAL INSTRUCTIONS

☐ It is very important that you take this medicine exactly as your doctor has prescribed and that you do not miss any doses. Try to take this medicine at the same time every day. Do not take extra tablets without your doctor's approval. Do not go without this medicine between prescription refills.

☐ If you forget to take a dose of this medicine and remember it within 1 hour of the missed dose, take it as soon as possible. Otherwise, do not take the missed dose but continue with your regular schedule.

☐ Some nonprescription drugs can aggravate your heart condition. Do not take any of the following without the approval of your doctor or pharmacist: cough, cold or sinus products; asthma and allergy products; or diet or weight-reducing medicines.

☐ In some people, this drug may cause dizziness or drowsiness. Do not drive a car or operate dangerous machinery or do jobs that require you to be alert until you know how you are going to react to this drug.

☐ Most people experience few or no side effects from their drugs. However, any medicine can sometimes cause unwanted effects. Call your doctor if you develop a sore throat, fever, mouth or gum sores, skin rash, easy bruising or nosebleeds, or symptoms of a cold (e.g. runny nose).

☐ Check with your doctor if you develop joint pain, joint stiffness, or painful breathing.

☐ Keep the container tightly closed and store in a cool, dry place. Do not store in the bathroom medicine cabinet or refrigerator because these areas are humid.

695

☐ Carry an identification card indicating that you are taking this medicine. Always tell your pharmacist, dentist, and other doctors who are treating you that you are taking this medicine.

* * * * *

Procarbazine HCl (*Oral Antineoplastic*)
United States: Matulane
Canada: Natulan

☐ This medicine is used in certain medical conditions to help slow down the growth and reproduction of some of the body's cells.

HOW TO USE THIS MEDICINE
☐ While taking this medicine and for at least 2 weeks after your treatment ends, you must be very careful about your diet. You must not eat any of the following foods or beverages because you could experience a very unpleasant reaction (severe headache, nausea, vomiting, or chest pains):
  • Aged and natural cheeses (for example, cheddar, blue, Camembert, Stilton, Gruyère, Brie, Swiss, and Emmenthaler). In general, avoid foods in which aging is used to increase the flavor. Cream cheese, processed cheese, and cottage cheese are safe to eat.
  • Sour cream or yogurt.
  • Wines, especially Chianti and other heavy red wines.
  • Alcoholic beverages, including sherry and beer. These beverages can cause flushing of the face and sweating in addition to the above reactions.
  • Canned figs or raisins.
  • Yeast extracts (such as Marmite or Bovril) or meat extracts.
  • Chicken livers.
  • Broad beans (also called fava beans).
  • Fermented sausage (such as fermented bolognas and salamis, pepperoni, and summer sausage).
  • Pickled or kippered herring.
  • Meats prepared with tenderizers.
  • Avocados, bananas.
  • Soya sauce.
  • Chocolate.
  • Excessive amounts of caffeine (for example, coffee, tea, cola beverages).

SPECIAL INSTRUCTIONS
☐ Always keep your doctor appointments so that your doctor can follow your progress.

☐ If your doctor has prescribed some other medicines for you, it is important that you take them in the right order and that you do not mix them.

☐ If you forget to take a dose, take it as soon as possible. However, if it is almost time for your next dose, do not take the missed dose. Instead, continue with your regular dosing schedule.

☐ Any medicine has a few unwanted side effects. Because this medicine takes a few weeks to work, the side effects are the only thing that tell the doctor that the drug is being absorbed. Most of these side effects will go away as your body adjusts to the medicine.

☐ In some people, this drug may cause dizziness, incoordination, or drowsiness. Do not drive a car or operate dangerous machinery or do jobs that require you to be alert until you know how you are going to react to this drug.

☐ If this medicine causes dizziness, you should be careful going up and down stairs and you should not change positions too quickly. Get out of bed slowly in the morning and dangle your feet over the edge of the bed for a few minutes before standing up. Sit or lie down at the first sign of dizziness. Tell your doctor you have been dizzy.

☐ It is important that you obtain the advice of your doctor or pharmacist before taking any other medicines, including pain relievers, sleeping pills, tranquilizers, medicines for depression, cough/cold or allergy medicines, or weight-reducing medicine.

☐ If your mouth becomes dry, suck a hard sour candy (sugarless) or ice chips, or chew gum. It is especially important to brush your teeth regularly if you develop a dry mouth.

☐ Men and women should take appropriate birth control measures to avoid conception while taking this medicine.

☐ If you become constipated, try increasing the amount of bulk in your diet (for example, bran and salads), exercising more often, or drinking more water.

☐ Call your doctor immediately if you develop frequent or severe headaches, chest pains, a rapid heart rate, or a stiff neck. If you cannot reach your doctor, call a hospital emergency department.

☐ Most people experience few or no side effects from their drugs. However, any medicine can sometimes cause unwanted effects. Call your doctor if you develop a skin rash, fever or infection, sore throat, mouth sores, fainting, a yellow color to the skin or eyes, or swelling of the legs and ankles.

☐ Do not stop taking this medicine suddenly without your doctor's approval. When your doctor tells you to stop this medicine, you must follow these precautions for 2 weeks since some of the medicine will still be in your body.

☐ Carry an identification card indicating that you are taking this medicine. Always tell your pharmacist, dentist, and other doctors who are treating you that you are taking this medicine. This is especially important if you plan to have surgery or any vaccinations.

* * * * *

697

Prochlorperazine (*Oral Antipsychotic-Antiemetic-Antianxiety*)
United States: Compazine
Canada: Stemetil

☐ This medicine is used to help relieve the symptoms of certain types of emotional problems. This drug has several other uses and the reason it was prescribed depends upon your condition. Check with your doctor if you do not fully understand why you are taking it.

☐ IMPORTANT: If you have ever had an allergic reaction to a phenothiazine medicine, tell your doctor or pharmacist before you take any of this medicine.

HOW TO USE THIS MEDICINE

☐ This medicine may be taken with food or a full glass of water.

☐ Do not take this medicine at the same time as antacids or diarrhea medicine. Try to space them at least 1 hour apart.

☐ Store the liquid medicines in a cool, dark place and do not get the liquid on your skin or clothing.

☐ These capsules must be swallowed whole. Do not open the capsules. (**United States:** Compazine Spansules; *Canada:* Stemetil Spansules)

☐ The effect of the medicine may not be noticed immediately but may take from 2 to 4 weeks. Be patient. Take the medicine regularly and try not to miss any doses.

☐ Do not stop taking this medicine suddenly without the approval of your doctor.

SPECIAL INSTRUCTIONS

☐ If you forget to take a dose, take it as soon as possible. However, if it is almost time for your next dose, do not take the missed dose. Instead, continue with your regular dosing schedule.

☐ Any medicine has a few unwanted side effects. Because this medicine takes a few weeks to work, the side effects show the doctor that the drug is being absorbed. Many of these side effects will go away as your body adjusts to the medicine.

☐ Women who are pregnant, breast-feeding, or planning to become pregnant should tell their doctor before taking this medicine.

☐ In some people, this drug may cause dizziness or drowsiness. Do not drive a car or operate dangerous machinery or do jobs that require you to be alert until you know how you are going to react to this drug.

☐ If this medicine causes dizziness, you should be careful going up and down stairs and you should not change positions too rapidly. Get out of bed slowly in the morning and dangle your feet over the edge of the bed for a few minutes before standing up. Sit down or lie down at the first sign of dizzi-

698

ness. Tell your doctor you have been dizzy. Avoid hot showers and baths because they could make you dizzy.

☐ Do not drink alcoholic beverages while taking this drug without the approval of your doctor.

☐ This medicine may make some people more sensitive to sunlight and sun-lamps. When you begin taking this medicine, try to avoid getting too much sun until you see how you are going to react. If your skin does become more sensitive to sunlight, tell your doctor and try to stay out of direct sunlight. While in the sun, wear protective clothing and sunglasses. You may wish to ask your pharmacist about suitable sunscreen products. Check with your doctor if you become sunburned.

☐ If your mouth becomes dry, suck a hard sour candy (sugarless) or ice chips, or chew gum. It is especially important to brush your teeth regularly if you develop a dry mouth.

☐ It is important that you obtain the advice of your doctor or pharmacist before taking **any** other medicines including pain relievers, sleeping pills, other tran-quilizers or medicines for depression, cough/cold or allergy medicines, weight-reducing medicines, or laxatives.

☐ This medicine may cause your urine to turn pink, red, or red-brown in color. This is not unusual.

☐ In hot weather or during exercise, be careful not to become overheated. You may be more sensitive to heat since this medicine may affect your body's ability to regulate temperature.

☐ If you become constipated, try increasing the amount of bulk in your diet (for example, bran and salads), exercising more often, or drinking more water. Call your doctor if the constipation continues.

☐ Call your doctor if you develop a sore throat, fever, mouth sores, skin rash, changes in eyesight, rapid heart rate, a yellow color in the eys or skin, un-usual weakness or unusual movements of the face, tongue, or hands, or difficulty in urinating ("passing your water"). Also call your doctor if you become restless or unable to sit still or sleep.

☐ Carry an identification card indicating that you are taking this medicine. Always tell your pharmacist, dentist, and other doctors who are treating you that you are taking this medicine.

* * * * *

Prochlorperazine (*Rectal Antipsychotic-Antiemetic-Antianxiety*)
United States: Compazine
Canada: Stemetil

☐ This medicine is used to help relieve the symptoms of certain types of emo-tional problems. This drug has several other uses and the reason it was prescribed depends upon your condition. Check with your doctor if you do not fully understand why you are taking it.

699

☐ IMPORTANT: If you have ever had an allergic reaction to a phenothiazine medicine, tell your doctor or pharmacist before you take any of this medicine.

HOW TO USE THIS MEDICINE

☐ Administration of SUPPOSITORIES
- Remove the wrapper from the suppository.
- Lie on your side and raise your knee to your chest.
- Insert the suppository with the tapered (pointed) end first into the rectum.
- Remain lying down for a few minutes so that the suppository will dissolve in the rectum.
- Try to avoid having a bowel movement for at least one hour so that the drug will have time to work.

☐ Store the suppositories in a cool place.

☐ Do not stop using this medicine suddenly without the approval of your doctor.

SPECIAL INSTRUCTIONS

☐ If you forget to use a dose, use it as soon as possible. However, if it is almost time for your next dose, do not use the missed dose. Instead, continue with your regular dosing schedule.

☐ Any medicine has a few unwanted side effects. Because this medicine takes a few weeks to work, the side effects show the doctor that the drug is being absorbed. Many of these side effects will go away as your body adjusts to the medicine.

☐ Women who are pregnant, breast-feeding, or planning to become pregnant should tell their doctor before taking this medicine.

☐ In some people, this drug may cause dizziness or drowsiness. Do not drive a car or operate dangerous machinery or do jobs that require you to be alert until you know how you are going to react to this drug.

☐ If this medicine causes dizziness, you should be careful going up and down stairs and you should not change positions too rapidly. Get out of bed slowly in the morning and dangle your feet over the edge of the bed for a few minutes before standing up. Sit down or lie down at the first sign of dizziness. Tell your doctor you have been dizzy. Avoid hot showers and baths because they could make you dizzy.

☐ Do not drink alcoholic beverages while taking this drug without the approval of your doctor.

☐ This medicine may make some people more sensitive to sunlight and sunlamps. When you begin taking this medicine, try to avoid getting too much sun until you see how you are going to react. If your skin does become more sensitive to sunlight, tell your doctor and try to stay out of direct sun-

700

light. While in the sun, wear protective clothing and sunglasses. You may wish to ask your pharmacist about suitable sunscreen products. Check with your doctor if you become sunburned.

☐ If your mouth becomes dry, suck a hard sour candy (sugarless) or ice chips, or chew gum. It is especially important to brush your teeth regularly if you develop a dry mouth.

☐ It is important that you obtain the advice of your doctor or pharmacist before taking **any** other medicines including pain relievers, sleeping pills, other tranquilizers or medicines for depression, cough/cold or allergy medicines, weight-reducing medicines, or laxatives.

☐ This medicine may cause your urine to turn pink, red, or red-brown in color. This is not unusual.

☐ In hot weather or during exercise, be careful not to become overheated. You may be more sensitive to heat since this medicine may affect your body's ability to regulate temperature.

☐ Call your doctor if you develop a sore throat, fever, mouth sores, skin rash, changes in eyesight, rapid heart rate, a yellow color in the eyes or skin, unusual weakness or unusual movements of the face, tongue or hands, or difficulty in urinating ("passing your water"). Also call your doctor if you become restless or unable to sit still or sleep.

☐ Carry an identification card indicating that you are taking this medicine. Always tell your pharmacist, dentist, and other doctors who are treating you that you are taking this medicine.

*   *   *   *   *

Procyclidine HCl (*Oral Antiparkinsonism Agent*)
United States: Kemadrin
Canada: Kemadrin, Procyclid

☐ This medicine is used to improve muscle control and to relieve muscle spasm in Parkinson's disease and certain other medical conditions.

HOW TO USE THIS MEDICINE
☐ Take this medicine with food or immediately after meals to help prevent stomach upset unless otherwise directed.

☐ If you forget to take a dose, take it as soon as possible. However, if your next dose is within 2 hours, do not take the missed dose but continue with your regular schedule.

SPECIAL INSTRUCTIONS
☐ If your mouth becomes dry, suck a hard sour candy (sugarless) or ice chips, or chew gum. It is especially important to brush your teeth regularly if you develop a dry mouth.

- ☐ In some people, this drug may cause dizziness, drowsiness, or blurred vision during the first 2 weeks of using this drug. This will usually go away as your body adjusts to this medicine. Do not drive a car or operate dangerous machinery or do jobs that require you to be alert until you know how you are going to react to this drug.

- ☐ If you become dizzy, you should be careful going up and down stairs. Sit or lie down at the first sign of dizziness.

- ☐ If your eyes become more sensitive to sunlight, it may help to wear sunglasses.

- ☐ Do not take antacids or diarrhea medicines within 1 hour of taking this medicine because they could make this medicine less effective.

- ☐ A desire to urinate ("pass your water") with an inability to do so is not an uncommon effect with this drug. Urinating each time before the drug is taken may help relieve this problem. Call your doctor if it continues.

- ☐ Do not drink alcoholic beverages while taking this drug without the approval of your doctor.

- ☐ It is important that you obtain the advice of your doctor or pharmacist before taking pain relievers, nonprescription drugs, sleeping pills, tranquilizers, or medicine for depression while you are taking this drug.

- ☐ You may become more sensitive to heat because your body may perspire less while you are taking this medicine. Be careful not to become overheated during exercise or in hot weather.

- ☐ Most people experience few or no side effects from their drugs. However, any medicine can sometimes cause unwanted effects. Call your doctor if you develop a skin rash, eye pain, dizziness or fainting, fast heartbeats, or constipation, or if you become confused.

* * * * *

Progestin Therapy (*Oral Contraceptive*)
United States: Micronor, Nor-Q.D., Ovrette
Canada: Micronor

- ☐ This medicine is a birth control measure.

HOW TO USE THIS MEDICINE
- ☐ Take this medicine at the same time each day: for example, after the evening meal or at bedtime. It is important to take this medicine regularly.

- ☐ During the first month of taking this medicine it is important to use some additional form of birth control to help prevent pregnancy.

- ☐ Instructions for use:
  - Take your first tablet on the very first day of menstruation.

702

- Take one tablet every day until the dispenser is empty.
- Start a new dispenser the next day. Do **not** miss a day even during menstrual bleeding.

☐ If you miss one daily dose, take it as soon as you remember and continue your regular schedule.

☐ If you miss two daily doses, take one of the missed tablets as soon as you remember as well as your regular tablet for that day. Resume your normal schedule. It is advisable to use some additional form of birth control for the next 14 days to help avoid pregnancy.

☐ If you miss more than 2 tablets, stop taking the medicine and use a non-hormonal method of birth control until menstruation begins or pregnancy has been ruled out.

SPECIAL INSTRUCTIONS

☐ Contact your doctor at least once every 6 to 12 months so that you can be examined.

☐ In the summer, it is best to take the tablet at bedtime so that the highest levels of the drug are in your body during the night. This will help protect your skin from the sunlight which sometimes causes discolorations in women on this medicine.

☐ Women who are pregnant, breast-feeding, or planning to become pregnant should tell their doctor before taking this medicine.

☐ It is recommended that you do not smoke while you are taking this medicine because smoking may increase the incidence of heart attacks.

☐ Contact your doctor if any of the following side effects occur:
- Severe or persistent headaches
- Vomiting, dizziness, or fainting
- Blurred vision or slurred speech
- Pain in the calves of the legs or numbness in an arm or leg
- Chest pain, shortness of breath, or coughing of blood
- Lumps in the breast
- Severe depression
- A yellow color to the skin or eyes or dark-colored urine
- Severe abdominal pain
- Breakthrough vaginal bleeding which persists after the third month of therapy. During the first 3 months of therapy, breakthrough bleeding may be expected, but you should keep taking the tablets and it will usually clear up in a day or two.
- If you miss 2 consecutive menstrual periods or if you think you are pregnant.

☐ Always tell your pharmacist, dentist, and other doctors who are treating you that you are taking this medicine.

*   *   *   *   *

Promazine HCl (*Oral Antipsychotic-Antiemetic-Antianxiety*)
Canada: Promanyl, Sparine

- [ ] This medicine is used to help relieve the symptoms of certain types of emotional problems. This drug has several other uses and the reason it was prescribed depends upon your condition. Check with your doctor if you do not fully understand why you are taking it.

- [ ] IMPORTANT: If you have ever had an allergic reaction to a phenothiazine medicine, tell your doctor or pharmacist before you take any of this medicine.

HOW TO USE THIS MEDICINE

- [ ] This medicine may be taken with food or a full glass of water.

- [ ] Do not take this medicine at the same time as antacids or diarrhea medicine. Try to space them at least 1 hour apart.

- [ ] Store the liquid medicines in a cool, dark place and do not get the liquid on your skin or clothing. (*Canada:* Sparine Syrup)

- [ ] The effect of the medicine may not be noticed immediately but may take from 2 to 4 weeks. Be patient. Take the medicine regularly and try not to miss any doses.

- [ ] Do not stop taking this medicine suddenly without the approval of your doctor.

SPECIAL INSTRUCTIONS

- [ ] If you forget to take a dose, take it as soon as possible. However, if it is almost time for your next dose, do not take the missed dose. Instead, continue with your regular dosing schedule.

- [ ] Any medicine has a few unwanted side effects. Because this medicine takes a few weeks to work, the side effects show the doctor that the drug is being absorbed. Many of these side effects will go away as your body adjusts to the medicine.

- [ ] Women who are pregnant, breast-feeding, or planning to become pregnant should tell their doctor before taking this medicine.

- [ ] In some people, this drug may cause dizziness or drowsiness. Do not drive a car or operate dangerous machinery or do jobs that require you to be alert until you know how you are going to react to this drug.

- [ ] If this medicine causes dizziness, you should be careful going up and down stairs and you should not change positions too rapidly. Get out of bed slowly in the morning and dangle your feet over the edge of the bed for a few minutes before standing up. Sit down or lie down at the first sign of dizziness. Tell your doctor you have been dizzy. Avoid hot showers and baths because they could make you dizzy.

☐ Do not drink alcoholic beverages while taking this drug without the approval of your doctor.

☐ This medicine may make some people more sensitive to sunlight and sunlamps. When you begin taking this medicine, try to avoid getting too much sun until you see how you are going to react. If your skin does become more sensitive to sunlight, tell your doctor and try to stay out of direct sunlight. While in the sun, wear protective clothing and sunglasses. You may wish to ask your pharmacist about suitable sunscreen products. Check with your doctor if you become sunburned.

☐ If your mouth becomes dry, suck a hard sour candy (sugarless) or ice chips, or chew gum. It is especially important to brush your teeth regularly if you develop a dry mouth.

☐ It is important that you obtain the advice of your doctor or pharmacist before taking **any** other medicines including pain relievers, sleeping pills, other tranquilizers or medicines for depression, cough/cold or allergy medicines, weight-reducing medicines, or laxatives.

☐ This medicine may cause your urine to turn pink, red or red-brown in color. This is not unusual.

☐ In hot weather or during exercise, be careful not to become overheated. You may be more sensitive to heat since this medicine may affect your body's ability to regulate temperature.

☐ If you become constipated, try increasing the amount of bulk in your diet (for example, bran and salads), exercising more often, or drinking more water. Call your doctor if the constipation continues.

☐ Call your doctor if you develop a sore throat, fever, mouth sores, skin rash, changes in eyesight, rapid heart rate, a yellow color in the eyes or skin, unusual weakness or unusual movements of the face, tongue or hands, or difficulty in urinating ("passing your water"). Also call your doctor if you become restless or unable to sit still or sleep.

☐ Carry an identification card indicating that you are taking this medicine. Always tell your pharmacist, dentist, and other doctors who are treating you that you are taking this medicine.

* * * * *

Promethazine (*Oral Antihistamine*)
United States: Phenergan, Remsed
Canada: Histanil, Phenergan

☐ This medicine is an antihistamine that has many uses, and the reason it was prescribed depends upon your condition. If you do not fully understand why you are taking it, check with your doctor.

705

HOW TO USE THIS MEDICINE

☐ This medicine may be taken with food or a glass of milk if it upsets your stomach.

SPECIAL INSTRUCTIONS

☐ Women who are pregnant, breast-feeding, or planning to become pregnant should tell their doctor before taking this medicine.

☐ If you forget to take a dose, take it as soon as possible. However, if it is almost time for your next dose, do not take the missed dose. Instead, continue with your regular dosing schedule.

☐ In some people, this drug may initially cause dizziness or drowsiness. Do not drive a car or operate dangerous machinery or do jobs that require you to be alert until you know how you are going to react to this drug. If you become dizzy, you should be careful going up and down stairs. Sit or lie down at the first sign of dizziness. Tell your doctor if it continues.

☐ Do not drink alcoholic beverages while taking this drug without the approval of your doctor.

☐ If your mouth becomes dry, suck a hard sour candy (sugarless) or ice chips, or chew gum. It is especially important to brush your teeth regularly if you develop a dry mouth.

☐ This medicine may make some people more sensitive to sunlight and sunlamps. When you begin taking this medicine, try to avoid getting too much sun until you see how you are going to react. If your skin does become more sensitive to sunlight, tell your doctor and try to stay out of direct sunlight. While in the sun, wear protective clothing and sunglasses. You may wish to ask your pharmacist about suitable sunscreen products. Check with your doctor if you become sunburned.

☐ It is important that you obtain the advice of your doctor or pharmacist before taking pain relievers, nonprescription drugs, sleeping pills or tranquilizers, or other medicines for allergies.

☐ Do not take this medicine more often or longer than recommended by your doctor.

☐ Most people experience few or no side effects from their drugs. However, any medicine can sometimes cause unwanted effects. Call your doctor if you develop a skin rash, fast heartbeats, blurred vision, stomach pain, or difficulty in urinating ("passing your water").

*   *   *   *   *

Promethazine HCl (*Topical Antihistamine*)
Canada: Phenergan Cream

☐ This medicine is used in the treatment of certain skin conditions.

706

HOW TO USE THIS MEDICINE
- ☐ INSTRUCTIONS FOR USE:
  - Each time you apply the medicine, wash your hands and gently cleanse the skin area well with water unless otherwise directed by your doctor. Do not allow the skin to dry completely. Pat with a clean towel until almost dry.
  - Apply a small amount of the drug to the affected area and spread lightly. Only the medicine that is actually touching the skin will work. A thick layer is not more effective than a thin layer. Do not bandage unless directed by your doctor.

SPECIAL INSTRUCTIONS
- ☐ This medicine may make some people more sensitive to sunlight and sunlamps. When you begin taking this medicine, try to avoid getting too much sun until you see how you are going to react. If your skin does become more sensitive to sunlight, tell your doctor and try to stay out of direct sunlight. While in the sun, wear protective clothing and sunglasses. You may wish to ask your pharmacist about suitable sunscreen products. Check with your doctor if you become sunburned.

- ☐ Call your doctor if the condition for which this drug is being used persists or becomes worse or if you have a constant irritation such as itching or burning that was not present before you started using this medicine.

- ☐ For external use only. Do not swallow.

* * * * *

Propantheline Bromide (*Oral Anticholinergic*)
United States: Giquel, Pro-Banthine, Robantaline, Ropanth
Canada: Banlin, Novopropanthil, Pro-Banthine, Propanthel

- ☐ This medicine is used to help relax muscles of the stomach, bowels, and bladder as well as to decrease the amount of acid formed in the stomach.

- ☐ IMPORTANT: If you have ever had an allergic reaction to atropine or bromides or any other drug used to relax the stomach or bowels, tell your doctor or pharmacist before you take any of this medicine.

HOW TO USE THIS MEDICINE
- ☐ Take this medicine approximately 30 minutes before a meal unless otherwise directed.

- ☐ This medicine must be swallowed whole. Do not crush, chew, or break it into pieces. (**United States:** Pro-Banthine PA)

- ☐ If you miss a dose of this medicine, do not take the missed dose and do not double the next dose.

SPECIAL INSTRUCTIONS

- ☐ If your mouth becomes dry, suck a hard sour candy (sugarless) or ice chips, or chew gum. It is especially important to brush your teeth regularly if you develop a dry mouth.

- ☐ In some people, this drug may cause dizziness or drowsiness. Do not drive a car or operate dangerous machinery or do jobs that require you to be alert until you know how you are going to react to this drug.

- ☐ If you become dizzy, you should be careful going up and down stairs. Sit or lie down at the first sign of dizziness. Tell your doctor you have been dizzy.

- ☐ A desire to urinate ("pass your water") with an inability to do so is not an uncommon effect with this drug. Urinating each time before taking the drug may help relieve this problem. Call your doctor if it continues.

- ☐ You may become more sensitive to heat because your body may perspire less while you are taking this drug. Be careful not to become overheated during exercise or in hot weather.

- ☐ Do not take antacids within 1 hour of taking this medicine because they could make this medicine less effective.

- ☐ If you become constipated, try increasing the amount of bulk in your diet (for example, bran and salads), exercising more often, or drinking more water. Call your doctor if the constipation continues.

- ☐ If your eyes become more sensitive to sunlight, it may help to wear sunglasses.

- ☐ Most people experience few or no side effects from their drugs. However, any medicine can sometimes cause unwanted effects. Call your doctor if you develop a skin rash, diarrhea, unusual restlessness, flushing, or eye pain.

*   *   *   *   *

Propoxyphene HCl (*Oral Analgesic*)

United States: Darvon, Dolene, Pargesic 65, Progesic-65, Proxagesic, SK-65, S-Pain-65

Canada: Algodex, Depronal SA, Novopropoxyn, Pro-65, 642

- ☐ This medicine is used to help relieve pain.

- ☐ IMPORTANT: If you have ever had an allergic reaction to a propoxyphene medicine, tell your doctor or pharmacist before you take any of this medicine.

HOW TO USE THIS MEDICINE

- ☐ This medicine may be taken with food or a glass of water.

- ☐ Do not take any more of this medicine than your doctor has prescribed. The

708

drug could become habit-forming or you could take an overdose if you take it more often or longer than prescribed.

☐ This medicine works best if you take it when the pain first becomes uncomfortable. Do not wait until the pain becomes severe. Call your doctor if you feel you need the medicine more often than was prescribed.

SPECIAL INSTRUCTIONS

☐ Women who are pregnant, breast-feeding, or planning to become pregnant should tell their doctor before taking this medicine.

☐ Do not drink alcoholic beverages while taking this drug without the approval of your doctor.

☐ It is important that you obtain the advice of your doctor or pharmacist before taking ANY other medicines including pain relievers, sleeping pills, tranquilizers or medicines for depression, cough/cold medicines or allergy medicines.

☐ In some people, this drug may cause dizziness or drowsiness. Do not drive a car or operate dangerous machinery or do jobs that require you to be alert until you know how you are going to react to this drug.

☐ If you become dizzy, you should be careful going up and down stairs. Sit or lie down at the first sign of dizziness.

☐ If you feel nauseated when you first start taking the medicine, it may help if you lie down for a few minutes.

☐ If you become constipated, try increasing the amount of bulk in your diet (for example, bran and salads), exercising more often, or drinking more water. Call your doctor if the constipation continues.

☐ Call your doctor immediately if you think you may be allergic to the medicine or if you develop a skin rash, hives, itching, swelling of the face, or difficulty in breathing. If you cannot reach your doctor, phone a hospital emergency department.

☐ Most people experience few or no side effects from their drugs. However, any medicine can sometimes cause unwanted effects. Call your doctor if you develop stomach pain, unusual tiredness or weakness, blurred vision or changes in eyesight, severe dizziness or drowsiness, seizures, confusion, or loss of consciousness.

☐ Carry an identification card indicating that you are taking this medicine. Always tell your pharmacist, dentist, and other doctors who are treating you that you are taking this medicine.

☐ Keep this medicine out of the reach of children.

* * * * *

Propoxyphene HCl-ASA-Caffeine (*Oral Analgesic*)
Canada: Novopropoxyn Compound, 692

Propoxyphene HCl-ASA

United States: Darvon w/ASA, Unigesic-A

- ☐ This medicine is used to help relieve pain.

- ☐ IMPORTANT: If you have a stomach ulcer or if you have ever had an allergic reaction to a propoxyphene medicine or aspirin, tell your doctor or pharmacist before you take any of this medicine.

HOW TO USE THIS MEDICINE

- ☐ This medicine may be taken with food or a glass of water.

- ☐ Do not take any more of this medicine than your doctor has prescribed. The drug could become habit-forming or you could take an overdose if you take it more often or longer than prescribed.

- ☐ This medicine works best if you take it when the pain first becomes uncomfortable. Do not wait until the pain becomes severe. Call your doctor if you feel you need the medicine more often than was prescribed.

- ☐ Do not take this medicine if it smells strongly like vinegar since this means that the aspirin in the medicine is not fresh.

SPECIAL INSTRUCTIONS

- ☐ Women who are pregnant, breast-feeding, or planning to become pregnant should tell their doctor before taking this medicine.

- ☐ Do not drink alcoholic beverages while taking this drug without the approval of your doctor.

- ☐ It is important that you obtain the advice of your doctor or pharmacist before taking ANY other medicines including pain relievers, sleeping pills, tranquilizers or medicines for depression, cough/cold medicines, or allergy medicines.

- ☐ In some people, this drug may cause dizziness or drowsiness. Do not drive a car or operate dangerous machinery or do jobs that require you to be alert until you know how you are going to react to this drug.

- ☐ If you become dizzy, you should be careful going up and down stairs. Sit or lie down at the first sign of dizziness.

- ☐ If you feel nauseated when you first start taking the medicine, it may help if you lie down for a few minutes.

- ☐ If you become constipated, try increasing the amount of bulk in your diet (for example, bran and salads), exercising more often, or drinking more water. Call your doctor if the constipation continues.

- ☐ Call your doctor immediately if you think you may be allergic to the medicine or if you develop a skin rash, hives, itching, swelling of the face, or difficulty in breathing. If you cannot reach your doctor, phone a hospital emergency department.

☐ Do not take extra aspirin while you are taking this medicine because it could result in too high a dose.

☐ Most people experience few or no side effects from their drugs. However, any medicine can sometimes cause unwanted effects. Call your doctor if you develop unusual tiredness or weakness, blurred vision or changes in eyesight, severe dizziness or drowsiness, seizures, confusion, or loss of consciousness. Also call your doctor if you develop "ringing" or "buzzing" in the ears, red or black stools, stomach pain, fever, or sweating.

☐ Carry an identification card indicating that you are taking this medicine. Always tell your dentist, pharmacist, and other doctors who are treating you that you are taking this medicine.

☐ Keep this medicine out of the reach of children.

* * * * *

Propoxyphene HCl-Acetaminophen
United States: Dolacet, Dolene-AP-65, Wygesic

☐ This medicine is used to help relieve pain.

☐ IMPORTANT: If you have ever had an allergic reaction to a propoxyphene, acetaminophen, or phenacetin medicine, tell your doctor or pharmacist before you take any of this medicine.

HOW TO USE THIS MEDICINE
☐ This medicine may be taken with food or a glass of water.

☐ Do not take any more of this medicine than your doctor has prescribed. The drug could become habit-forming or you could take an overdose if you take it more often or longer than prescribed.

☐ This medicine works best if you take it when the pain first becomes uncomfortable. Do not wait until the pain becomes severe. Call your doctor if you feel you need the medicine more often than was prescribed.

SPECIAL INSTRUCTIONS
☐ Women who are pregnant, breast-feeding, or planning to become pregnant should tell their doctor before taking this medicine.

☐ Do not drink alcoholic beverages while taking this drug without the approval of your doctor.

☐ It is important that you obtain the advice of your doctor or pharmacist before taking ANY other medicines including pain relievers, sleeping pills, tranquilizers or medicines for depression, cough/cold medicines, or allergy medicines.

☐ In some people, this drug may cause dizziness or drowsiness. Do not drive a

car or operate dangerous machinery or do jobs that require you to be alert until you know how you are going to react to this drug.

☐ If you become dizzy, you should be careful going up and down stairs. Sit or lie down at the first sign of dizziness.

☐ If you feel nauseated when you first start taking the medicine, it may help if you lie down for a few minutes.

☐ If you become constipated, try increasing the amount of bulk in your diet (for example, bran and salads), exercising more often, or drinking more water. Call your doctor if the constipation continues.

☐ Do not take any other medicines containing acetaminophen while you are taking this medicine because it could result in too high a dose.

☐ Call your doctor immediately if you think you may be allergic to the medicine or if you develop a skin rash, hives, itching, swelling of the face, or difficulty in breathing. If you cannot reach your doctor, phone a hospital emergency department.

☐ Most people experience few or no side effects from their drugs. However, any medicine can sometimes cause unwanted effects. Call your doctor if you develop stomach pain, unusual tiredness or weakness, blurred vision or changes in eyesight, severe dizziness or drowsiness, seizures, confusion, or loss of consciousness. Also call your doctor if you develop a sore throat or fever, easy bruising or bleeding, a yellow color to the skin or eyes, or diarrhea.

☐ Carry an identification card indicating that you are taking this medicine. Always tell your dentist, pharmacist, and other doctors who are treating you that you are taking this medicine.

☐ Keep this medicine out of the reach of children.

* * * * *

Propoxyphene HCl-ASA-Caffeine-Phenacetin (*Oral Analgesic*)
United States: Darvon Compound-65, Dolene Compound-65, SK-65 Compound

☐ This medicine is used to help relieve pain.

☐ IMPORTANT: If you have a stomach ulcer or if you have ever had an allergic reaction to propoxyphene, aspirin, acetaminophen, phenacetin, or caffeine, tell your doctor or pharmacist before you take any of this medicine.

HOW TO USE THIS MEDICINE
☐ This medicine may be taken with food or a glass of water.

☐ Do not take any more of this medicine than your doctor has prescribed. The

712

drug could become habit-forming or you could take an overdose if you take it more often or longer than prescribed.

☐ This medicine works best if you take it when the pain first becomes uncomfortable. Do not wait until the pain becomes severe. Call your doctor if you feel you need the medicine more often than was prescribed.

☐ Do not take this medicine if it smells strongly like vinegar since this means that the aspirin in the medicine is not fresh.

SPECIAL INSTRUCTIONS

☐ Women who are pregnant, breast-feeding, or planning to become pregnant should tell their doctor before taking this medicine.

☐ Do not drink alcoholic beverages while taking this drug without the approval of your doctor.

☐ It is important that you obtain the advice of your doctor or pharmacist before taking ANY other medicines including pain relievers, sleeping pills, tranquilizers or medicines for depression, cough/cold medicines, or allergy medicines.

☐ In some people, this drug may cause dizziness or drowsiness. Do not drive a car or operate dangerous machinery or do jobs that require you to be alert until you know how you are going to react to this drug.

☐ If you become dizzy, you should be careful going up and down stairs. Sit or lie down at the first sign of dizziness.

☐ If you feel nauseated when you first start taking the medicine, it may help if you lie down for a few minutes.

☐ If you become constipated, try increasing the amount of bulk in your diet (for example, bran and salads), exercising more often, or drinking more water. Call your doctor if the constipation continues.

☐ Do not take extra aspirin or acetaminophen while you are taking this medicine because it could result in too high a dose.

☐ Call your doctor immediately if you think you may be allergic to the medicine or if you develop a skin rash, hives, itching, swelling of the face, or difficulty in breathing. If you cannot reach your doctor, phone a hospital emergency department.

☐ Most people experience few or no side effects from their drugs. However, any medicine can sometimes cause unwanted effects. Call your doctor if you develop unusual tiredness or weakness, blurred vision or changes in eyesight, severe dizziness or drowsiness, seizures, confusion, or loss of consciousness. Also call your doctor if you develop "ringing" or "buzzing" in the ears, red or black stools, stomach pain, sore throat or fever, sweating, easy bruising or bleeding, a yellow color in the skin or eyes, or swelling of the legs or ankles.

☐ Carry an identification card indicating that you are taking this medicine.

Always tell your dentist, pharmacist, and other doctors who are treating you that you are taking this medicine.

☐ Keep this medicine out of the reach of children.

*　*　*　*　*

Propoxyphene Napsylate (*Oral Analgesic*)
United States: Darvon-N
Canada: Darvon-N

☐ This medicine is used to help relieve pain.

☐ IMPORTANT: If you have ever had an allergic reaction to a propoxyphene medicine, tell your doctor or pharmacist before you take any of this medicine.

HOW TO USE THIS MEDICINE
☐ This medicine may be taken with food or a glass of water.

☐ For LIQUID MEDICINE
  • Shake the bottle well before using so that you can measure an accurate dose. (**United States:** Darvon-N Suspension)

☐ Do not take any more of this medicine than your doctor has prescribed. The drug could become habit-forming or you could take an overdose if you take it more often or longer than prescribed.

☐ This medicine works best if you take it when the pain first becomes uncomfortable. Do not wait until the pain becomes severe. Call your doctor if you feel you need the medicine more often than was prescribed.

SPECIAL INSTRUCTIONS
☐ Women who are pregnant, breast-feeding, or planning to become pregnant should tell their doctor before taking this medicine.

☐ Do not drink alcoholic beverages while taking this drug without the approval of your doctor.

☐ It is important that you obtain the advice of your doctor or pharmacist before taking ANY other medicines including pain relievers, sleeping pills, tranquilizers or medicines for depression, cough/cold medicines, or allergy medicines.

☐ In some people, this drug may cause dizziness or drowsiness. Do not drive a car or operate dangerous machinery or do jobs that require you to be alert until you know how you are going to react to this drug.

☐ If you become dizzy, you should be careful going up and down stairs. Sit or lie down at the first sign of dizziness.

714

- ☐ If you feel nauseated when you first start taking the medicine, it may help if you lie down for a few minutes.

- ☐ If you become constipated, try increasing the amount of bulk in your diet (for example, bran and salads), exercising more often, or drinking more water. Call your doctor if the constipation continues.

- ☐ Call your doctor immediately if you think you may be allergic to the medicine or if you develop a skin rash, hives, itching, swelling of the face, or difficulty in breathing. If you cannot reach your doctor, phone a hospital emergency department.

- ☐ Most people experience few or no side effects from their drugs. However, any medicine can sometimes cause unwanted effects. Call your doctor if you develop stomach pain, unusual tiredness or weakness, blurred vision or changes in eyesight, severe dizziness or drowsiness, seizures, confusion, or loss of consciousness.

- ☐ Carry an identification card indicating that you are taking this medicine. Always tell your dentist, pharmacist, and other doctors who are treating you that you are taking this medicine.

- ☐ Keep this medicine out of the reach of children.

* * * * *

Propoxyphene Napsylate-ASA (*Oral Analgesic*)
United States: Darvon-N with ASA
Canada: Darvon-N with ASA

Propoxyphene Napsylate-ASA-Caffeine
Canada: Darvon-N Compound

- ☐ This medicine is used to help relieve pain.

- ☐ IMPORTANT: If you have a stomach ulcer or if you have ever had an allergic reaction to a propoxyphene medicine or aspirin, tell your doctor or pharmacist before you take any of this medicine.

HOW TO USE THIS MEDICINE
- ☐ This medicine may be taken with food or a glass of water.

- ☐ Do not take any more of this medicine than your doctor has prescribed. The drug could become habit-forming or you could take an overdose if you take it more often or longer than prescribed.

- ☐ This medicine works best if you take it when the pain first becomes uncomfortable. Do not wait until the pain becomes severe. Call your doctor if you feel you need the medicine more often than was prescribed.

- ☐ Do not take this medicine if it smells strongly like vinegar since this means that the aspirin in the medicine is not fresh.

715

SPECIAL INSTRUCTIONS

- ☐ Women who are pregnant, breast-feeding, or planning to become pregnant should tell their doctor before taking this medicine.

- ☐ Do not drink alcoholic beverages while taking this drug without the approval of your doctor.

- ☐ It is important that you obtain the advice of your doctor or pharmacist before taking ANY other medicines including pain relievers, sleeping pills, tranquilizers or medicines for depression, cough/cold medicines or allergy medicines.

- ☐ In some people, this drug may cause dizziness or drowsiness. Do not drive a car or operate dangerous machinery or do jobs that require you to be alert until you know how you are going to react to this drug.

- ☐ If you become dizzy, you should be careful going up and down stairs. Sit or lie down at the first sign of dizziness.

- ☐ If you feel nauseated when you first start taking the medicine, it may help if you lie down for a few minutes.

- ☐ If you become constipated, try increasing the amount of bulk in your diet (for example, bran and salads), exercising more often, or drinking more water. Call your doctor if the constipation continues.

- ☐ Call your doctor immediately if you think you may be allergic to the medicine or if you develop a skin rash, hives, itching, swelling of the face, or difficulty in breathing. If you cannot reach your doctor, phone a hospital emergency department.

- ☐ Do not take extra aspirin while you are taking this medicine because it could result in too high a dose.

- ☐ Most people experience few or no side effects from their drugs. However, any medicine can sometimes cause unwanted effects. Call your doctor if you develop unusual tiredness or weakness, blurred vision or changes in eyesight, severe dizziness or drowsiness, seizures, confusion, or loss of consciousness. Also call your doctor if you develop "ringing" or "buzzing" in the ears, red or black stools, stomach pain, fever, or sweating.

- ☐ Carry an identification card indicating that you are taking this medicine. Always tell your pharmacist, dentist, and other doctors who are treating you that you are taking this medicine.

- ☐ Keep this medicine out of the reach of children.

*   *   *   *   *

Propoxyphene Napsylate-Acetaminophen
United States: Darvocet-N, Darvocet-N 100

- ☐ This medicine is used to help relieve pain.

- ☐ IMPORTANT: If you have ever had an allergic reaction to a propoxyphene, acetaminophen, or phenacetin medicine, tell your doctor or pharmacist before you take any of this medicine.

HOW TO USE THIS MEDICINE

- ☐ This medicine may be taken with food or a glass of water.

- ☐ Do not take any more of this medicine than your doctor has prescribed. The drug could become habit-forming or you could take an overdose if you take it more often or longer than prescribed.

- ☐ This medicine works best if you take it when the pain first becomes uncomfortable. Do not wait until the pain becomes severe. Call your doctor if you feel you need the medicine more often than was prescribed.

SPECIAL INSTRUCTIONS

- ☐ Women who are pregnant, breast-feeding, or planning to become pregnant should tell their doctor before taking this medicine.

- ☐ Do not drink alcoholic beverages while taking this drug without the approval of your doctor.

- ☐ It is important that you obtain the advice of your doctor or pharmacist before taking ANY other medicines including pain relievers, sleeping pills, tranquilizers or medicines for depression, cough/cold medicines, or allergy medicines.

- ☐ In some people, this drug may cause dizziness or drowsiness. Do not drive a car or operate dangerous machinery or do jobs that require you to be alert until you know how you are going to react to this drug.

- ☐ If you become dizzy, you should be careful going up and down stairs. Sit or lie down at the first sign of dizziness.

- ☐ If you feel nauseated when you first start taking the medicine, it may help if you lie down for a few minutes.

- ☐ If you become constipated, try increasing the amount of bulk in your diet (for example, bran and salads), exercising more often, or drinking more water. Call your doctor if the constipation continues.

- ☐ Do not take any other medicines containing acetaminophen while you are taking this medicine because it could result in too high a dose.

- ☐ Call your doctor immediately if you think you may be allergic to the medicine or if you develop a skin rash, hives, itching, swelling of the face, or difficulty in breathing. If you cannot reach your doctor, phone a hospital emergency department.

717

☐ Most people experience few or no side effects from their drugs. However, any medicine can sometimes cause unwanted effects. Call your doctor if you develop stomach pain, unusual tiredness or weakness, blurred vision or changes in eyesight, severe dizziness or drowsiness, seizures, confusion, or loss of consciousness. Also call your doctor if you develop a sore throat or fever, easy bruising or bleeding, a yellow color to the skin or eyes, or diarrhea.

☐ Carry an identification card indicating that you are taking this medicine. Always tell your pharmacist, dentist, and other doctors who are treating you that you are taking this medicine.

☐ Keep this medicine out of the reach of children.

*   *   *   *   *

Propranolol (*Oral Angina Pectoris and Cardiac Arrhythmia Therapy*)

United States: Inderal

Canada: Inderal

☐ This medicine is usually used to treat heart conditions or high blood pressure, but it has many other uses. Make sure you understand why you are taking it.

☐ IMPORTANT: If you have a history of allergies, tell your doctor or pharmacist before taking any of this medicine.

☐ It may be necessary for you to take this medicine for a long time in spite of the fact that you may feel better. It is very important that you take the medicine as your doctor has prescribed and that you do not miss any doses. Otherwise, you cannot expect the drug to work for you.

HOW TO USE THIS MEDICINE

☐ Depending upon your doctor's instructions, this medicine can be taken with a glass of water before or after meals or on an empty stomach (1 hour before or 2 hours after meals). It is important to always take it in the same way each day.

SPECIAL INSTRUCTIONS

☐ If you forget to take a dose, take it as soon as possible. However, if your next dose is within 4 hours, do not take the missed dose. Instead continue with your regular dosing schedule.

☐ Women who are pregnant, breast-feeding, or planning to become pregnant should tell their doctor before taking this medicine.

☐ In some people, this drug may cause dizziness or drowsiness. Do not drive a car or operate dangerous machinery or do jobs that require you to be alert until you know how you are going to react to this drug.

☐ If this medicine causes dizziness, you should be careful going up and down

718

stairs and you should not change positions too rapidly. Get out of bed slowly in the morning and dangle your feet over the edge of the bed for a few minutes before standing up. Sit down or lie down at the first sign of dizziness. Tell your doctor you have been dizzy. Do not drive a car or operate dangerous machinery if you are dizzy.

☐ If your mouth becomes dry, suck a hard sour candy (sugarless) or ice chips, or chew gum. It is especially important to brush your teeth regularly if you develop a dry mouth.

☐ Some nonprescription drugs can aggravate your condition. Do not take any of the following without the approval of your doctor or pharmacist: cough, cold, or sinus products; asthma or allergy products; or diet or weight-reducing medicines.

☐ Most people experience few or no side effects from their drugs. However, any medicine can sometimes cause unwanted effects. Call your doctor if you develop a skin rash, shortness of breath, fever or sore throat, easy bruising, or if your pulse becomes slower than normal (less than 60 beats per minute). Also call your doctor if you develop nightmares, or headaches, or if you become depressed.

☐ It is recommended that patients receiving this drug should stop smoking.

☐ Carry an identification card indicating that you are taking this medicine. Always tell your pharmacist, dentist, and other doctors who are treating you that you are taking this medicine.

☐ Do not stop taking this medicine without your doctor's approval and do not go without medicine between prescription refills. Call your pharmacist 2 or 3 days before you will run out of the medicine.

*   *   *   *   *

Propylhexedrine (*Nasal Decongestant*)
United States: Benzedrex
Canada: Benzedrex

☐ This medicine is used to help relieve nasal stuffiness.

HOW TO USE THIS MEDICINE
☐ For NASAL INHALATION
- Blow your nose gently.
- Sit upright with your head slightly back.
- Insert inhaler into one nostril and close the other nostril by pressing your finger on the side.
- Breathe in deeply.

☐ This inhaler will be good for approximately 2 to 3 months of normal use. After this time, the active ingredient will be exhausted and a new inhaler will be required.

719

SPECIAL INSTRUCTIONS

☐ Do not use this medicine more often or longer than recommended by your doctor. If used for too long, this medicine may actually cause a type of congestion.

☐ Rinse the dropper in hot water after each use.

☐ If you forget to use the medicine, use it as soon as possible. However, if it is almost time for your next dose, do not use the missed dose but continue with your regular schedule.

☐ Do not use this medicine at the same time as any other nasal medicine without the approval of your doctor. Some medicines cannot be mixed.

☐ Contact your doctor if the condition for which you are using this medicine does not improve. Also call your doctor if you develop fast heartbeats, headache, dizziness, trembling, blurred vision, or drowsiness.

☐ Check with your doctor if you develop a stinging sensation which does not go away as your body adjusts to the medicine.

☐ For external use only. Do not swallow.

*   *   *   *   *

Propylthiouracil (*Oral Hyperthyroidism Therapy*)
United States: Propacil
Canada: Propyl-Thyracil

☐ This medicine is used to treat an overactive thyroid gland and also is used before thyroid surgery.

HOW TO USE THIS MEDICINE

☐ This medicine may be taken with meals or on an empty stomach. To make sure that you always get the same effect, always take it the same way.

☐ If you miss a dose of this medicine, take it as soon as you remember.

SPECIAL INSTRUCTIONS

☐ It is very important that you take this medicine exactly as your doctor has prescribed and that you do not miss any doses. Try to take this medicine at the same time every day. Do not take extra tablets without your doctor's approval. Do not stop taking this medicine without the approval of your doctor.

☐ Women who are pregnant, breast-feeding, or planning to become pregnant should tell their doctor before taking this medicine.

☐ Check with your doctor or pharmacist before taking any nonprescription drugs that contain iodides (for example, some cough, cold, or asthma products).

- [ ] Call your doctor immediately if you become sick or develop a fever, sore throat, skin abscess, or other symptoms of an infection.
- [ ] Most people experience few or no side effects from their drugs. However, any medicine can sometimes cause unwanted effects. Call your doctor if you develop a sore throat, fever or mouth sores, skin rash, dark-colored urine or a yellow color to the skin or eyes, easy bruising or bleeding, swelling of the legs, swollen glands, changes in urination ("passing your water"), fast heartbeats, or unusual tiredness.

*   *   *   *   *

Protokylol HCl (*Oral Bronchodilator*)
United States: Ventaire

- [ ] This medicine is used to help open up the bronchioles (air passages in the lungs) to make breathing easier.
- [ ] IMPORTANT: If you have ever had an allergic reaction to any cough/cold, allergy, heart, or weight-reducing medicines, tell your doctor or pharmacist before you take any of this medicine.

HOW TO USE THIS MEDICINE
- [ ] This tablet may be taken with food or a glass of water.

SPECIAL INSTRUCTIONS
- [ ] Do not change the dose of your regular asthma or bronchitis medicines except on the advice of your doctor.
- [ ] It is not unusual to have a little flushing of the face or a faster heartbeat just after you take the medicine.
- [ ] Call your doctor if the medicine does not relieve your breathing problems.
- [ ] Most people experience few or no side effects from their drugs. However, any medicine can sometimes cause unwanted effects. Call your doctor if you develop swollen glands, skin rash, dizziness, sweating, or chest pain.

*   *   *   *   *

Protriptyline HCl (*Oral Antidepressant*)
United States: Vivactil
Canada: Triptil

- [ ] This medicine is used to help relieve the symptoms of depression. It is important that you take the medicine regularly and that you do not miss any doses. The full effect of the medicine will not be noticed immediately but may take from a few days to several weeks. Early signs of improvement are increased appetite, better sleep, increased energy, and later improved

721

mood. DO NOT STOP TAKING the medicine when you first feel better or you may feel worse in 3 or 4 days.

HOW TO USE THIS MEDICINE

☐ This medicine may be taken with food unless otherwise directed.

SPECIAL INSTRUCTIONS

☐ If you forget to take a dose, take it as soon as possible. However, if it is almost time for your next dose, do not take the missed dose. Instead, continue with your regular dosing schedule.

☐ Any medicine has a few unwanted side effects. Because this medicine takes a few weeks to work, the side effects are the only thing that tell the doctor that the drug is being absorbed. Most of these side effects will go away as your body adjusts to the medicine.

☐ In some people, this drug may cause dizziness or drowsiness. Do not drive a car or operate dangerous machinery or do jobs that require you to be alert until you know how you are going to react to this drug.

☐ If this medicine causes dizziness, you should be careful going up and down stairs and you should not change positions too quickly. Get out of bed slowly in the morning and dangle your feet over the edge of the bed for a few minutes before standing up. Sit or lie down at the first sign of dizziness. Tell your doctor you have been dizzy and he may adjust your dose.

☐ Do not drink alcoholic beverages while taking this drug without the approval of your doctor.

☐ It is important that you obtain the advice of your doctor or pharmacist before taking any other medicines, including pain relievers, sleeping pills, tranquilizers, other medicines for depression, cough/cold or allergy medicines, or weight-reducing medicines.

☐ If your mouth becomes dry, suck a hard sour candy (sugarless) or ice chips, or chew gum. It is especially important to brush your teeth regularly if you develop a dry mouth.

☐ If you become constipated, try increasing the amount of bulk in your diet (for example, bran and salads), exercising more often, or drinking water.

☐ Call your doctor if you develop a sore throat, fever, mouth sores, eye pain or blurred vision, difficulty in urinating ("passing your water"), fast heartbeats, or a skin rash.

☐ Do not stop taking this medicine suddenly without your doctor's approval. When your doctor tells you to stop this medicine, you must follow these precautions for 1 week since some of the medicine will still be in your body.

☐ Carry an identification card indicating that you are taking this medicine. Always tell your dentist, pharmacist, and other doctors who are treating you that you are taking this medicine.

*   *   *   *   *

Pseudoephedrine HCl (*Bronchodilator-Decongestant*)

United States: Novafed, Sudafed, Sudadrine

Canada: Eltor, Pseudofrin, Robidrine, Sudafed

☐ This medicine is used to help relieve nasal stuffiness and make breathing easier. It is also used to relieve ear congestion.

☐ IMPORTANT: If you have ever had an allergic reaction to any cough/cold, allergy, heart, or weight-reducing medicines, tell your doctor or pharmacist before you take any of this medicine.

HOW TO USE THIS MEDICINE

☐ This medicine may be taken with food or a glass of milk in order to prevent stomach upset.

☐ Do not take this medicine more often than your doctor has prescribed.

☐ This medicine must be swallowed whole. Do not crush, chew, or break it into pieces. (*United States:* Novaphed Timed Release, Sudafed Timeceles, Sudafed S.A.)

☐ If you forget to take a dose, take it as soon as possible. However, if it is almost time for your next dose, do not take the missed dose. Instead, continue with your regular dosing schedule.

SPECIAL INSTRUCTIONS

☐ Women who are breast-feeding should tell their doctor before taking this medicine.

☐ Do not take this medicine within 2 hours of bedtime. It could cause insomnia (difficulty in falling asleep) if you take it too close to bedtime.

☐ It is important that you obtain the advice of your doctor before taking pain relievers, nonprescription drugs, sleeping pills, tranquilizers, or medicines for depression while you are taking this drug.

☐ Call your doctor if you do not feel better within 5 days or if you have a fever.

☐ Most people experience few or no side effects from their drugs. However, any medicine can sometimes cause unwanted effects. Call your doctor if you develop unusual restlessness, difficulty in urinating ("passing your water"), a fast heartbeat, shortness of breath, headache, dizziness, or sweating.

* * * * *

Psyllium Hydrophilic Muciloid (*Oral Laxative*)

United States: Effersyllium, Metamucil, Modane Bulk, Mucilose

Canada: Metamucil, Novo-Mucilax

☐ This medicine is a bulk-producing agent useful both in constipation, caused by inadequate fiber in the diet, and in diarrhea.

723

HOW TO USE THIS MEDICINE

- ☐ This medicine may be stirred into milk, orange juice, or prune juice, or it can be placed on the tongue and swallowed with water, or it may be sprinkled on cereals and eaten. (**United States:** Mucilose)

- ☐ Put the prescribed dose of powder into an 8 oz. glass and then slowly add cool water. Drink immediately. (**United States:** Metamucil Instant Mix, Effersyllium Instant Mix; **Canada:** Metamucil Instant Mix)

- ☐ Unless otherwise directed, stir the prescribed dose of powder into an 8 oz. glass of cool water or other cool liquid. (**United States:** Metamucil Powder, Modane Bulk; **Canada:** Metamucil Powder, Novo-Mucilax

SPECIAL INSTRUCTIONS

- ☐ Do not take this medicine if you have stomach pain, nausea, or vomiting.

- ☐ It may be necessary to take this medicine for 2 or 3 days before you notice its full effect.

- ☐ Call your doctor if you develop a fever or if your symptoms are not relieved.

*   *   *   *   *

Pyrantel Pamoate (*Oral Anthelmintic*)

United States: Antiminth
Canada: Combantrin

- ☐ This medicine is used to treat intestinal worm infections.

HOW TO USE THIS MEDICINE

- ☐ This medicine may be taken with milk or fruit juice either with food or on an empty stomach.

- ☐ Shake the liquid preparation well before using in order to get an accurate dose.

SPECIAL INSTRUCTIONS

- ☐ In some people, this drug may cause dizziness or drowsiness. Do not drive a car or operate dangerous machinery or do jobs that require you to be alert until you know how you are going to react to this drug.

- ☐ If you become dizzy, you should be careful going up and down stairs. Sit or lie down at the first sign of dizziness.

- ☐ It is not necessary to take a laxative or change your diet unless your doctor recommends that you do so.

- ☐ Store the medicine in a cool, dark place.

- ☐ Most people experience few or no side effects from their drugs. However, any medicine can sometimes cause unwanted effects. Call your doctor if you develop a skin rash, stomach cramps, or severe headache.

724

GENERAL INSTRUCTIONS

- [ ] Good personal hygiene is very important to prevent reinfection.

- [ ] It is recommended that you have a shower every morning in order to remove any eggs in the anal area that have appeared during the night.

- [ ] Wash your hands frequently, especially before handling food or anything that will be put into the mouth. Wash the hands after urination and bowel movements.

- [ ] Keep the nails short and clean and avoiding biting them. Do not put your fingers in your mouth or nose.

- [ ] On the day of therapy, change the bed linen, underwear, and nightclothes. Wash or dry-clean them immediately.

- [ ] Do not scratch the affected area.

- [ ] Disinfect the toilet seat and bathtub daily.

* * * * *

Pyridostigmine Bromide (*Oral Antimyasthenic-Cholinergic*)
United States: Mestinon Bromide
Canada: Mestinon

- [ ] This medicine is used to treat the fatigue and muscular weakness of myasthenia gravis.

HOW TO USE THIS MEDICINE

- [ ] This medicine may be taken with food or a glass of water.

- [ ] This medicine must be swallowed whole. Do not crush, chew, or break it into pieces. (***United States:*** Mestinon Bromide Timespans; ***Canada:*** Mestinon Supraspans)

SPECIAL INSTRUCTIONS

- [ ] If you forget to take a dose, take it as soon as possible. However, if it is almost time for your next dose, do not take the missed dose. Instead, continue with your regular dosing schedule.

- [ ] In some people, this drug may cause "double vision." Do not drive a car or operate dangerous machinery or do jobs that require you to be alert until you know how you are going to react to this drug.

- [ ] It is important that you obtain the advice of your doctor or pharmacist before taking pain relievers, nonprescription drugs, sleeping pills or tranquilizers, or medicines for depression while you are taking this drug.

- [ ] It is a good idea to keep a diary of "peaks and valleys" of your muscle strength. This will help your doctor in designing your treatment.

725

☐ Most people experience few or no side effects from their drugs. However, any medicine can sometimes cause unwanted effects. Call your doctor if you develop slow or fast heartbeats, changes in vision, muscle cramps, nausea, vomiting or diarrhea, difficulty in breathing, fainting spells or dizziness, convulsions, unusual sweating, or if you urinate ("pass your water") more frequently than usual.

*   *   *   *   *

Pyrilamine Maleate (Oral Antihistamine)
United States: Allertoc, Zem-Histine

☐ This medicine is used to help relieve the symptoms of certain types of allergic conditions, coughs and colds, and certain skin conditions.

HOW TO USE THIS MEDICINE
☐ This medicine may be taken with food or a glass of milk if it upsets your stomach.

SPECIAL INSTRUCTIONS
☐ If you forget to take a dose, take it as soon as possible. However, if it is almost time for your next dose, do not take the missed dose. Instead, continue with your regular dosing schedule.

☐ In some people, this drug may initially cause dizziness or drowsiness. Do not drive a car or operate dangerous machinery or do jobs that require you to be alert until you know how you are going to react to this drug. If you become dizzy, you should be careful going up and down stairs. Sit or lie down at the first sign of dizziness. Tell your doctor if it continues.

☐ Do not drink alcoholic beverages while taking this drug without the approval of your doctor.

☐ If your mouth becomes dry, suck a hard sour candy (sugarless) or ice chips, or chew gum. It is especially important to brush your teeth regularly if you develop a dry mouth.

☐ It is important that you obtain the advice of your doctor or pharmacist before taking pain relievers, nonprescription drugs, sleeping pills or tranquilizers, or other medicines for allergies.

☐ Do not take this medicine more often or longer than recommended by your doctor.

☐ Most people experience few or no side effects from their drugs. However, any medicine can sometimes cause unwanted effects. Call your doctor if you develop a skin rash, fast heartbeats, blurred vision, stomach pain, or difficulty in urinating ("passing your water").

*   *   *   *   *

Pyrimethamine (*Oral Antimalarial*)
United States: Daraprim
Canada: Daraprim

☐ This medicine is used to treat malaria and certain types of infections.

HOW TO USE THIS MEDICINE
☐ This medicine may be taken with meals or food to help prevent stomach upset.

SPECIAL INSTRUCTIONS
☐ It is very important that you take this medicine exactly as your doctor has prescribed and that you do not miss any doses. Try to take this medicine at the same time every day. Do not take extra tablets without your doctor's approval.

☐ Most people experience few or no side effects from their drugs. However, any medicine can sometimes cause unwanted effects. Call your doctor if you develop persistent vomiting, diarrhea, sore throat, fever, sore tongue, or a skin rash.

*   *   *   *   *

Pyrvinium Pamoate (*Oral Oxyuriasis Therapy*)
United States: Povan
Canada: Pamovin, Pyr-Pam, Vanquin

☐ This medicine is used to treat worm infections.

HOW TO USE THIS MEDICINE
☐ Take this medicine before or after meals.

☐ Shake the liquid preparation well before using in order to get an accurate dose. (**United States:** Povan Suspension; **Canada:** Pyr-Pam, Vanquin Suspensions)

☐ Do not crush, suck, or chew the tablets. Swallow the tablets whole to avoid staining the teeth red.

SPECIAL INSTRUCTIONS
☐ Women who are pregnant, breast-feeding, or planning to become pregnant should tell their doctor before taking this medicine.

☐ This medicine may cause the stools to turn red. This is not unusual.

☐ Avoid spilling this medicine on clothing or fabrics as it will stain them and the color is difficult to remove.

☐ It is not necessary to take a laxative or change your diet unless your doctor recommends that you do so.

727

☐ Most people experience few or no side effects from their drugs. However, any medicine can sometimes cause unwanted effects. Call your doctor if you develop a skin rash, hives or itching, or severe stomach cramps.

☐ Store the medicine in a cool place.

GENERAL INSTRUCTIONS

☐ Good personal hygiene is very important to prevent reinfection.

☐ It is recommended that you have a shower every morning in order to remove any eggs in the anal area that have appeared during the night.

☐ Wash your hands frequently especially before handling food or anything that will be put into the mouth. Wash the hands after urination and bowel movements.

☐ Keep the nails short and clean and avoid biting them. Do not put your fingers in your mouth or nose.

☐ On the day of therapy, change the bed linen, underwear, and nightclothes. Wash or dry-clean them immediately.

☐ Do not scratch the affected area.

☐ Disinfect the toilet seat and bathtub daily.

*   *   *   *   *

Quinacrine (*Oral Antimalarial-Antiparasitic*)
United States: Atabrine
Canada: Atabrine

☐ This medicine is used in the treatment of malaria and intestinal worm infestations.

HOW TO USE THIS MEDICINE

☐ Take the drug exactly as prescribed by your doctor.

SPECIAL INSTRUCTIONS

☐ This medicine may cause the urine and skin to turn yellow in color. This is a temporary effect and usually disappears within 2 weeks after your treatment is finished.

☐ In some people, this drug may cause dizziness. Do not drive a car or operate dangerous machinery or do jobs that require you to be alert until you know how you are going to react to this drug.

☐ If you become dizzy, you should be careful going up and down stairs. Sit or lie down at the first sign of dizziness.

☐ Most people experience few or no side effects from their drugs. However, any medicine can sometimes cause unwanted effects. Call your doctor if you

728

develop blurred vision, "double" vision, a skin rash, or nightmares, or if you become depressed.

☐ Keep this medicine well out of the reach of children.

* * * * *

Quinestrol (Oral Estrogen)
United States: Estrovis

☐ This medicine is a hormone and is used to help relieve the symptoms of menopause or is used if the ovaries have been removed.

HOW TO USE THIS MEDICINE
☐ Take the medicine with a glass of water. Try not to miss any doses.

SPECIAL INSTRUCTIONS
☐ Women who are pregnant, breast-feeding, or planning to become pregnant should tell their doctor before taking this medicine.

☐ It is recommended that you do not smoke while you are taking this medicine because smoking may increase the incidence of heart attacks.

☐ Contact your doctor if any of the following side effects occur:
- Severe or persistent headaches
- Vomiting, dizziness, or fainting
- Blurred vision or slurred speech
- Pain in the calves of the legs or numbness in an arm or leg
- Chest pain, shortness of breath, or coughing up of blood
- Lumps in the breast
- Severe depression
- A yellow color to the skin or eyes or dark-colored urine
- Severe abdominal pain
- Vaginal bleeding

☐ Carry an identification card indicating that you are taking this medicine. Always tell your pharmacist, dentist, and other doctors who are treating you that you are taking this medicine.

* * * * *

Quinethazone (Oral Diuretic-Antihypertensive)
United States: Hydromox
Canada: Aquamox

☐ This medicine is used to help rid the body of excess water and to decrease swelling. It is also used to treat high blood pressure. It is commonly called a "water pill."

☐ IMPORTANT: If you have ever had an allergic reaction to sulfa drugs or thiazide diuretics, tell your doctor or pharmacist before taking any of this medicine.

HOW TO USE THIS MEDICINE

☐ Take the medicine with food, meals, or milk.

☐ Try to take it at the same time(s) every day so that you have a constant level of the medicine in your body. Do not miss any doses. Otherwise, you cannot expect the drug to work as well.

☐ When you first start taking this medicine, you will probably urinate ("pass your water") more often and in larger amounts than usual. Therefore, if you are to take one dose every day, take it in the morning after breakfast. If you are to take more than one dose every day, take the last dose 6 hours before bedtime so that you will not have to get up during the night to go to the bathroom. This effect will usually lessen after you have taken the drug for awhile.

SPECIAL INSTRUCTIONS

☐ If you forget to take a dose, take it as soon as possible. However, if it is almost time for your next dose, do not take the missed dose. Instead, continue with your regular dosing schedule.

☐ Women who are pregnant, breast-feeding, or planning to become pregnant should tell their doctor before taking this medicine.

☐ This medicine normally causes your body to lose potassium. The body has warning signs to let you know if too much potassium is being lost. Call your doctor if you become unusually thirsty or if you develop leg cramps, unusual weakness, fatigue, vomiting, confusion, or irregular pulse.

☐ If your doctor recommends that you eat foods which are high in potassium, one or more of the foods listed in Appendix A should be eaten daily. All of these foods are rich in potassium. Your goal should be to take in 1000 to 2000 mg. of potassium (approximately 25.6 to 51 mEq) each day. The calorie content and sodium content are included for your convenience in meal planning. CHANGE YOUR DIET ONLY IF YOUR DOCTOR TELLS YOU TO.

☐ If this medicine causes dizziness, you should be careful going up and down stairs and you should not change positions too rapidly. Get out of bed slowly in the morning and dangle your feet over the edge of the bed for a few minutes before standing up. Sit down or lie down at the first sign of dizziness. Tell your doctor you have been dizzy. Be careful drinking alcoholic beverages while taking this medicine because they could make the dizziness worse. Do not drive a car or operate dangerous machinery or do jobs that require you to be alert if you are dizzy.

☐ In order to help prevent dizziness and fainting, your doctor may also recommend that you avoid strenuous exercises, standing for long periods of time (especially in hot weather), or hot showers or hot baths.

- [ ] This medicine may make some people more sensitive to sunlight and sunlamps. When you begin taking this medicine, try to avoid getting too much sun until you see how you are going to react. If your skin does become more sensitive to sunlight, tell your doctor and try to stay out of direct sunlight. While in the sun, wear protective clothing and sunglasses. You may wish to ask your pharmacist about suitable sunscreen products. Check with your doctor if you become sunburned.

- [ ] Call your doctor immediately if you think you may be allergic to the medicine or if you develop a skin rash, hives, itching, swelling of the face, or difficulty in breathing. If you cannot reach your doctor, phone a hospital emergency department.

- [ ] Most people experience few or no side effects from their drugs. However, any medicine can sometimes cause unwanted effects. Call your doctor if you develop a sore throat, fever, sharp stomach pain, chest pain, sharp joint pain, easy bruising or bleeding, a yellow color to the skin or eyes, or a sudden weight gain of 5 pounds or more.

* * * * *

Quinidine Polygalacturonate (*Oral Anti-arrhythmic*)
United States: Cardioquin
Canada: Cardioquin

Quinidine Gluconate
United States: Quinaglute Dura-Tabs
Canada: Quinaglute Dura-Tabs, Quinate

Quinidine Bisulfate
Canada: Biquin Durules

Quinidine Sulfate
United States: Cin-Quin, Kinidine, Quinora, Quinidex Extentabs

- [ ] This medicine is used to help make your heart beat at a regular and normal rate.

- [ ] IMPORTANT: If you have ever had an allergic reaction to quinine or quinidine, tell your doctor or pharmacist before you take any of this medicine.

HOW TO USE THIS MEDICINE
- [ ] It is best to take this medicine on an empty stomach 1 hour before (or 2 hours after) eating food. However, if it upsets your stomach, take the medicine with some food or milk.

- [ ] This medicine must be swallowed whole. It must not be chewed, crushed, or broken into pieces. (**United States:** Quinaglute Dura-Tabs, Quinidex Extentabs; **Canada:** Biquin Durules, Quinaglute Dura-Tabs)

731

SPECIAL INSTRUCTIONS

- [ ] It is very important that you take this medicine exactly as your doctor has prescribed and that you do not miss any doses. Try to take this medicine at the same time every day. Do not take extra tablets without your doctor's approval. Do not go without this medicine between prescription refills.

- [ ] Women who are pregnant, breast-feeding, or planning to become pregnant should tell their doctor before taking this medicine.

- [ ] If you forget to take a dose and remember it within 2 hours of the missed dose, take it as soon as possible. Otherwise, do not take the missed dose and continue with your regular schedule.

- [ ] Some nonprescription drugs can interfere with this medicine or aggravate your heart condition. Do not take any of the following without the approval of your doctor or pharmacist: antacids or baking soda; cough, cold, or sinus products; asthma or allergy products; or diet or weight-reducing medicines.

- [ ] Tell your doctor if you become dizzy or feel faint. Sit or lie down at the first sign of dizziness and do not drive a car, operate dangerous machinery, or do jobs that require you to be alert.

- [ ] Most people experience few or no side effects from their drugs. However, any medicine can sometimes cause unwanted effects. Call your doctor if you develop "ringing" or "buzzing" in the ears or any loss of hearing, blurred vision, a skin rash, fever, severe headaches, vomiting, troublesome diarrhea, shortness of breath, or unusual bruising.

- [ ] Carry an identification card indicating that you are taking this medicine. Always tell your pharmacist, dentist, and other doctors who are treating you that you are taking this medicine.

* * * * *

Quinine (*Oral Antimalarial*)
United States: Coco-Quinine, Quinine Sulfate
Canada: Kinine

- [ ] This medicine has many uses and the reason it was prescribed depends upon your condition. If you do not understand why you are taking it, check with your doctor.

- [ ] IMPORTANT: If you have ever had an allergic reaction to a quinine or quinidine medicine, tell your doctor or pharmacist before you take any of this medicine.

HOW TO USE THIS MEDICINE

- [ ] Take this medicine immediately before or after meals or with food in order to help prevent stomach upset.

☐ For LIQUID MEDICINE
- Shake the bottle well before using so that you can measure an accurate dose. (**United States:** Coco-Quinine)

☐ It is very important that you take this medicine exactly as your doctor has prescribed and that you do not miss any doses. Try to take this medicine at the same time every day. Do not take extra tablets without your doctor's approval. Take the medicine for the full treatment.

SPECIAL INSTRUCTIONS
☐ If you forget to take a dose, take it as soon as possible. However, if it is almost time for your next dose, do not take the missed dose. Instead, continue with your regular dosing schedule.

☐ Women who are pregnant, breast-feeding, or planning to become pregnant should tell their doctor before taking this medicine

☐ Most people experience few or no side effects from their drugs. However, any medicine can sometimes cause unwanted effects. Call your doctor if you develop a sore throat, fever or mouth sores, a skin rash, dizziness or fainting spells, changes in vision, "ringing" or "buzzing" in the ears, shortness of breath, or stomach pain.

* * * * *

Rescinnamine (*Oral Antihypertensive*)
United States: Cinnasil, Moderil

☐ This medicine is used to lower blood pressure and relieve anxiety.

☐ Hypertension (high blood pressure) is a long-term condition and it will probably be necessary for you to take the drug for a long time in spite of the fact that you feel better. It is very important that you take this medicine as your doctor has directed and that you do not miss any doses. Otherwise, you cannot expect the drug to keep your blood pressure down.

☐ IMPORTANT: If you have allergies, tell your doctor or pharmacist before you take any of this medicine.

HOW TO USE THIS MEDICINE
☐ Take this medicine with food, meals, or milk.

☐ Try to take the medicine at the same time(s) every day.

SPECIAL INSTRUCTIONS
☐ If you forget to take a dose, take it as soon as possible. However, if it is almost time for your next dose, do not take the missed dose. Instead, continue with your regular dosing schedule.

☐ Women who are pregnant, breast-feeding, or planning to become pregnant should tell their doctor before taking this medicine.

☐ In some people, this drug may cause dizziness or drowsiness. Do not drive a car or operate dangerous machinery or do jobs that require you to be alert until you know how you are going to react to this drug.

☐ In a few people, this medicine may cause dizziness or fainting if you get up quickly from a lying or sitting position. Get up slowly, especially in the morning. It is advisable to dangle your feet over the edge of the bed for a few minutes before standing up. Sit or lie down at the first sign of dizziness. Tell your doctor that you have been dizzy.

☐ In order to help prevent dizziness and fainting, it is also recommended that you avoid strenuous exercise, standing for long periods of time (especially in hot weather), and hot showers or hot baths.

☐ If you develop a stuffy nose, tell your doctor.

☐ Some nonprescription drugs can aggravate your condition. Do not take any of the following without the approval of your doctor or pharmacist: cough, cold, or sinus products; asthma or allergy products; or diet or weight reducing medicines.

☐ Most people experience few or no side effects from their drugs. However, any medicine can sometimes cause unwanted effects. Call your doctor if you develop severe diarrhea (loose bowel movements), stomach pain, a skin rash, nightmares, loss of appetite or depression, swelling of the legs or ankles, sudden weight gain of 5 pounds or more, chest pains, or difficulty in breathing.

☐ Carry an identification card indicating that you are taking this medicine. Always tell your pharmacist, dentist, and other doctors who are treating you that you are taking this medicine.

☐ Do not stop taking this medicine without your doctor's approval and do not go without medicine between prescription refills. Call your pharmacist 2 or 3 days before you will run out of the medicine.

* * * * *

Reserpine (*Oral Antihypertensive-Antipsychotic*)
　　United States: Alkarau, Hiserpia, Lemiserp, Rauloydin, Raurine, Rau-Sed, Resercen, Reserpoid, Rolserp, Sandril, Serpalan, Serpanray, Serpasil, Serpate, SK-Reserpine, Tri-Serp, Vio-Serpine
　　Canada: Neo-Serp, Reserfia, Reserpanca, Serpasil

☐ This medicine is used to lower blood pressure and relieve anxiety.

☐ Hypertension (high blood pressure) is a long-term condition and it will probably be necessary for you to take the drug for a long time in spite of the fact that you feel better. It is very important that you take this medicine as your doctor has directed and that you do not miss any doses. Otherwise, you cannot expect the drug to keep your blood pressure down.

- ☐ IMPORTANT: If you have allergies, tell your doctor or pharmacist before you take any of this medicine.

HOW TO USE THIS MEDICINE
- ☐ Take this medicine with food, meals, or milk.
- ☐ Try to take the medicine at the same time(s) every day.

SPECIAL INSTRUCTIONS
- ☐ If you forget to take a dose, take it as soon as possible. However, if it is almost time for your next dose, do not take the missed dose. Instead, continue with your regular dosing schedule.

- ☐ Women who are pregnant, breast-feeding, or planning to become pregnant should tell their doctor before taking this medicine.

- ☐ In some people, this drug may cause dizziness or drowsiness. Do not drive a car or operate dangerous machinery or do jobs that require you to be alert until you know how you are going to react to this drug.

- ☐ In a few people, this medicine may cause dizziness or fainting if you get up quickly from a lying or sitting position. Get up slowly, especially in the morning. It is advisable to dangle your feet over the edge of the bed for a few minutes before standing up. Sit or lie down at the first sign of dizziness. Tell your doctor that you have been dizzy.

- ☐ In order to help prevent dizziness and fainting, it is also recommended that you avoid strenuous exercise, standing for long periods of time (especially in hot weather), and hot showers or hot baths.

- ☐ If you develop a stuffy nose, tell your doctor.

- ☐ Some nonprescription drugs can aggravate your condition. Do not take any of the following without the approval of your doctor or pharmacist: cough, cold, or sinus products; asthma or allergy products; or diet or weight-reducing medicines.

- ☐ Most people experience few or no side effects from their drugs. However, any medicine can sometimes cause unwanted effects. Call your doctor if you develop severe diarrhea (loose bowel movements), stomach pain, a skin rash, nightmares, loss of appetite or depression, swelling of the legs or ankles, sudden weight gain of 5 pounds or more, chest pains, or difficulty in breathing.

- ☐ Carry an identification card indicating that you are taking this medicine. Always tell your pharmacist, dentist, and other doctors who are treating you that you are taking this medicine.

- ☐ Do not stop taking this medicine without your doctor's approval and do not go without medicine between prescription refills. Call your pharmacist 2 or 3 days before you will run out of the medicine.

* * * * *

Reserpine-Benzthiazide (*Oral Antihypertensive*)
United States: Exna-R

Reserpine-Chlorothiazide
United States: Chloroserpine, Diupres, Ro-Chloro-Serp, Thiaserp
Canada: Diupres-250

Reserpine-Chlorthalidone
United States: Regroton
Canada: Hygroton-Reserpine

Reserpine-Hydrochlorothiazide
United States: Hydropres, Hydroserp, Hydroserpine, Hydrotensin,
   Loquapres, Serpasil-Esidrex, Thia-Serp
Canada: Hydropres, Serpasil-Esidrix

Reserpine-Hydroflumethiazide
United States: Salutensin

Reserpine-Trichlormethiazide
United States: Metatensin, Naquival

☐ This medicine is used to help lower the blood pressure.

☐ Hypertension (high blood pressure) is a long-term condition and it will probably be necessary for you to take the drug for a long time in spite of the fact
that you feel better. It is very important that you take this medicine as your
doctor has directed and that you do not miss any doses. Otherwise, you
cannot expect the drug to keep your blood pressure down.

☐ IMPORTANT: If you have allergies, tell your doctor or pharmacist before you
take any of this medicine.

HOW TO USE THIS MEDICINE
☐ Take this medicine with food, meals, or milk.

☐ Try to take the medicine at the same time(s) every day.

SPECIAL INSTRUCTIONS
☐ If you forget to take a dose, take it as soon as possible. However, if it is
almost time for your next dose, do not take the missed dose. Instead, continue with your regular dosing schedule.

☐ Women who are pregnant, breast-feeding, or planning to become pregnant
should tell their doctor before taking this medicine.

☐ This medicine normally causes your body to lose potassium. The body has warning signs to let you know if too much potassium is being lost. Call your doctor if you become unusually thirsty or if you develop leg cramps, unusual weakness, fatigue, vomiting, confusion, or an irregular pulse.

☐ If your doctor recommends that you eat foods which are high in potassium, one or more of the foods listed in Appendix A should be eaten daily. All of these foods are rich in potassium. CHANGE YOUR DIET ONLY IF YOUR DOCTOR TELLS YOU TO.

☐ This medicine may make some people more sensitive to sunlight and sunlamps. When you begin taking this medicine, try to avoid getting too much sun until you see how you are going to react. If your skin does become more sensitive to sunlight, tell your doctor and try to stay out of direct sunlight. While in the sun, wear protective clothing and sunglasses. You may wish to ask your pharmacist about suitable sunscreen products. Check with your doctor if you become sunburned.

☐ In some people, this drug may cause dizziness or drowsiness. Do not drive a car or operate dangerous machinery or do jobs that require you to be alert until you know how you are going to react to this drug.

☐ This medicine may cause dizziness or fainting if you get up quickly from a lying or sitting position. Get up slowly, especially in the morning. It is advisable to dangle your feet over the edge of the bed for a few minutes before standing up. Sit or lie down at the first sign of dizziness. Tell your doctor that you have been dizzy.

☐ In order to help prevent dizziness and fainting, it is also recommended that you avoid strenuous exercise, standing for long periods of time (especially in hot weather), and hot showers or hot baths.

☐ If you develop a stuffy nose, tell your doctor.

☐ Some nonprescription drugs can aggravate your condition. Do not take any of the following without the approval of your doctor or pharmacist: cough, cold, or sinus products; asthma or allergy products; or diet or weight-reducing medicines.

☐ Most people experience few or no side effects from their drugs. However, any medicine can sometimes cause unwanted effects. Call your doctor if you develop severe diarrhea (loose bowel movements), stomach pain, a skin rash, nightmares, loss of appetite or depression, swelling of the legs or ankles, sudden weight gain of 5 pounds or more, chest pains, or difficulty in breathing. Also call your doctor if you develop sharp joint pain, easy bruising or bleeding, or a yellow color to the skin or eyes.

☐ Carry an identification card indicating that you are taking this medicine. Always tell your pharmacist, dentist, and other doctors who are treating you that you are taking this medicine.

☐ Do not stop taking this medicine without your doctor's approval and do not go without medicine between prescription refills. Call your pharmacist 2 or 3 days before you will run out of the medicine.

* * * * *

Reserpine-Hydralazine (*Oral Antihypertensive*)
United States: Dralserp, Serpasil-Apresoline
Canada: Serpasil-Apresoline

☐ This medicine is used to help lower the blood pressure.

☐ Hypertension (high blood pressure) is a long-term condition, and it will probably be necessary for you to take the drug for a long time in spite of the fact that you feel better. It is very important that you take this medicine as your doctor has directed and that you do not miss any doses. Otherwise, you cannot expect the drug to keep your blood pressure down.

☐ IMPORTANT: If you have allergies, tell your doctor or pharmacist before you take any of this medicine.

HOW TO USE THIS MEDICINE
☐ Take this medicine with food, meals, or milk.

☐ Try to take the medicine at the same time(s) every day.

SPECIAL INSTRUCTIONS
☐ If you forget to take a dose, take it as soon as possible. However, if it is almost time for your next dose, do not take the missed dose. Instead, continue with your regular dosing schedule.

☐ Women who are pregnant, breast-feeding, or planning to become pregnant should tell their doctor before taking this medicine.

☐ Headaches may occur during the first few days of therapy and will usually disappear within the first week of treatment. If they continue, call your doctor.

☐ Do not drink alcoholic beverages while taking this drug without the approval of your doctor.

☐ In some people, this drug may cause dizziness or drowsiness. Do not drive a car or operate dangerous machinery or do jobs that require you to be alert until you know how you are going to react to this drug.

☐ This medicine may cause dizziness or fainting if you get up quickly from a lying or sitting position. Get up slowly, especially in the morning. It is advisable to dangle your feet over the edge of the bed for a few minutes before standing up. Sit or lie down at the first sign of dizziness. Tell your doctor that you have been dizzy.

☐ In order to help prevent dizziness and fainting, it is also recommended that

738

you avoid strenuous exercise, standing for long periods of time (especially in hot weather), and hot showers or hot baths.

☐ If you develop a stuffy nose, tell your doctor.

☐ Some nonprescription drugs can aggravate your condition. Do not take any of the following without the approval of your doctor or pharmacist: cough, cold, or sinus products; asthma or allergy products; or diet or weight-reducing medicines.

☐ Most people experience few or no side effects from their drugs. However, any medicine can sometimes cause unwanted effects. Call your doctor if you develop severe diarrhea (loose bowel movements), stomach pain, a skin rash, nightmares, loss of appetite or depression, swelling of the legs or ankles, sudden weight gain of 5 pounds or more, chest pains or difficulty in breathing, sore throat, muscle or joint pain, or numbness or tingling of the hands or feet.

☐ Carry an identification card indicating that you are taking this medicine. Always tell your pharmacist, dentist, and other doctors who are treating you that you are taking this medicine.

☐ Do not stop taking this medicine without your doctor's approval and do not go without medicine between prescription refills. Call your pharmacist 2 or 3 days before you will run out of the medicine.

*   *   *   *   *

Retinoic Acid (See Tretinoin)

*   *   *   *   *

Rifampin (Oral Antituberculous Antibiotic)
United States: Rifadin, Rimactane
Canada: Rifadin, Rimactane, Rofact

☐ This medicine is used to prevent or help the body overcome tuberculosis. Because tuberculosis (TB) heals very slowly, it may be necessary for you to take this medicine for a long time.

☐ Some patients who carry meningitis bacteria may be prescribed this medicine to help prevent them from spreading the bacteria to others.

☐ It is very important that you keep taking this medicine for the full length of time that your doctor has prescribed. Do not stop taking the medicine earlier than your doctor has recommended in spite of the fact that you may feel better. DO NOT MISS ANY DOSES and DO NOT RUN OUT OF THIS MEDICINE.

☐ The most important thing you can do to protect others from catching your TB is to take your medicine regularly and to cover your coughs and sneezes with a double-ply tissue. This will reduce the spray of germs into the air. Covering your mouth with the bare hand does no good.

HOW TO USE THIS MEDICINE

☐ It is best to take this medicine on an empty stomach 1 hour before (or 2 hours after) meals or food unless otherwise directed. Take it at the proper time even if you skip a meal.

☐ Take the medicine with a full glass of water.

SPECIAL INSTRUCTIONS

☐ If you forget to take a dose, take it as soon as you can remember and then continue with your regular schedule. However, if it is almost time for your next dose, do not take the dose you forgot.

☐ Women who are pregnant, breast-feeding, or planning to become pregnant should tell their doctor before taking this medicine.

☐ It is recommended that you avoid the use of alcoholic beverages while you are taking this medicine.

☐ In some people, this drug may cause dizziness or drowsiness. Do not drive a car or operate dangerous machinery or do jobs that require you to be alert until you know how you are going to react to this drug.

☐ This medicine may cause the urine, stools, saliva, sputum, sweat, and tears to turn orange-red in color. This is not an unusual effect. However, if you wear soft contact lenses, it is best not to wear them while you are on this medicine as they may become stained.

☐ Birth control pills may not work as well when you are taking this medicine. Check with your doctor or pharmacist about a different method of birth control.

☐ Stop taking the medicine and call your doctor if you develop a loss of appetite, severe diarrhea, fever, chills, nausea or vomiting, unusual weakness or tiredness, bone pain, or "flu-like" symptoms.

☐ Most people experience few or no side effects from their drugs. However, any medicine can sometimes cause unwanted effects. Call your doctor if you develop a skin rash, dark-colored urine, a yellow color in the skin or eyes, easy bruising, shortness of breath, or if you urinate ("pass your water") less frequently or in smaller amounts than normal.

*   *   *   *   *

Salbutamol (*Oral Bronchilator*)
Canada: Ventolin

☐ This medicine is used to help open the bronchioles (air passages in the lungs) to make breathing easier.

☐ IMPORTANT: If you have ever had an allergic reaction to any cough/cold, allergy, heart, or weight-reducing medicines, tell your doctor or pharmacist before you take any of this medicine.

HOW TO USE THIS MEDICINE
☐ This medicine may be taken with food or a glass of water.

SPECIAL INSTRUCTIONS
☐ Do not change the dose of your regular asthma or bronchitis medicines except on the advice of your doctor.

☐ Call your doctor if the medicine does not relieve your breathing problems, or if your sputum turns yellow or green in color.

☐ Most people experience few or no side effects from their drugs. However, any medicine can sometimes cause unwanted effects. Call your doctor if you develop chest pain, headaches, palpitations, or dizziness.

*   *   *   *   *

Salbutamol (*Inhalation Bronchodilator*)
Canada: Ventolin

☐ This medicine is used to help open the bronchioles (air passages in the lungs) to take breathing easier.

☐ IMPORTANT: If you have ever had an allergic reaction to any cough/cold, allergy, heart, or weight-reducing medicines, tell your doctor or pharmacist before you take any of this medicine.

HOW TO USE THIS MEDICINE
☐ INSTRUCTIONS FOR USE
- If troubled with sputum, try to clear your chest as completely as possible before using this medicine. This will help the drug to reach the lungs and will allow more thorough clearing of mucus during subsequent coughing.
- Hold the inhaler upright during use so that the mouthpiece is at the bottom.
- Shake the canister.
- Breathe out fully and place the lips tightly around the mouthpiece and tilt the head slightly back.

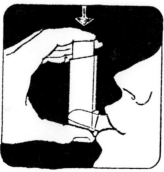

- Start to breathe in slowly and press down firmly and fully on the valve at the middle of or early during inspiration ("breathing in") to release a "puff." Take the inhaler out of the mouth and close the lips.
- Hold your breath for a few seconds. Breathe out through your nose slowly.

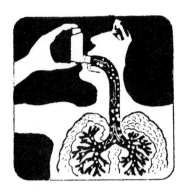

- If your doctor has prescribed a second dose, wait at least 30 seconds before shaking the container again and repeating this procedure.
- Rinse your mouth with warm water after you have inhaled the medicine. This will help prevent your mouth and throat from becoming dry.
- The mouthpiece of the inhaler should be kept clean and dry. The metal canister must be fully and firmly positioned in the outer "shell" and rotated occasionally.
- Failure to follow these instructions carefully can result in inadequate treatment.

SPECIAL INSTRUCTIONS

☐ Do not change the dose of your regular asthma or bronchitis medicines except on the advice of your doctor.

☐ Store the container in a cool place. Do not place the container in hot water or near radiators, stoves, or other sources of heat. Do not puncture, burn, or incinerate the container (even when it is empty).

☐ Call your doctor if the medicine does not relieve your breathing problems, or if your sputum turns yellow or green in color.

☐ Most people experience few or no side effects from their drugs. However, any medicine can sometimes cause unwanted effects. Call your doctor if you develop chest pain, headaches, palpitations, or dizziness.

*   *   *   *   *

Salicylamide (*Oral Analgesic-Antipyretic-Antirheumatic*)
United States: Salrin

742

Salicylamide-Acetaminophen

United States: Arthralgen, Dapase, Duoprin, Panritis

Canada: Arthralgen

☐ This medicine is used to help relieve pain, reduce fever, and relieve redness and swelling in certain kinds of arthritis.

☐ IMPORTANT: If you have a stomach ulcer or if you have ever had an allergic reaction to aspirin or acetaminophen, tell your doctor or pharmacist before you take any of this medicine.

HOW TO USE THIS MEDICINE

☐ This medicine may be taken with food or a full glass of water.

☐ For LIQUID MEDICINE

  • Shake the bottle well before using so that you can measure an accurate dose.

☐ Do not take this medicine if it smells strongly like vinegar since this means the medicine is not fresh.

☐ Do not take this medicine regularly for more than 10 days without consulting your doctor and do not administer it to children under 12 years of age for more than 5 days without your doctor's approval.

SPECIAL INSTRUCTIONS

☐ Women who are pregnant, breast-feeding, or planning to become pregnant should tell their doctor before taking this medicine.

☐ Do not take any other medicines containing aspirin while you are taking this medicine because it could result in too high a dose.

☐ If you are taking this medicine for arthritis, it is very important that you take it regularly and that you DO NOT MISS ANY DOSES. If you miss a dose, the level of the medicine in your body will fall and the drug will not be as effective. Only if the level of drug is high enough can it decrease the inflammation in your joints and help prevent further damage. If you forget a dose, take it as soon as possible. However, if it is almost time for your next dose, do not take the missed dose. Instead, continue with your regular dosing schedule.

☐ It is best not to drink alcoholic beverages while you are taking this medicine since the combination can cause stomach problems.

☐ In some people, this drug may cause dizziness or drowsiness. Do not drive a car or operate dangerous machinery or do jobs that require you to be alert until you know how you are going to react to this drug.

☐ Most people experience few or no side effects from their drugs. However, any medicine can sometimes cause unwanted effects. Call your doctor if you develop "ringing" or "buzzing" in the ears, skin rash, stomach pain, red or

743

black stools, dizziness, fever, sweating, wheezing or shortness of breath, unusual weakness, a yellow color in the skin or eyes, or easy bruising.

☐ Call your doctor if the medicine does not relieve your symptoms.

* * * * *

Secobarbital Sodium (*Oral Sedative-Hypnotic*)
United States: Seconal Sodium
Canada: Secogen, Seconal Sodium, Seral

☐ This medicine is used to cause sleep.

☐ IMPORTANT: If you have ever had an allergic reaction to a barbiturate medicine, tell your doctor or pharmacist before you take any of this medicine.

HOW TO USE THIS MEDICINE
☐ This medicine may be taken with food or a full glass of water.

SPECIAL INSTRUCTIONS
☐ Sleeping medicines are only useful for a short time. If used for too long, they lose their effectiveness. Do not take any more of this medicine than your doctor has prescribed and do not stop taking this medicine suddenly without the approval of your doctor.

☐ Women who are pregnant, breast-feeding, or planning to become pregnant should tell their doctor before taking this medicine.

☐ In some people, this drug may cause dizziness or drowsiness. Do not drive a car or operate dangerous machinery or do jobs that require you to be alert until you know how you are going to react to this drug.

☐ If you become dizzy, you should be careful going up and down stairs. Sit or lie down at the first sign of dizziness.

☐ Do not drink alcoholic beverages while taking this drug without the approval of your doctor.

☐ It is important that you obtain the advice of your doctor or pharmacist before taking ANY other medicines including pain relievers, sleeping pills, tranquilizers or medicines for depression, cough/cold medicines, or allergy medicines.

☐ Since you are taking this medicine to help you sleep, take it about 20 minutes before you want to go to sleep. Go to bed after you have taken it. Do not smoke in bed after you have taken it.

☐ Do not store this medicine at the bedside and keep it out of the reach of children.

☐ Call your doctor immediately if you think you may be allergic to the medicine or if you develop a skin rash, hives, itching, swelling of the face, or difficulty

744

in breathing. If you cannot reach your doctor, phone a hospital emergency department.

☐ Most people experience few or no side effects from their drugs. However, any medicine can sometimes cause unwanted effects. Call your doctor if you develop a sore throat, bothersome sleepiness or laziness during the day, nightmares, staggering walk, unusual nervousness, a yellow color to the skin or eyes, easy bruising, or slow heartbeats.

* * * * *

Secobarbital Sodium (*Rectal Sedative-Hypnotic*)
United States: Seconal Sodium

☐ This medicine is used to cause sleep.

☐ IMPORTANT: If you have ever had an allergic reaction to a barbiturate medicine, tell your doctor or pharmacist before you take any of this medicine.

HOW TO USE THIS MEDICINE
☐ Administration of SUPPOSITORIES
  • Remove the wrapper from the suppository.
  • Lie on your side and raise your knee to your chest.
  • Insert the suppository with the tapered (pointed) end first into the rectum.
  • Remain lying down for a few minutes so that the suppository will dissolve in the rectum.
  • Try to avoid having a bowel movement for at least one hour so that the drug will have time to work.

☐ Store these suppositories in a cool place.

SPECIAL INSTRUCTIONS
☐ Sleeping medicines are only useful for a short time. If used for too long, they lose their effectiveness. Do not use any more of this medicine than your doctor has prescribed and do not stop using this medicine suddenly without the approval of your doctor.

☐ Women who are pregnant, breast-feeding, or planning to become pregnant should tell their doctor before taking this medicine.

☐ In some people, this drug may cause dizziness or drowsiness. Do not drive a car or operate dangerous machinery or do jobs that require you to be alert until you know how you are going to react to this drug.

☐ If you become dizzy, you should be careful going up and down stairs. Sit or lie down at the first sign of dizziness.

☐ Do not drink alcoholic beverages while taking this drug without the approval of your doctor.

☐ It is important that you obtain the advice of your doctor or pharmacist before taking ANY other medicines including pain relievers, sleeping pills, tranquilizers or medicines for depression, cough/cold medicines, or allergy medicines.

☐ Since you are using this medicine to help you sleep, use it about 20 minutes before you want to go to bed. Go to bed after you have used it. Do not smoke in bed after you have used it.

☐ Call your doctor immediately if you think you may be allergic to the medicine or if you develop a skin rash, hives, itching, swelling of the face, or difficulty in breathing. If you cannot reach your doctor, phone a hospital emergency department.

☐ Most people experience few or no side effects from their drugs. However, any medicine can sometimes cause unwanted effects. Call your doctor if you develop a sore throat, bothersome sleepiness or laziness during the day, nightmares, a staggering walk, unusual nervousness, a yellow color to the skin or eyes, easy bruising, or slow heartbeats.

* * * * *

Selenium Sulfide (*Topical Antiseborrheic Agent*)
United States: Exsel, Selsun, Selsun Blue
Canada: Exsel, Sebusan, Selsun Suspension

☐ This medicine is used to treat dandruff and scalp conditions.

HOW TO USE THIS MEDICINE
☐ Instructions for use:
  - Shake well before using. (*United States:* Exsel, Selsun, Selsun Blue Lotions; *Canada:* Exsel, Selsun Lotions)
  - Wet hair and work 1 or 2 teaspoonfuls of lotion into the scalp using warm water to form a lather.
  - Allow the medicine to stay on the scalp for about $2\frac{1}{2}$ minutes.
  - Rinse with water and repeat.
  - Rinse hair thoroughly after shampooing and wash your hands well.

SPECIAL INSTRUCTIONS
☐ It is important to rinse hair thoroughly after shampooing. Incomplete rinsing of the hair may cause gray or white hair to become discolored yellow or orange. Allow at least 48 hours between tinting hair and treatment with this medicine.

☐ Keep this medicine out of the eyes and off the eyelids.

☐ Discontinue using this medicine if an irritation develops.

☐ Keep out of the reach of children.

☐ For external use only. Do not swallow.

*   *   *   *   *

Senna Preparations (*Oral Laxative*)
United States: Casafru, Glyssenid, Senokot, Senolax
Canada: Glysennid Norsenna, Senokot

Senna-Docusate Sodium
United States: Gentlax S, Senokap D.S.S., Senokot-S
Canada: Senokot-S

Senna-Psyllium
United States: Senokot with Psyllium

☐ This medicine is a laxative used to help relieve constipation.

HOW TO USE THIS MEDICINE
☐ Take the medicine in the evening or before breakfast with a full glass of water.

☐ Do not take mineral oil while you are taking this medicine. (*United States:* Gentlax S, Senokap D.S.S., Senokot-S; *Canada:* Senokot-S)

☐ Take this medicine with a full glass of water. (*United States:* Senokot with Psyllium)

SPECIAL INSTRUCTIONS
☐ Do not take this medicine more often or longer than your doctor has pre-scribed as your bowels may become dependent upon it. If you feel you require this medicine every day and cannot have a bowel movement without it, call your doctor.

☐ Women who are breast-feeding should tell their doctor before taking this medicine.

☐ Unless otherwise directed, you should also try increasing the amount of bulk foods in your diet (for example, bran, fresh fruits, and salads), exercising more often, and drinking 6 to 8 glasses of water every day.

☐ This medicine may cause your urine to turn yellow-brown or red in color. This is not unusual.

☐ Do not take this medicine if you have any stomach pain, nausea, or vomiting.

☐ Call your doctor if your constipation is not relieved or if you develop rectal bleeding, muscle cramps, unusual weakness, or dizziness.

*   *   *   *   *

Senna Preparations (*Rectal Laxative*)
Canada: Senokot

☐ This medicine is a laxative used to help relieve constipation.

HOW TO USE THIS MEDICINE
☐ Administration of SUPPOSITORIES
  - Remove the wrapper from the suppository.
  - Lie on your side and raise your knee to your chest.
  - Insert the suppository with the tapered (pointed) end first into the rectum.
  - Remain lying down for a few minutes so that the suppository will dissolve in the rectum.
  - Try to avoid having a bowel movement for at least one hour so that the drug will have time to work.

☐ Store the suppositories in a cool place.

SPECIAL INSTRUCTIONS
☐ Do not use this medicine more often or longer than your doctor has prescribed as your bowels may become dependent upon it. If you feel you require this medicine every day and cannot have a bowel movement without it, call your doctor.

☐ Unless otherwise directed, you should also try increasing the amount of bulk foods in your diet (for example, bran, fresh fruits, and salads), exercising more often, and drinking 6 to 8 glasses of water every day.

☐ Do not use this medicine if you have any stomach pain, nausea, or vomiting.

☐ Call your doctor if your constipation is not relieved or if you develop rectal bleeding, muscle cramps, unusual weakness, or dizziness.

☐ This medicine may cause the urine to turn yellow-brown or red in color. This is not unusual.

*   *   *   *   *

Sodium Aurothiomalate (*Rheumatoid Arthritis Therapy*)
United States: Myochrysine
Canada: Myochrysine

Aurothioglucose
United States: Solganal

☐ This medicine is used in the treatment of rheumatoid arthritis.

☐ Your doctor will initially inject a small test dose of the drug to determine whether you are allergic to the drug. If you are not allergic to it, he will inject

748

the drug at weekly intervals and gradually increase the dose of the drug. Once a certain dose of the drug has been reached, the doctor will inject the drug at monthly intervals.

☐ It will take a few weeks before you will begin to notice an effect. The drug has been very effective in many patients; however, it can cause side effects. In order to help prevent these side effects, your doctor will do both blood and urine tests.

SPECIAL INSTRUCTIONS

☐ Women who are breast-feeding should tell their doctor before taking this medicine.

☐ This medicine may make some people more sensitive to sunlight and sunlamps. When you begin taking this medicine, try to avoid getting too much sun until you see how you are going to react. If your skin does become more sensitive to sunlight, tell your doctor and try to stay out of direct sunlight. While in the sun, wear protective clothing and sunglasses. You may wish to ask your pharmacist about suitable sunscreen (protective) products. Check with your doctor if you become sunburned.

☐ Most people experience few or no side effects from their drugs. However, any medicine can sometimes cause unwanted effects. Call your doctor if you develop a skin rash, itching, metallic taste, sore mouth, stomach upset, fever or chills, a yellow-color to the skin or eyes, easy bruising or bleeding, nosebleeds, unusual weakness, or blood in the urine.

*   *   *   *   *

Sodium Fluoride (*Oral—Dental Caries Prophylaxis*)

United States: Flo-Tabs, Flura-Drops, Fluoritab, Fluorident, Karidium, Luride, Pediaflur, Solu-Flur

Canada: Fluor-A-Day, Fluorinse, Karidium, Pedi-Dent

☐ This medicine is used to help prevent tooth decay.

HOW TO USE THIS MEDICINE

☐ Drops may be placed directly on the tongue or mixed with water or fruit juices. Your pharmacist will explain the correct methods of using the dropper. (*United States:* Flura-Drops, Fluoritab Liquid, Karidium, Luride Drops, Pediaflur; *Canada:* Karidium, Fluorinse, Pedi-Dent)

☐ It is best to avoid putting the medicine in glass tumblers because it causes etching of the glass. It is best to use plastic tumblers or dishes.

☐ Chew the tablets completely before swallowing. (*United States:* Flo-Tabs Chewable, Luride Lozi-Tabs, Luride-SF Lozi-Tabs; *Canada:* Fluor-A-Day)

749

☐ If you move to another city or if your water supply is changed, check with your doctor or dentist to determine if any additional fluoride is needed.

☐ Do not exceed the recommended dosage.

☐ Discontinue using this medicine if you should notice a change in the color of your teeth or if you develop a skin rash, nausea, vomiting, or diarrhea.

☐ Keep this medicine out of the reach of children.

* * * * *

Sodium Levothyroxine (*Oral Hypothyroidism Therapy*)
United States: Levoid, Synthroid
Canada: Eltroxin, Synthroid

☐ This medicine is a hormone used to treat conditions in which the body is not producing enough thyroid hormone.

HOW TO USE THIS MEDICINE

☐ It is very important that you take this medicine exactly as your doctor has prescribed and that you do not miss any doses. Try to take this medicine at the same time every day.

☐ If you forget to take a dose, take it as soon as possible. However, if it is almost time for your next dose, do not take the missed dose. Instead, continue with your regular dosing schedule.

☐ Do not take any more of this medicine than your doctor has prescribed and do not stop taking this medicine suddenly without the approval of your doctor.

SPECIAL INSTRUCTIONS

☐ It is important that you obtain the advice of your doctor or pharmacist before taking ANY other medicines including pain relievers, sleeping pills, tranquilizers or medicines for depression, cough/cold or allergy medicines, or weight-reducing medicines.

☐ Most people experience few or no side effects from their drugs. However, any medicine can sometimes cause unwanted effects. Call your doctor if you develop chest pain, shortness of breath, leg cramps, a skin rash, fast heartbeats, trembling, diarrhea, sensitivity to heat, unusual nervousness, sweating, or weight loss.

* * * * *

Sodium Nitroprusside Reagent (*Ketonuria Diagnostic Reagent*)
United States: Acetest
Canada: Acetest

☐ This preparation is used to test for the presence of ketones in the urine.

☐ DIRECTIONS FOR USE:
   - Place the tablet on a clean surface, preferably a piece of white paper.
   - Put **one** drop of urine on the tablet.
   - Compare urine-ketone test results with the color chart supplied with the tablets at 30 seconds.

   NOTE: To test the reliability of the tablets, place a drop of urine on a tablet. The drop of urine should be completely absorbed into the tablet within a 30-second period. If absorption of the urine into the tablet takes longer than 30 seconds, the tablet has been exposed to moisture and may give a faulty reading. Purchase a new bottle of Acetest tablets.

   - **Negative result:** Tablet color is unchanged or turns cream colored.
   Positive result: Tablet color will change from lavender to deep purple within 30 seconds, depending upon the amount of ketone bodies present in the specimen. Results may be recorded as "small," "moderate," or "large" amounts.

☐ For further information, refer to the package insert which accompanies this medication.*

* * * * *

Sodium Nitroprusside Reagent (*Ketone Diagnostic Aid*)
United States: Ketostix
Canada: Ketostix

☐ This preparation is used to test for the presence of ketones in the urine.

☐ DIRECTIONS FOR USE:
   - Dip a test area in a fresh specimen of urine. Remove immediately.
   - Tap the edge of the strip against the container to remove excess specimen.
   - Fifteen seconds after wetting, compare the color of the test area closely with the color chart.
   - The test is positive if a purple color develops. The shade of purple

---

*Acetest (Package Insert), Ames Company Division, Miles Laboratories, Ltd. Rexdale, Ontario.

developed after 15 seconds indicates varying amounts of ketones in the urine.

light = small amount
medium = moderate amount
dark = large amount

☐ For further information, refer to the package insert which accompanies this medicine.*

* * * * *

Sodium Salicylate (*Oral Analgesic-Antipyretic-Antirheumatic*)
United States: Uracel

☐ This medicine is used to help relieve pain, reduce fever, and relieve redness and swelling in certain kinds of arthritis.

☐ IMPORTANT: If you have a stomach ulcer or if you have ever had an allergic reaction to aspirin, tell your doctor or pharmacist before you take any of this medicine.

HOW TO USE THIS MEDICINE

☐ This medicine may be taken with food or a full glass of water.

☐ This medicine has a special coating to help prevent stomach upset. It must be swallowed whole. Do not crush, chew, or break it into pieces and do not take chipped tablets.

☐ Do not take this medicine regularly for more than 10 days without consulting your doctor and do not administer it to children under 12 years of age for more than 5 days without your doctor's approval.

SPECIAL INSTRUCTIONS

☐ This medicine contains sodium, and it is important to tell your doctor or pharmacist if you are on a sodium-restricted diet.

☐ Do not take any other medicines containing aspirin while you are taking this medicine because it could result in too high a dose.

☐ Women who are pregnant, breast-feeding, or planning to become pregnant should tell their doctor before using this medicine.

☐ If you are taking this medicine for arthritis, it is very important that you take it regularly and that you DO NOT MISS ANY DOSES. If you miss a dose, the level of the medicine in your body will fall and the drug will not be as effective. Only if the level of drug is high enough can it decrease the inflammation in your joints and help prevent further damage. If you forget a dose, take it

---

*Ketostix (Package Insert), Ames Company Division, Miles Laboratories, Ltd., Rexdale, Ontario.

752

as soon as possible. However, if it is almost time for your next dose, do not take the missed dose. Instead, continue with your regular dosing schedule.

☐ It is best not to drink alcoholic beverages while you are taking this medicine since the combination can cause stomach problems.

☐ Most people experience few or no side effects from their drugs. However, any medicine can sometimes cause unwanted effects. Call your doctor if you develop "ringing" or "buzzing" in the ears, a skin rash, stomach pain, red or black stools, dizziness, fever, sweating, wheezing, or shortness of breath.

☐ Call your doctor if the medicine does not relieve your symptoms.

*   *   *   *   *

Sodium Sulfacetamide (*Ophthalmic Antibacterial*)
United States: Bleph, Cetamide, Isopto Cetamide, Sodium Sulamyd, Sulfacel-15, Sulf-10
Canada: Bleph-10 Liquifilm, Cetamide, Isopto Cetamide, Optosulfex, Sodium Sulamyd, Sulf-10, Sulf-30

☐ This medicine is an antibiotic used to treat certain types of eye and eyelid infections.

☐ IMPORTANT: If you have ever had an allergic reaction to sulfa or sulfonamide medicines, tell your doctor or pharmacist before you use any of this drug.

HOW TO USE THIS MEDICINE
☐ For EYE DROPS

INSTILLATION OF EYE DROPS

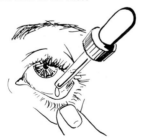

• The person administering the eye drops should wash his hands with soap and water.
• The eye drops must be kept clean. Do not touch the dropper against the face or anything else.
• Lie down or tilt your head backward and look at the ceiling.
• Gently pull down the lower lid of your eye to form a pouch.
• Hold the dropper in your other hand and approach the eye from the

753

side. Place the dropper as close to the eye as possible without touching it.
- Place the prescribed number of drops into the pouch of the eye.
- Close your eyes. Do not rub them.
- Apply gentle pressure for a minute with your fingers to the bridge of the nose (inside corner of the eye) to prevent the eye drops from being drained from the eye.
- Blot excess solution around the eye with a tissue.
- If necessary, have someone else administer the eye drops for you.
- Do not use the eye drops if they have changed in color or have changed in any way since being purchased.
- Keep the eye drop bottle tightly closed when not in use.

☐ For EYE OINTMENT

INSTILLATION OF EYE OINTMENT

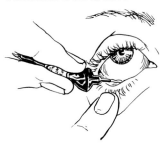

- The person administering the eye ointment should wash his hands with soap and water.
- The eye ointment must be kept clean. Do not touch the tube against the face or anything else.
- Lie down or tilt your head backward and look at the ceiling.
- Gently pull down the lower lid of your eye to form a pouch.
- Hold the tube in your other hand and place the tube as close as possible to the eye without touching it.
- Squeeze the prescribed amount of ointment (usually $\frac{1}{2}$ inch in adults) from the tube along the pouch.
- Close your eyes. Do not rub them.
- Wipe off any excess ointment around the eye with a tissue.
- Clean the tip of the ointment tube with a tissue.
- If necessary, have someone else administer the eye ointment for you.
- Keep the eye ointment tube tightly closed when not in use.
- Do not use the drug more frequently or in larger quantities than prescribed by your doctor.

SPECIAL INSTRUCTIONS

☐ Vision may be blurred for a few minutes after using the eye medicine. Do not drive a car or operate dangerous machinery or do jobs that require you to be alert until your vision has cleared.

754

- [ ] It is important to use **all** of this medicine, plus any refills that your doctor told you to use. Do not stop using it earlier than your doctor has recommended in spite of the fact that your symptoms seem to have improved. Otherwise, the infection may return.

- [ ] If you forget to use the medicine, use it as soon as possible. However, if it is almost time for your next dose, do not use the missed dose but continue with your regular schedule.

- [ ] Contact your doctor if the condition for which you are using this medicine does not improve or if the eye becomes irritated by it for more than a few minutes. Many eye medicines sting for a short time immediately after use.

- [ ] Do not use this medicine at the same time as any other eye medicine without the approval of your doctor. Some medicines cannot be mixed.

- [ ] For external use only. Do not swallow.

- [ ] The ointment must be stored away from heat. (**United States:** Cetamide, Sodium Sulamyd Ophthalmic Ointments; **Canada:** Cetamide, Sodium Sulamyd Ophthalmic Ointments)

- [ ] Store the solution in a cool place. (**United States:** Bleph, Isopto Cetamide, Sodium Sulamyd; **Canada:** Bleph-10 Liquifilm, Isopto Cetamide, Sodium Sulamyd, Sulf-30)

- [ ] For external use only.

* * * * *

Spironolactone (*Oral Diuretic-Antihypertensive*)
United States: Aldactone
Canada: Aldactone

Spironolactone-Hydrochlorothiazide (*Oral Diuretic-Antihypertensive*)
United States: Aldactazide
Canada: Aldactazide

- [ ] This medicine is used to help rid the body of excess water and to decrease swelling. It is also used to treat high blood pressure. It is commonly called a "water pill."

HOW TO USE THIS MEDICINE
- [ ] Take the medicine with food, meals, or milk.

- [ ] Try to take it at the same time(s) every day so that you have a constant level of the medicine in your body. Do not miss any doses. Otherwise, you cannot expect the drug to work as well.

SPECIAL INSTRUCTIONS

☐ It will usually take 3 days before you feel the full effect of this drug. If you are to take more than one dose every day, take the last dose 6 hours before bedtime so that you will not have to get up during the night to go to the bathroom. This effect will usually lessen after you have taken the drug for awhile.

☐ If you forget to take a dose, take it as soon as possible. However, if it is almost time for your next dose, do not take the missed dose. Instead, continue with your regular dosing schedule.

☐ Women who are pregnant, breast-feeding, or planning to become pregnant should tell their doctor before taking this medicine.

☐ Do not take large doses of aspirin or other salicylates without the approval of your doctor while you are taking this drug.

☐ If you become drowsy, do not drive a car, operate machinery, or do jobs that require you to be alert. Tell your doctor you are drowsy.

☐ Most people experience few or no side effects from their drugs. However, any medicine can sometimes cause unwanted effects. Call your doctor if you develop a fever, a dry mouth (or if you are very thirsty), nausea, fatigue, skin rash, weakness, swelling of the legs or ankles, stomach cramps, a sudden weight gain of 5 pounds or more, or swelling and tenderness of the breasts.

☐ Also call your doctor if you develop joint pain, easy bruising or bleeding, or a yellow color to the skin or eyes. (**United States** and **Canada:** Aldactazide)

*   *   *   *   *

Stanozolol (*Oral Anabolic Steroid*)
United States: Winstrol
Canada: Winstrol

☐ This medicine is similar to a hormone which is normally produced by the body. This medicine has many uses and the reason it was prescribed depends upon your condition. If you do not understand why you are taking it, check with your doctor.

HOW TO USE THIS MEDICINE

☐ Take the drug after meals or with a snack if it upsets your stomach.

☐ It is very important that you take this drug as your doctor has prescribed.

SPECIAL INSTRUCTIONS

☐ Women who are pregnant, breast-feeding, or planning to become pregnant should tell their doctor before taking this medicine.

☐ Diabetic patients should regularly check the sugar in the urine and report any abnormal results to their doctor.

☐ Carry an identification card indicating that you are taking this medicine. Always tell your pharmacist, dentist, and other doctors who are treating you that you are taking this medicine.

☐ Most people experience few or no side effects from their drugs. However, any medicine can sometimes cause unwanted effects. Call your doctor if you develop swelling of the hands, legs or ankles, sore throat and fever, acne, unusual restlessness, dark-colored urine, or a yellow color to the skin or eyes. Women should call their doctor if they develop menstrual problems, hoarseness or a deepening of the voice, baldness, or increased facial hair.

* * * * *

Streptokinase-Streptodornase (Oral Fibrinolytic Enzymes)
United States: Varidase
Canada: Varidase

☐ This medicine is used to reduce inflammation and help relieve pain and swelling.

HOW TO USE THIS MEDICINE
☐ This medicine may be taken with food or a glass of water.

SPECIAL INSTRUCTIONS
☐ If you forget to take a dose, take it as soon as possible. However, if it is almost time for your next dose, do not take the missed dose. Instead, continue with your regular dosing schedule.

☐ Most people experience few or no side effects from their drugs. However, any medicine can sometimes cause unwanted effects. Call your doctor if you develop a skin rash, vomiting, or diarrhea.

* * * * *

Succinylsulfathiazole (Oral Antibacterial)
Canada: Sulfasuxidine

☐ This medicine is used to treat conditions of the intestines.

☐ IMPORTANT: If you have ever had an allergic reaction to sulfa drugs, thiazide "water pills," or diabetes or glaucoma medicine that you take by mouth, tell your doctor or pharmacist before you take any of this medicine.

HOW TO USE THIS MEDICINE
☐ Take the medicine with a glass of water.

☐ If you forget to take a dose, take it as soon as you remember and then continue with your regular schedule.

757

□ Women who are pregnant, breast-feeding, or planning to become pregnant should tell their doctor before taking this medicine.

□ Do not take mineral oil while taking this medicine.

□ Do not take strong laxatives while taking this medicine. Check with your pharmacist.

□ Call your doctor immediately if you think you may be allergic to the medicine or if you develop a skin rash, hives, itching, swelling of the face, or difficulty in breathing. If you cannot reach your doctor, phone a hospital emergency department.

□ Most people experience few or no side effects from their drugs. However, any medicine can sometimes cause unwanted effects. Call your doctor if you develop a sore throat, fever or mouth sores, easy bruising, a yellow color to the skin or eyes, or blood in the urine.

* * * * *

Sulfasalazine (*Oral Ulcerative Colitis Therapy*)
United States: Azulfidine, S.A.S.-500
Canada: Salazopyrin, S.A.S.-500

□ This medicine is used to treat certain conditions of the intestines involving diarrhea (loose bowel movements).

□ IMPORTANT: If you have ever had an allergic reaction to sulfa drugs, thiazide "water pills," diabetes medicine that you take by mouth, or glaucoma medicine that you take by mouth, tell your doctor or pharmacist before you take any of this medicine.

HOW TO USE THIS MEDICINE

□ It is best to take this medicine with food or after meals to help lessen stomach upset. Call your doctor if you continue to have stomach upset. Take the medicine with a full glass of water and try to drink eight 8-ounce glasses of water or other fluids every day unless otherwise directed by your doctor.

□ This medicine has a special coating and must be swallowed whole. Do not crush, chew, or break it into pieces. (**United States:** Azulfidine En-Tabs; **Canada:** Salazopyrin En Tablets)

SPECIAL INSTRUCTIONS

□ It is important to take **all** of this medicine plus any refills that your doctor told you to take. Do not stop taking it earlier than your doctor has recommended in spite of the fact that you may feel better. Otherwise, the infection may return.

□ Take this medicine at regular intervals during a 24-hour period. The time between your night-time and morning dose should not be longer than 8 hours unless otherwise directed.

□ If you forget to take a dose, take it as soon as you remember and then continue with your regular schedule. However, if it is almost time for your next dose, do not take the missed dose.

□ Women who are pregnant, breast-feeding, or planning to become pregnant should tell their doctor before taking this medicine.

□ This medicine may make some people more sensitive to sunlight and sunlamps. When you begin taking this medicine, try to avoid getting too much sun until you see how you are going to react. If your skin does become more sensitive to sunlight, tell your doctor and try to stay out of direct sunlight. While in the sun, wear protective clothing and sunglasses. You may wish to ask your pharmacist about suitable sunscreen products. Check with your doctor if you become sunburned.

□ In some people, this drug may cause dizziness or drowsiness. Do not drive a car or operate dangerous machinery or do jobs that require you to be alert until you know how you are going to react to this drug.

□ This medicine may cause the urine to turn orange-yellow in color. This is not an unusual effect.

□ Most people experience few or no side effects from their drugs. However, any medicine can sometimes cause unwanted effects. Call your doctor if you develop a sore throat, fever, mouth sores, easy bruising, skin blisters, a yellow color to the skin and eyes, constant headache, unusual joint or back pain, or pain while urinating ("passing your water").

□ Call your doctor immediately if you think you may be allergic to the medicine or if you develop a skin rash, hives, itching, swelling of the face, or difficulty in breathing. If you cannot reach your doctor, phone a hospital emergency department.

□ If for some reason you cannot take all of the medicine, throw away the unused portion by flushing it down the toilet. Do not take or save old medicine.

*   *   *   *   *

Sulfinpyrazone (*Oral Uricosuric*)
United States: Anturane
Canada: Anturan, Zynol

□ This medicine is used in the treatment of gout and in other conditions in which the body has high levels of uric acid. It is also used to help prevent painful blood clots from forming in some conditions.

759

HOW TO USE THIS MEDICINE

☐ It is best to take this medicine with food or a glass of milk to help prevent stomach upset. Call your doctor if you continue to have stomach upset.

SPECIAL INSTRUCTIONS

☐ If you forget to take a dose, take it as soon as possible. However, if it is almost time for your next dose, do not take the missed dose. Instead, continue with your regular dosing schedule.

☐ It is very important that you take this medicine exactly as your doctor prescribed and that you do not miss any doses. Otherwise, you cannot expect the medicine to help you.

☐ Try to drink at least 8 to 10 glasses of water or other liquids every day while you are taking this medicine unless otherwise directed.

☐ Do not take vitamin C, aspirin or salicylates, or alcohol while you are taking this medicine without the approval of your doctor.

☐ Most people experience few or no side effects from their drugs. However, any medicine can sometimes cause unwanted effects. Call your doctor if you develop a skin rash, sore throat and fever, easy bruising or bleeding, blood in the urine, lower back pain or pain when you urinate ("pass your water"), severe stomach pain, or unusual tiredness or weakness.

*　*　*　*　*

Sulfisoxazole (*Eye/Ear Antibacterial-Sulfonamide*)
United States: Gantrisin Ophthalmic Solution & Ointment
Canada: Gantrisin Ear Solution, Gantrisin Eye Solution

☐ This medicine is used to treat certain types of infections.

☐ IMPORTANT: If you have ever had an allergic reaction to sulfa or sulfonamide medicines, tell your doctor or pharmacist before you use any of this drug.

HOW TO USE THIS MEDICINE
☐ For EYE DROPS

INSTILLATION OF EYE DROPS

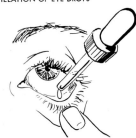

- The person administering the eye drops should wash his hands with soap and water.
- The eye drops must be kept clean. Do not touch the dropper against the face or anything else.
- Lie down or tilt your head backward and look at the ceiling.
- Gently pull down the lower lid of your eye to form a pouch.
- Hold the dropper in your other hand and approach the eye from the side. Place the dropper as close to the eye as possible without touching it.
- Place the prescribed number of drops into the pouch of the eye.
- Close your eyes. Do not rub them.
- Apply gentle pressure for a minute with your fingers to the bridge of the nose (inside corner of the eye) to prevent the eye drops from being drained from the eye.
- Blot excess solution around the eye with a tissue.
- If necessary, have someone else administer the eye drops for you.
- Do not use the eye drops if they have changed in color or have changed in any way since you purchased them.
- Keep the eye drop bottle tightly closed when not in use.

□ For EYE OINTMENT

INSTILLATION OF EYE OINTMENT

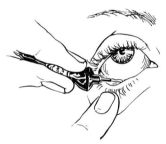

- The person administering the eye ointment should wash his hands with soap and water.
- The eye ointment must be kept clean. Do not touch the tube against the face or anything else.
- Lie down or tilt your head backward and look at the ceiling.
- Gently pull down the lower lid of your eye to form a pouch.
- Hold the tube in your other hand and place the tube as close as possible to the eye without touching it.
- Squeeze the prescribed amount of ointment (usually $\frac{1}{2}$ inch in adults) from the tube along the pouch.
- Close your eyes. Do not rub them.
- Wipe off any excess ointment around the eye with a tissue.
- Clean the tip of the ointment tube with a tissue.
- If necessary, have someone else administer the eye ointment for you.
- Keep the eye ointment tube tightly closed when not in use.
- Do not use the drug more frequently or in larger quantities than prescribed by your doctor.

☐ For EAR DROPS

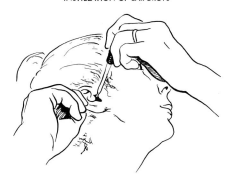

- Warm the ear drops to body temperature by holding the bottle in your hands for a few minutes. Do NOT heat the drops in hot water.
- The person administering the ear drops should wash his hands with soap and water.
- The ear drops must be kept clean. Do not touch the dropper against the ear or anything else.
- Tilt your head or lie on your side so that the ear to be treated is facing up.
- In ADULTS, hold the ear lobe up and back.
- In CHILDREN, hold the ear lobe down and back.
- Place the prescribed number of drops into the ear. Do not insert the dropper into the ear as it may cause injury.
- Remain in the same position for a short time (2 minutes) after you have administered the drops.
- Dry the ear lobe if there are any drops on it.
- If necessary, have someone else administer the ear drops for you.
- Do not use the ear drops if they have changed in color or have changed in any way since you purchased them.
- Keep the bottle tightly closed when not in use.

SPECIAL INSTRUCTIONS

☐ Vision may be blurred for a few minutes after using the eye medicine. Do not drive a car or operate dangerous machinery or do jobs that require you to be alert until your vision has cleared.

☐ It is important to use **all** of this medicine, plus any refills that your doctor told you to use. Do not stop using it earlier than your doctor has recommended in spite of the fact that your symptoms seem to have improved. Otherwise, the infection may return.

☐ If you forget to use the medicine, use it as soon as possible. However, if it is almost time for your next dose, do not use the missed dose but continue with your regular schedule.

☐ Call your doctor if the condition for which you are using this medicine persists or becomes worse or if the medicine causes itching or burning for more than a few minutes after instillation.

☐ Do not use this medicine at the same time as any other eye or ear medicine without the approval of your doctor. Some medicines cannot be mixed.

☐ For external use only. Do not swallow.

*   *   *   *   *

Sulfonamide Preparations (*Oral Antibacterial Sulfonamide*)

Sulfachlorpyridazine
United States: Sonilyn

Sulfacytine
United States: Renoquid

Sulfadiazine
United States: Microsulfon

Sulfadiazine-Trimethoprim
Canada: Coptin

Sulfadimethoxine
Canada: Madribon

Sulfameter
United States: Sulla
Canada: Sulla

Sulfamethizole
United States: Microsul, Proklar, Sulfstat Forte, Thiosulfil, Unisul, Urifon
Canada: Thiosulfil

Sulfamethoxazole
United States: Gantanol
Canada: Gantanol

Sulfamethoxazole-Trimethoprim
United States: Bactrim, Septra
Canada: Bactrim, Septra

763

Sulfamethoxypyridazine

United States: Midicel

Sulfapyridine

Canada: Dagenan

Sulfisoxazole

United States: Gantrisin, Lipo-Gantrisin, Rosoxol, SK-Soxazole, Sulfalar
Canada: Gantrisin, Novosoxazole, Sulfizole

☐ This medicine is an antibiotic used to treat certain types of infections.

☐ IMPORTANT: If you have ever had an allergic reaction to sulfa drugs, thia-zide "water pills," diabetes medicine that you take by mouth, or glaucoma medicine that you take by mouth, tell your doctor or pharmacist before you take any of this medicine.

HOW TO USE THIS MEDICINE

☐ Take the medicine with a full glass of water and try to drink eight 8-ounce glasses of water or other fluids every day unless otherwise directed by your doctor.

☐ It is recommended that this medicine be taken after breakfast. (*United States* and *Canada:* Sulla)

☐ For LIQUID MEDICINE
  • Shake the bottle well before using so that you can measure an accurate dose. (*United States:* Bactrim, Coco-Diazine, Gantanol, Gantrisin, Proklar, Septra Suspensions; *Canada:* Bactrim, Coptin, Gantanol, Gantrisin, Madribon, Septra Suspensions)

SPECIAL INSTRUCTIONS

☐ It is important to take *all* of this medicine plus any refills that your doctor told you to take. Do not stop taking it earlier than your doctor has recommended in spite of the fact that you may feel better. Otherwise, the infection may return.

☐ If you forget to take a dose, take it as soon as you remember and then continue with your regular schedule.

☐ Women who are pregnant, breast-feeding, or planning to become pregnant should tell their doctor before taking this medicine.

☐ This medicine may make some people more sensitive to sunlight and sunlamps. When you begin taking this medicine, try to avoid getting too much sun until you see how you are going to react. If your skin does become more sensitive to sunlight, tell your doctor and try to stay out of direct sun-light. While in the sun, wear protective clothing and sunglasses. You may

764

wish to ask your pharmacist about suitable sunscreen products. Check with your doctor if you become sunburned.

☐ In some people, this drug may cause dizziness or drowsiness. Do not drive a car or operate dangerous machinery or do jobs that require you to be alert until you know how you are going to react to this drug.

☐ Most people experience few or no side effects from their drugs. However, any medicine can sometimes cause unwanted effects. Call your doctor if you develop a sore throat, fever, mouth sores, easy bruising, skin blisters, a yellow color to the skin or eyes, unusual joint or back pain, or pain while urinating ("passing your water").

☐ Call your doctor immediately if you think you may be allergic to the medicine or if you develop a skin rash, hives, itching, swelling of the face, or difficulty in breathing. If you cannot reach your doctor, phone a hospital emergency department.

☐ If for some reason you cannot take all of the medicine, throw away the unused portion by flushing it down the toilet. Do not take or save old medicine.

* * * * *

Sulfonamide-Phenazopyridine Preparations (*Oral Urinary Anti-infective*)

Sulfamethizole-Phenazopyridine
United States: Azo-Sulfstat, Signa Sul-A, Thiosulfil-A, Thiosulfil-A Forte, Uremide
Canada: Thiosulfil-A, Thiosulfil-A Forte, Thiosulfil Duo-Pak

Sulfamethoxazole-Phenazopyridine
United States: Azo-Gantanol
Canada: Uro Gantanol

Sulfisoxazole-Phenazopyridine
United States: Azo-Gantrisin, Azo-Soxazole, Azosul, Suldiazo
Canada: Azo-Gantrisin

☐ This medication is used to treat and relieve pain of urinary tract infections.

☐ IMPORTANT: If you have ever had an allergic reaction to sulfa drugs, thiazide "water pills," diabetes medicine that you take by mouth, or glaucoma medicine that you take by mouth, tell your doctor or pharmacist before you take any of this medicine.

765

HOW TO USE THIS MEDICINE

☐ Take the medicine with a full glass of water and try to drink eight 8-ounce glasses of water or other fluids every day unless otherwise directed by your doctor.

SPECIAL INSTRUCTIONS

☐ It is important to take **all** of this medicine plus any refills that your doctor told you to take. Do not stop taking it earlier than your doctor has recommended in spite of the fact that you may feel better. Otherwise, the infection may return.

☐ If you forget to take a dose, take it as soon as you remember and then continue with your regular schedule.

☐ Women who are pregnant, breast-feeding, or planning to become pregnant should tell their doctor before taking this medicine.

☐ This medicine may make some people more sensitive to sunlight and sunlamps. When you begin taking this medicine, try to avoid getting too much sun until you see how you are going to react. If your skin does become more sensitive to sunlight, tell your doctor and try to stay out of direct sunlight. While in the sun, wear protective clothing and sunglasses. You may wish to ask your pharmacist about suitable sunscreen products. Check with your doctor if you become sunburned.

☐ In some people, this drug may cause dizziness or drowsiness. Do not drive a car or operate dangerous machinery or do jobs that require you to be alert until you know how you are going to react to this drug.

☐ This medicine may cause the urine to turn orange-red in color. This is not an unusual effect. Protect your undergarments while you are taking this medicine as your urine could cause staining.

☐ Most people experience few or no side effects from their drugs. However, any medicine can sometimes cause unwanted effects. Call your doctor if you develop a sore throat, fever, mouth sores, easy bruising, skin blisters, a yellow color to the skin or eyes, unusual joint or back pain, or pain while urinating ("passing your water").

☐ Call your doctor immediately if you think you may be allergic to the medicine or if you develop a skin rash, hives, itching, swelling of the face, or difficulty in breathing. If you cannot reach your doctor, phone a hospital emergency department.

☐ If for some reason you cannot take all of the medicine, throw away the unused portion by flushing it down the toilet. Do not take or save old medicine.

* * * * *

Sulfonamide Preparations (*Vaginal Anti-infective*)

Sulfisoxazole
United States: Gantrisin Cream
Canada: Gantrisin Cream

Triple Sulfa Cream
United States: Sultrin
Canada: Sultrin

☐ This medicine is used to treat infections of the vagina.

☐ IMPORTANT: If you have ever had an allergic reaction to sulfa or sulfonamide medicine, tell your doctor or pharmacist before you use any of this drug.

HOW TO USE THIS MEDICINE

☐ Use this medicine at the times specified by your doctor.

☐ For VAGINAL CREAM

    • Remove the cap from the tube of medicine.
    • Screw the applicator to the tube.

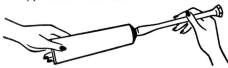

    • Squeeze the tube until the applicator plunger is fully extended. The applicator will now be filled with medicine. If your doctor has ordered a smaller dose, use as he has directed.

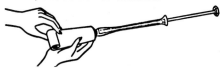

    • Unscrew the applicator by the cylinder. Apply a small amount of cream to the outside of the applicator and gently insert it into the vaginal canal as far as it will comfortably go.
    • While still holding the cylinder, press the plunger gently to deposit the medicine.

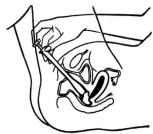

767

- While keeping the plunger depressed, remove the applicator from the vagina.
- After *each* use, take the applicator apart by holding the cylinder of the plunger and turning the cap counterclockwise.
- Wash thoroughly with warm water and soap and rinse thoroughly.
- Reassemble by dropping the plunger back into the cylinder as far as it will go. Place the cap on the end of the plunger and turn until the cap is tight.

☐ Wash the applicator with warm water and soap after each use.

SPECIAL INSTRUCTIONS

☐ It is important to use *all* of this medicine, plus any refills that your doctor told you to use. Do not stop using it earlier than your doctor has recommended in spite of the fact that your symptoms seem to have improved. Otherwise, the infection may return.

☐ If you forget to apply the medicine, apply it as soon as possible. However, if it is almost time for your next dose, do not apply the missed dose but continue with your regular schedule.

☐ Call your doctor if the condition for which this drug is being used persists or becomes worse or if you develop a constant irritation such an itching or burning that was not present before you started using this medicine.

☐ For external use only. Do not swallow.

* * * * *

Sulfoxone Sodium (*Oral Antibacterial Sulfone*)
United States: Diasone Sodium

☐ This medicine is used in the treatment of certain types of skin conditions.

HOW TO USE THIS MEDICINE

☐ Take the medicine with food or a glass of water.

☐ It is very important that you take this medicine exactly as your doctor has prescribed and that you do not miss any doses. Try to take this medicine at the same time every day. Do not take extra tablets without your doctor's approval.

☐ This medicine has a special coating and must be swallowed whole. Do not crush, chew, or break it into pieces.

SPECIAL INSTRUCTIONS

☐ If you forget to take a dose, take it as soon as possible. However, if it is almost time for your next dose, do not take the missed dose. Instead, continue with your regular dosing schedule.

- [ ] Most people experience few or no side effects from their drugs. However, any medicine can sometimes cause unwanted effects. Call your doctor if you develop a sore throat, fever or mouth sores, numbness, swelling or pain in the hands or feet, muscle weakness, joint pain, a yellow color to the skin or eyes, unusual tiredness, or blood in the urine.

* * * * *

Sulindac (*Oral Anti-inflammatory–Analgesic*)
United States: Clinoril
Canada: Clinoril

- [ ] This medicine is used to help relieve pain, redness, stiffness, and swelling in certain kinds of arthritis and other medical conditions.

- [ ] IMPORTANT: If you have ever had an allergic reaction to aspirin or any other medicine for arthritis, tell your doctor or pharmacist before you take any of this medicine.

- [ ] It is very important that you take this medicine regularly and that you DO NOT MISS ANY DOSES. If you miss a dose, the level of the medicine in your body will fall and the drug will not be as effective. Only if the level of the drug is high enough can it decrease the inflammation and swelling in your joints and help prevent further damage.

- [ ] The full benefit of this medicine may not be noticed immediately but may take from 1 to 2 weeks.

- [ ] Do not take any more of this medicine than your doctor has prescribed and do not stop taking this medicine suddenly without the approval of your doctor.

HOW TO USE THIS MEDICINE
- [ ] Always take this medicine with food or a glass of milk or immediately after meals to help prevent stomach upset.

SPECIAL INSTRUCTIONS
- [ ] In some people, this drug may cause dizziness. Do not drive a car or operate dangerous machinery or do jobs that require you to be alert until you know how you are going to react to this drug.

- [ ] If you become dizzy, you should be careful going up and down stairs. Sit or lie down at the first sign of dizziness.

- [ ] If you forget to take a dose, take it as soon as possible. However, if it is almost time for your next dose, do not take the missed dose. Instead, continue with your regular dosing schedule.

- [ ] While you are taking this medicine, do not drink alcoholic beverages or take aspirin without the permission of your doctor. It is usually safe to take acetaminophen for the occasional headache. Check with your pharmacist.

- [ ] Do not self-medicate with products containing aspirin because they can make this medicine less effective.

- [ ] Do not take antacids containing large amounts of sodium while you are taking this medicine. Check with your pharmacist.

- [ ] If your mouth becomes dry, suck a hard sour candy (sugarless) or ice chips, or chew gum. It is especially important to brush your teeth regularly if you develop a dry mouth.

- [ ] Call your doctor immediately if you think you may be allergic to the medicine or if you develop a skin rash, hives, itching, swelling of the face, or difficulty in breathing. If you cannot reach your doctor, phone a hospital emergency department.

- [ ] Most people experience few or no side effects from their drugs. However, any medicine can sometimes cause unwanted effects. Call your doctor if you develop "ringing" or "buzzing" in the ears, swelling of the legs or ankles or a sudden weight gain, stomach pain, red or black stools, easy bruising, changes in your hearing or eyesight, or depression.

- [ ] Carry an identification card indicating that you are taking this medicine. Always tell your pharmacist, dentist, and other doctors who are treating you that you are taking this medicine.

* * * * *

Talbutal (*Oral Sedative-Hypnotic*)
United States: Lotusate Caplets

- [ ] This medicine is used to cause sleep.

- [ ] IMPORTANT: If you have ever had an allergic reaction to a barbiturate medicine, tell your doctor or pharmacist before you take any of this medicine.

HOW TO USE THIS MEDICINE
- [ ] This medicine may be taken with food or a full glass of water.

SPECIAL INSTRUCTIONS
- [ ] Sleeping medicines are only useful for a short time. If used for too long, they lose their effectiveness. Do not take any more of this medicine than your doctor has prescribed, and do not stop taking this medicine suddenly without the approval of your doctor.

- [ ] Women who are pregnant, breast-feeding, or planning to become pregnant should tell their doctor before taking this medicine.

- [ ] In some people, this drug may cause dizziness or drowsiness. Do not drive a car or operate dangerous machinery or do jobs that require you to be alert until you know how you are going to react to this drug.

770

- [ ] If you become dizzy, you should be careful going up and down stairs. Sit or lie down at the first sign of dizziness.

- [ ] Do not drink alcoholic beverages while taking this drug without the approval of your doctor.

- [ ] It is important that you obtain the advice of your doctor or pharmacist before taking ANY other medicines including pain relievers, sleeping pills, tranquilizers or medicines for depression, cough/cold medicines, or allergy medicines.

- [ ] Since you are taking this medicine to help you sleep, take it about 20 minutes before you want to go to sleep. Go to bed after you have taken it. Do not smoke in bed after you have taken it.

- [ ] Do not store this medicine at the bedside and keep it out of the reach of children.

- [ ] Call your doctor immediately if you think you may be allergic to the medicine or if you develop a skin rash, hives, itching, swelling of the face, or difficulty in breathing. If you cannot reach your doctor, phone a hospital emergency department.

- [ ] Most people experience few or no side effects from their drugs. However, any medicine can sometimes cause unwanted effects. Call your doctor if you develop a sore throat, bothersome sleepiness or laziness during the day, nightmares, a staggering walk, unusual nervousness, a yellow color to the skin or eyes, easy bruising, or slow heartbeats.

*   *   *   *   *

Tamoxifen (*Oral Antineoplastic*)
United States: Nolvadex
Canada: Nolvadex

- [ ] This medicine is used in certain medical conditions to help slow down the growth and reproduction of some of the body's cells.

HOW TO USE THIS MEDICINE

- [ ] It is best to take this medicine on an empty stomach at least 1 hour before (or 2 hours after) eating food. Take it at the proper time even if you skip a meal.

- [ ] It is very important that you take this medicine exactly as your doctor has prescribed and that you do not miss any doses. Try to take this medicine at the same time every day. Do not take extra tablets without your doctor's approval.

- [ ] Even if you become nauseated, do not stop taking the medicine until you check with your doctor.

771

SPECIAL INSTRUCTIONS

- ☐ Always keep your doctor appointments so that your doctor can watch your progress.

- ☐ Always tell your pharmacist, dentist, and other doctors who are treating you that you are taking this medicine.

- ☐ It is recommended that you take appropriate birth control measures while taking this medicine and for at least 2 months after the medicines has been stopped.

- ☐ If you miss a dose of this medicine, do not take the missed dose and do not double your next dose. Check with your doctor.

- ☐ Most people experience few or no side effects from their drugs. However, any medicine can sometimes cause unwanted effects. Call your doctor if you develop pain or swelling in the legs or ankles, shortness of breath, sudden weight gain, skin rash, headache, unusual weakness or drowsiness, or unusual vaginal bleeding.

*　*　*　*　*

Terbutaline (*Oral Bronchodilator*)

United States: Brethine, Bricanyl
Canada: Bricanyl

- ☐ This medicine is used to help open the bronchioles (air passages in the lungs) to make breathing easier.

- ☐ IMPORTANT: If you have ever had an allergic reaction to any cough/cold, allergy, heart, or weight-reducing medicines, tell your doctor or pharmacist before you take any of this medicine.

HOW TO USE THIS MEDICINE

- ☐ This medicine may be taken with food or a glass of water.

SPECIAL INSTRUCTIONS

- ☐ Do not change the dose of your regular asthma or bronchitis medicines except on the advice of your doctor.

- ☐ Call your doctor if the medicine does not relieve your breathing problems, or if your sputum turns yellow or green in color.

- ☐ Most people experience few or no side effects from their drugs. However, any medicine can sometimes cause unwanted effects. Call your doctor if you develop chest pain, headaches, sweating, palpitations, or dizziness.

*　*　*　*　*

Testolactone (*Oral Antineoplastic*)
United States: Teslac

☐ This medicine is used in certain medical conditions to help slow down the growth and reproduction of some of the body's cells.

HOW TO USE THIS MEDICINE

☐ It is best to take this medicine on an empty stomach at least 1 hour before (or 2 hours after) eating food. Take it at the proper time even if you skip a meal.

☐ It is very important that you take this medicine exactly as your doctor has prescribed and that you do not miss any doses. Try to take this medicine at the same time every day. Do not take extra tablets without your doctor's approval.

☐ Even if you become nauseated, do not stop taking the medicine until you check with your doctor.

SPECIAL INSTRUCTIONS

☐ If you forget to take a dose, take it as soon as possible. However, if it is almost time for your next dose, do not take the missed dose. Instead, continue with your regular dosing schedule.

☐ It is recommended that you take appropriate birth control measures to avoid conception while taking this medicine.

☐ Always keep your doctor appointments so that your doctor can watch your progress.

☐ Always tell your pharmacist, dentist, and other doctors who are treating you that you are taking this medicine.

☐ Most people experience few or no side effects from their drugs. However, any medicine can sometimes cause unwanted effects. Call your doctor if you develop pain or swelling in the legs or ankles, sudden weight gain, or severe vomiting. Also call your doctor if you become unusually thirsty, drowsy, or confused, or if you urinate ("pass your water") more frequently than usual.

*   *   *   *   *

Testosterone Propionate (*Oral Anabolic Steroid*)
United States: Oreton Propionate

☐ This medicine is similar to a hormone which is normally produced by the body. This medicine has many uses and the reason it was prescribed depends upon your condition. If you do not understand why you are taking it, check with your doctor.

HOW TO USE THIS MEDICINE

☐ It is very important that you take this drug as your doctor has prescribed.

773

□ For BUCCAL TABLETS

  • Place the tablets in the pouch of the cheek (between the outside of the teeth and the cheek) and let the tablet dissolve. DO NOT SWALLOW until the tablet has dissolved and the taste of the drug has disappeared. Avoid eating, drinking, or smoking immediately after taking the tablet. Change the place in the cheek where you place the tablet with each dose.

SPECIAL INSTRUCTIONS

□ Women who are pregnant, breast-feeding, or planning to become pregnant should tell their doctor before taking this medicine.

□ Diabetic patients should regularly check the sugar in the urine and report any abnormal results to their doctor.

□ Carry an identification card indicating that you are taking this medicine. Always tell your pharmacist, dentist, and other doctors who are treating you that you are taking this medicine.

□ Most people experience few or no side effects from their drugs. However, any medicine can sometimes cause unwanted effects. Call your doctor if you develop swelling of the hands, legs or ankles, sore throat and fever, acne, unusual restlessness, dark-colored urine, or a yellow color to the skin or eyes. Women should call their doctor if they develop menstrual problems, hoarseness or a deepening of the voice, baldness, or increased facial hair.

*　*　*　*　*

Tetracaine HCl (*Topical Anesthetic*)
United States: Pontocaine
Canada: Pontocaine

□ This medicine is used to help relieve pain and itching of the skin.

□ IMPORTANT: If you have ever had an allergic reaction to tetracaine or any "caine" type of medicine, tell your doctor or pharmacist before you use any of this drug.

HOW TO USE THIS MEDICINE

□ For CREAM and OINTMENT

  • Each time you apply the medicine, wash your hands and gently cleanse the skin area well with water unless otherwise directed by your doctor. Do not allow the skin to dry completely. Pat with a clean towel until almost dry.
  • Apply a small amount of the drug to the affected area and spread lightly. Only the medicine that is actually touching the skin will work. A thick layer is not more effective than a thin layer. Do not bandage unless directed by your doctor.

774

- ☐ Do not use the drug more frequently, in larger quantities, or for a longer period of time than prescribed by your doctor.

SPECIAL INSTRUCTIONS

- ☐ Call your doctor if the condition for which this drug is being used persists or becomes worse or if you have a constant irritation such as itching or burning that was not present before you started using this medicine. Also call your doctor if you develop a slow heartbeat, fainting, or tremors.

- ☐ For external use only. Do not swallow.

*　*　*　*　*

Tetracycline HCl (*Ophthalmic Antibiotic*)
United States: Achromycin
Canada: Achromycin

- ☐ This medicine is an antibiotic used to treat certain types of eye infections.

- ☐ IMPORTANT: If you have ever had an allergic reaction to tetracycline or any antibiotic medicine, tell your doctor or pharmacist before you use any of this drug.

HOW TO USE THIS MEDICINE
- ☐ For EYE OINTMENT

INSTILLATION OF EYE OINTMENT

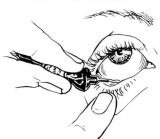

- The person administering the eye ointment should wash his hands with soap and water.
- The eye ointment must be kept clean. Do not touch the tube against the face or anything else.
- Lie down or tilt your head backward and look at the ceiling.
- Gently pull down the lower lid of your eye to form a pouch.
- Hold the tube in your other hand and place the tube as close as possible to the eye without touching it.
- Squeeze the prescribed amount of ointment (usually $\frac{1}{2}$ inch in adults) from the tube along the pouch.
- Close your eyes. Do not rub them.
- Wipe off any excess ointment around the eye with a tissue.

- Clean the tip of the ointment tube with a tissue.
- If necessary, have someone else administer the eye ointment for you.
- Keep the eye ointment tube tightly closed when not in use.

□ For EYE DROPS

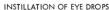

INSTILLATION OF EYE DROPS

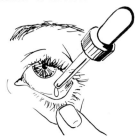

- The person administering the eye drops should wash his hands with soap and water.
- The eye drops must be kept clean. Do not touch the dropper against the face or anything else.
- Lie down or tilt your head backward and look at the ceiling.
- Shake the bottle well before using.
- Gently pull down the lower lid of your eye to form a pouch.
- Hold the dropper in your other hand and approach the eye from the side. Place the dropper as close to the eye as possible without touching it.
- Place the prescribed number of drops into the pouch of the eye.
- Close your eyes. Do not rub them.
- Apply gentle pressure for a minute with your fingers to the bridge of the nose (inside corner of the eye) to prevent the eye drops from being drained from the eye.
- Blot excess solution around the eye with a tissue.
- If necessary, have someone else administer the eye drops for you.
- Do not use the eye drops if they have changed in color or have changed in any way since you purchased them.
- Keep the eye drop bottle tightly closed when not in use.

SPECIAL INSTRUCTIONS

□ Vision may be blurred for a few minutes after using the eye medicine. Do not drive a car or operate dangerous machinery or do jobs that require you to be alert until your vision has cleared.

□ Eye medicines should be used as prescribed by your doctor. Often eye infections clear rapidly after a few days of use of the medicine but do not always clear completely. It is important to use *all* of this medicine, plus any refills that your doctor told you to use. Do not stop using it earlier than your doctor has recommended in spite of the fact that your symptoms seem to have improved. Otherwise, the infection may return.

☐ If you forget to use the medicine, use it as soon as possible. However, if it is almost time for your next dose, do not use the missed dose but continue with your regular schedule.

☐ Do not use this medicine at the same time as any other eye medicine without the approval of your doctor. Some medicines cannot be mixed.

☐ Contact your doctor if the condition for which you are using this medicine does not improve or if the eye becomes irritated by it for more than a few minutes. Many eye medicines sting for a short time immediately after use.

☐ For external use only. Do not swallow.

*　　*　　*　　*　　*

Tetracycline HCl (*Topical Antibiotic*)
United States: Achromycin, Topicycline
Canada: Achromycin

☐ This medicine is an antibiotic used to treat infections of the skin and to help control acne.

☐ IMPORTANT: If you have ever had an allergic reaction to a tetracycline or any antibiotic medicine, tell your doctor or pharmacist before you use any of this drug.

HOW TO USE THIS MEDICINE
☐ For OINTMENT
- Each time you apply the medicine, wash your hands and gently cleanse the skin area well with water unless otherwise directed by your doctor. Do not allow the skin to dry completely. Pat with a clean towel until almost dry.
- Apply a small amount of the drug to the affected area and spread lightly. Only the medicine that is actually touching the skin will work. A thick layer is not more effective than a thin layer. Do not bandage unless directed by your doctor.

☐ For TOPICAL SOLUTION (***United States:*** Topicycline)
- Cleanse the affected area well with water unless otherwise directed.
- Tilt the bottle and rub the applicator top over the skin while gently applying pressure.
- Apply the medicine generously until the skin is thoroughly wet. This may cause a stinging or burning sensation for a few minutes.
- Discard any unused medicine after 2 months.
- Cosmetics may be applied after the solution has dried.

☐ Do not apply cosmetics or lotions on top of the drug unless your doctor approves

☐ Do not use the drug more frequently or in larger quantities than prescribed by your doctor.

SPECIAL INSTRUCTIONS

☐ It is important to use **all** of this medicine, plus any refills that your doctor told you to use. Do not stop using it earlier than your doctor has recommended in spite of the fact that your symptoms seem to have improved. Otherwise, the infection may return or your acne may not improve.

☐ If you forget to apply the medicine, apply it as soon as possible. However, if it is almost time for your next dose, do not apply the missed dose but continue with your regular schedule.

☐ Keep this preparation away from the eyes. If you should accidentally get some in your eyes, wash it away with water immediately.

☐ A slight yellow color on the skin may be removed easily by washing. If you are exposed to ultraviolet light (such as in discotheques), the treated skin areas will appear bright yellow. (**United States:** Topicycline)

☐ Call your doctor if the condition for which this drug is being used persists or becomes worse or if you develop a constant irritation such as itching or burning that was not present before you started using this medicine. Also call your doctor if you develop pain, redness, swelling, or sensitivity to sunlight.

☐ For external use only. Do not swallow.

* * * * *

Tetracycline HCl (*Oral Antibiotic*)

United States: Achromycin V, Bristacycline, Centet, Cyclopar, G-Mycin, Maytrex, Nor-Tet, Paltet, Panmycin, Piracaps, Retet, Robitet, SK-Tetracycline, Sumycin, Tetrachel, Tetracyn, Tetrex, T-250

Canada: Achromycin V, Bio-Tetra, Cefracycline, Medicycline, Neo-Tetrine, Novotetra, Sumycin, T-Caps, Tetracrine, Tetracyn, Tetralean, Tetrex

☐ This medicine is an antibiotic used to treat certain types of infections and to help control acne.

☐ IMPORTANT: If you have ever had an allergic reaction to tetracycline or any other antibiotic, tell your doctor or pharmacist before you take any of this medicine.

HOW TO USE THIS MEDICINE

☐ It is best to take this medicine on an empty stomach 1 hour before eating food or 2 hours after eating food. Take it at the proper time even if you skip a meal. If this medicine upsets your stomach, take it with some crackers (not with dairy products). Call your doctor if you continue to have stomach upset.

778

- [ ] Take this medicine with a full glass of water.

- [ ] Do not drink milk or eat cheese, cottage cheese, ice cream, or other dairy products 1 hour before or 2 hours after you have taken a dose of this medicine.

- [ ] For LIQUID MEDICINE
    - Shake the bottle well before using so that you can measure an accurate dose. (**Canada:** Cefracycline, Novotetra, Tetracyn Suspensions).

SPECIAL INSTRUCTIONS

- [ ] It is important that you take **all** of this medicine plus any refills that your doctor told you to take. Do not stop taking this medicine earlier than your doctor has recommended in spite of the fact that you may feel better. Otherwise, the infection may return or your skin condition may get worse.

- [ ] If you forget to take a dose, take it as soon as you remember and then continue with your regular schedule.

- [ ] Women who are pregnant, breast-feeding, or planning to become pregnant should tell their doctor before taking this medicine.

- [ ] Some antacids and some laxatives can make this medicine less effective if they are taken at the same time. If you must take them, they should be taken at least 2 to 3 hours after this medicine. If you have any questions, ask your pharmacist.

- [ ] If you must take iron products or vitamins containing iron, take them 2 hours before (or 3 hours after) this medicine.

- [ ] This medicine may make some people more sensitive to sunlight or sunlamps. When you begin taking this medicine, try to avoid getting too much sun until you see how you are going to react. If your skin does become more sensitive, try to stay out of direct sunlight. While in the sun, wear protective clothing and sunglasses. You may wish to ask your pharmacist about suitable sunscreen products. You may remain sensitive to sunlight and sunlamps for several weeks after you have stopped taking the drug. Check with your doctor if you become sunburned.

- [ ] Most people experience few or no side effects from their drugs. However, any medicine can sometimes cause unwanted effects. Call your doctor if you develop a dark-colored tongue, sore mouth, yellow-green stools or, in women, a vaginal discharge that was not present before you started taking this medicine.

- [ ] Store the medicine in a cool, dark place and keep tightly closed.

- [ ] If for some reason you cannot take all of the medicine, discard the unused portion by flushing it down the toilet. Do not save this medicine for future use. Outdated tetracycline can be harmful.

* * * * *

Tetrahydrozoline HCl (*Ophthalmic Decongestant*)

United States: Murine 2, Visine

Canada: Soothe

☐ This medicine is used to treat eye conditions to help relieve burning, itching, or smarting of the eye.

HOW TO USE THIS MEDICINE

☐ For EYE DROPS

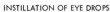

INSTILLATION OF EYE DROPS

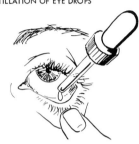

- The person administering the eye drops should wash his hands with soap and water.
- The eye drops must be kept clean. Do not touch the dropper against the face or anything else.
- Lie down or tilt your head backward and look at the ceiling.
- Gently pull down the lower lid of your eye to form a pouch.
- Hold the dropper in your other hand and approach the eye from the side. Place the dropper as close to the eye as possible without touching it.
- Place the prescribed number of drops into the pouch of the eye.
- Close your eyes. Do not rub them.
- Apply gentle pressure for a minute with your fingers to the bridge of the nose (inside corner of the eye) to prevent the eye drops from being drained from the eye.
- Blot excess solution around the eye with a tissue.

☐ If necessary, have someone else administer the eye drops for you.

☐ Do not use the eye drops if they have changed in color or have changed in any way since being purchased.

☐ Keep the eye drop bottle tightly closed when not in use.

☐ Do not use the drug more frequently or in larger quantities than prescribed by your doctor.

SPECIAL INSTRUCTIONS

☐ Vision may be blurred for a few minutes after using the eye medicine. Do not drive a car or operate dangerous machinery or do jobs that require you to be alert until your vision has cleared.

780

- [ ] If you forget to use the medicine, use it as soon as possible. However, if it is almost time for your next dose, do not use the missed dose but continue with your regular schedule.

- [ ] Do not use this medicine at the same time as any other eye medicine without the approval of your doctor. Some medicines cannot be mixed.

- [ ] Check with your doctor if you develop a headache which does not go away as your body adjusts to the medicine.

- [ ] Contact your doctor if the condition for which you are using this medicine does not improve or if the eye becomes irritated by it for more than a few minutes. Many eye medicines sting for a short time immediately after use. Also call your doctor if you develop fast heartbeats, trembling, or excessive sweating.

- [ ] Store the solution in a cool dark place because it is sensitive to heat and light.

- [ ] For external use only. Do not swallow.

*　*　*　*　*

Tetrahydrozoline HCl (Nasal Decongestant)
United States: Tyzine

- [ ] This medicine is used to help relieve nasal stuffiness.

HOW TO USE THIS MEDICINE
- [ ] For NASAL SPRAY
  - Blow your nose gently
  - Sit upright with your head slightly back.
  - Place the atomizer at the entrance of the nostril and close the other nostril by pressing your finger on the side.
  - Squeeze the atomizer the prescribed number of times.
  - Repeat for the other nostril if necessary.

- [ ] For NOSE DROPS

INSTILLATION OF NOSE DROPS

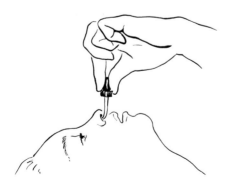

781

- Blow your nose gently before administration of the drops.
- Sit in a chair and tilt your head backward, or lie down on a bed with your head extending over the edge of the bed, or lie down and place a pillow under the shoulders so that the head is tipped backward.
- Insert the dropper into the nostril about $\frac{1}{3}$ inch and drop the prescribed number of drops into the nose.
- Try not to touch the inside of the nose with the dropper as it will probably make you sneeze and will contaminate the dropper.
- Remain in the same position for at least 5 minutes.

SPECIAL INSTRUCTIONS

☐ Do not use this medicine more often or longer than recommended by your doctor. If used for too long, this medicine may actually cause a type of congestion.

☐ Rinse the dropper in hot water after each use.

☐ If you forget to use the medicine, use it as soon as possible. However, if it is almost time for your next dose, do not use the missed dose but continue with your regular schedule.

☐ Do not use this medicine at the same time as any other nasal medicine without the approval of your doctor. Some medicines cannot be mixed.

☐ Contact your doctor if the condition for which you are using this medicine does not improve. Also call your doctor if you develop fast heartbeats, headache, dizziness, trembling, blurred vision, or drowsiness.

☐ Check with your doctor if you develop a stinging sensation which does not go away as your body adjusts to the medicine.

☐ For external use only. Do not swallow.

*   *   *   *   *

Theophylline (*Oral Bronchodilator*)

United States: Aerolate, Elixophyllin, Lanophyllin, Somophyllin-T, Sustaire, Theobid, Theo-Dur, Theolair, Theolixir

Canada: Acet-Am, Asthmophylline, Elixophyllin, Theocyne, Theolixir, Theo-Dur, Theolair, Theophyl-225

Theophylline-Guaifenesin

United States: Quibron, Theo-Guaia

Canada: Acet-AM Expectorant, Entair, Quibron

☐ This medicine is used to help open up the bronchioles (air passages in the lungs) to make breathing easier.

782

☐ IMPORTANT: If you have ever had an allergic reaction to caffeine or any medicine for lung conditions, tell your doctor or pharmacist before you take any of this medicine.

HOW TO USE THIS MEDICINE

☐ It is best to take this medicine on an empty stomach with a glass of water. However, if it upsets your stomach, it may be taken with a glass of milk or a snack. Call your doctor if the stomach upset continues.

☐ It is very important that you take this medicine exactly as your doctor has prescribed and that you do not miss any doses. Try to take this medicine at the same time every day. Do not take extra tablets without your doctor's approval.

☐ This medicine must be swallowed whole. Do not crush, chew, or break it into pieces. (**United States:** Aerolate, Elixophyllin SR, Sustaire, Theobid Dura-caps, Theo-Dur, Theolair-SR; **Canada:** Theo-Dur).

SPECIAL INSTRUCTIONS

☐ Do not change the dose of any other asthma or bronchitis medicines except on the advice of your doctor.

☐ If you forget to take a dose, take it as soon as possible. However, if it is almost time for your next dose, do not take the missed dose. Instead, continue with your regular dosing schedule.

☐ Women who are breast-feeding should tell their doctor before taking this medicine.

☐ In some people, this drug may cause dizziness or drowsiness. Do not drive a car or operate dangerous machinery or do jobs that require you to be alert until you know how you are going to react to this drug.

☐ If you become dizzy, you should be careful going up and down stairs. Sit or lie down at the first sign of dizziness.

☐ It is important that you obtain the advice of your doctor or pharmacist before taking ANY other medicines, including pain relievers, sleeping pills, tranquilizers or medicines for depression, cough/cold or allergy medicines, or weight-reducing medicines.

☐ Do not smoke while you are on this medicine because smoking can make the drug less effective.

☐ Avoid drinking large amounts of coffee, tea, cocoa, or cola drinks because you could be more sensitive to the caffeine in these beverages.

☐ Most people experience few or no side effects from their drugs. However, any medicine can sometimes cause unwanted effects. Call your doctor if you develop a skin rash, vomiting, stomach pain or red or black stools, fast heartbeats, confusion, unusual tiredness, restlessness or thirst, or increased urination ("passing your water").

* * * * *

Theophylline-Ephedrine-Phenobarbital (*Oral Antiasthmatic*)
United States: Asminyl, Tedral, Tedral SA, Theotabs
Canada: Asthmagyl, Chemfedral, Neo-Asma, Tedral, T.E.P.

Theophylline-Ephedrine-Amobarbital
United States: Amesec
Canada: Amesec

☐ This medicine is used to help open up the bronchioles (air passages in the lungs) to make breathing easier.

☐ IMPORTANT: If you have ever had an allergic reaction to caffeine, barbiturate medicine, or any medicine for lung conditions, tell your doctor or pharmacist before you take any of this medicine.

HOW TO USE THIS MEDICINE

☐ It is best to take this medicine on an empty stomach with a glass of water. However, if it upsets your stomach, it may be taken with a glass of milk or a snack. Call your doctor if the stomach upset continues.

☐ It is very important that you take this medicine exactly as your doctor has prescribed and that you do not miss any doses. Try to take this medicine at the same time every day. Do not take extra tablets without your doctor's approval.

SPECIAL INSTRUCTIONS

☐ Do not change the dose of any other asthma or bronchitis medicines except on the advice of your doctor.

☐ If you forget to take a dose, take it as soon as possible. However, if it is almost time for your next dose, do not take the missed dose. Instead, continue with your regular dosing schedule.

☐ Women who are pregnant, breast-feeding, or planning to become pregnant should tell their doctor before taking this medicine.

☐ In some people, this drug may cause dizziness or drowsiness. Do not drive a car or operate dangerous machinery or do jobs that require you to be alert until you know how you are going to react to this drug.

☐ If you become dizzy, you should be careful going up and down stairs. Sit or lie down at the first sign of dizziness.

☐ It is important that you obtain the advice of your doctor or pharmacist before taking ANY other medicines including pain relievers, sleeping pills, tranquilizers or medicines for depression, cough/cold or allergy medicines, or weight-reducing medicines.

☐ Do not smoke while you are on this medicine because smoking can make the drug less effective.

784

- [ ] Avoid drinking large amounts of coffee, tea, cocoa, or cola drinks because you could be more sensitive to the caffeine in these beverages.

- [ ] Most people experience few or no side effects from their drugs. However, any medicine can sometimes cause unwanted effects. Call your doctor if you develop a skin rash, vomiting, stomach pain or red or black stools, fast heart-beats, confusion, unusual tiredness, restlessness or thirst, or increased urination ("passing your water"). Also call your doctor if you develop a yellow-color to the skin or eyes, easy bruising, or nightmares.

* * * * *

Theophylline (*Rectal Bronchodilator*)
United States: Aqualin Suprettes

- [ ] This medicine is used to help open up the bronchioles (air passages in the lungs) to make breathing easier.

- [ ] IMPORTANT: If you have ever had an allergic reaction to caffeine or any medicine for lung conditions, tell your doctor or pharmacist before you use any of this medicine.

HOW TO USE THIS MEDICINE
- [ ] Administration of SUPPOSITORIES
    - Remove the wrapper from the suppository.
    - Lie on your side and raise your knee to your chest.
    - Insert the suppository with the tapered (pointed) end first into the rectum.
    - Remain lying down for a few minutes so that the suppository will dissolve in the rectum
    - Try to avoid having a bowel movement for at least one hour so that the drug will have time to work.

- [ ] It is very important that you use this medicine exactly as your doctor has prescribed and that you do not miss any doses. Do not use extra suppositories without your doctor's approval.

SPECIAL INSTRUCTIONS
- [ ] Do not change the dose of any other asthma or bronchitis medicines except on the advice of your doctor.

- [ ] Women who are breast-feeding should tell their doctor before taking this medicine.

- [ ] If you forget a dose, insert it as soon as possible. However, if it is almost time for your next dose, do not use the missed dose. Instead, continue with your regular dosing schedule.

- [ ] In some people, this drug may cause dizziness or drowsiness. Do not drive

785

a car or operate dangerous machinery or do jobs that require you to be alert until you know how you are going to react to this drug.

- [ ] If you become dizzy, you should be careful going up and down stairs. Sit or lie down at the first sign of dizziness.

- [ ] It is important that you obtain the advice of your doctor or pharmacist before taking ANY other medicines including pain relievers, sleeping pills, tranquilizers or medicines for depression, cough/cold or allergy medicines, or weight-reducing medicines.

- [ ] Do not smoke while you are on this medicine because smoking can make the drug less effective.

- [ ] Avoid drinking large amounts of coffee, tea, cocoa, or cola drinks because you could be more sensitive to the caffeine in these beverages.

- [ ] Most people experience few or no side effects from their drugs. However, any medicine can sometimes cause unwanted effects. Call your doctor if you develop a skin rash, vomiting, stomach pain or red or black stools, fast heartbeats, confusion, unusual tiredness, restlessness or thirst, or increased urination ("passing your water"), or if you develop rectal burning or pain that was not present before you used the medicine.

*   *   *   *   *

Thiabendazole (*Oral Anthelmintic*)
United States: Mintezol
Canada: Mintezol

- [ ] This medicine is used to treat intestinal worm infestations.

HOW TO USE THIS MEDICINE
- [ ] This medicine should be taken with food, preferably after a meal.

- [ ] Shake the liquid preparation well before using. (**United States:** Mintezol Oral Suspension)

- [ ] The tablets should be chewed well before swallowing.

- [ ] Take the medicine with a glass of water.

SPECIAL INSTRUCTIONS
- [ ] Do not take any more of this medicine than your doctor has prescribed, but it is important that you do not miss any doses. Otherwise, the infection will not be eliminated.

- [ ] In some people, this drug may cause dizziness or drowsiness. Do not drive a car or operate dangerous machinery or do jobs that require you to be alert until you know how you are going to react to this drug.

786

- ☐ If you become dizzy, you should be careful going up and down stairs. Sit or lie down at the first sign of dizziness.

- ☐ This medicine may cause the urine to have a different odor. This is not an unusual effect.

- ☐ It is not necessary to take a laxative or change your diet unless your doctor recommends that you do so.

- ☐ Most people experience few or no side effects from their drugs. However, any medicine can sometimes cause unwanted effects. Call your doctor if you develop a skin rash, fainting spells, a yellow color to the skin or eyes, unusual tiredness, or joint pains.

GENERAL INSTRUCTIONS

- ☐ Good personal hygiene is very important to prevent reinfection.

- ☐ It is recommended that you have a shower every morning in order to remove any eggs in the anal area that have appeared during the night.

- ☐ Wash your hands frequently, especially before handling food or anything that will be put into the mouth. Wash the hands after urination and bowel movements.

- ☐ Keep the nails short and clean and avoid biting them. Do not put your fingers in your mouth or nose.

- ☐ On the day of therapy, change the bed linen, underwear, and nightclothes. Wash or dry-clean them immediately.

- ☐ Do not scratch the affected area.

- ☐ Disinfect the toilet seat and bathtub daily.

* * * * *

Thiethylperazine (*Oral Antivertigo-Antiemetic*)
United States: Torecan
Canada: Torecan

- ☐ This medicine is used to help prevent and treat nausea and vomiting.

HOW TO USE THIS MEDICINE
- ☐ Take the tablets with a little water.

SPECIAL INSTRUCTIONS
- ☐ In some people, this drug may cause dizziness or drowsiness. Do not drive a car or operate dangerous machinery or do jobs that require you to be alert until you know how you are going to react to this drug.

- ☐ If you become dizzy, you should be careful going up and down stairs. Sit

787

or lie down at the first sign of dizziness. Get up slowly after you have been sitting or lying down.

☐ If your mouth becomes dry, suck a hard sour candy (sugarless) or ice chips, or chew gum. It is especially important to brush your teeth regularly if you develop a dry mouth.

☐ Do not drink alcoholic beverages while taking this drug without the approval of your doctor.

☐ It is important that you obtain the advice of your doctor or pharmacist before taking pain relievers, nonprescription drugs, sleeping pills, tranquilizers, or medicines for depression while you are taking this drug.

☐ This medicine may make some people more sensitive to sunlight and sunlamps. When you begin taking this medicine, try to avoid getting too much sun until you see how you are going to react. If your skin does become more sensitive to sunlight, tell your doctor and try to stay out of direct sunlight. While in the sun, wear protective clothing and sunglasses. You may wish to ask your pharmacist about suitable sunscreen products. Check with your doctor if you become sunburned.

☐ Most people experience few or no side effects from their drugs. However, any medicine can sometimes cause unwanted effects. Call your doctor if you develop unusual restlessness or movements of the hands, face or tongue, a shuffling walk, dark-colored urine or a yellow color to the skin or eyes, sore throat, fever, mouth sores, or severe constipation.

* * * * *

Thiethylperazine (*Rectal Antivertigo-Antiemetic*)
United States: Torecan
Canada: Torecan

☐ This medicine is used to help prevent and treat nausea and vomiting.

HOW TO USE THIS MEDICINE
☐ Administration of SUPPOSITORIES
  • Remove the wrapper from the suppository.
  • Lie on your side and raise your knee to your chest.
  • Insert the suppository with the tapered (pointed) end first into the rectum.
  • Remain lying down for a few minutes so that the suppository will dissolve in the rectum.
  • Try to avoid having a bowel movement for at least one hour so that the drug will have time to work.

☐ Store the suppositories in a cool place.

788

SPECIAL INSTRUCTIONS

☐ In some people, this drug may cause drowsiness or dizziness. Do not drive a car or operate dangerous machinery or do jobs that require you to be alert until you know how you are going to react to this drug.

☐ If you become dizzy, you should be careful going up and down stairs. Sit or lie down at the first sign of dizziness. Get up slowly after you have been sitting or lying down.

☐ If your mouth becomes dry, suck a hard sour candy (sugarless) or ice chips, or chew gum. It is especially important to brush your teeth regularly if you develop a dry mouth.

☐ Do not drink alcoholic beverages while you are on this drug without the approval of your doctor.

☐ It is important that you obtain the advice of your doctor or pharmacist before taking pain relievers, nonprescription drugs, sleeping pills, tranquilizers, or medicines for depression while you are taking this drug.

☐ This medicine may make some people more sensitive to sunlight and sunlamps. When you begin taking this medicine, try to avoid getting too much sun until you see how you are going to react. If your skin does become more sensitive to sunlight, tell your doctor and try to stay out of direct sunlight. While in the sun, wear protective clothing and sunglasses. You may wish to ask your pharmacist about suitable sunscreen products. Check with your doctor if you become sunburned.

☐ Most people experience few or no side effects from their drugs. However, any medicine can sometimes cause unwanted effects. Call your doctor if you develop unusual restlessness or movements of the hands, face or tongue, a shuffling walk, dark-colored urine or a yellow color to the skin or eyes, sore throat, fever or mouth sores, or severe constipation.

*   *   *   *   *

Thimerosal (*Topical Antiseptic-Disinfectant*)
United States: Merthiolate
Canada: Merthiolate

☐ This medicine is used to treat certain types of skin infections.

HOW TO USE THIS MEDICINE
☐ INSTRUCTIONS FOR USE:
- Cleanse the skin area to be treated with water unless otherwise directed by your doctor.
- Apply the medicine to the area, but do **not** cover the treated area with a bandage until the medicine has dried.

☐ Do not use iodine with or immediately after using this medicine.

789

- [ ] Call your doctor if the condition for which this drug is being used persists or becomes worse or if you develop a constant irritation such as itching or burning that was not present before you started using this medicine.

- [ ] For external use only. Do not swallow.

*   *   *   *   *

Thioguanine (*Oral Antineoplastic*)
United States: Thioguanine
Canada: Lanvis

- [ ] This medicine is used in certain medical conditions to help slow down the growth and reproduction of some of the body's cells.

- [ ] This drug is sometimes called 6-Thioguanine. "6" is part of the name and has nothing to do with the dosage.

HOW TO USE THIS MEDICINE

- [ ] It is best to take this medicine on an empty stomach at least 1 hour before (or 2 hours after) eating food. Take it at the proper time even if you skip a meal.

- [ ] It is very important that you take this medicine exactly as your doctor has prescribed and that you do not miss any doses. Try to take this medicine at the same time every day.

- [ ] Even if you become nauseated, do not stop taking the medicine but check with your doctor.

- [ ] If you miss a dose of this medicine, do not take the missed dose and do not double your next dose. Check with your doctor.

SPECIAL INSTRUCTIONS

- [ ] Always keep your doctor appointments so that your doctor can watch your progress.

- [ ] If your doctor has prescribed some other medicines for you, it is important that you take them in the right order and that you do not miss them.

- [ ] Unless otherwise directed, drink plenty of fluids (2 to 3 quarts daily) while you are taking this medicine. This will help your kidneys handle the medicine and help prevent kidney problems.

- [ ] Men and women should take appropriate birth control measures to avoid conception while taking this medicine and for at least 2 months after the medicine has been stopped.

- [ ] Always tell your pharmacist, dentist, and any other doctors who are treating you that you are taking this medicine. This is especially important if you plan to have surgery or any vaccinations.

☐ This is a very strong medicine. In addition to its benefits, there may be some unwanted effects, even for a short time after you stop taking the medicine. Call your doctor if you develop unusual brusing or bleeding, black "tarry" stools, a sore throat, fever, a skin rash, swelling of the legs or ankles, shortness of breath, a yellow color to the skin or eyes, stomach or joint pain, decrease in frequency of urinating ("passing your water"), nausea, severe vomiting, or loss of appetite.

* * * * *

Thiopropazate Dihydrochloride (*Oral Antipsychotic-Antianxiety*)
Canada: Dartal

☐ This medicine is used to treat certain types of emotional conditions.

☐ IMPORTANT: If you have ever had an allergic reaction to a phenothiazine medicine or a medicine that you took for the same reason, tell your doctor or pharmacist before you take any of this medicine.

HOW TO USE THIS MEDICINE
☐ This medicine may be taken with food or a full glass of water.

SPECIAL INSTRUCTIONS
☐ The full benefit of the medicine may not be noticed immediately but may take a few weeks. Be patient. Take the medicine regularly and try not to miss any doses.

☐ If you forget to take a dose, take it as soon as possible. However, if it is almost time for your next dose, do not take the missed dose. Instead, continue with your regular dosing schedule.

☐ Do not stop taking the medicine suddenly without the approval of your doctor.

☐ If your mouth becomes dry, suck a hard sour candy (sugarless) or ice chips, or chew gum. It is especially important to brush your teeth regularly if you develop a dry mouth.

☐ Do not drink alcoholic beverages while taking this drug without the approval or your doctor.

☐ It is important that you obtain the advice of your doctor or pharmacist before taking ANY other medicines including pain relievers, sleeping pills, tranquilizers or medicines for depression, cough/cold or allergy medicines, or weight-reducing medicines.

☐ If this medicine causes dizziness, you should be careful going up and down stairs and you should not change positions too rapidly. Get out of bed slowly in the morning and dangle your feet over the edge of the bed for a few minutes before standing up. Sit down or lie down at the first sign of dizzi-

791

ness. Tell your doctor you have been dizzy. Avoid hot showers and baths because they could make you dizzy.

☐ Most people experience few or no side effects from their drugs. However, any medicine can sometimes cause unwanted effects. Call your doctor if you develop a skin rash, sore throat, fever or mouth sores, unusual movements of the face, hands or tongue, a staggering walk, difficulty in urinating ("passing your water"), changes in your eyesight, dark-colored urine, or a yellow color to the skin or eyes.

☐ Carry an identification card indicating that you are taking this medicine. Always tell your pharmacist, dentist, and other doctors who are treating you that you are taking this medicine.

* * * * *

Thioproperazine Mesylate
Canada: Majeptil

☐ This medicine is used to treat certain types of emotional conditions.

☐ IMPORTANT: If you have ever had an allergic reaction to a phenothiazine medicine, tell your doctor or pharmacist before you take any of this medicine.

HOW TO USE THIS MEDICINE
☐ This medicine may be taken with food or a full glass of water.

☐ Do not take this medicine at the same time as antacids or diarrhea medicine. Try to space them at least 1 hour apart.

☐ The effect of the medicine may not be noticed immediately, but may take from 2 to 4 weeks. Be patient. Take the medicine regularly and try not to miss any doses.

☐ Do not stop taking this medicine suddenly without the approval of your doctor.

SPECIAL INSTRUCTIONS
☐ If you forget to take a dose, take it as soon as possible. However, if it is almost time for your next dose, do not take the missed dose. Instead, continue with your regular dosing schedule.

☐ Any medicine has a few unwanted side effects. Because this medicine takes a few weeks to work, the side effects show the doctor that the drug is being absorbed. Many of these side effects will go away as your body adjusts to the medicine.

☐ Women who are pregnant, breast-feeding, or planning to become pregnant should tell their doctor before taking this medicine.

☐ In some people, this drug may cause dizziness or drowsiness. Do not drive a

792

car or operate dangerous machinery or do jobs that require you to be alert until you know how you are going to react to this drug.

☐ If this medicine causes dizziness, you should be careful going up and down stairs and you should not change positions too rapidly. Get out of bed slowly in the morning and dangle your feet over the edge of the bed for a few minutes before standing up. Sit down or lie down at the first sign of dizziness. Tell your doctor you have been dizzy. Avoid hot showers and baths because they could make you dizzy.

☐ Do not drink alcoholic beverages while taking this drug without the approval of your doctor.

☐ This medicine may make some people more sensitive to sunlight and sunlamps. When you begin taking this medicine, try to avoid getting too much sun until you see how you are going to react. If your skin does become more sensitive to sunlight, tell your doctor and try to stay out of direct sunlight. While in the sun, wear protective clothing and sunglasses. You may wish to ask your pharmacist about suitable sunscreen products. Check with your doctor if you become sunburned.

☐ If your mouth becomes dry, suck a hard sour candy (sugarless) or ice chips, or chew gum. It is especially important to brush your teeth regularly if you develop a dry mouth.

☐ It is important that you obtain the advice of your doctor or pharmacist before taking **any** other medicines including pain relievers, sleeping pills, tranquilizers or medicines for depression, cough/cold or allergy medicines, weight-reducing medicines, or laxatives.

☐ This medicine may cause your urine to turn pink, red, or red-brown in color. This is not unusual.

☐ In hot weather or during exercise, be careful not to become overheated. You may be more sensitive to heat since this medicine may affect your body's ability to regulate temperature.

☐ If you become constipated, try increasing the amount of bulk in your diet (for example, bran and salads), exercising more often, or drinking more water. Call your doctor if the constipation continues.

☐ Call your doctor if you develop a sore throat, fever, mouth sores, skin rash, changes in eyesight, rapid heartrate, a yellow color in the eyes or skin, unusual weakness or unusual movements of the face, tongue or hands, or difficulty in urinating ("passing your water"). Also call your doctor if you become restless or unable to sit still or sleep.

☐ Carry an identification card indicating that you are taking this medicine. Always tell your pharmacist, dentist, and other doctors who are treating you that you are taking this medicine.

* * * * *

Thioridazine HCl (*Oral Antipsychotic-Antianxiety*)
United States: Mellaril
Canada: Mellaril, Novoridazine, Thioril

☐ This medicine is used to help relieve the symptoms of certain types of emotional problems. This drug has several other uses and the reason it was prescribed depends upon your condition. Check with your doctor if you do not fully understand why you are taking it.

☐ IMPORTANT: If you have ever had an allergic reaction to a phenothiazine medicine, tell your doctor or pharmacist before you take any of this medicine.

HOW TO USE THIS MEDICINE

☐ This medicine may be taken with food or a full glass of water.

☐ Do not take this medicine at the same time as antacids or diarrhea medicine. Try to space them at least 1 hour apart.

☐ If a dropper is used to measure the dose and you do not fully understand how to use it, check with your pharmacist. (**Canada:** Mellaril Solution)

☐ Store the liquid medicines in a cool, dark place and do not get the liquid on your skin or clothing. (**United States** and **Canada:** Mellaril)

☐ Shake the bottle well each time you use it so that you get an accurate dose. (**Canada:** Mellaril Suspension)

☐ The effect of the medicine may not be noticed immediately but may take from 2 to 4 weeks. Be patient. Take the medicine regularly and try not to miss any doses.

☐ Do not stop taking this medicine suddenly without the approval of your doctor.

SPECIAL INSTRUCTIONS

☐ If you forget to take a dose, take it as soon as possible. However, if it is almost time for your next dose, do not take the missed dose. Instead, continue with your regular dosing schedule.

☐ Any medicine has a few unwanted side effects. Because this medicine takes a few weeks to work, the side effects show the doctor that the drug is being absorbed. Many of these side effects will go away as your body adjusts to the medicine.

☐ Women who are pregnant, breast-feeding, or planning to become pregnant should tell their doctor before taking this medicine.

☐ In some people, this drug may cause dizziness or drowsiness. Do not drive a car or operate dangerous machinery or do jobs that require you to be alert until you know how you are going to react to this drug.

794

☐ If this medicine causes dizziness, you should be careful going up and down stairs and you should not change positions too rapidly. Get out of bed slowly in the morning and dangle your feet over the edge of the bed for a few minutes before standing up. Sit down or lie down at the first sign of dizziness. Tell your doctor you have been dizzy. Avoid hot showers and baths because they could make you dizzy.

☐ Do not drink alcoholic beverages while taking this drug without the approval of your doctor.

☐ This medicine may make some people more sensitive to sunlight and sunlamps. When you begin taking this medicine, try to avoid getting too much sun until you see how you are going to react. If your skin does become more sensitive to sunlight, tell your doctor and try to stay out of direct sunlight. While in the sun, wear protective clothing and sunglasses. You may wish to ask your pharmacist about suitable sunscreen products. Check with your doctor if you become sunburned.

☐ If your mouth becomes dry, suck a hard sour candy (sugarless) or ice chips, or chew gum. It is especially important to brush your teeth regularly if you develop a dry mouth.

☐ It is important that you obtain the advice of your doctor or pharmacist before taking **any** other medicines including pain relievers, sleeping pills, other tranquilizers or medicines for depression, cough/cold or allergy medicines, weight-reducing medicines, or laxatives.

☐ This medicine may cause your urine to turn pink, red, or red-brown in color. This is not unusual.

☐ In hot weather or during exercise, be careful not to become overheated. You may be more sensitive to heat since this medicine may affect your body's ability to regulate temperature.

☐ If you become constipated, try increasing the amount of bulk in your diet (for example, bran and salads), exercising more often, or drinking more water. Call your doctor if the constipation continues.

☐ Call your doctor if you develop a sore throat, fever, mouth sores, skin rash, changes in eyesight, rapid heart rate, a yellow color in the eyes or skin, unusual weakness or unusual movements of the face, tongue or hands, or difficulty in urinating ("passing your water"). Also call your doctor if you become restless or unable to sit still or sleep.

☐ Carry an identification card indicating that you are taking this medicine. Always tell your pharmacist, dentist, and other doctors who are treating you that you are taking this medicine.

* * * * *

795

Thiothixene (*Oral Antipsychotic*)
United States: Navane
Canada: Navane

□ This medicine is used to treat certain types of emotional conditions.

□ IMPORTANT: If you have ever had an allergic reaction to a medicine that you took for the same reason, tell your doctor or pharmacist before you take any of this medicine.

HOW TO USE THIS MEDICINE

□ This medicine may be taken with food or a full glass of water.

□ Do not take this medicine at the same time as antacids or diarrhea medicine. Try to space them at least 1 hour apart.

□ The effect of the medicine may not be noticed immediately but may take from 2 to 4 weeks. Be patient. Take the medicine regularly and try not to miss any doses.

□ Do not stop taking this medicine suddenly without the approval of your doctor.

SPECIAL INSTRUCTIONS

□ If you forget to take a dose, take it as soon as possible. However, if it is almost time for your next dose, do not take the missed dose. Instead, continue with your regular dosing schedule.

□ Any medicine has a few unwanted side effects. Because this medicine takes a few weeks to work, the side effects show the doctor that the drug is being absorbed. Many of these side effects will go away as your body adjusts to the medicine.

□ In some people, this drug may cause dizziness or drowsiness. Do not drive a car or operate dangerous machinery or do jobs that require you to be alert until you know how you are going to react to this drug.

□ If this medicine causes dizziness, you should be careful going up and down stairs and you should not change positions too rapidly. Get out of bed slowly in the morning and dangle your feet over the edge of the bed for a few minutes before standing up. Sit down or lie down at the first sign of dizziness. Tell your doctor you have been dizzy. Avoid hot showers and baths because they could make you dizzy.

□ Do not drink alcoholic beverages while taking this drug without the approval of your doctor.

□ This medicine may make some people more sensitive to sunlight and sunlamps. When you begin taking this medicine, try to avoid getting too much sun until you see how you are going to react. If your skin does become more sensitive to sunlight, tell your doctor and try to stay out of direct sun-

light. While in the sun, wear protective clothing and sunglasses. You may wish to ask your pharmacist about suitable sunscreen products. Check with your doctor if you become sunburned.

☐ If your mouth becomes dry, suck a hard sour candy (sugarless) or ice chips, or chew gum. It is especially important to brush your teeth regularly if you develop a dry mouth.

☐ It is important that you obtain the advice of your doctor or pharmacist before taking **any** other medicines including pain relievers, sleeping pills, other tranquilizers or medicines for depression, cough/cold or allergy medicines, weight-reducing medicines, or laxatives.

☐ In hot weather or during exercise, be careful not to become overheated. You may be more sensitive to heat since this medicine may affect your body's ability to regulate temperature.

☐ Call your doctor if you develop a sore throat, fever, mouth sores, skin rash, changes in eyesight, rapid heart rate, dark-colored urine or a yellow color in the eyes or skin, unusual weakness or unusual movements of the face, tongue or hands, difficulty in urinating ("passing your water"). Also call your doctor if you become restless or unable to sit still or sleep.

☐ Carry an identification card indicating that you are taking this medicine. Always tell your pharmacist, dentist, and other doctors who are treating you that you are taking this medicine.

*　*　*　*　*

Thyroglobulin (*Oral Hypothyroidism Therapy*)
United States: Proloid, Thyroglobulin
Canada: Proloid

☐ This medicine is a hormone which is used to treat conditions in which the body is not producing enough thryoid hormone.

HOW TO USE THIS MEDICINE
☐ Take this medicine with some water.

☐ It is very important that you take this medicine exactly as your doctor has prescribed and that you do not miss any doses. Try to take this medicine at the same time every day.

☐ If you forget to take a dose, take it as soon as possible. However, if it is almost time for your next dose, do not take the missed dose. Instead, continue with your regular dosing schedule.

☐ Do not take any more of this medicine than your doctor has prescribed and do not stop taking this medicine suddenly without the approval of your doctor.

SPECIAL INSTRUCTIONS

□ It is important that you obtain the advice of your doctor or pharmacist before taking ANY other medicines including pain relievers, sleeping pills, tranquilizers or medicines for depression, cough/cold or allergy medicines, or weight-reducing medicines.

□ Most people experience few or no side effects from their drugs. However, any medicine can sometimes cause unwanted effects. Call your doctor if you develop chest pain, shortness of breath, leg cramps, skin rash, fast heartbeats, trembling, diarrhea, sensitivity to heat, unusual nervousness, sweating, or weight loss.

*   *   *   *   *

Thyroid (*Oral Hypothyroidism Therapy*)
United States: Armour Thyroid, Thyrocrine, Thyroid

□ This medicine is a hormone which is used to treat conditions in which the body is not producing enough thyroid hormone.

HOW TO USE THIS MEDICINE

□ Take this medicine with some water.

□ This medicine must be swallowed whole. Do not crush, chew, or break it into pieces. (*United States:* Thyroid Enteric Coated, Thyroid Timed Release)

□ It is very important that you take this medicine exactly as your doctor has prescribed and that you do not miss any doses. Try to take this medicine at the same time every day.

□ If you forget to take a dose, take it as soon as possible. However, if it is almost time for your next dose, do not take the missed dose. Instead, continue with your regular dosing schedule.

□ Do not take any more of this medicine than your doctor has prescribed and do not stop taking this medicine suddenly without the approval of your doctor.

SPECIAL INSTRUCTIONS

□ It is important that you obtain the advice of your doctor or pharmacist before taking ANY other medicines including pain relievers, sleeping pills, tranquilizers or medicines for depression, cough/cold or allergy medicines, or weight-reducing medicines.

□ Most people experience few or no side effects from their drugs. However, any medicine can sometimes cause unwanted effects. Call your doctor if you develop chest pain, shortness of breath, leg cramps, skin rash, fast heartbeats, trembling, diarrhea, sensitivity to heat, unusual nervousness, sweating, or weight loss.

*   *   *   *   *

Timolol (*Ophthalmic Glaucoma Therapy*)
United States: Timoptic
Canada: Timoptic

☐ This medicine is used in the treatment of glaucoma.

HOW TO USE THIS MEDICINE
☐ For EYE DROPS

INSTILLATION OF EYE DROPS

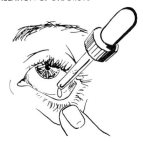

- The person administering the eye drops should wash his hands with soap and water.
- The eye drops must be kept clean. Do not touch the dropper against the face or anything else.
- Lie down or tilt your head backward and look at the ceiling.
- Gently pull down the lower lid of your eye to form a pouch.
- Hold the dropper in your other hand and approach the eye from the side. Place the dropper as close to the eye as possible without touching it.
- Place the prescribed number of drops into the pouch of the eye.
- Close your eyes. Do not rub them.
- Apply gentle pressure for a minute with your fingers to the bridge of the nose (inside corner of the eye) to prevent the eye drops from being drained from the eye.
- Blot excess solution around the eye with a tissue.

☐ If necessary, have someone else administer the eye drops for you.

☐ Do not use the eye drops if they have changed in color or have changed in any way since you purchased them.

☐ Keep the eye drop bottle tightly closed when not in use.

☐ Do not use the drug more frequently or in larger quantities than prescribed by your doctor.

SPECIAL INSTRUCTIONS
☐ If you forget to use the medicine, use it as soon as possible. However, if it is almost time for your next dose, do not use the missed dose but continue with your regular dosing schedule.

□ Do not use this medicine at the same time as any other eye medicine without the approval of your doctor. Some medicines cannot be mixed.

□ Contact your doctor if the condition for which you are using this medicine does not improve or if the eye becomes irritated by it for more than a few minutes. Many eye medicines sting for a short time immediately after use.

□ Always tell any future doctors who are treating you that you have used this medicine.

□ For external use only. Do not swallow.

* * * * *

Timolol Maleate (*Oral Antianginal—Antihypertensive*)
Canada: Blocadren

□ This medicine is used to help relieve chest pain (angina), and it is sometimes used to treat high blood pressure.

□ IMPORTANT: If you have a history of allergies, tell your doctor or pharmacist before taking any of this medicine.

□ It may be necessary for you to take this medicine for a long time in spite of the fact that you may feel better. It is very important that you take the medicine as your doctor has prescribed and that you do not miss any doses. Otherwise, you cannot expect the drug to work for you.

HOW TO USE THIS MEDICINE
□ This medicine may be taken with food or a glass of water.

□ Try to take the medicine at the same time(s) every day.

SPECIAL INSTRUCTIONS
□ If you forget to take a dose, take it as soon as possible. However, if your next dose is within 4 hours, do not take the missed dose. Instead continue with your regular dosing schedule.

□ In some people, this drug may cause dizziness or drowsiness. Do not drive a car or operate dangerous machinery or do jobs that require you to be alert until you know how you are going to react to this drug. Sit down or lie down at the first sign of dizziness. Tell your doctor you have been dizzy.

□ In order to help prevent dizziness and fainting, your doctor may also recommend that you avoid strenuous exercises, standing for long periods of time (especially in hot weather), or hot showers or hot baths.

□ If your mouth becomes dry, suck a hard sour candy (sugarless) or ice chips, or chew gum. It is especially important to brush your teeth regularly if you develop a dry mouth.

□ Some nonprescription drugs can aggravate your condition. Do not take any

800

of the following without the approval of your doctor or pharmacist: cough, cold, or sinus products; asthma or allergy products; or diet or weight-reducing medicines.

☐ Most people experience few or no side effects from their drugs. However, any medicine can sometimes cause unwanted effects. Call your doctor if you develop a skin rash, shortness of breath, fever or sore throat, easy bruising, swelling of the hands or feet, sudden weight gain, earache, or mouth sores.

☐ It is recommended that patients receiving this drug stop smoking.

☐ Carry an identification card indicating that you are taking this medicine. Always tell your pharmacist, dentist, and other doctors who are treating you that you are taking this medicine.

☐ Do not stop taking this medicine without your doctor's approval and do not go without medicine between prescription refills. Call your pharmacist 2 or 3 days before you will run out of the medicine.

* * * * *

Tolazoline HCl (*Oral Vasodilator*)
United States: Priscoline, Tolzol
Canada: Priscoline

☐ This medicine is used to improve the circulation of blood in the body.

HOW TO USE THIS MEDICINE
☐ For ORAL TABLETS
- Take this medicine after meals or with a glass of milk to help prevent stomach upset.
- If you forget to take a dose, take it as soon as possible. However, if it is almost time for your next dose, do not take the missed dose. Instead, continue with your regular dosing schedule.

☐ For SUSTAINED RELEASE MEDICINE
- These tablets must be swallowed whole. Do not crush, chew, or break them into pieces. (***United States:*** Priscoline Lontabs)
- If you forget to take a dose, take it as soon as possible. However, if your next dose is within 6 hours, do not take the missed dose but continue with your regular schedule.

SPECIAL INSTRUCTIONS
☐ This medicine commonly produces flushing of the face and a feeling of warmth. This is normal and you should not become concerned.

☐ The activity of this drug is improved if you keep warm. Avoid getting cold or exposing yourself to a cold environment.

☐ If this medicine causes dizziness, you should be careful going up and down stairs and you should not change positions too rapidly. Get out of bed slowly in the morning and dangle your feet over the edge of the bed for a few minutes before standing up. Sit down or lie down at the first sign of dizziness. Tell your doctor you have been dizzy. Do not drive a car or operate dangerous machinery if you are dizzy. Avoid hot showers and baths because they could make you dizzy.

☐ Do not drink alcoholic beverages while taking this drug without the approval of your doctor.

☐ Some nonprescription drugs can aggravate your condition. Do not take any of the following without the approval of your doctor or pharmacist: cough, cold, or sinus products; asthma or allergy products; or diet or weight-reducing medicines.

☐ Most people experience few or no side effects from their drugs. However, any medicine can sometimes cause unwanted effects. Call your doctor if you develop a sore throat, fever or mouth sores, fainting spells, a rapid pulse, severe headache, or sharp stomach pain.

* * * * *

Tolbutamide (*Oral Hypoglycemic*)

United States: Orinase, Tolbutamide

Canada: Mellitol, Mobenol, Neo-Dibetic, Novobutamide, Oramide, Orinase, Tolbutone

☐ This medicine is used in the treatment of diabetes. When you have diabetes, the body either is not producing enough insulin or is not able to use what is produced. Insulin is needed for the body's proper use of food, especially sugar. In a diabetic, the sugar in the blood can build up to dangerous levels and is passed out in the urine. Your doctor has prescribed this medicine to help keep your blood sugar at nearly normal levels.

HOW TO USE THIS MEDICINE

☐ This medicine may be taken with food to help prevent stomach upset.

☐ It is very important that you take this medicine exactly as your doctor has prescribed. Do not miss any doses. Try to take this medicine at the same time every day. Do not take extra tablets without your doctor's approval.

☐ Do not take this medicine at bedtime unless your doctor tells you to.

☐ If you forget to take a dose, take as soon as possible. However, if it is almost time for your next dose, do not take the missed dose. Instead, continue with your regular dosing schedule.

SPECIAL INSTRUCTIONS

☐ Women who are pregnant, breast-feeding, or planning to become pregnant should tell their doctor before taking this medicine.

☐ This medicine may make some people more sensitive to sunlight and sunlamps. When you begin taking this medicine try to avoid getting too much sun until you see how you are going to react. If your skin does become more sensitive to sunlight, tell your doctor and try to stay out of direct sunlight. While in the sun, wear protective clothing and sunglasses. You may wish to ask your pharmacist about suitable sunscreen products. Check with your doctor if you become sunburned.

☐ Most people experience few or no side effects from their drugs. However, any medicine can sometimes cause unwanted effects. Call your doctor if you develop a skin rash, sore throat, fever, mouth sores, dark-colored urine, a yellow color to the skin or eyes, easy bruising or bleeding, unusual tiredness, diarrhea, or light-colored stools.

GENERAL INSTRUCTIONS FOR DIABETIC PATIENTS

☐ Keep a regular schedule of daily activities. Eat, exercise, and take your insulin at approximately the same time every day.

☐ The diet that your doctor has prescribed has been carefully planned especially for you. It is to your advantage to follow it very closely.

☐ Test your urine regularly for sugar and, if your doctor recommends, test it for acetone.

☐ Learn the signs of hypoglycemia (low blood sugar). When this happens, your urine sugar will be negative. Hypoglycemia may occur if you delay or skip a meal, exercise too much, become sick or emotionally upset, take too much insulin, drink alcohol, or take certain drugs. If you develop sweating, drowsiness, unusual hunger, dizziness, nausea, nervousness, blurred vision, weakness, shaking, or trembling, eat or drink any of the following:
- 2 sugar cubes or 2 teaspoons of sugar in water
- 4 ounces orange juice
- 4 ounces regular ginger ale, cola beverages or any other sweetened carbonated beverage. Do not use low-calorie or diet beverages.
- 2-3 teaspoons honey or corn syrup
- 4 Lifesaver candies

Artificial sweeteners are of no use. Call your doctor if one of these does not relieve your symptoms in about 15 minutes.

☐ Always carry sugar cubes or hard candy in case you have a hypoglycemic (low blood sugar) reaction.

☐ Before you purchase any nonprescription medicine (for example, cough and cold medicines), ask your pharmacist if the medicine is safe for diabetic patients to use. Some nonprescription medicines have very high sugar contents which could interfere with the control of your diabetes. Aspirin and medicines containing salicylates or vitamin C could affect your urine test results. Check with your pharmacist.

☐ Ask your doctor if it is safe for you to drink alcoholic beverages because the combination may cause low blood sugar as well as a pounding headache, flushing, upset stomach, dizziness, or sweating.

803

□ Take special care of your feet.
- Wash your feet daily and dry them well.
- Check your feet daily for minor injuries. Bring these to the attention of your doctor immediately.
- Wear clean shoes and stockings and choose shoes that fit well.
- If you develop corns or calluses, soak your feet in lukewarm water for about 10 minutes. Then rub them off gently with a pumice stone. Never use a knife to cut corns or calluses on your feet. Do NOT use commercial corn removers, or commercial arch supports.
- Soften dry skin by rubbing with oil or lotion.
- Trim your toenails straight across with a file or a nail cutter. Do not cut your own toenails if your eyesight is poor.
- Do now wear garters or socks with tight elastic tops. Do not sit with your knees crossed.
- Do not warm your feet with a hot water bottle or a heating pad. Use loose bed socks instead. If your feet are cold under normal conditions, tell your doctor. Your circulation may be poor and your doctor can offer advice.
- Call your doctor if you injure your toes or feet. Cuts and scratches in the diabetic can become infected easily and take longer to heal. Do not apply iodine or strong antiseptics to the feet at any time.

□ Call your doctor immediately if you develop any of the following symptoms of hyperglycemia (high blood sugar): high urine sugar, acetone in the urine, drowsiness, hunger, unusual thirst, fast breathing, nausea, confusion, a flushed dry skin, increase in urination ("passing your water"), or a fruity odor to the breath. These symptoms may occur if you are taking too little insulin, miss a dose, overeat, or if you have a fever or infection.

□ Call your doctor if you become sick and have a fever, an infection, nausea, or vomiting.

□ Carry an identification card or wear a bracelet indicating that you are a diabetic and that you are taking this medicine. Always tell your pharmacist, dentist, and other doctors who are treating you that you are taking this medicine.

* * * * *

Tolmetin
United States: Tolectin
Canada: Tolectin

□ This medicine is used to help relieve pain, redness, stiffness, and swelling in certain kinds of arthritis.

□ IMPORTANT: If you have ever had an allergic reaction to aspirin or any other medicine for arthritis, tell your doctor or pharmacist before you take any of this medicine.

☐ It is very important that you take this medicine regularly and that you DO NOT MISS ANY DOSES. If you miss a dose, the level of the medicine in your body will fall and the drug will not be as effective. Only if the level of the drug is high enough can it decrease the inflammation and swelling in your joints and help prevent further damage.

☐ The full benefit of this medicine may not be noticed immediately but may take from a few days to 1 week.

HOW TO USE THIS MEDICINE

☐ It is best to take this medicine on an empty stomach at least 1 hour before (or 2 hours after) food unless otherwise directed. If you develop stomach upset, take the medicine with food or immediately after meals. Call your doctor if you continue to have stomach upset.

SPECIAL INSTRUCTIONS

☐ Women who are pregnant, breast-feeding, or planning to become pregnant should tell their doctor before taking this medicine.

☐ In some people, this drug may cause dizziness or drowsiness. Do not drive a car or operate dangerous machinery or do jobs that require you to be alert until you know how you are going to react to this drug.

☐ If you become dizzy, you should be careful going up and down stairs. Sit or lie down at the first sign of dizziness.

☐ If you forget to take a dose, take as soon as possible. However, if it is almost time for your next dose, do not take the missed dose. Instead, continue with your regular dosing schedule.

☐ While you are taking this medicine, do not drink alcoholic beverages or take aspirin without the permission of your doctor. It is usually safe to take acetaminophen for the occasional headache. Check with your pharmacist.

☐ Call your doctor immediately if you think you may be allergic to the medicine or if you develop a skin rash, hives, itching, swelling of the face, or difficulty in breathing. If you cannot reach your doctor, phone a hospital emergency department.

☐ Most people experience few or no side effects from their drugs. However, any medicine can sometimes cause unwanted effects. Call your doctor if you develop a skin rash, sore throat or fever, "ringing" or "buzzing" in the ears, fast heartbeats, swelling of the legs or ankles or sudden weight gain, blurred vision or changes in your eyesight, red or black stools, or severe stomach pain.

☐ Carry an identification card indicating that you are taking this medicine. Always tell your pharmacist, dentist, and other doctors who are treating you that you are taking this medicine.

*   *   *   *   *

Tolnaftate (*Topical Antifungal*)
United States: Tinactin
Canada: Tinactin

☐ This medicine is used to treat fungal infections of the skin and nails.

HOW TO USE THIS MEDICINE
☐ For SOLUTION
- Cleanse the affected area well with water unless otherwise directed by your doctor. Dry the skin well.
- Drop the prescribed amount of medicine onto the affected area, massage gently, and allow it to dry.
  Note: Two drops are sufficient for an area as large as a hand and 2 to 3 drops are enough to cover the toes and in between the toes.

☐ For POWDER
- Cleanse the affected area well with water unless otherwise directed by your doctor. Dry the skin well.
- Apply a small amount of powder to the affected area and rub in gently.
- The powder may also be dusted (ever 3 to 4 weeks) into the socks and shoes to help prevent further infection.

☐ For CREAM
- Cleanse the affected area well with water unless otherwise directed by your doctor. Dry the skin well.
- Apply a small amount of cream to the affected area and massage gently until it disappears.

SPECIAL INSTRUCTIONS
☐ Consult your doctor if the condition for which this medicine is being used persists or becomes worse, or if the medicine causes an irritation such as itching or burning.

☐ For external use only. Do not swallow.

* * * * *

Tranylcypromine (*Oral Antidepressant*)
United States: Parnate
Canada: Parnate

☐ This medicine is used to help relieve the symptoms of depression. It is important that you take the medicine regularly and that you do not miss any doses. The full effect of the medicine will not be noticed immediately but may take from a few days to several weeks. Early signs of improvement are increased appetite, better sleep, increased energy and, later, improved mood. DO NOT STOP TAKING the medicine when you first feel better or you may feel worse in 3 or 4 days.

HOW TO USE THIS MEDICINE

☐ It is best to take this medicine with a glass of water.

☐ While taking this medicine and for at least 2 weeks after your treatment ends, you must be very careful about your diet. You must not eat any of the following foods or beverages because you could experience a very unpleasant reaction (severe headache, nausea, vomiting, and chest pains):

- Aged and natural cheeses (for example, cheddar, blue, Camembert, Stilton, Gruyère, Brie, Swiss, and Emmenthaler). In general, avoid foods in which aging is used to increase the flavor. Cream cheese, processed cheese, and cottage cheese are safe to eat.
- Sour cream or yogurt.
- Wines, especially Chianti and other heavy red wines.
- Alcoholic beverages, including sherry and beer.
- Canned figs or raisins.
- Yeast extracts (such as Marmite or Bovril) or meat extracts.
- Chicken livers.
- Broad beans (also called fava beans)
- Fermented sausage (such as fermented bolognas and salamis, pepperoni, and summer sausage).
- Pickled or kippered herring.
- Meats prepared with tenderizers.
- Avocados, bananas.
- Soya sauce.
- Chocolate.
- Excessive amounts of caffeine (for example, coffee, tea, cola beverages).

SPECIAL INSTRUCTIONS

☐ If you forget to take a dose, take it as soon as possible. However, if your next dose is within 2 hours, do not take the missed dose but continue with your regular schedule.

☐ Any medicine has a few unwanted side effects. Because this medicine takes a few weeks to work, the side effects are the only thing that tell the doctor that the drug is being absorbed. Most of these side effects will go away as your body adjusts to the medicine.

☐ In some people, this drug may cause dizziness or drowsiness. Do not drive a car or operate dangerous machinery or do jobs that require you to be alert until you know how you are going to react to this drug.

☐ If this medicine causes dizziness, you should be careful going up and down stairs and you should not change positions too rapidly. Get out of bed slowly in the morning and dangle your feet over the edge of the bed for a few minutes before standing up. Sit or lie down at the first sign of dizziness. Tell your doctor you have been dizzy.

☐ It is important that you obtain the advice of your doctor or pharmacist before taking any other medicines, including pain relievers, sleeping pills, tranquilizers, other medicines for depression, cough/cold or allergy medicines, or weight-reducing medicine.

☐ If your mouth becomes dry, suck a hard sour candy (sugarless) or ice chips, or chew gum. It is especially important to brush your teeth regularly if you develop a dry mouth.

☐ This medicine may make some people more sensitive to sunlight or sunlamps. When you begin taking this medicine, try to avoid getting too much sun until you see how you are going to react. If your skin does become more sensitive to sunlight, tell your doctor and try to stay out of direct sunlight. While in the sun, wear protective clothing and sunglasses. You may wish to ask your pharmacist about suitable sunscreen products. Check with your doctor if you become sunburned.

☐ If you become constipated, try increasing the amount of bulk in your diet (for example, bran and salads), exercising more often or drinking water.

☐ Call your doctor immediately if you develop frequent or severe headaches, chest pains, rapid heartrate, nausea, or vomiting. If you cannot reach your doctor call a hospital emergency department.

☐ Most people experience few or no side effects from their drugs. However, any medicine can sometimes cause unwanted effects. Call your doctor if you develop a skin rash, fever, fainting, difficulty in urinating ("passing your water"), swelling of the legs and ankles, eye pain, or changes in ability to see red and green colors.

☐ Do not stop taking this medicine suddenly without your doctor's approval. Have your prescriptions refilled before you are completely out of this medicine so that you will not miss any doses. When your doctor tells you to stop this medicine, you must follow these precautions for 2 weeks since some of the medicine will still be in your body.

☐ Carry an identification card indicating that you are taking this medicine. Always tell your pharmacist, dentist, and other doctors who are treating you that you are taking this medicine.

*   *   *   *   *

Tretinoin (*Topical Acne Therapy*)
United States: Retin-A
Canada: Aquasol A Cream, Vitamin A Acid Gel

☐ This cream is used to treat skin conditions.

HOW TO USE THIS MEDICINE
☐ For CREAM or SOLUTION
  • Cleanse the skin area well with water unless otherwise directed by your doctor. Pat the skin with a clean towel until almost dry.
  • Apply the medicine and spread lightly.

808

□ For SWABS
   • Cleanse the skin area well with water unless otherwise directed. Pat dry.
   • Gently wipe the affected areas with the swab.
   • Do not use a swab more than once.

SPECIAL INSTRUCTIONS

□ Do not use this medicine at the same time as any other skin medicine without the approval of your doctor. Some medicines cannot be mixed.

□ If you forget to apply the medicine, apply it as soon as possible. However, if it is almost time for your next dose, do not apply the missed dose but continue with your regular schedule.

□ While using this medicine, your skin may become more sensitive to sunlight. Do not use sunlamps and wear protective clothing. Call your doctor if you get a sunburn.

□ When you apply this medicine, you may have a mild stinging sensation or redness. This is not unusual. After a few days, you can expect some peeling to occur.

□ Call your doctor if the condition for which this drug is being used persists or becomes worse or if you develop a constant irritation such as itching or burning that was not present before you started using this medicine.

□ Keep this preparation away from the eyes. If you should accidentally get some in your eyes, wash it away with water immediately.

□ For external use only. Do not swallow.

*   *   *   *   *

Triacetin (*Topical Antifungal*)
United States: Enzactin, Fungacetin

□ This medicine is used to treat fungal infections of the skin.

HOW TO USE THIS MEDICINE

□ For CREAM and OINTMENT: (**United States:** Enzactin Cream, Fungacetin Ointment)
   • Cleanse the affected area well with water unless otherwise directed by your doctor. Pat the skin with a clean towel until almost dry.
   • Apply a small amount of medicine to the affected and surrounding areas and massage gently until it disappears.

□ For AEROSOL: (**United States:** Enzactin Aerosol)

   • Cleanse the affected area well with water unless otherwise directed by your doctor.
   • Shake the container well.

- Spray the medicine on the affected area. Keep away from the eyes and mouth.
- Do not inhale the vapors from the spray.

SPECIAL INSTRUCTIONS

☐ Keep the medicine away from rayon and rayon fabrics as it may damage them.

☐ If you have a fungal infection of the feet, it is important to dry your feet (especially between the toes) well after washing.

☐ Consult your doctor if the condition for which you are using this medicine persists or becomes worse, or if the drug causes an irritation.

☐ Do not place the medicine container in hot water or near radiators, stoves, or other sources of heat. Do not puncture or incinerate the container (even when empty). Do not store at temperatures greater than 120°F. (49°C) (**United States:** Enzactin Aerosol)

☐ For external use only.

*   *   *   *   *

Triamcinolone (Oral Corticosteroid)

United States: Aristocort, SK-Triamcinolone, Spencort

Canada: Aristocort, Aristospan, Kenacort

☐ This medicine is similar to cortisone, which is a hormone normally produced by the body. This medicine is used to help decrease inflammation; this then relieves pain, redness, and swelling. It is used in the treatment of certain kinds of arthritis, severe allergies, or skin conditions.

HOW TO USE THIS MEDICINE

☐ Take this medicine with food or a glass of milk in order to help prevent stomach upset. Call your doctor if you develop stomach upset or stomach pain or heartburn (especially if it awakens you during the night). Do not try to treat this yourself.

☐ If your doctor has prescribed only ONE dose of this medicine every day, it is best to take it before 9 A.M. or with breakfast.

☐ If you forget to take a dose, take it as soon as possible. However, if it is almost time for your next dose, do not take the missed dose. Instead, continue with your regular dosing schedule.

☐ Shake the bottle well before using so that you can measure an accurate dose. (**Canada:** Aristospan Oral Suspension)

SPECIAL INSTRUCTIONS

☐ Women who are pregnant, breast-feeding, or planning to become pregnant should tell their doctor before taking this medicine.

810

- [ ] It is best not to drink alcoholic beverages while you are taking this medicine because the combination can cause stomach problems.

- [ ] Do not take any more of this medicine than your doctor has prescribed and do not stop taking this medicine suddenly without the approval of your doctor. It may be necessary for your doctor to slowly reduce your dose since your body becomes used to this medicine. It might be harmful if you suddenly did not receive this medicine.

- [ ] Do not take aspirin or medicines containing aspirin without the approval of your doctor.

- [ ] While you are taking this medicine you may gain some weight. This could be due to an increase in your appetite or to increased water in your system. Your doctor may prescribe a special diet to decrease the number of calories you eat and/or to lower the amount of sodium or increase the amount of potassium in your diet. Follow any diet that your doctor may order.

- [ ] You may find that you bruise more easily. Try to protect yourself from all injuries to prevent bruising.

- [ ] Diabetic patients should regularly check the sugar in their urine and report any unusual levels to their doctor.

- [ ] Carry an identification card indicating that you are taking this medicine. Always tell your pharmacist, dentist, and other doctors who are treating you that you are taking this medicine. If you have an acute infection, injury, operation, or dental surgery within 1 year of taking this medicine, it is important to tell your doctor.

- [ ] Most people experience few or no side effects from their drugs. However, any medicine can sometimes cause unwanted effects. Call your doctor if you develop stomach pain, sore throat, fever, swelling of the legs or ankles, a wound which does not heal, eye pain or blurred vision, frequent urination ("passing your water"), nightmares or depression, muscle cramps, red or black stools, puffing of the face, or menstrual problems.

*   *   *   *   *

Triamcinolone Acetonide (*Dental Paste—Dental Corticosteroid*)
United States: Kenalog in Orabase
Canada: Kenalog in Orabase

- [ ] This medicine is used to help relieve pain, redness, and swelling in certain types of mouth and gum problems.

HOW TO USE THIS MEDICINE
- [ ] For DENTAL PASTE
  - Clean the affected area as directed by your doctor.
  - Apply a small dab of the paste (about $\frac{1}{4}$ inch) to the affected area and **press** until a smooth, thin film forms. Do not rub the paste in.

811

- It is best to apply this medicine at bedtime so that it can work during the night. If you apply it during the day, apply it after meals and, if possible, do not eat or drink for a few hours.

☐ Do not use the drug more frequently or in larger quantities than prescribed by your doctor.

SPECIAL INSTRUCTIONS

☐ If you forget to apply the medicine, apply it as soon as possible. However, if it is almost time for your next dose, do not apply the missed dose but continue with your regular schedule.

☐ Do not use this medicine for any other mouth and gum problems without checking with your doctor or dentist.

☐ Call your doctor if the condition for which this drug is being used persists or becomes worse or if you have a constant irritation such as itching or burning that was not present before you started using this medicine.

☐ Call your doctor if you develop a sore throat, fever, stomach pain, or an infection.

☐ Keep the container tightly closed.

* * * * *

Triamcinolone Acetonide (*Topical Corticosteroid*)

United States: Aristocort, Aristogel, Kenalog, Tramacin

Canada: Aristocort, Kenalog, Kenalog-E, Triamalone, Trimacort, Viaderm-TA

Triamcinolone Acetonide-Clioquinol

Canada: Aristoform, Aristoform D, Aristoform R

☐ This medicine is used to help relieve redness, swelling, itching, and inflammation of certain types of skin conditions.

☐ IMPORTANT: If you have ever had an allergic reaction to iodine medicine, tell your doctor or pharmacist before you use any of this drug. (**Canada:** Aristoform, Aristoform D, Aristoform R)

HOW TO USE THIS MEDICINE

☐ For CREAM, OINTMENT, and LOTION
- Each time you apply the medicine, wash your hands and gently cleanse the skin area well with water unless otherwise directed by your doctor. Do not allow the skin to dry completely. Pat with a clean towel until slightly damp.
- Apply a small amount of the drug to the affected area and spread lightly. Only the medicine that is actually touching the skin will work.

812

A thick layer is not more effective than a thin layer. Do not bandage unless directed by your doctor.

☐ Shake the liquid preparation well before using. (**United States** and **Canada:** Kenalog Lotion)

☐ The liquid preparation may cause a slight temporary stinging sensation after it is applied.

☐ Do not use the drug more frequently or in larger quantities than prescribed by your doctor. Overuse of this medicine may cause you to absorb too much of the drug and increase the risk of side effects.

☐ Keep the medicine away from the eyes, nose, and mouth.

☐ Keep this medicine away from the hair, nails, and clothing because it may cause staining. (**Canada:** Kenalog Lotion)

SPECIAL INSTRUCTIONS

☐ If you forget to apply the medicine, apply it as soon as possible. However, if it is almost time for your next dose, do not apply the missed dose but continue with your regular schedule.

☐ Do not use this medicine for any other skin problems without checking with your doctor.

☐ Do not apply cosmetics or lotions on top of the drug unless your doctor approves.

☐ Call your doctor if the condition for which this drug is being used persists or becomes worse or if you develop a constant irritation such as itching or burning that was not present before you started using this medicine. Also call your doctor if you develop abnormal lines or thinning of the skin, especially under the arms or between the legs.

☐ Store in a cool place but do not freeze.

☐ For external use only. Do not swallow.

☐ Tell future doctors that you have used this medicine.

*　*　*　*　*

Triamterene (*Oral Diuretic*)
United States: Dyrenium
Canada: Dyrenium

Triamterene-Hydrochlorothiazide
United States: Dyazide
Canada: Dyazide

☐ This medicine is used to help rid the body of excess water and to decrease swelling. It is also used to treat high blood pressure. It is commonly called a "water pill."

HOW TO USE THIS MEDICINE

☐ Take the medicine with food, meals, or milk.

☐ Try to take it at the same time(s) every day so that you have a constant level of the medicine in your body. Do not miss any doses. Otherwise, you cannot expect the drug to work as well.

SPECIAL INSTRUCTIONS

☐ If you forget to take a dose, take it as soon as possible. However, if it is almost time for your next dose, do not take the missed dose. Instead, continue with your regular dosing schedule.

☐ Women who are pregnant, breast-feeding, or planning to become pregnant should tell their doctor before taking this medicine.

☐ If you are to take more than one dose every day, take the last dose 6 hours before bedtime so that you will not have to get up during the night to go to the bathroom. This effect will usually lessen after you have taken the drug for awhile.

☐ If you become drowsy, do not drive a car or operate machinery or do jobs that require you to be alert. Tell your doctor you are drowsy.

☐ If you become dizzy, you should be careful going up and down stairs. Sit or lie down at the first sign of dizziness.

☐ This medicine may make some people more sensitive to sunlight and sunlamps. When you begin taking this medicine, try to avoid getting too much sun until you see how you are going to react. If your skin does become more sensitive to sunlight, tell your doctor and try to stay out of direct sunlight. While in the sun, wear protective clothing and sunglasses. You may wish to ask your pharmacist about suitable sunscreen products. Check with your doctor if you become sunburned.

☐ Most people experience few or no side effects from their drugs. However, any medicine can sometimes cause unwanted effects. Call your doctor if you develop a skin rash, fever, sore throat, mouth sores, nausea or vomiting, dry mouth (or if you are very thirsty), weakness, irregular pulse, stomach cramps, swelling of the legs or ankles, or a sudden weight gain of 5 pounds or more.

☐ Also call your doctor if you develop joint pain, easy bruising or bleeding, or a yellow color to the skin or eyes. (*United States* and *Canada:* Dyazide)

*   *   *   *   *

Triazolam (*Oral Hypnotic*)
United States: Halcion
Canada: Halcion

☐ This medicine is used to cause sleep.

814

☐ IMPORTANT: If you have ever had an allergic reaction to a benzodiazepine medicine, tell your doctor or pharmacist before you take any of this medicine.

HOW TO USE THIS MEDICINE

☐ This medicine may be taken with food or a full glass of water.

SPECIAL INSTRUCTIONS

☐ Women who are pregnant, breast-feeding, or planning to become pregnant should tell their doctor before taking this medicine.

☐ In some people, this drug may cause dizziness or drowsiness. Do not drive a car or operate dangerous machinery or do jobs that require you to be alert until you know how you are going to react to this drug.

☐ If you become dizzy, you should be careful going up and down stairs. Sit or lie down at the first sign of dizziness.

☐ Do not drink alcoholic beverages while taking this drug without the approval of your doctor.

☐ It is important that you obtain the advice of your doctor or pharmacist before taking ANY other medicines including pain relievers, sleeping pills, tranquilizers or medicines for depression, cough/cold or allergy medicines, or weight-reducing medicines.

☐ Do not take any more of this medicine than your doctor has prescribed and do not stop taking this medicine suddenly without the approval of your doctor.

☐ Most people experience few or no side effects from their drugs. However, any medicine can sometimes cause unwanted effects. Call your doctor if you develop a sore throat, fever or mouth sores, a staggering walk, a yellow color to the skin or eyes, fast heartbeats, stomach pain, or changes in vision.

* * * * *

Trichlormethiazide (*Oral Diuretic-Antihypertensive*)
United States: Aquex, Diurese, Kirkrinal, Metahydrin, Naqua

☐ This medicine is used to help rid the body of excess water and to decrease swelling. It is also used to treat high blood pressure. It is commonly called a "water pill."

☐ IMPORTANT: If you have ever had an allergic reaction to sulfa drugs or thiazide diuretics, tell your doctor or pharmacist before taking any of this medicine.

HOW TO USE THIS MEDICINE

☐ Take the medicine with food, meals, or milk.

☐ Try to take it at the same time(s) every day so that you have a constant level of the medicine in your body. Do not miss any doses. Otherwise, you can-not expect the drug to work as well.

☐ When you first start taking this medicine, you will probably urinate ("pass your water") more often and in larger amounts than usual. Therefore, if you are to take one dose every day, take it in the morning after breakfast. If you are to take more than one dose every day, take the last dose 6 hours before bedtime so that you will not have to get up during the night to go to the bathroom. This effect will usually lessen after you have taken the drug for awhile.

SPECIAL INSTRUCTIONS

☐ If you forget to take a dose, take it as soon as possible. However, if it is almost time for your next dose, do not take the missed dose. Instead, con-tinue with your regular dosing schedule.

☐ Women who are pregnant, breast-feeding, or planning to become pregnant should tell their doctor before taking this medicine.

☐ This medicine normally causes your body to lose potassium. The body has warning signs to let you know if too much potassium is being lost. Call your doctor if you become unusually thirsty or if you develop leg cramps, unusual weakness, fatigue, vomiting, confusion, or irregular pulse.

☐ If your doctor recommends that you eat foods which are high in potassium, one or more of the foods listed in Appendix A should be eaten daily. All of these foods are rich in potassium. Your goal should be to take in 1000 to 2000 mg. of potassium (approximately 25.6 to 51 mEq) each day. The calo-rie content and sodium content are included for your convenience in meal planning. CHANGE YOUR DIET ONLY IF YOUR DOCTOR TELLS YOU TO.

☐ If this medicine causes dizziness, you should be careful going up and down stairs and you should not change positions too rapidly. Get out of bed slowly in the morning and dangle your feet over the edge of the bed for a few minutes before standing up. Sit down or lie down at the first sign of dizzi-ness. Tell your doctor you have been dizzy. Be careful drinking alcoholic beverages while taking this medicine because they could make the dizziness worse. Do not drive a car or operate dangerous machinery or do jobs that require you to be alert if you are dizzy.

☐ In order to help prevent dizziness and fainting, your doctor may also recom-mend that you avoid strenuous exercises, standing for long periods of time (especially in hot weather), or hot showers or hot baths.

☐ This medicine may make some people more sensitive to sunlight and sunlamps. When you begin taking this medicine, try to avoid getting too much sun until you see how you are going to react. If your skin does become more sensitive to sunlight, tell your doctor and try to stay out of direct sun-light. While in the sun, wear protective clothing and sunglasses. You may wish to ask your pharmacist about suitable sunscreen products. Check with your doctor if you become sunburned.

□ Call your doctor immediately if you think you may be allergic to the medicine or if you develop a skin rash, hives, itching, swelling of the face, or difficulty in breathing. If you cannot reach your doctor, phone a hospital emergency department.

□ Most people experience few or no side effects from their drugs. However, any medicine can sometimes cause unwanted effects. Call your doctor if you develop a sore throat, fever, sharp stomach pain, chest pain, sharp joint pain, easy bruising or bleeding, a yellow color to the skin or eyes, or a sudden weight gain of 5 pounds or more.

* * * * *

Triclofos Sodium
United States: Triclos

□ This medicine is used to cause sleep and for certain types of nervous tension.

HOW TO USE THIS MEDICINE
□ Take the medicine with a full glass of water, fruit juice or ginger ale to help prevent stomach upset.

SPECIAL INSTRUCTIONS
□ Sleeping medicines are only useful for a short time. If used for too long, they lose their effectiveness. Do not take any more of this medicine than your doctor has prescribed and do not stop taking this medicine suddenly without the approval of your doctor.

□ Women who are pregnant, breast-feeding, or planning to become pregnant should tell their doctor before taking this medicine.

□ In some people, this drug may cause dizziness or drowsiness. Do not drive a car or operate dangerous machinery or do jobs that require you to be alert until you know how you are going to react to this drug.

□ If you become dizzy, you should be careful going up and down stairs. Sit or lie down at the first sign of dizziness.

□ Do not drink alcoholic beverages while taking this drug without the approval of your doctor.

□ It is important that you obtain the advice of your doctor or pharmacist before taking ANY other medicines including pain relievers, sleeping pills, tranquilizers or medicines for depression, cough/cold medicines, or allergy medicines.

□ If you are taking this medicine to help you sleep, take it about 20 minutes before you want to go to sleep. Go to bed after you have taken it. Do not smoke in bed after you have taken it.

□ Call your doctor immediately if you think you may be allergic to the medicine or if you develop a skin rash, hives, itching, swelling of the face, or difficulty

in breathing. If you cannot reach your doctor, phone a hospital emergency department.

☐ Most people experience few or no side effects from their drugs. However, any medicine can sometimes cause unwanted effects. Call your doctor if you develop slow heartbeats, bothersome sleepiness or laziness during the day, stomach pain, vomiting, or unusual nervousness.

* * * * *

Tridihexethyl Chloride (*Oral Antispasmodic*)
United States: Pathilon

☐ This medicine is used to help relax muscles of the stomach and bowels and to decrease the amount of acid formed in the stomach.

☐ IMPORTANT: If you have ever had an allergic reaction to atropine or any other drug used to relax the stomach or bowels, tell your doctor or pharmacist before you take any of this medicine.

HOW TO USE THIS MEDICINE

☐ Take this medicine approximately 30 minutes before a meal unless otherwise directed.

☐ This medicine must be swallowed whole. Do not crush, chew, or break it into pieces. (**United States:** Pathilon Sequels)

SPECIAL INSTRUCTIONS

☐ If your mouth becomes dry, suck a hard sour candy (sugarless) or ice chips, or chew gum. It is especially important to brush your teeth regularly if you develop a dry mouth.

☐ In some people, this drug may cause dizziness or drowsiness. Do not drive a car or operate dangerous machinery or do jobs that require you to be alert until you know how you are going to react to this drug.

☐ If you become dizzy, you should be careful going up and down stairs. Sit or lie down at the first sign of dizziness. Tell your doctor you have been dizzy.

☐ A desire to urinate ("pass your water") with an inability to do so is not an uncommon effect with this drug. Urinating each time before taking the drug may help relieve this problem. Call your doctor if it continues.

☐ You may become more sensitive to heat because your body may perspire less while you are taking this drug. Be careful not to become overheated during exercise or in hot weather.

☐ Do not take antacids within 1 hour of taking this medicine as they could make this medicine less effective.

☐ If you become constipated, try increasing the amount of bulk in your diet (for example, bran and salads), exercising more often, or drinking more water. Call your doctor if the constipation continues.

818

- ☐ If your eyes become more sensitive to sunlight, it may help to wear sunglasses.

- ☐ Most people experience few or no side effects from their drugs. However, any medicine can sometimes cause unwanted effects. Call your doctor if you develop a skin rash, diarrhea, unusual restlessness, flushing, or eye pain.

* * * * *

Trifluoperazine HCl (*Oral Antipsychotic-Antiemetic-Antianxiety*)

United States: Stelazine

Canada: Clinazine, Novoflurazine, Pentazine, Solazine, Stelazine, Terfluzine, Triflurin, Tripazine

- ☐ This medicine is used to help relieve the symptoms of certain types of emotional problems. This drug has several other uses and the reason it was prescribed depends upon your condition. Check with your doctor if you do not fully understand why you are taking it.

- ☐ IMPORTANT: If you have ever had an allergic reaction to a phenothiazine medicine, tell your doctor or pharmacist before you take any of this medicine.

HOW TO USE THIS MEDICINE

- ☐ This medicine may be taken with food or a full glass of water.

- ☐ Do not take this medicine at the same time as antacids or diarrhea medicine. Try to space them at least 1 hour apart.

- ☐ The effect of the medicine may not be noticed immediately but may take from 2 to 4 weeks. Be patient. Take the medicine regularly and try not to miss any doses.

- ☐ Do not stop taking this medicine suddenly without the approval of your doctor.

SPECIAL INSTRUCTIONS

- ☐ If you forget to take a dose, take it as soon as possible. However, if it is almost time for your next dose, do not take the missed dose. Instead, continue with your regular dosing schedule.

- ☐ Any medicine has a few unwanted side effects. Because this medicine takes a few weeks to work, the side effects show the doctor that the drug is being absorbed. Many of these side effects will go away as your body adjusts to the medicine.

- ☐ Women who are pregnant, breast-feeding, or planning to become pregnant should tell their doctor before taking this medicine.

- ☐ In some people, this drug may cause dizziness or drowsiness. Do not drive a

car or operate dangerous machinery or do jobs that require you to be alert until you know how you are going to react to this drug.

- [ ] If this medicine causes dizziness, you should be careful going up and down stairs and you should not change positions too rapidly. Get out of bed slowly in the morning and dangle your feet over the edge of the bed for a few minutes before standing up. Sit down or lie down at the first sign of dizziness. Tell your doctor you have been dizzy. Avoid hot showers and baths because they could make you dizzy.

- [ ] Do not drink alcoholic beverages while taking this drug without the approval of your doctor.

- [ ] This medicine may make some people more sensitive to sunlight and sunlamps. When you begin taking this medicine, try to avoid getting too much sun until you see how you are going to react. If your skin does become more sensitive to sunlight, tell your doctor and try to stay out of direct sunlight. While in the sun, wear protective clothing and sunglasses. You may wish to ask your pharmacist about suitable sunscreen products. Check with your doctor if you become sunburned.

- [ ] If your mouth becomes dry, suck a hard sour candy (sugarless) or ice chips, or chew gum. It is especially important to brush your teeth regularly if you develop a dry mouth.

- [ ] It is important that you obtain the advice of your doctor or pharmacist before taking **any** other medicines including pain relievers, sleeping pills, other tranquilizers or medicines for depression, cough/cold or allergy medicines, weight-reducing medicines, or laxatives.

- [ ] This medicine may cause your urine to turn pink, red, or red-brown in color. This is not unusual.

- [ ] In hot weather or during exercise, be careful not to become overheated. You may be more sensitive to heat since this medicine may affect your body's ability to regulate temperature.

- [ ] If you become constipated, try increasing the amount of bulk in your diet (for example, bran and salads), exercising more often, or drinking more water. Call your doctor if the constipation continues.

- [ ] Call your doctor if you develop a sore throat, fever, mouth sores, skin rash, changes in eyesight, rapid heartrate, a yellow color in the eyes or skin, unusual weakness or unusual movements of the face, tongue or hands, or difficulty in urinating ("passing your water"). Also call your doctor if you become restless or unable to sit still or sleep.

- [ ] Carry an identification card indicating that you are taking this medicine. Always tell your pharmacist, dentist, and other doctors who are treating you that you are taking this medicine.

*   *   *   *   *

820

Triflupromazine (*Oral Antipsychotic-Antiemetic-Antianxiety*)
United States: Vesprin

- [ ] This medicine is used to help relieve the symptoms of certain types of emotional problems. This drug has several other uses and the reason it was prescribed depends upon your condition. Check with your doctor if you do not fully understand why you are taking it.

- [ ] IMPORTANT: If you have ever had an allergic reaction to a phenothiazine medicine, tell your doctor or pharmacist before you take any of this medicine.

HOW TO USE THIS MEDICINE

- [ ] This medicine may be taken with food or a full glass of water.

- [ ] Do not take this medicine at the same time as antacids or diarrhea medicine. Try to space them at least 1 hour apart.

- [ ] Shake the bottle well each time you use it so that you can measure an accurate dose. (**United States:** Vesprin Suspension)

- [ ] Store the liquid medicines in a cool, dark place and do not get the liquid on your skin or clothing.

- [ ] The effect of the medicine may not be noticed immediately but may take from 2 to 4 weeks. Be patient. Take the medicine regularly and try not to miss any doses.

- [ ] Do not stop taking this medicine suddenly without the approval of your doctor.

SPECIAL INSTRUCTIONS

- [ ] If you forget to take a dose, take it as soon as possible. However, if it is almost time for your next dose, do not take the missed dose. Instead, continue with your regular dosing schedule.

- [ ] Any medicine has a few unwanted side effects. Because this medicine takes a few weeks to work, the side effects show the doctor that the drug is being absorbed. Many of these side effects will go away as your body adjusts to the medicine.

- [ ] Women who are pregnant, breast-feeding, or planning to become pregnant should tell their doctor before taking this medicine.

- [ ] In some people, this drug may cause dizziness or drowsiness. Do not drive a car or operate dangerous machinery or do jobs that require you to be alert until you know how you are going to react to this drug.

- [ ] If this medicine causes dizziness, you should be careful going up and down stairs and you should not change positions too rapidly. Get out of bed slowly in the morning and dangle your feet over the edge of the bed for a few minutes before standing up. Sit down or lie down at the first sign of dizzi-

ness. Tell your doctor you have been dizzy. Avoid hot showers and baths because they could make you dizzy.

☐ Do not drink alcoholic beverages while taking this drug without the approval of your doctor.

☐ This medicine may make some people more sensitive to sunlight and sunlamps. When you begin taking this medicine, try to avoid getting too much sun until you see how you are going to react. If your skin does become more sensitive to sunlight, tell your doctor and try to stay out of direct sunlight. While in the sun, wear protective clothing and sunglasses. You may wish to ask your pharmacist about suitable sunscreen products. Check with your doctor if you become sunburned.

☐ If your mouth becomes dry, suck a hard sour candy (sugarless) or ice chips, or chew gum. It is especially important to brush your teeth regularly if you develop a dry mouth.

☐ It is important that you obtain the advice of your doctor or pharmacist before taking *any* other medicines including pain relievers, sleeping pills, other tranquilizers or medicines for depression, cough/cold or allergy medicines, weight-reducing medicines, or laxatives.

☐ This medicine may cause your urine to turn pink, red, or red-brown in color. This is not unusual.

☐ In hot weather or during exercise, be careful not to become overheated. You may be more sensitive to heat since this medicine may affect your body's ability to regulate temperature.

☐ If you become constipated, try increasing the amount of bulk in your diet, (for example, bran and salads), exercising more often, or drinking more water. Call your doctor if the constipation continues.

☐ Call your doctor if you develop a sore throat, fever, mouth sores, skin rash, changes in eyesight, rapid heartrate, a yellow color in the eyes or skin, unusual weakness or unusual movements of the face, tongue or hands, or difficulty in urinating ("passing your water"). Also call your doctor if you become restless or unable to sit still or sleep.

☐ Carry an identification card indicating that you are taking this medicine. Always tell your pharmacist, dentist, and other doctors who are treating you that you are taking this medicine.

* * * * *

Trifluoperazine HCl (*Rectal Antipsychotic-Antiemetic-Antianxiety*)
Canada: Stelazine

☐ This medicine is used to help relieve the symptoms of certain types of emotional problems. This drug has several other uses and the reason it was

822

prescribed depends upon your condition. Check with your doctor if you do not fully understand why you are using it.

☐ IMPORTANT: If you have ever had an allergic reaction to a phenothiazine medicine, tell your doctor or pharmacist before you use any of this medicine.

HOW TO USE THIS MEDICINE

☐ Administration of SUPPOSITORIES
- Remove the wrapper from the suppository.
- Lie on your side and raise your knee to your chest.
- Insert the suppository with the tapered (pointed) end first into the rectum.
- Remain lying down for a few minutes so that the suppository will dissolve in the rectum.
- Try to avoid having a bowel movement for at least one hour so that the drug will have time to work.

☐ Store the suppositories in a cool place.

☐ Do not stop using this medicine suddenly without the approval of your doctor.

SPECIAL INSTRUCTIONS

☐ If you forget to use a dose, use it as soon as possible. However, if it is almost time for your next dose, do not use the missed dose. Instead, continue with your regular dosing schedule.

☐ Any medicine has a few unwanted side effects. Because this medicine takes a few weeks to work, the side effects show the doctor that the drug is being absorbed. Many of these side effects will go away as your body adjusts to the medicine.

☐ Women who are pregnant, breast-feeding, or planning to become pregnant should tell their doctor before using this medicine.

☐ In some people, this drug may cause dizziness or drowsiness. Do not drive a car or operate dangerous machinery or do jobs that require you to be alert until you know how you are going to react to this drug.

☐ If this medicine causes dizziness, you should be careful going up and down stairs and you should not change positions too rapidly. Get out of bed slowly in the morning and dangle your feet over the edge of the bed for a few minutes before standing up. Sit down or lie down at the first sign of dizziness. Tell your doctor you have been dizzy. Avoid hot showers and baths because they could make you dizzy.

☐ Do not drink alcoholic beverages while using this drug without the approval of your doctor.

☐ This medicine may make some people more sensitive to sunlight and sunlamps. When you begin using this medicine, try to avoid getting too much sun until you see how you are going to react. If your skin does become more sensitive to sunlight, tell your doctor and try to stay out of direct sunlight. While in the sun, wear protective clothing and sunglasses. You may wish to ask your pharmacist about suitable sunscreen products. Check with your doctor if you become sunburned.

☐ If your mouth becomes dry, suck a hard sour candy (sugarless) or ice chips, or chew gum. It is especially important to brush your teeth regularly if you develop a dry mouth.

☐ It is important that you obtain the advice of your doctor or pharmacist before taking **any** other medicines including pain relievers, sleeping pills, other tranquilizers or medicines for depression, cough/cold or allergy medicines, weight-reducing medicines, or laxatives.

☐ This medicine may cause your urine to turn pink, red, or red-brown in color. This is not unusual.

☐ In hot weather or during exercise, be careful not to become overheated. You may be more sensitive to heat since this medicine may affect your body's ability to regulate temperature.

☐ Call your doctor if you develop a sore throat, fever, mouth sores, skin rash, changes in eyesight, rapid heartrate, a yellow color in the eyes or skin, unusual weakness or unusual movements of the face, tongue or hands, or difficulty in urinating ("passing your water"). Also call your doctor if you become restless or unable to sit still or sleep.

☐ Carry an identification card indicating that you are taking this medicine. Always tell your pharmacist, dentist and other doctors who are treating you that you are taking this medicine.

*   *   *   *   *

Trihexyphenidyl HCl (*Oral Antispasmodic*)

United States: Artane, Hexyphen, T.H.P., Tremin, Trihexane, Trihexidyl

Canada: Aparkane, Artane, Novohexidyl, Trixyl

☐ This medicine is used to improve muscle control and relieve muscle spasm in Parkinson's disease and certain other medical conditions.

HOW TO USE THIS MEDICINE

☐ This medicine may be taken before or after meals. If you have excessive salivation, you may prefer to take the drug after meals. If you have a very dry mouth, you may prefer to take the medicine before meals.

☐ This medicine must be swallowed whole. Do not crush, chew, or break it into pieces. (**United States** and **Canada:** Artane Sequels)

824

☐ If you forget to take a dose, take it as soon as possible. However, if your next dose is within 2 hours, do not take the missed dose but continue with your regular schedule.

SPECIAL INSTRUCTIONS

☐ If your mouth becomes dry, suck a hard sour candy (sugarless) or ice chips or chew gum. It is espcially important to brush your teeth regularly if you develop a dry mouth.

☐ In some people, this drug may cause dizziness, drowsiness, or blurred vision during the first 2 weeks of using this drug. This will usually go away as your body adjusts to this medicine. Do not drive a car or operate dangerous machinery or do jobs that require you to be alert until you know how you are going to react to this drug.

☐ If you become dizzy, you should be careful going up and down stairs. Sit or lie down at the first sign of dizziness.

☐ If your eyes become more sensitive to sunlight, it may help to wear sunglasses.

☐ Do not take antacids or diarrhea medicines within 1 hour of taking this medicine as they could make this medicine less effective.

☐ A desire to urinate ("pass your water") with an inability to do so is not an uncommon effect with this drug. Urinating each time before the drug is taken may help relieve this problem. Call your doctor if it continues.

☐ Do not drink alcoholic beverages while taking this drug without the approval of your doctor.

☐ It is important that you obtain the advice of your doctor or pharmacist before taking pain relievers, nonprescription drugs, sleeping pills, tranquilizers, or medicine for depression while you are taking this drug.

☐ You may become more sensitive to heat because your body may perspire less while you are taking this medicine. Be careful not to become overheated during exercise or in hot weather.

☐ Most people experience few or no side effects from their drugs. However, any medicine can sometimes cause unwanted effects. Call your doctor if you develop a skin rash, eye pain, dizziness or fainting, fast heartbeats, constipation, or confusion.

*   *   *   *   *

Trimeprazine Tartrate (*Oral Antihistamine*)
United States: Temaril
Canada: Panectyl

☐ This medicine is used to help relieve the symptoms of certain types of allergic conditions, coughs and colds, and certain skin conditions.

HOW TO USE THIS MEDICINE

□ This medicine may be taken with food or a glass of milk if it upsets your stomach.

□ This medicine must be swallowed whole. Do not crush, chew, or break it into pieces. (**United States:** Temaril Spansules)

SPECIAL INSTRUCTIONS

□ If you forget to take a dose, take it as soon as possible. However, if it is almost time for your next dose, do not take the missed dose. Instead, continue with your regular dosing schedule.

□ Women who are pregnant, breast-feeding, or planning to become pregnant should tell their doctor before taking this medicine.

□ In some people, this drug may initially cause dizziness or drowsiness. Do not drive a car or operate dangerous machinery or do jobs that require you to be alert until you know how you are going to react to this drug. If you become dizzy, you should be careful going up and down stairs. Sit or lie down at the first sign of dizziness. Tell your doctor if it continues.

□ Do not drink alcoholic beverages while taking this drug without the approval of your doctor.

□ If your mouth becomes dry, suck a hard sour candy (sugarless) or ice chips, or chew gum. It is especially important to brush your teeth regularly if you develop a dry mouth.

□ It is important that you obtain the advice of your doctor or pharmacist before taking pain relievers, nonprescription drugs, sleeping pills or tranquilizers, or other medicines for allergies.

□ Do not take this medicine more often or longer than recommended by your doctor.

□ This medicine may make a few people more sensitive to sunlight or sunlamps. When you begin taking this medicine, try to avoid getting too much sun until you see how you are going to react. If your skin does become more sensitive to sunlight, tell your doctor and try to stay out of direct sunlight.

□ Most people experience few or no side effects from their drugs. However, any medicine can sometimes cause unwanted effects. Call your doctor if you develop a skin rash, sore throat, fever or mouth sores, a yellow color to the skin or eyes, unusual movements of the head, face, or neck, a shuffling walk, or difficulty in urinating ("passing your water").

* * * * *

Trimethadione (*Oral Anticonvulsant*)
United States: Tridione
Canada: Trimedone

☐ This medicine is used to help control convulsions and seizures. It is commonly used in the treatment of epilepsy.

☐ IMPORTANT: If you have ever had an allergic reaction to an anticonvulsant or seizure medicine, tell your doctor or pharmacist before you take any of this medicine.

HOW TO USE THIS MEDICINE

☐ Take this medicine with food if it upsets your stomach. Call your doctor if you continue to have stomach upset.

☐ Chew these tablets well before swallowing. (*United States:* Tridione Chewable)

☐ It is very important that you take this medicine regularly and that you do not miss any doses. Try to take the medicine at the same time(s) every day. This is the only way that you can receive the full benefit of the medicine. If you forget to take this medicine, the amount of medicine in your blood will go down and you may have seizures.

SPECIAL INSTRUCTIONS

☐ If you forget to take a dose, take it as soon as possible. However, if it is almost time for your next dose, do not take the missed dose. Instead, continue with your regular dosing schedule. Do not double doses.

☐ Do not stop taking this medicine suddenly or change the amount you are taking without the approval of your doctor.

☐ Avoid swimming alone or taking part in high-risk sports in which a sudden seizure could cause injury.

☐ In some people, this drug may cause dizziness or drowsiness. Do not drive a car or operate dangerous machinery or do jobs that require you to be alert until you know how you are going to react to this drug. If you become dizzy, you should be careful going up and down stairs. Sit or lie down at the first sign of dizziness.

☐ If this medicine is for a child, do not let him (her) ride a bike or climb trees until you can determine how he (she) is going to react to the medicine. Children could hurt themselves if they participated in these activities when they were dizzy.

☐ Do not drink alcoholic beverages while taking this drug without the approval of your doctor.

☐ It is important that you obtain the advice of your doctor or pharmacist before taking pain relievers, nonprescription drugs, sleeping pills, tranquilizers, or medicines for depression while you are taking this drug.

- [ ] This medicine may cause your eyes to become more sensitive to sunlight and changes in the brightness of light. Wearing sunglasses during the day may help. Be careful driving a car at night if you find the bright lights of cars irritating to your eyes.

- [ ] Women who are pregnant, breast-feeding, or planning to become pregnant should tell their doctor before taking this medicine.

- [ ] Most people experience few or no side effects from their drugs. However, any medicine can sometimes cause unwanted effects. Call your doctor if you develop a sore throat, fever or mouth sores, skin rash, swelling of the hands, legs or face, joint pain, easy bruising or bleeding, yellow color to the skin or eyes, dark-colored urine, or swollen glands.

- [ ] Do not go without this medicine between prescription refills. Call your pharmacist 2 or 3 days before you will run out of the medicine.

- [ ] Carry an identification card indicating that you are taking this medicine. Always tell your pharmacist, dentist, and other doctors who are treating you that you are taking this medicine.

*   *   *   *   *

Trimethobenzamide (*Oral Antiemetic*)
United States: Tigan
Canada: Tigan

- [ ] This medicine is used to help control nausea and vomiting.

HOW TO USE THIS MEDICINE
- [ ] Take the medicine with a little water.

SPECIAL INSTRUCTIONS
- [ ] In some people, this drug may cause drowsiness. Do not drive a car or operate dangerous machinery or do jobs that require you to be alert until you know how you are going to react to this drug.

- [ ] Do not drink alcoholic beverages while taking this drug without the approval of your doctor.

- [ ] It is important that you obtain the advice of your doctor or pharmacist before taking pain relievers, nonprescription drugs, sleeping pills, tranquilizers, or medicines for depression while you are taking this drug.

- [ ] Call your doctor immediately if you think you may be allergic to the medicine or if you develop a skin rash, hives, itching, swelling of the face, or difficulty in breathing. If you cannot reach your doctor, phone a hospital emergency department.

- [ ] Most people experience few or no side effects from their drugs. However, any medicine can sometimes cause unwanted effects. Call your doctor if you develop a sore throat, fever or mouth sores, muscle cramps, blurred vision, vomiting, dark-colored urine, a yellow color to the skin or eyes, unusual movements of the hands or face, or depression.

* * * * *

Trimethobenzamide (*Rectal Antiemetic*)
United States: Tigan

☐ This medicine is used to help control nausea and vomiting.

HOW TO USE THIS MEDICINE
☐ Administration of SUPPOSITORIES
  • Remove the wrapper from the suppository.
  • Lie on your side and raise your knee to your chest.
  • Insert the suppository with the tapered (pointed) end first into the rectum.
  • Remain lying down for a few minutes so that the suppository will dissolve in the rectum.
  • Try to avoid having a bowel movement for at least one hour so that the drug will have time to work.

☐ Store the suppositories in a cool place.

SPECIAL INSTRUCTIONS
☐ In some people, this drug may cause drowsiness. Do not drive a car or operate dangerous machinery or do jobs that require you to be alert until you know how you are going to react to this drug.

☐ Do not drink alcoholic beverages while taking this drug without the approval of your doctor.

☐ It is important that you obtain the advice of your doctor or pharmacist before taking pain relievers, nonprescription drugs, sleeping pills, tranquilizers, or medicines for depression while you are using this drug.

☐ Call your doctor immediately if you think you may be allergic to the medicine or if you develop a skin rash, hives, itching, swelling of the face, or difficulty in breathing. If you cannot reach your doctor, phone a hospital emergency department.

☐ Most people experience few or no side effects from their drugs. However, any medicine can sometimes cause unwanted effects. Call your doctor if you develop a sore throat, fever or mouth sores, muscle cramps, blurred vision, vomiting, dark-colored urine, a yellow color to the skin or eyes, unusual movements of the hands or face, or depression.

* * * * *

Trimipramine (*Oral Antidepressant*)
United States: Surmontil
Canada: Surmontil

☐ This medicine is used to help relieve the symptoms of depression. It is important that you take the medicine regularly and that you do not miss any doses. The full effect of the medicine may not be noticed immediately but may take from a few days to 4 weeks. Early signs of improvement are increased appetite, better sleep, increased energy, and later improved mood. DO NOT STOP TAKING the medicine when you first feel better or you will feel worse in 3 or 4 days.

☐ This medicine has also been used in children to treat bed-wetting.

HOW TO USE THIS MEDICINE
☐ This medicine may be taken with food unless otherwise directed.

SPECIAL INSTRUCTIONS
☐ If you forget to take a dose, take it as soon as possible. However, if it is almost time for your next dose, do not take the missed dose. Instead, continue with your regular dosing schedule.

☐ Any medicine has a few unwanted side effects. Because this medicine takes a few weeks to work, the side effects are the only thing that tell the doctor that the drug is being absorbed. Most of these side effects will go away as your body adjusts to the medicine.

☐ In some people, this drug may cause dizziness or drowsiness. Do not drive a car or operate dangerous machinery or do jobs that require you to be alert until you know how you are going to react to this drug.

☐ If this medicine causes dizziness, you should be careful going up and down stairs and you should not change positions too quickly. Get out of bed slowly in the morning and dangle your feet over the edge of the bed for a few minutes before standing up. Sit or lie down at the first sign of dizziness. Tell your doctor you have been dizzy.

☐ Do not drink alcoholic beverages while taking this drug without the approval of your doctor.

☐ It is important that you obtain the advice of your doctor or pharmacist before taking any other medicines, including pain relievers, sleeping pills, tranquilizers, other medicines for depression, cough/cold or allergy medicines, or weight-reducing medicine.

☐ If your mouth becomes dry, suck a hard sour candy (sugarless) or ice chips, or chew gum. It is especially important to brush your teeth regularly if you develop a dry mouth.

☐ This medicine may make some people more sensitive to sunlight and sunlamps. When you begin taking this medicine, try to avoid getting too much sun until you see how you are going to react. If your skin does become more sensitive to sunlight, tell your doctor and try to stay out of direct sunlight. While in the sun, wear protective clothing and sunglasses. You may wish to ask your pharmacist about suitable sunscreen products. Check with your doctor if you become sunburned.

☐ If you become constipated, try increasing the amount of bulk in your diet (for example, bran and salads), exercising more often, or drinking water.

☐ Call your doctor if you develop a sore throat, fever, mouth sores, eye pain or blurred vision, difficulty in urinating ("passing your water"), fast heartbeats, dark-colored urine or a yellow color to the skin or eyes, a skin rash, or nightmares.

☐ Do not stop taking this medicine suddenly without your doctor's approval. When your doctor tells you to stop this medicine, you must follow these precautions for 2 weeks since some of the medicine may still be in your body.

☐ Carry an identification card indicating that you are taking this medicine. Always tell your pharmacist, dentist, and other doctors who are treating you that you are taking this medicine.

*   *   *   *   *

Trioxsalen (*Oral Melanizing Agent*)
United States: Trisoralen
Canada: Trisoralen

☐ This medicine is used to help increase the pigmentation (color) of the skin and to increase tolerance to sunlight.

HOW TO USE THIS MEDICINE

☐ This is a **potent drug.** Do not increase dosage and exposure time that have been recommended by your doctor. Overdosage and/or overexposure may result in serious burning and blistering.

☐ Take the medicine with milk or after a meal.

SPECIAL INSTRUCTIONS

☐ Sunglasses should be worn during exposure, and the lips should be protected with a light-screening lipstick.

☐ Do not eat limes, figs, parsley, parsnips, mustard, carrots, or celery while you are taking this medicine.

*   *   *   *   *

831

Tripelennamine (*Oral Antihistamine*)
United States: PBZ-SR, Pyribenzamine, Ro-Hist
Canada: Pyribenzamine

☐ This medicine is used to help relieve the symptoms of certain types of allergic conditions, coughs and colds, and certain skin conditions.

HOW TO USE THIS MEDICINE
☐ This medicine may be taken with food or a glass of milk if it upsets your stomach.

☐ This medicine must be swallowed whole. Do not crush, chew, or break it into pieces. (**United States:** PBZ-SR, Pyribenzamine Lontabs; **Canada:** Pyribenzamine Lontabs)

SPECIAL INSTRUCTIONS
☐ If you forget to take a dose, take it as soon as possible. However, if it is almost time for your next dose, do not take the missed dose. Instead, continue with your regular dosing schedule.

☐ In some people, this drug may initially cause dizziness or drowsiness. Do not drive a car or operate dangerous machinery or do jobs that require you to be alert until you know how you are going to react to this drug. If you become dizzy, you should be careful going up and down stairs. Sit or lie down at the first sign of dizziness. Tell your doctor if it continues.

☐ Do not drink alcoholic beverages while taking this drug without the approval of your doctor.

☐ If your mouth becomes dry, suck a hard sour candy (sugarless) or ice chips, or chew gum. It is especially important to brush your teeth regularly if you develop a dry mouth.

☐ It is important that you obtain the advice of your doctor or pharmacist before taking pain relievers, nonprescription drugs, sleeping pills or tranquilizers, or other medicines for allergies.

☐ Do not take this medicine more often or longer than recommended by your doctor.

☐ Most people experience few or no side effects from their drugs. However, any medicine can sometimes cause unwanted effects. Call your doctor if you develop a skin rash, fast heartbeats, blurred vision, stomach pain, or difficulty in urinating ("passing your water").

*   *   *   *   *

Triprolidine HCl (*Oral Antihistamine*)
United States: Actidil
Canada: Actidil

Triprolidine HCl-Pseudoephedrine (*Oral Antihistamine-Decongestant*)
United States: Actifed
Canada: Actifed

☐ This medicine is used to help relieve the symptoms of certain types of allergic conditions, coughs and colds, and certain skin conditions.

HOW TO USE THIS MEDICINE
☐ This medicine may be taken with food or a glass of milk if it upsets your stomach.

SPECIAL INSTRUCTIONS
☐ If you forget to take a dose, take it as soon as possible. However, if it is almost time for your next dose, do not take the missed dose. Instead, continue with your regular dosing schedule.

☐ In some people, this drug may initially cause dizziness or drowsiness. Do not drive a car or operate dangerous machinery or do jobs that require you to be alert until you know how you are going to react to this drug. If you become dizzy, you should be careful going up and down stairs. Sit or lie down at the first sign of dizziness. Tell your doctor if it continues.

☐ Do not drink alcoholic beverages while taking this drug without the approval of your doctor.

☐ If your mouth becomes dry, suck a hard sour candy (sugarless) or ice chips, or chew gum. It is especially important to brush your teeth regularly if you develop a dry mouth.

☐ It is important that you obtain the advice of your doctor or pharmacist before taking pain relievers, nonprescription drugs, sleeping pills or tranquilizers, or other medicines for allergies.

☐ Do not take this medicine more often or longer than recommended by your doctor.

☐ Most people experience few or no side effects from their drugs. However, any medicine can sometimes cause unwanted effects. Call your doctor if you develop a skin rash, fast heartbeats, blurred vision, stomach pain or difficulty in urinating ("passing your water").

* * * * *

Troleandomycin (*Oral Antibiotic*)
United States: TAO

☐ This medicine is an antibiotic used to treat certain types of infections.

☐ IMPORTANT: If you have ever had an allergic reaction to erythromycin or

833

any other antibiotics, tell your doctor or pharmacist before you take any of this medicine.

HOW TO USE THIS MEDICINE

☐ This medicine may be taken with meals or on an empty stomach.

☐ For LIQUID MEDICINE

☐ If you were prescribed a SUSPENSION, shake the bottle well before using so that you can measure an accurate dose. (**United States:** TAO Suspension)

SPECIAL INSTRUCTIONS

☐ It is important to take **all** of this medicine plus any refills that your doctor told you to take. Do not stop taking this medicine earlier than your doctor has recommended in spite of the fact that you may feel better. Otherwise, the infection may return.

☐ If you forget to take a dose, take it as soon as you remember and then continue with your regular schedule.

☐ Most people experience few or no side effects from their drugs. However, any medicine may cause unwanted effects. Call your doctor if you develop a dark-colored tongue, yellow-green stools or, in women, a vaginal discharge that was not present before you started taking the medicine. Also call your doctor if you develop a yellow color to the skin or eyes, dark-colored urine, or stomach pain.

☐ Call your doctor immediately if you think you may be allergic to the medicine or if you develop a skin rash, hives, itching, swelling of the face, or difficulty in breathing. If you cannot reach your doctor, phone a hospital emergency department.

☐ If for some reason you cannot take all of the medicine, discard the unused portion by flushing it down the toilet. Do not take or save old medicine.

* * * * *

Undecylenic Acid (*Topical Antifungal*)
United States: Desenex

Calcium Undecylenate
United States: Caldesene, Cruex, Jockex

Zinc Undecylenate

Undecylenic Acid Compound
United States: Desenex Ointment

☐ This medicine is used to treat fungal infections of the skin.

834

HOW TO USE THIS MEDICINE

☐ Instructions for use:

- Cleanse the skin area well with water unless otherwise specified by your doctor.
- Apply the preparation and spread lightly.

SPECIAL INSTRUCTIONS

☐ Consult your doctor if the condition for which this medicine is being used persists or becomes worse, or if the medicine causes an irritation such as itching or burning.

☐ Avoid inhaling the powder and keep away from the eyes, nose, and mouth. (**United States:** Caldesene, Cruex, Desenex, Jockex Powders)

☐ For external use only. Do not swallow.

*   *   *   *   *

Uracil Mustard (*Oral Antineoplastic*)
United States: Uracil Mustard

☐ This medicine is used in certain medical conditions to help slow down the growth and reproduction of some of the body's cells.

HOW TO USE THIS MEDICINE

☐ It is best to take this medicine 1 hour before breakfast or 2 hours after supper in order to help prevent nausea or vomiting.

☐ It is very important that you take this medicine exactly as your doctor has prescribed and that you do not miss any doses. Try to take this medicine at the same time every day.

☐ Even if you become nauseated or lose your appetite, do not stop taking the medicine but check with your doctor.

☐ If you miss a dose of this medicine, do not take the missed dose and do not double your next dose. Check with your doctor.

SPECIAL INSTRUCTIONS

☐ Always keep your appointments so that your doctor can watch your progress.

☐ If your doctor has prescribed some other medicines for you, it is important that you take them in the right order and that you do not miss them.

☐ Men and women should take appropriate birth control measures to avoid conception while taking this medicine.

☐ Unless otherwise directed, drink plenty of fluids (2 to 3 quarts daily) while you are taking this medicine. This will help your kidneys handle the medicine and help prevent kidney problems.

□ This medicine may cause a temporary loss of hair. Brush your hair gently and no more often than necessary. After your treatment is finished, your hair should grow back in.

□ Always tell your pharmacist, dentist, and any other doctors who are treating you that you are taking this medicine. This is especially important if you plan to have surgery or any vaccinations.

□ This is a very strong medicine. In addition to its benefits, there may be some unwanted effects, even for a short time after you stop taking the medicine. Call your doctor if you develop unusual bruising or bleeding, sore throat, fever, a skin rash, swelling of the legs or ankles, stomach or joint pain, or difficulty or pain in urinating ("passing your water").

* * * * *

Urine-Sugar Analysis Paper (*Diagnostic Aid*)
United States: Tes-Tape
Canada: Tes-Tape

□ This preparation is used to test for glucose (sugar) in the urine.*

□ Testing procedure:
1. Lift top lid of dispenser and withdraw approximately 3 cm. (1½ inches) of tape.
2. While keeping a slight tension on the tape, close the lid and hold. Tear the tape by pulling straight out.
3. Dip part of the tape into the urine specimen; remove immediately. The strip should be moistened uniformly, but the end of the tape held between the fingers should be kept dry.
4. Wait for one minute. Calibrated color development in the moistened tape is accomplished in one minute. Yellow color indicates urine is sugar-free.
5. Then immediately compare the darkest area on the test strip with the color chart on the dispenser. If the tape indicates ½% or higher, wait one additional minute and make the final comparison.

□ *Precautions:*
1. Do not use tape if it has turned brown.
2. The activity of Tes-Tape must be checked periodically, especially if it is in use over a prolonged period of time. If the urine tests are consistently negative or if a reduction in insulin dosage based on negative readings of Tes-Tape is instructed by the doctor, the following Coca-Cola test should be used to confirm the activity of Tes-Tape.

*Tes-Tape (Package Insert), Eli Lilly & Company (Canada) Limited, Toronto, Ontario.

a. Dip a piece of Tes-Tape in a properly prepared glucose solution. (If a properly prepared glucose solution is not available, Coca-Cola from a freshly opened bottle is satisfactory. Coca-Cola is a well-controlled, carefully standardized product that can be relied upon to give the same reaction as a properly prepared glucose solution.) The tape should be removed immediately as one would when testing a urine specimen. After 2 minutes have elapsed, the reading obtained when the tape is compared with the color chart should be approximately 2%. If such a reading is not obtained, the tape has apparently deteriorated and should not be used. PURCHASE A NEW PACKAGE OF TES-TAPE.

3. Protect from direct light, excessive moisture, and heat. Do not store in a hot or humid room such as a kitchen or bathroom.

☐ *What to do if the tape breaks inside the dispenser:*

1. Open lid. Insert the tip of the blade under the ridge next to the black arrow on the direction label.
2. Tilt the blade handle upward to loosen the tape holder from case; slide out as you would open a drawer.
3. Place the loose end of the tape over the raised platform on the holder. Slide the holder back into the case.

* * * * *

Uristix (*Diagnostic Aid*)
United States: Uristix
Canada: Uristix

☐ This preparation is used to test for glucose (sugar) and protein in the urine.

☐ Directions for use

• Dip the strip in the urine or briefly pass it through the urine stream.
• Touch the tip of the strip against the edge of the container to remove any excess urine.
• Compare test areas with color charts at the correct times.
   Protein—read immediately
   Glucose—wait 10 seconds

☐ For further information, refer to the package insert which accompanies this medicine.*

* * * * *

*Uristix (Package Insert), Ames Company Division, Miles Laboratories, Ltd., Rexdale, Ontario.

Valproic Acid (*Oral Anticonvulsant*)
United States: Depakene
Canada: Depakene

☐ This medicine is used to help control convulsions and seizures. It is commonly used in the treatment of epilepsy.

HOW TO USE THIS MEDICINE

☐ Take this medicine with food if it upsets your stomach. Call your doctor if you continue to have stomach upset.

☐ The capsules should be swallowed whole without chewing in order to prevent irritation of the mouth and throat.

☐ It is very important that you take this medicine regularly and that you do not miss any doses. Try to take the medicine at the same time(s) every day. This is the only way that you can receive the full benefit of the medicine. If you forget to take this medicine, the amount of medicine in your blood will go down and you may have seizures.

SPECIAL INSTRUCTIONS

☐ If you forget to take a dose, take it as soon as possible. However, if your next dose is within 6 hours, do not take the missed dose but continue with your regular schedule.

☐ Do not stop taking this medicine suddenly or change the amount you are taking without the approval of your doctor.

☐ Avoid swimming alone or taking part in high-risk sports in which a sudden seizure could cause injury.

☐ In some people, this drug may cause dizziness or drowsiness. Do not drive a car or operate dangerous machinery or do jobs that require you to be alert until you know how you are going to react to this drug. If you become dizzy, you should be careful going up and down stairs. Sit or lie down at the first sign of dizziness.

☐ If this medicine is for a child, do not let him (her) ride a bike or climb trees until you can determine how he (she) is going to react to the medicine. Children could hurt themselves if they participated in these activities when they were dizzy.

☐ Do not drink alcoholic beverages while taking this drug without the approval of your doctor.

☐ It is important that you obtain the advice of your doctor or pharmacist before taking pain relievers, nonprescription drugs, sleeping pills, tranquilizers, or medicines for depression while you are taking this drug.

☐ Women who are pregnant, breast-feeding, or planning to become pregnant should tell their doctor before taking this medicine.

☐ Most people experience few or no side effects from their drugs. However, any medicine can sometimes cause unwanted effects. Call your doctor if you develop a skin rash, easy bruising or bleeding, dark-colored urine or a yellow color to the skin or eyes, fast eye movements or changes in vision, nightmares, or depression.

☐ Do not go without this medicine between prescription refills. Call your pharmacist 2 or 3 days before you will run out of the medicine.

☐ Carry an identification card indicating that you are taking this medicine. Always tell your pharmacist, dentist, and other doctors who are treating you that you are taking this medicine.

* * * * *

Vidarabine (*Ophthalmic Antiviral*)
United States: Vira-A
Canada: Vira-A

☐ This medicine is used to treat viral infections of the eye.

HOW TO USE THIS MEDICINE
☐ For EYE OINTMENT

INSTILLATION OF EYE OINTMENT

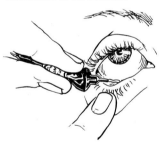

- The person administering the eye ointment should wash his hands with soap and water.
- The eye ointment must be kept clean. Do not touch the tube against the face or anything else.
- Lie down or tilt your head backward and look at the ceiling.
- Gently pull down the lower lid of your eye to form a pouch.
- Hold the tube in your other hand and place the tube as close as possible to the eye without touching it.
- Squeeze the prescribed amount of ointment (usually $\frac{1}{2}$ inch in adults) from the tube along the pouch.
- Close your eyes. Do not rub them.
- Wipe off any excess ointment around the eye with a tissue.
- Clean the tip of the ointment tube with a tissue.

839

- ☐ If necessary, have someone else administer the eye ointment for you.

- ☐ Keep the eye ointment tube tightly closed when not in use.

- ☐ Do not use the drug more frequently or in larger quantities than prescribed by your doctor.

SPECIAL INSTRUCTIONS

- ☐ Vision may be blurred for a few minutes after using the eye medicine. Do not drive a car or operate dangerous machinery or do jobs that require you to be alert until your vision has cleared.

- ☐ If you forget to use the medicine, use it as soon as possible. However, if it is almost time for your next dose, do not use the missed dose but continue with your regular schedule.

- ☐ Do not use this medicine at the same time as any other eye medicine without the approval of your doctor. Some medicines cannot be mixed.

- ☐ The eyes may become sensitive to sunlight while using this medicine. Wearing sunglasses in brightly lit areas will help to relieve this problem.

- ☐ It is important to keep the eye surface covered with this medicine. Use the medicine regularly and EXACTLY as your doctor advises.

- ☐ Continue to use this medicine until your doctor tells you otherwise, despite the fact that the infection may appear to have cleared.

- ☐ Contact your doctor if the condition for which you are using this medicine does not improve or if the eye becomes irritated by it for more than a few minutes. Many eye medicines sting for a short time immediately after use. Call your doctor if you develop eye pain.

- ☐ For external use only. Do not swallow.

*   *   *   *   *

Vitamins: Multivitamin and Vitamin B Complex Preparations

GENERAL INSTRUCTIONS

Be sure to check the label of each vitamin preparation to be certain of the contents. Establish the presence or absence of such ingredients as iron and fluoride. Pay particular attention to those ingredients that apply to your vitamin preparation.

- ☐ Take this medicine with meals.

- ☐ Vitamin products should be treated as drugs. Excessive doses of vitamins can be dangerous and the label instructions should always be followed. If you feel you need medical attention, contact your doctor. **Do not self-medicate.**

- [ ] Eat well-balanced meals. Do **not** depend on fortified foods or vitamin products to balance your diet.

- [ ] If the medicine is a liquid, it may be taken directly or mixed with milk, fruit juices, formula, cereal, or other foods.

- [ ] Vitamins with an iron supplement are to improve the quality of your blood and help make you feel better. This medicine may cause the stools to turn black. This is not an unusual effect. Take this medicine with meals.

- [ ] Medicines that have a special coating must be swallowed whole. Do not crush or chew.

- [ ] If your vitamin supplement contains a drug to help relieve anxiety and tension, then it deserves special attention. It is suggested that patients taking this medicine avoid the use of alcohol. If this medicine produces drowsiness or impairs physical coordination, you should not drive a car or operate machinery.

- [ ] Store vitamin preparations (especially those containing iron) out of the reach of children. Children may think they are candy and could become seriously ill if they swallowed several of the tablets.

*   *   *   *   *

Vitamin A (*Oral Vitamin*)
United States: Acon, Alphalin, Aquasol A, Dispatabs
Canada: Afaxin, Aquasol A

- [ ] This medicine is a vitamin A supplement.

HOW TO USE THIS MEDICINE
- [ ] Do not take mineral oil, especially when taking this medicine.

SPECIAL INSTRUCTIONS
- [ ] Women who are pregnant, breast-feeding, or planning to become pregnant should tell their doctor before taking this medicine.

- [ ] Do not take any more of this vitamin than your doctor has prescribed.

- [ ] The body has warning signs if you take too much of this medicine. Call your doctor if you develop nausea, vomiting, loss of appetite, skin rash, or cracking of the skin or lips.

*   *   *   *   *

Vitamin A Acid (*See Tretinoin*)

*   *   *   *   *

Vitamin A-D Preparations (*Oral Vitamin*)

United States: Cod Liver Oil, Super D Cod Liver Oil, Super D Perles
Canada: Alphamettes, Aquasol A & D

☐ This medicine is a vitamin supplement.

HOW TO USE THIS MEDICINE

☐ Do not take mineral oil while taking this medicine.

☐ The liquid medicine may be mixed in milk, formula, juices, cereals, or placed directly on the tongue. (*United States:* Cod Liver Oil, Super D Cod Liver Oil; *Canada:* Aquasol A & D)

SPECIAL INSTRUCTIONS

☐ Women who are pregnant, breast-feeding, or planning to become pregnant should tell their doctor before taking this medicine.

☐ Do not take any more of this vitamin than your doctor has prescribed.

☐ The body has warning signs if you take too much of this medicine. Call your doctor if you develop nausea, vomiting, loss of appetite, skin rash or cracking of the skin or lips, diarrhea, or weakness.

☐ Store this medicine in a cool place.

*　*　*　*　*

Vitamin B Complex (*Oral Vitamin*)

United States: B Complex, Beplete, Betalin, Lederplex, Taka-Combex
Canada: Brewers Yeast, Vibelan

☐ This medicine is a vitamin B supplement.

SPECIAL INSTRUCTIONS

☐ Do not take any more of this vitamin than your doctor has recommended.

☐ If you develop flu-like symptoms while taking this preparation, contact your doctor.* (*Canada:* Brewers Yeast)

*　*　*　*　*

*Jensen, D. P. et al: Fever of unknown origin secondary to Brewers Yeast ingestion, **Arch. Intern. Med. 136:**332 (March) 1976.

Vitamin B₁ (Thiamine) (*Oral Vitamin*)

United States: Betalin S
Canada: Bewon

☐ This drug is a vitamin. The reason it was prescribed depends upon your condition. Check with your doctor.

SPECIAL INSTRUCTIONS

☐ Do not take any more of this vitamin than your doctor has prescribed.

☐ Most people experience few or no side effects from their drugs. However, any medicine can sometimes cause unwanted effects. Call your doctor if you develop a skin rash, difficulty in breathing, or tightness of the throat.

*   *   *   *   *

Vitamin B₆ (Pyridoxine) (*Oral Vitamin*)

United States: Hexabetalin
Canada: Hexabetalin, Hexavibex

Vitamin B₆-Vitamin B₁ (*Oral Vitamin*)

Canada: Fortior-2B

☐ This drug is a vitamin. The reason it was prescribed depends upon your condition. Check with your doctor.

SPECIAL INSTRUCTIONS

☐ Do not take any more of this vitamin than your doctor has prescribed.

☐ Most people experience few or no side effects from their drugs. However, any medicine can sometimes cause unwanted effects. Call your doctor if you develop numbness in the hands or feet.

☐ Store the medicine in a cool dark place.

*   *   *   *   *

Vitamin B₁₂ (*Oral Hematopoietic*)

United States: Redisol, Rhodavite
Canada: Redisol, Rubramin

☐ This medicine is used to treat anemia.

SPECIAL INSTRUCTIONS

☐ Do not take any more of this medicine than your doctor has recommended.

☐ Most people experience few or no side effects from their drugs. However, any medicine can sometimes cause unwanted effects. Call your doctor if you develop a skin rash, swelling, or difficulty in breathing.

☐ Store the medicine in a cool dark place.

* * * * *

Vitamin C (Ascorbic Acid) *(Oral Vitamin)*

United States: Ascorbicap, Best C Caps, Cecon, Cemill, Cetane Timed, Cevalin, Ce-Vi-Sol, C-Long Granucap, Saro-C, Tega-C-Tabs

Canada: Adenex, Ascoril, Ce-Vi-Sol, Erivit C, Redoxon

☐ This medicine is a vitamin C supplement. The reason it was prescribed depends upon your condition.

HOW TO USE THIS MEDICINE

☐ These tablets may be chewed, swallowed whole, or allowed to dissolve in the mouth. (**Canada:** Adenex, Ascoril)

☐ Dissolve the tablet completely in a glass of water and drink the solution immediately. (**Canada:** Redoxon Effervescent Tablets)

☐ Swallow this medicine whole. (**United States:** Ascorbicap, Best C Caps, Cemill, Cetane Timed, C-Long Granucaps, Saro-C)

SPECIAL INSTRUCTIONS

☐ Do not take any more of this vitamin than your doctor has recommended.

☐ This medicine can sometimes interact with other medicines. Always tell any other doctors who are treating you that you are taking vitamin C.

☐ Call your doctor if you develop low back pain or pain during urination ("passing your water").

* * * * *

Vitamin D *(Oral Vitamin)*

United States: Calciferol, Deltalin, Drisdol, Geltabs

Canada: Drisdol, Ostoforte, Radiostol

☐ This drug has many uses and the reason it was prescribed depends upon your condition. Check with your doctor.

HOW TO USE THIS MEDICINE

☐ This medicine should always be taken in milk. (**Canada:** Drisdol)

844

SPECIAL INSTRUCTIONS

- ☐ Do not take mineral oil, especially while taking this medicine.

- ☐ Contact your doctor if you develop nausea, vomiting, drowsiness or diarrhea.

- ☐ Store in a cool dark place.

*　*　*　*　*

Vitamin E (*Oral Vitamin*)

United States: Aquasole E, E-Ferol, Eprolin, Kell-E, Lethopherol, Maxi-E, Tokols

Canada: Aquasol E, Daltose

- ☐ This medicine contains vitamin E. This drug has many uses and the reason it was prescribed depends upon your condition. Check with your doctor.

HOW TO USE THIS MEDICINE

- ☐ Do not take mineral oil while taking this medicine.

- ☐ This medicine may be chewed. (**United States:** Maxi-E)

- ☐ These tablets have a special coating and must be swallowed whole. Do not crush, chew, or break them into pieces. Do not take milk or antacids within 1 hour of taking these tablets. (**Canada:** Daltose)

SPECIAL INSTRUCTIONS

- ☐ Keep the container tightly capped and store in a cool dark place.

*　*　*　*　*

Warfarin Potassium (*Oral Anticoagulant*)

United States: Athrombin-K

Canada: Athrombin-K

Warfarin Sodium

United States: Coumadin, Panwarfin

Canada: Coumadin, Warfilone, Warnerin

- ☐ This medicine is used to help prevent harmful blood clots from forming. It is commonly called a "blood thinner."

HOW TO USE THIS MEDICINE

- ☐ Take this medicine **exactly** as your doctor has prescribed. Try to take the medicine at the same time every day and do not miss any doses. Do not take extra tablets without your doctor's approval because overtreatment will cause bleeding.

☐ Regular blood tests, called "prothrombin times," are necessary in order for your doctor to prescribe the correct dose for you. Your dose may change from time to time depending on these tests.

☐ It is best to take this medicine with a glass of water. Do not take it with food or other drugs unless otherwise directed.

☐ If you forget to take a dose, take it as soon as possible. However, if it is almost time for your next dose, do not take the missed dose. Instead, continue with your regular dosing schedule. Record the date of the missed dose so that you can tell your doctor the next time you see him for a blood test. Call your doctor if you miss more than 1 dose.

SPECIAL INSTRUCTIONS

☐ Do not take any other drugs or stop taking any drugs you are currently taking without first consulting with your doctor. This even includes many products that you can buy without a prescription such as pain relievers and antacids. Always check with your pharmacist before you take or buy ANY nonprescription products.

☐ Do not take aspirin or medicines containing aspirin or salicylates. It is usually safe to take acetaminophen as a substitute for aspirin for occasional headaches and pain. Check with your pharmacist.

☐ It is best to avoid alcoholic beverages while you are taking this medicine because the combination may cause undesirable side effects. Ask your doctor if he feels it is safe for you to have the occasional drink.

☐ Do not eat unusually large amounts of leafy, green vegetables or change your diet without telling your doctor.

☐ If you have a tendency to cut yourself while shaving, you may wish to use an electric razor to avoid possible bleeding.

☐ Try to avoid contact sports or activities in which you could become injured because they could result in internal bleeding.

☐ If your body gets more medicine than it needs, bleeding may occur. Call your doctor if you notice any of the following signs of bleeding which you cannot explain or are unusual for you: nosebleeds, bruising or heavy menstrual bleeding, bleeding from the gums after brushing the teeth, heavy bleeding from cuts, red or black stools, red or dark brown urine, or vomiting or coughing up blood. Your doctor will do some blood tests and adjust your dose.

☐ Women who are pregnant, breast-feeding, or planning to become pregnant should tell their doctor before taking this medicine.

☐ Most people experience few or no side effects from their drugs. However, any medicine can sometimes cause unwanted effects. Call your doctor if you

develop stomach or back pain, unusual headaches, changes in eyesight, constipation or diarrhea, dizziness, a skin rash, sore throat, fever, mouth sores, a yellow color to the skin or eyes, or unusual tiredness.

☐ Carry an identification card indicating that you are taking this medicine. Always tell your pharmacist, dentist, and other doctors who are treating you that you are taking this medicine.

☐ Do not go without this medicine between prescription refills. Call your pharmacist 2 or 3 days before you will run out of the medicine.

☐ After you stop taking the medicine, it will take your body some time to return to normal. Your doctor or pharmacist will tell you how long you must follow these instructions AFTER you have stopped taking this medicine.

* * * * *

Xylometazoline HCl (*Nasal Decongestant*)
United States: Neosynephrine II, Otrivin
Canada: Otrivin, Sinutab Sinus Spray

☐ This medicine is used to help relieve nasal stuffiness and associated headaches.

HOW TO USE THIS MEDICINE
☐ For NASAL SPRAY
  • Blow your nose gently.
  • Sit upright with your head slightly back.
  • Place the atomizer at the entrance of the nostril and close the other nostril by pressing your finger on the side.
  • Squeeze the atomizer the prescribed number of times.
  • Repeat for the other nostril if necessary.

☐ For NOSE DROPS

INSTILLATION OF NOSE DROPS

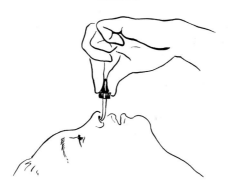

- Blow your nose gently before administration of drops.
- Sit in a chair and tilt your head backward, or lie down on a bed with your head extending over the edge of the bed, or lie down and place a pillow under the shoulders so that the head is tipped backward.
- Insert the dropper into the nostril about $\frac{1}{3}$ inch and drop the prescribed number of drops into the nose.
- Try not to touch the inside of the nose with the dropper as it will probably make you sneeze and will contaminate the dropper.
- Remain in the same position for at least 5 minutes.

SPECIAL INSTRUCTIONS

☐ Do not use this medicine more often or longer than recommended by your doctor. If used for too long, this medicine may actually cause a type of congestion.

☐ Rinse the dropper in hot water after each use.

☐ If you forget to use the medicine, use it as soon as possible. However, if it is almost time for your next dose, do not use the missed dose but continue with your regular schedule.

☐ Do not use this medicine at the same time as any other nasal medicine without the approval of your doctor. Some medicines cannot be mixed.

☐ Contact your doctor if the condition for which you are using this medicine does not improve. Also call your doctor if you develop fast heartbeats, headache, dizziness, trembling, blurred vision, or drowsiness.

☐ Check with your doctor if you develop a stinging sensation which does not go away as your body adjusts to the medicine.

☐ For external use only. Do not swallow.

* * * * *

Zinc Sulfate-Phenylephrine HCl (*Eye Astringent-Decongestant*)
United States: Eyephrine, Neozin, Phenylzin, Prefrin-Z, Zincfrin
Canada: Zincfrin

Zinc Sulfate-Antazoline-Naphazoline
Canada: Zincfrin-A

☐ This medicine is used to help relieve eye irritations.

848

HOW TO USE THIS MEDICINE

☐ For EYE DROPS

INSTILLATION OF EYE DROPS

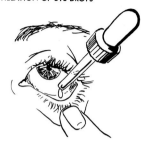

- The person administering the eye drops should wash his hands with soap and water.
- The eye drops must be kept clean. Do not touch the dropper against the face or anything else.
- Lie down or tilt your head backward and look at the ceiling.
- Gently pull down the lower lid of your eye to form a pouch.
- Hold the dropper in your other hand and approach the eye from the side. Place the dropper as close to the eye as possible without touching it.
- Place the prescribed number of drops into the pouch of the eye.
- Close your eyes. Do not rub them.
- Apply gentle pressure for a minute with your fingers to the bridge of the nose (inside corner of the eye) to prevent the eye drops from being drained from the eye.
- Blot excess solution around the eye with a tissue.

☐ If necessary, have someone else administer the eye drops for you.

☐ Do not use the eye drops if they have changed in color or have changed in any way since you purchased them.

☐ Keep the eye drop bottle tightly closed when not in use.

☐ Do not use the drug more frequently or in larger quantities than prescribed by your doctor.

SPECIAL INSTRUCTIONS

☐ Vision may be blurred for a few minutes after using the eye medicine. Do not drive a car or operate dangerous machinery or do jobs that require you to be alert until your vision has cleared.

☐ Do not use this medicine at the same time as any other eye medicine without the approval of your doctor. Some medicines cannot be mixed.

☐ Contact your doctor if the condition for which you are using this medicine does not improve or if the eye becomes irritated by it for more than a few minutes. Many eye medicines sting for a short time immediately after use.

Also call your doctor if you develop fast heartbeats, trembling, or excessive sweating.

☐ Keep the container tightly closed.

☐ For external use only. Do not swallow.

*   *   *   *   *

Zinc Undecylenate (*See Undecylenic Acid*)

*   *   *   *   *

Selected Potassium-Rich and Sodium-Rich Foods

Foods	Average Portion	Potassium (in mg.)	Calories	Sodium (in mg.)
FRUITS				
☐ Orange	1 medium	360 mg	95	0.8
☐ Grapefruit	1 cup	380 mg	75	1.0
☐ Banana	1 medium	630 mg	130	0.8
☐ Strawberries	1 cup	270 mg	55	1.2
☐ Avocado	one half	380 mg	275	3.4
☐ Apricots	3 medium	500 mg	55	0.7
☐ Dates	1 cup	1390 mg	500	1.8
☐ Watermelon	one-half slice	380 mg	95	1.0
☐ Cantaloupe	one-half melon	880 mg	75	46.0
☐ Raisins	1 cup	1150 mg	425	34.0
☐ Prunes	4 large	240 mg	90	2.4
JUICES				
☐ Orange	8-oz. glass	440 mg	105	9.0
☐ Grapefruit	8-oz. glass	370 mg	130	1.0
☐ Prune	8-oz. glass	620 mg	170	5.0
☐ Pineapple	8-oz. glass	340 mg	120	1.2
MEAT				
☐ Hamburger	3 ounces	290 mg	310	92.0
☐ Beef chuck	3 ounces	310 mg	260	44.0
☐ Beef round	3 ounces	340 mg	200	58.0
☐ Rib roast	3 ounces	290 mg	270	92.0
☐ Turkey	4 ounces	350 mg	300	46.0
VEGETABLES				
☐ Tomato	1 medium	340 mg	30	4.5
☐ Artichoke	1 medium	210 mg	30	22.0
☐ Brussels sprouts	1 cup	300 mg	35	11.0

*Courtesy Merck Sharp & Dohme Canada Limited

Cholesterol Content of Selected Foods*

To the Patient:
This diet guide will help you to avoid high-cholesterol foodstuffs. For some patients, your doctor may also prescribe drug therapy which, to be effective, requires that it be taken regularly, just as you must maintain your diet. Although you will probably not feel any specific benefits, do not reduce the dosage or discontinue your medicine without first consulting your doctor.

	Low-Cholesterol Foodstuffs	High-Cholesterol Foodstuffs
Beverages	Skim milk, buttermilk, coffee, tea, postum, cacao, carbonated drinks, fruit and vegetable juices	Whole milk (pasteurized or homogenized), cream
Cereals	All cereals and grain products, such as rice, noodles, macaroni, and spaghetti	Egg noodles
Bread	All types of bread, biscuits, soda crackers	All baked goods made with butter, fat, egg yolk, cream, whole milk, including muffins, croissants, waffles
Soups	Bouillon and consommé (without fat), noodle and vegetable soups and soups made with skim milk or vegetable oil	All cream and pea soups
Meats Poultry Fish	Lean meats, beef, lamb, veal, chicken, turkey, ham, pork, well-trimmed steaks and chops	Fat meats, goose, duck, bacon, brain, heart, liver, tongue, sweetbread, kidney, hotdogs, corned beef, caviar, shrimps, oysters
Cheeses	Defatted cottage cheese	All others
Eggs	Egg white only	Egg yolk
Potatoes	Boiled, baked, or mashed potatoes (without butter and cream)	Potato chips, fried potatoes, mashed potatoes

*Courtesy Ayerst Laboratories

	Low-Cholesterol Foodstuffs	High-Cholesterol Foodstuffs
Vegetables	All	None
Fruits	All	None
Desserts	Angel food cakes, tea or graham biscuits, all gelatin or milk desserts without cream, mousse made with egg white only, fruit ice	All desserts and cakes made with butter, fat, egg yolk, whole milk, such as pâtisseries, ice cream, yogurt
Sweets	Sugar, hard candies, marshmallows, mints, molasses, honey, jelly, marmalade, syrups	All chocolates, candies made with cream and butter, butterscotch candies
Fats	Corn oil margarine, corn oil, peanut oil, olive oil	Butter, all margarines (except corn oil), cream, mayonnaise, sandwich spreads
Miscellaneous	Salt, pepper, spices, herbs, mustard	Sauces, coconut

APPENDIX C

Alternate Method of Using Pressurized Aerosol Inhalers

The Standards Committee of the Canadian Thoracic Society* made the following recommendations regarding the use of pressurized aerosol inhalers:

1. Place the tip of the pressurized inhaler approximately 2 finger breadths in front of the widely opened mouth.
2. Breathe in a normal relaxed manner.
3. Following relaxed expiration, breathe in as slowly and as deeply as possible. Approximately one third of the way through inspiration, release one puff of the bronchodilator and continue breathing to the maximum.

*Originally published in *Canadian Medical Association Journal,* Vol. 121, September 22, 1979.

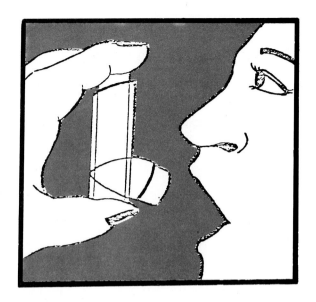

4. Hold the breath for as long as possible (approximately 5 to 10 seconds) and then breathe out in a normal, relaxed manner.

5. If 2 puffs are required, repeat with the second puff released approximately 30 seconds after the first. This will also allow the inhaler valve pressure to be relieved.

Explanation:

The Standards Committee of the Canadian Thoracic Society recommended that the inhaler be held approximately 8 to 10 cm. from the pharynx to minimize the jetting effect and impaction of medication at the back of the throat. The mouth is held wide open in order to obtain a maximum flow of aerosol into the lungs and to minimize the baffle-like effect of the tongue and palate. Expiration should be relaxed rather than full since the latter could collapse some of the airways and result in poorer distribution of the aerosol when inspired. The aerosol should be released toward the middle of full inspiration since the airways are widely dilated at that time. This should result in more even distribution of the aerosol and better penetration into the lungs. If the aerosol were released at the beginning of inspiration, it would be distributed primarily to the upper lobes of the lungs. This effect is greatest if inspiration follows full expiration.

854

A Method to Determine the Approximate Amount of Active Ingredient in an Aerosol Inhaler*

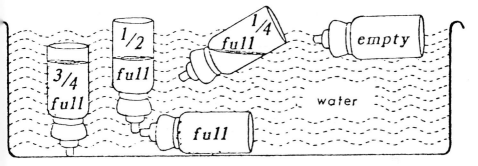

The amount of active ingredient remaining in an aerosol container may be checked by a simple method. (1) Immerse the aerosol inhaler in a container of water which is at room temperature. (2) If the aerosol inhaler is full, it will sink to the bottom. If it is empty, it will float on top of the water. (3) A partially filled aerosol inhaler will float at an angle, as shown in the diagram.

Patients should be advised to shake the aerosol inhaler prior to each use so that the active ingredient is delivered accurately.

*Grainger, J.R.: Aerosol Inhalers. *Canadian Pharmaceutical Journal*, 15:319–322, Oct. 1976.

Guidelines on Alcohol for Professional Use in Counseling Diabetics‡

The decision whether a diabetic should use alcohol must be determined between the diabetic person and the physician. Alcohol may be contraindicated in some individuals for whom diabetes is complicated by other

‡Courtesy of The Canadian Diabetes Association, Toronto, Ontario

considerations: (1) Several conditions are aggravated by alcohol (e.g., hypertriglyceridemia, liver disease, alcoholism), and (2) certain drugs interact adversely with alcohol (e.g., chlorpropamide in some persons).

Alcohol is a concentrated source of energy (Table I) and should be avoided during weight reduction. However, under conditions of well-controlled diabetes and normal weight, the occasional, moderate use of alcohol will not adversely affect the diabetic state.

Table I. Comparison of Energy Values

Nutrient	kilocalories per gram	kilojoules* per gram
	(kcal/g)	(kj/g)
Carbohydrate	4	16.7
Protein	4	16.7
Alcohol	7	29.3
Fat	9	37.7

*1 kilocalorie = 4.184 kilojoules

Points to stress in counseling when alcohol is permitted:

1. Use alcohol only in moderation. Sip slowly and make a drink last a long time.
2. Types of Alcohol:
   - Avoid those which contain large amounts of rapidly absorbed carbohydrate, e.g., liqueurs, sweet wines, sweet mixes.
   - Use in moderation those which do not contain significant sugar, e.g., whiskey, Scotch, rye, vodka, gin, cognac, dry brandy, dry sherry, dry wine.
   - Beer and ale contain malt sugar which must be substituted for carbohydrate in the meal plan (Table II).
   - *Canada:* In most provinces the carbohydrate content of wines is indicated as a Liquor Board rating on a list displayed in the store (e.g. wines rated "0" to "3" would have 0 to 3% sugar content and would be considered dry).
   - *United States:* When you purchase wine, check with the vendor to determine the amount of sugar the wine contains.
3. Alcohol does not contribute sugar into the blood stream, but it is a very concentrated source of energy (kilocalories or kilojoules). If alcohol is used daily, the energy value of the alcohol should be included in the total energy intake. Care should be taken to provide balanced nutrition before adding the energy value of the alcohol. Occasional use of carbohydrate-free alcohol for the normal-

weight person in whom diabetes is controlled may be regarded as an extra.

4. Counsel the person to take precautions to avoid hypoglycemia, especially when drinking before meals or during a peak insulin action period. Advise the person never to drink on an empty stomach—always drink with food, preferably during a meal or after a meal. (Protein foods slow down the rate of alcohol absorption.) Within the social context of a pre-meal drink, the meal may be delayed sufficiently to create the risk of hypoglycemia. The symptoms of hypoglycemia are so similar to those of intoxication that the diabetic person and others around him or her may fail to recognize and treat an insulin reaction.

5. Visible identification should be worn when the diabetic person is drinking away from home.

6. Alcohol can have a relaxing effect and may dull judgment. Counsel the individual with diabetes to ensure that meals and snacks are taken on time and are selected with usual care.

Table II. Comparison of Alcoholic Beverages and Mixes*‡

	Amount	CHO† Content	Alcohol Content	Total Energy Kilocalories
Beer				(kcal)
Canadian beer or ales	340 ml (12 oz)	10–12 g	13 g	140
American beer	340 ml (12 oz)	13 g	12 g	140
Dietetic beer (Holsten-Brauerei, Dia Malt Beverage)	340 ml (12 oz)	4 g	17 g	138
Distilled Alcohol and Wine				
Distilled Alcohol (rye, gin)	43 ml (1.5 oz)	–	15 g	105
Brandy or cognac	43 ml (1.5 oz)	–	15 g	105
Dry red or white wine	100 ml (3.5 oz)	–	9 g	63
Dry sherry	57 ml (2 oz)	–	9 g	63
Mixes Containing Sugar				
Regular sweetened soft drink	300 ml (10 oz tin)	34 g	–	136
	360 ml (12 oz tin)	41 g	–	163
Tom Collins mix bitter lemon	300 ml (10 oz tin)	40 g	–	160
	360 ml (12 oz tin)	48 g	–	192
Tonic water	300 ml (10 oz tin)	30 g	–	120
	360 ml (12 oz tin)	36 g	–	144
Soda water or club soda	any amount	–	–	–
Unsweetened orange juice	250 ml (8 oz)	26 g	–	108
Tomato juice	250 ml (8 oz)	10 g	–	40

*Values are for averages rounded to the nearest whole number. In the United States, the usual volume of the soft drink mixes is 12 oz.

†One serving of fruit (1 FRUIT EXCHANGE) contains 10 grams of simple carbohydrate (as sugars).

‡Adapted from The Canadian Diabetes Association, Toronto, Ontario.

Index of Drug Names

Generic drug names are listed in *italics.*

860

861

Butone, 652

C3, 69
C4, 69
Cafergot, 317
Cafermine, 317
Cafertrate, 317
Calciferol, 844
Calcitriol, 148
Calcium Chloride Powder, 148
Calcium-Eri, 148
Calcium Preparations, 148
Calcium-Rougier, 148
Calcium-Sandoz, 148
Calcium Undecylenate, 834
Caldesene, 834
Calora, 148
Calusterone, 149
Camalox, 475
Camoquin HCl, 87
Campain, 58
Candex, 591
Canesten, 218
Cantil, 489
Capital, 57
Capital W/Codeine, 59
Caquin Cream, 207
Carbacel Ophthalmic, 150
Carbachol, 150
Carbamazepine, 151
Carbarsone, 153
Carbenicillin Idanyl Sodium, 154
Carbimazole, 155
Carbinoxamine Maleate, 156
Carbolith, 468
Cardabid, 580
Cardilate, 317, 319
Cardioquin, 731
Carisoprodol, 157
Carphenazine Maleate, 158
Casafru, 747
Casanthranol-Docusate Sodium, 160
Cascara Sagrada, 160
Cas-Evac, 160
Castor Oil, 161
Catapres, 215
Ceclor, 161
Cecon, 844
Cedilanid, 282
CeeNu, 469
Cefaclor, 161
Cefadroxil, 162
Cefracycline, 778
Celestoderm-V, 131
Celestoderm-V/2, 131
Celestone, 127
Celontin, 525
Cemill, 844
Centet, 778

Cephalexin Monohydrate, 163
Cephaloglycin, 164
Cephradine, 165
Cephulac, 459
Ceporex, 163
Cerevon, 354
C.E.S., 332
Cetacort, 414
Cetamide, 753
Cetane Timed, 844
Cetapred, 687
Cetasal, 65
Cevalin, 844
Ce-Vi-Sol, 844
Chemdrox, 475
Chemfedral, 784
Chemgastric, 476
Chemgel Antacid, 77
Chemlox, 475
Chemphyl, 82
Children's Aspirin, 65
Children's 217 Tablets, 65
Chlophedianol HCl, 166
Chloral Betaine, 166
Chloral Hydrate, 167, 169
Chloralex, 167
Chloralvan, 167
Chlorambucil, 170
Chloramphenicol, 171, 174
Chlordantoin, 175
Chlordiazepoxide HCl, 176
Chlordiazepoxide-Clidinium, 177
Chlormezanone, 178
Chloromide, 192
Chloromycetin, 171
Chloromycetin Cream, 174
Chloromycetin Ophthalmic, 171
Chloromycetin Otic, 171
Chloronase, 192
Chlorophenoxamine HCl, 179
Chloroptic, 171
Chloroptic S.O.P., 171
Chloroquine Phosphate, 180
Chloroserpine, 736
Chlorothiazide, 181
Chlorotrianisene, 183
Chlorophen, 188
Chlorphenesin, 185
Chlorphenesin Carbamate, 184
Chlorpheniramine Maleate, 186
Chlorpheniramine Maleate-
  Phenylephrine, 186
Chlorpheniramine-Phenylpropanolamine,
  187
Chlorpheniramine-
  Phenylpropanolamine-Isopropamide,
  187
Chlorphentermine HCl, 188
Chlorprom, 188

863

865

873

877

878

883

Undecylenic Acid, 834
Undecylenic Acid Compound, 834
Unicort, 414
Unigesic-A, 710
Unipen, 556
Unisoil, 161
Unisul, 763
Unitensen, 231
Univol, 475
Uracel, 752
Uracil Mustard, 835
Urazide, 121
Urecholine, 133
Uremide, 765
Urex, 513
Uridon, 200
Urifon, 763
Urine-Sugar Analysis Paper, 836
Urispas, 355
Uristix, 837
Uritol, 378
Uro Gantanol, 765
Urodine, 640
Urozide, 403
Utibid, 601
Uticillin VK, 626
Uticort, 129
Utimox, 88

Vacon, 655
Valadol, 57
Valisone, 131
Valisone Scalp Lotion, 131
Valium, 269
Vallestril, 505
Valmid, 339
Valpin, 97
Valpin 50, 97
Valproic Acid, 838
Vancenase, 113
Vanceril Inhaler, 111
Vanceril Oral Inhaler, 111
Vanoxide, 119
Vanquin, 727
Varidase, 757
Vaso-80 Unicelles, 627
Vasocon, 558
Vasocon A, 558
Vasocon Regular, 558
Vasodilan, 454
Vasoprine, 454
Vasosulf, 656
V-Cillin Drops, 626
V-Cillin K, 626
VC-K 500, 626
Vectrin, 550
Veetids, 626
Velosef, 165

Veltane, 138
Ventaire, 721
Ventolin, 740, 741
Veracillin, 272
Vercyte, 669
Vermizine, 667
Vermox, 481
Versapen, 397
Versapen-K, 397
Verstran, 681
Vertiban, 288
Vesprin, 821
Viaderm-F.A., 362
Viaderm-N, 591
Viaderm-TA, 812
Vibelan, 842
Vibramycin, 303
Vidarabine, 839
Vimicon, 243
Vioform, 207
Vioform-Hydrocortisone, 207
Viokase, 616
Vio-Serpine, 734
Vira-A, 839
Virilon, 538
Viscephen, 276
Viscerol, 274
Visculose, 527
Visine, 780
Visken, 664
Vistaril, 422
Vitalone, 509
Vitamin A, 841
Vitamin A Acid, 841
Vitamin A Acid Gel, 808
Vitamin A-D Preparations, 842
Vitamin B Complex, 842
Vitamin B_1 (Thiamine), 843
Vitamin B_6 (Pyridoxine), 843
Vitamin B_6-Vitamin B_1, 843
Vitamin B_{12}, 843
Vitamin C (Ascorbic Acid), 844
Vitamin D, 844
Vitamin E, 845
Vitamin Preparations, 840
Vitron-C, 352
Vivactil, 721
Vivol, 269
Voranil, 217

Wampocap, 575
Warfarin Potassium, 845
Warfarin Sodium, 845
Warfilone, 845
Warnerin, 845
Wesco-Hex, 398
Westadone, 504
Westcort, 414